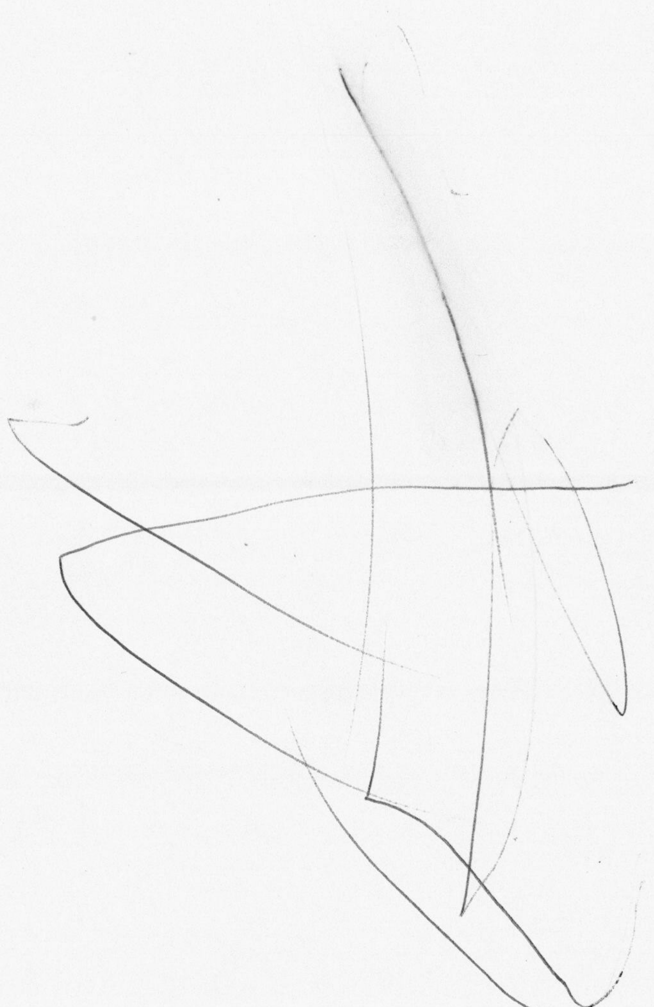

Principles and Applications of Assessment in Counseling

Third Edition

Susan C. Whiston
Indiana University

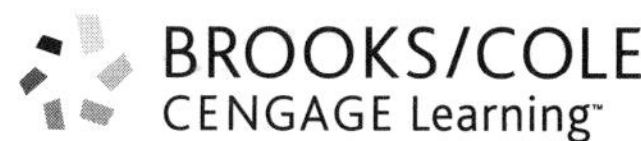

Australia • Brazil • Japan • Korea • Mexico • Singapore • Spain • United Kingdom • United States

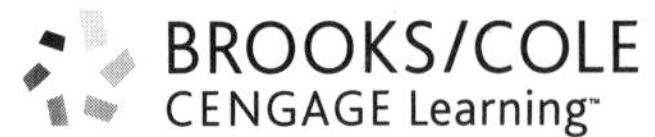

Principles and Applications of Assessment in Counseling: Third Edition
Susan C. Whiston

Publisher/Executive Editor: Marcus Boggs

Acquisitions Editor: Seth Dobrin

Assistant Editor: Allison Bowie

Editorial Assistant: Diane Mars

Technology Project Manager: Andrew Keay

Marketing Manager: Karin Sandberg

Marketing Assistant: Ting Jian Yap

Marketing Communications Manager: Shemika Britt

Project Manager, Editorial Production: Abigail Greshik

Creative Director: Rob Hugel

Art Director: Vernon Boes, Cate Barr

Print Buyer: Karen Hunt

Permissions Editor: Mardell Glinski-Schultz

Production Service: Pre-Press PMG

Copy Editor: Sarah Wales-McGrath

Cover Designer: Ross Carron

Compositor: Pre-Press PMG

Library of Congress Control Number: 2008924468

Student Edition:

ISBN-13: 978-0-495-50197-8

ISBN-10: 0-495-50197-2

Brooks/Cole, Cengage Learning
10 Davis Drive
Belmont, CA 94002-3098
USA

Cengage Learning products are represented in Canada by Nelson Education, Ltd.

For your course and learning solutions, visit **academic.cengage.com**

Purchase any of our products at your local college store or at our preferred online store **www.ichapters.com**

Printed in the United States of America
4 5 6 7 12 11 10

To Jen, Michael, and Matt

Brief Contents

Contents

Preface

Consistent with previous editions of *Principles and Applications of Assessment in Counseling*, this edition is based on the premise that counselors functioning in almost all clinical or school settings must have a sound understanding of assessment. I will argue that assessment is an integral part of the counseling process and that all practitioners need refined assessment skills. In my opinion, selecting a treatment or determining the appropriate counseling theory should be based on a sound and comprehensive assessment of the client. In assessment, it is important to emphasize the terms *sound* and *comprehensive*. A sound assessment occurs when a counselor gathers accurate information and interprets and uses that information in an appropriate manner. The importance of sound assessment procedures applies to both formal and informal assessment techniques. Furthermore, counselors need to consider the whole person and understand that people are complex; hence, assessment procedures must be comprehensive. The goals of this book are, first, to provide a foundation in assessment so clinicians can select and use sound assessment techniques and, second, to expose counselors to a variety of assessment areas and issues.

Principles of Assessment

Section I of this book focuses on the underlying principles of any type of psychological assessment. This section is designed so that clinicians can understand basic concepts of measurement and the fundamental methods used in assessment. To evaluate and use any assessment, a clinician needs to understand these foundational concepts. Although the intent of this book is not to turn readers into statisticians, there are a few formulas. However, readers are encouraged to focus more on concepts than on mathematical calculations. For example, in most instrument manuals, there will be standard deviation(s), and counselors will not need to calculate a standard deviation. They will, however, need to understand how the standard deviation was calculated and what it means. Chapter 1 introduces assessment terms and briefly describes some of the historical influences on assessment practices and procedures. To use many assessment instruments properly, counselors need an understanding of some basic statistics that *describe* individuals' scores. Therefore, Chapter 2 includes a discussion of the two basic types of assessment instruments (i.e., norm-referenced and criterion-referenced) and the scoring methods and approaches.

Clinicians also need to understand the psychometric qualities of assessment instruments. In general, the psychometric qualities considered by experts in assessment to be of primary importance are *reliability* and *validity*. In counseling, these psychometric qualities are important as they influence whether an instrument should be used. Chapters 3 and 4 cover these two topics as well as how they are important in both evaluating instruments and determining the meaning of the assessment results. Chapter 5 focuses on selecting, administering, scoring, and communicating assessment results.

Overview of Assessment Areas

Section II builds on the foundations established in the first section by exploring specific methods and areas of client assessment. Clinicians can use numerous methods of client assessment, such as interviews, informal tools, and standardized instruments. No matter what type of assessment strategies a counselor selects, however, the tools must be both reliable and sound. Chapter 6, which discusses initial assessment in counseling, focuses on topics related to the initial interview and to assessment methods that can be used during the first session with a client. Chapters 7 and 8 address the assessment of human cognitive abilities—Chapter 7, the measure of intelligence or general ability; and Chapter 8, achievement and aptitude assessment. Counselors are expected to be knowledgeable in these areas and to be able to interpret the results from instruments that measure them. Rapid changes in our society are leading many individuals to seek career counseling. Because assessment is often a part of career counseling, this area is addressed in Chapter 9. Chapter 10 discusses personality assessment and many of the methods used to assess personality. The last chapter in this section, Chapter 11, focuses on assessing couples and families and describing the dynamics that occur within families.

Applications and Issues

In the last section of the book, the focus shifts from specific areas of assessment to the application of assessment in counseling and issues that surround the process. The premise of these final chapters is that assessment has a role throughout the entire counseling process. Therefore, clinicians need to continually incorporate sound and ethical assessment practices. Assessment serves three major purposes in counseling.

First, an important primary step in the counseling process is often assessment and diagnosis. Accurate diagnosis of client issues and problems is central to the counseling process—if a counselor misdiagnoses or does not properly assess the client's issues in the initial stages, then the chances of providing efficient counseling services are diminished. Hence, this third section begins with a chapter that addresses diagnosis and commonly used diagnostic systems. In many mental health settings, counselors must have refined diagnostic skills. Therefore, Chapter 12 is designed as an introduction to the *Diagnostic and Statistical Manual of Mental Disorders*—Fourth Edition-Text Revision (*DSM-IV-TR*), a commonly used diagnostic system.

Second, counselors often use assessment information to make treatment-planning decisions during the treatment process. This area concerns using assessment as a therapeutic intervention rather than as a technique. As an example, clients frequently enter counseling for assistance in making a major decision (e.g., what career to pursue, whether to get a divorce, whether to quit drinking). Assessment results can be an integral part of the information-gathering phase necessary for effective decision making. Chapter 13 begins with an overview of assessment and treatment planning and then goes on to address the use of assessments during the counseling process.

The third area in which assessment results play a crucial role in counseling is in *evaluating* the services provided to clients. Because there are increasing demands for counselors to provide accountability information, they often use assessment instruments to produce that data and information. Furthermore, assessing the effectiveness of counseling can provide insight into how to improve counseling services in the future. For this reason, Chapter 13 also includes an overview of methods for evaluating and assessing counseling services.

Because the professional responsibilities associated with assessment are substantial, any professional counselor must have comprehensive knowledge of ethical practices and professional standards related to counseling assessment. Chapter 14 addresses the ethical and legal issues of counseling, with a focus on the importance of assessment knowledge and ethical integrity. In addition, competent assessment requires knowledge about the influence of background and culture, particularly as it relates to race and ethnicity. Because counselors must have specific knowledge of issues related to assessing individuals from diverse backgrounds, Chapter 15 provides an introduction to assessment of special populations.

Finally, in the past 10 years, changes in technology have had a significant influence on many aspects of counseling; this is particularly true of assessment. The last chapter of this book examines technology's influence on assessment. I conclude with some projections about future trends related to assessment in counseling.

Acknowledgments

I wrote the first edition of this book while on sabbatical at the University of Nevada, Las Vegas. As I wrote this edition, I often remembered my colleagues and friends and the significance of my time at UNLV. I consistently say that there is no better place to learn about mental health issues than Las Vegas. Although many people from Las Vegas contributed to the first edition of this book, one of my colleagues, Fred Kirschner, deserves a special note of gratitude.

In all editions of this book, I have attempted to write from a student perspective. This was easier for the second edition of the book because I had an excellent doctoral student, Jen Bouwkamp, assisting me. Instrumental in both the second and third editions of this book was Marquita Flemming. Marquita was the editor of the second edition and provided substantial support and understanding in my writing of the third edition. A special thank you should also be extended to Abby Greshik who made the publication process of this edition bearable and often fun.

Sometimes we have times in our lives when life becomes more challenging and some individuals are incredibly helpful and supportive. I am grateful to many remarkable individuals who helped me through a difficult transition. The third edition of this book could not have been written without the support from those friends. Finally, the third edition of this book is dedicated to Jen, Michael, and Matt, who are all maturing into wonderful people in spite of their mother. It is not always easy to live with a mother who is continually quoting counseling and psychological research.

Susan C. Whiston
Indiana University

SECTION I

Principles of Assessment

CHAPTER 1

Assessment in Counseling

By their very nature, humans are complex and the more pieces of the human puzzle clinicians can access, the more likely it is that they will have a more complete picture. As with a jigsaw puzzle, if counselors have only a few pieces of the puzzle, they will have a hard time determining what the whole picture is. Formal and informal assessment techniques can assist counselors in gathering "puzzle pieces," thus facilitating a more comprehensive view of clients. Counselors with numerous methods for accessing client information have more material to use in a therapeutic manner than do those who have limited assessment skills.

As a counselor, you will regularly assess clients. This assessment may address what the client's issues are, the magnitude of his or her problems, the client's strengths and level of motivation, or whether counseling can be beneficial. Assessing people is probably not entirely new to you. Chances are you have been doing assessment on an informal basis for many years. When you walk into a class for the first time, you may begin to casually assess your fellow classmates. You may have also assessed personalities or interests of people at a social gathering. Assessing other individuals is part of everyday life; it is also part of the counseling process. In the 1930s and 1940s, many people viewed the terms *counseling* and *assessment* as being synonymous and, during this period, most of the public thought counseling always involved the use of tests (Hood & Johnson, 2007). Most clinicians currently do not see counseling and assessment as synonymous; however, client assessment does continue to play a crucial role in the counseling process.

What Is Assessment?

Before further pursuing the topic of assessment in counseling, it is important to discuss the precise meaning of *assessment*. A term closely associated with assessment is

psychological test, which Anastasi and Urbina (1997) defined as an objective and standardized measure of a sample of behavior. Cronbach's (1990) definition is similar, with a test being a systematic procedure for observing behavior and describing it with the aid of numerical scales or fixed categories. As these two similar definitions suggest, many of the definitions of assessment have some commonalities. They all discuss getting a *measure* or using some type of measurement. In assessment, counselors often want an indication of quantity. (E.g., How depressed is the client? Are the test scores high enough to get into an Ivy League school?) In simple terms, in assessment we are often attempting to determine whether there is a lot of "something" or just a little.

The issue of quantity leads to the next topic: the something that is being measured. In counseling, practitioners are often interested in human constructs such as emotions, career interests, personality factors, abilities, and aptitudes. These constructs, however, are difficult to measure directly. For example, individuals cannot give a pint of emotions in the same way they can a pint of blood. Humans, for the most part, indicate their emotions by their behavior, their statements, or even the answers they give on a questionnaire. It is important to remember that speaking and responding to a questionnaire are behaviors. Even when people take a test or assessment, their answers are just a sample of behaviors in that area. Thus, for most of the areas in which counselors want to gather information, all that they can truly gather are *samples of behavior* (although in very rare instances, a clinician may use a physiological measure, such as pulse rate as a measure of anxiety). In addition, when assessing clients, counselors observe a sample of behavior and then *infer* certain meanings from those behaviors. Hence, when first beginning to observe or assess a client, a counselor should consider their observations as a sample of behavior and then reflect on two important questions: first, is the sample of behavior indicative of how the person usually behaves and, second, are the inferences being made about the client correct?

If the intent is to obtain a sample of behaviors and make some inferences or clinical decisions, then it makes sense for counselors to be careful about the manner in which they obtain the behavior samples. Being careful during the assessment process is particularly important when the intent of the assessment process is to compare individuals and make decisions (e.g., determine who gets a scholarship or whether a client has a substance abuse problem). This care is related to the third common point in the definitions of assessment—an objective or systematic measure of behavior. For example, if a counselor wants to work only with motivated clients, then she would need to gather samples of behaviors that reflect each client's level of motivation. The counselor might decide that a direct approach is good, so she would ask each client about level of motivation. To the first client, she might ask, "Are you motivated to try some different things in counseling?" To the second client, she might ask, "Are you motivated?" With the third client, she might say, "You do not seem very motivated. Are you?" This counselor's way of gathering samples of behavior will probably affect the behaviors of the clients, so their answers may be quite different depending on the way she asks the question. This illustrates how important it is that, in assessment, the manner of gathering behavior samples be objective, standardized, and systematic.

Although this book's focus is on assessment and appraisal in counseling, it does adhere to the traditional definition of psychological assessment. To be fair to all clients, assessments need to be systematic and objective. With assessment in counseling, clinicians are, in essence, gathering samples of client behaviors and making inferences based on those behaviors. Therefore, when considering assessment strategies, clinicians should focus on the methods or procedures used for gathering the samples of behavior. For example, a counselor interviewing a client should consider what behaviors are being sampled and whether these behaviors are typical of that client. The counselor also needs to consider the inferences he makes about the client and the evidence (or validity) of those inferences.

The final aspect of assessment is measurement. When assessing a client, a counselor is attempting to measure some aspect of the client. Even if the question is whether or not the client has some particular attribute, the assessment involves measurement. For instance, determining whether a client is suicidal involves measuring the degree to which suicidal indicators are present. One of the challenges in assessment is finding methods for obtaining meaningful measures of many psychological constructs. For example, we cannot say a client has one liter of anxiety.

A distinction is sometimes made among the words **assessment**, **appraisal**, and **testing**. The *Standards for Educational and Psychological Testing* (American Educational Research Association (AERA), American Psychological Association (APA), & National Council on Measurement in Education (NCME), 1999), which is one of the primary authoritative sources related to assessment, distinguishes between the terms *test* and *assessment*. It defines assessment as "a broader term, commonly referring to a process that integrates test information with information from other sources (e.g., information from the individual's social, educational, employment, or psychological history)" (p. 3). In this book, the terms *assessment* and *appraisal* are used interchangeably, based on the opinion that they both include the use of formal and informal techniques, not just standardized tests. Assessment and appraisal are not just formal psychological evaluations; in this book, they are defined as procedures for gathering client information that is then used to facilitate clinical decisions and provide information to clients. A distinction, however, does need to be made between **tests** and **instruments**. The term *test* is often reserved for an individual instrument in which the focus is on evaluation, such as a test that is graded in a class. Many instruments that counselors use, such as scales, checklists, and inventories, are designed to provide information and are not evaluative. In this book, the term *instrument* includes tests, scales, checklists, and inventories. As you read this book, there may be terms with which you are unfamiliar; in such a case, the glossary at the end of the book may be helpful.

Do Counselors Need to Know About Assessment?

Counselors must know about assessment because the American Counseling Association's (2005a) *Code of Ethics* devoted an entire section (Section E) to evaluation, assessment, and interpretation. Furthermore, the Council for Accreditation of Counseling and Related Educational Programs (CACREP, 2001) stipulated that eight common core areas are required of all students in accredited programs, one of which is assessment. Hence, there are professional expectations that all counselors have training and knowledge in assessment and in the appropriate use of assessment instruments and techniques.

Numerous research studies indicate that counselors in a variety of settings (e.g., schools, community agencies, mental health facilities) view formal assessment strategies as a significant aspect of their work. Ekstrom, Elmore, Schafer, Trotter, and Webster (2004) surveyed school counselors. Ninety-one percent indicated they interpreted scores from tests/assessments and used the information in counseling. These researchers also found that 81% communicated and interpreted test/assessment information to parents and 80% had communicated and interpreted test/assessment information to teachers, school administrators, and other professionals. In a survey of nationally certified counselors, Sampson, Vacc, and Loesch (1998) found that work behaviors related to assessment were considered fundamental to the general practice of counseling. Frauenhoffer, Ross, Gfeller, Searight, and Piotrowski (1998) found that mental health counselors frequently used the Minnesota Multiphasic Personality Inventory-2 (MMPI-2), Beck Depression Inventory, Wechsler Intelligence Scale for Children-III (WISC-III), Wechsler Adult Intelligence Scale-Revised (WAIS-R), some projective tests (e.g., House-Tree-Person, human figure drawings, sentence completion tests), and the Wide Range Achievement Test 3 (WRAT3).

Refined assessment skills can often assist counselors in providing treatment more quickly and efficiently. Meyer et al. (2001) compared the empirical evidence concerning psychological assessments and medical testing and found that psychological assessments are comparable to medical tests in terms of accuracy. Impara and Plake (1995) found that teachers and school administrators typically consider the school counselor as the "test expert," with whom they would consult if they had questions about testing.

In addition, the public expects that counselors understand assessment and are able to interpret assessment results. Both mental health and school counselors work with other professionals in multidisciplinary teams where other team members (e.g., psychologists) will quickly lose respect for a counselor who has limited knowledge of psychometric principles and common assessment instruments. Moreover, for some clients, formal assessment strategies have an influence above and beyond a counselor's verbal comments. For these clients, assessment results presented either on a computer screen or printed on paper have greater credibility than what they know themselves or what the counselors may be telling them. For example, I have worked with career counseling clients who could articulate career preferences but who did not see those interests as being legitimate until the results of an interest inventory confirmed their preferences. In addition, a counselor can quickly tarnish her reputation by not being adequately prepared in assessment. As an example, a school counselor can quickly lose credibility with a student's parents by not being able to interpret the results from an achievement test.

Counselor credibility is important and there is considerable support of Strong's (1968) theory of social influence, which proposes that clients are more likely to accept a counselor's feedback and less likely to discredit a counselor if they perceive the counselor to be expert, attractive, and trustworthy (Heppner & Claiborn, 1989). Research in this area indicates that several counselor characteristics contribute to a counselor being perceived as an expert; hence, counselors should consider each client and the factors that may contribute to perceptions that they have credible knowledge and skills. For some clients, the counselor's conduct during a formal assessment will positively influence their perception of the clinician's expertness.

Assessment Is Integral to Counseling

Some counseling students may view assessment as using only formal instruments and see it as a distinct activity separate from the counseling process. Consider for a moment the counseling process and the essential steps included in it. Although the counseling process is quite complex, it encompasses the following four broad steps:

1. Assessing the client problem(s)
2. Conceptualizing and defining the client problem(s)
3. Selecting and implementing effective treatment(s)
4. Evaluating the counseling

The following is a discussion of how assessment is an integral part of the counseling process. Sometimes clinicians think of assessment only as formal tests that are expensive and time consuming. I have a broader view of assessment that is focused on gathering information holistically and using different assessment tools throughout the counseling process.

1. Assessing the Client Problem(s)

In the initial stage of counseling, a counselor needs to *assess* the client problem because there is "no one-size-fits-all" approach to the therapeutic process. It is important that counselors skillfully assess the client's problem. For if the assessment process is incomplete or inaccurate, the entire counseling process can be negatively affected. Furthermore, if counselors have limited assessment skills, they may miss or underestimate important client issues. If problems are delineated in an efficient manner, treatment can be initiated sooner.

Epperson, Bushway, and Warman (1983) found that clients are more likely to continue in counseling if they and the counselor agree on the nature of the problem. Hood and Johnson (2007) recommended combining different types of assessment data (e.g., formal and informal) to maximize the strengths and minimize the limitations of different strategies. Meyer et al. (2001) found substantial empirical support for the practice of using multimethod assessment batteries and found that clinicians who use interviewing exclusively often have incomplete client information. Assessment skills, however, are not needed solely in this first stage of counseling; they are important throughout the entire therapeutic process.

2. Conceptualizing and Defining the Client Problem(s)

A counselor may be extraordinarily skilled at initial assessment, but if she refrains from gathering additional information, then the process will be hampered. During conceptualizing, the second stage of the process, counselors need to continually assess a client to ensure that they maintain an adequate understanding of the client's needs and problems. Distinguishing between simple and complex problems is critical in the selection of treatment and the effectiveness of the counseling. Mohr (1995) found that one of the most robust predictors of negative outcomes in counseling and psychotherapy is the clinician underestimating the severity of the client's problems.

Dawes (1994) presented some compelling evidence that counselors are not always objective in their perceptions and analyses of client issues. There is research supporting the notion that counselors do have a tendency toward *confirmatory bias* (Spengler, Strohmer, Dixon, & Shivy, 1995), which entails the tendency to seek evidence that confirms an individual's preferred hypothesis. For example, if a counselor believes that substance abuse is rampant in our society, that clinician may have a tendency to perceive many clients' issues as being related to their abuse of substances. Grove, Zald, Lebow, Snitz, and Nelson (2000) compared *clinical* judgments made by health care and human services personnel with *mechanical* judgments that involved statistical and actuarial prediction. On average, mechanical predictions were slightly more accurate than clinical predictions.

Fredman and Sherman (1987) proposed that clients often benefit from formal assessments because they can provide counselors with a different avenue for reaching the client. They contended that counselors should occasionally get away from relying completely on auditory experience and add visual, kinesthetic, and tactile dimensions to their sessions. They suggested that testing can provide a visual experience that often inspires more confidence in the information than do spoken words. In addition, this visual experience often motivates clients to take action about a conflict or problem. Thus, I assert that assessment skills are necessary for adequately conceptualizing the client's concerns, identifying contextual factors that may be contributing to the problems, and ascertaining factors that may be helpful in the treatment phase of counseling.

3. *Selecting and Implementing Effective Treatment(s)*

The third step in counseling involves implementing treatment that is based on the previous assessments; however, assessment does not stop once clinical treatment begins. Rather, the assessment process continues throughout the treatment phase of counseling. This is the stage of counseling where a counselor might use either informal or formal assessment to answer a therapeutic question.

Clients often come to counseling for assistance in answering questions such as: Should I drop out of school? Should I get a divorce? or Should I change careers? Increasing the amount of information a client can use in decision making usually enhances their decision-making process. Selecting instruments that generate information about occupational choices, career interests, and family dynamics can often assist clients in making major decisions. Using assessment information to aid clients in decision making, however, does not always necessitate administering tests. Counselors can often use assessment instruments that clients have taken during previous educational experiences or in other situations. As an example, one client, who had taken the American College Testing (ACT) exam two years earlier, made his decision to pursue a new job after reviewing his scores from that test. Campbell (2000) argued that tests in counseling should provide new information and that counselors can use assessment results to encourage client learning and insight.

Sometimes clinicians believe that assessment is used only to identify problems or pathologies. This seems somewhat inconsistent with counseling's developmental and preventative foundation. Rather than using tests to diagnose pathologies or identify limitations, counselors can use an instrument's assessment to reveal strengths. Lopez, Snyder, and Rasmussen (2003) argued that clinicians must strike a vital balance between assessing strengths and limitations. Drawing from the substantial research supporting positive psychology, these authors contended that psychological assessment is currently slanted toward identifying limitations, even though there is compelling empirical evidence that constructs such as hope, resiliency, learned optimism, and courage are intimately tied with well-being and performance. Hence, if practitioners want to build on positive processes, outcomes, and environments, they should also assess the degree to which these positive factors are present. Wright and Lopez (2002) suggested a four-pronged approach to positive psychological assessment. In this approach, counselors should identify (1) undermining characteristics of the client, (2) client strengths and assets, (3) missing and destructive aspects of the client's environment, and (4) resources and opportunities within the environment. Counselors can also use positive psychological assessment to chart changes during the counseling process and to measure the development of client strengths.

In addition, during the third step in counseling, counselors need to continually monitor whether they have comprehensively understood the client and the client's situation. Furthermore, practitioners need to scrutinize whether progress is being made and adjust the counseling process if the client is not making progress toward the therapeutic goals. Because the matching of effective treatment to specific clients is not always a simple task, counselors must continually reassess the client and the efficacy of the counseling services they are providing.

4. *Evaluating the Counseling*

Finally, once the treatment phase is completed, counselors need to assess or evaluate whether it was effective. Once again, just as counselors need effective communication skills to help clients, they also need effective assessment and appraisal skills related to evaluation. Outcome assessment can provide clinicians information about their own effectiveness and, if gathered by all clients, can provide information to administrators, appropriate boards (e.g., a school board), and other relevant organizations (e.g., a governmental organization that controls grant funding). Hence, assessment is an integral part of the entire counseling process and it should not be viewed as a distinct area in which counselors simply administer tests.

In the counseling profession, clinicians are frequently more interested in helping individuals than in showing that the services they provide are effective. This approach, however, puts many clinicians at risk, because there are increasing demands from legislators, administrators, foundations, managed-care providers, clients, and parents for tangible documentation showing that counseling is both helpful and cost-effective. In these times of budgetary constraints, when school counseling positions could be cut, school counselors need to have accountability information readily available to document their usefulness (Dahir & Stone, 2003; Hughes & James, 2001; Myrick, 2003). Savin and Kiesling (2000) documented the necessity for community agencies and health care organizations to have well-designed accountability systems. Not only do counselors need knowledge of assessment to meet the accountability demands, but outcome information can also be used in the counseling process. Some clients finding it very empowering to view assessment results that indicate they have made positive changes (e.g., feel less depressed).

Assessment Can Be Therapeutic

The view that assessment can be used in a therapeutic manner is sometimes contrary to how professionals think of testing and assessment. Counselors can, however, use assessment results to stimulate clients' self-awareness and exploration. Finn and Tonsager (1992, 1997) suggested a model in which the assessment itself is considered to be a therapeutic intervention. This *therapeutic assessment model* is compared with the traditional *information-gathering model,* in which assessment is viewed as a way to collect information that will guide subsequent treatment. The intent of therapeutic assessment is to promote positive changes in clients through the *use* of assessment instruments. The assessor's primary task is to be sensitive, attentive, and responsive to clients and to foster opportunities for clients to gain information about themselves. The therapeutic assessment process involves establishing a relationship with the client and then working collaboratively to define individualized assessment goals. The assessment results are then shared and explored with the client. Finn and Tonsager (1997) suggested that in feedback sessions, clinicians begin with the feedback that most closely matches clients' preconceived notions and then move on to more discrepant information.

In the past, little attention was paid to the therapeutic effect of assessment, but recent research is encouraging. Two studies (Finn & Tonsager, 1992; Newman & Greenway, 1997) found that those who received therapeutic assessment with the MMPI-2 reported better outcomes than those who received supportive, nondirective counseling. A number of case studies also support Finn and Tonsager's model (Clair & Prendergast, 1994; Dorr, 1981; Waiswol, 1995). Hanson, Claiborn, and Kerr (1997) found some differences between career counseling clients who received an interactive interpretation and those who received a delivered interpretation. The clients who received the interactive interpretation considered their sessions to be deeper and rated the counselor as being more expert, trustworthy, and attractive.

Michel (2002) provided some examples of using assessments therapeutically with clients who have eating disorders. She argued that for these clients, assessments can provide self-verifying information, which can be very therapeutic. In addition, she indicated that "joining" or aligning with the clients' families can be facilitated by providing assessment information that acknowledges the difficulties of their situation. She recommended the following assessment strategies:

1. Continue to nurture and maintain the therapeutic alliance throughout the evaluation.
2. Present all findings in a helpful context, emphasizing that the results reflect the patient's communication.
3. Recognize that defensive protocols are useful, and attempt to discern the reasons for such responding.

4. Encourage and allow the patient to respond affectively, and give/modify examples of findings.
5. Tie the findings to the adaptive functions of the eating disorder.
6. Use examples from the assessment process and test findings to provide education about eating disorders to help normalize the patient's feelings.
7. Use psychological test results in the same manner with family members to enlist family involvement. (p. 476)

In counseling, assessment results can also be used in a therapeutic manner by helping clients make effective decisions. Counselors can use information gained from assessment to help clients weigh the pros and cons of a decision and examine the probabilities of expected outcomes. This manner of using assessment information, which is common in career counseling, can also be used with assessment results related to other issues.

What Do Counselors Need to Know About Assessment?

Because assessment is an integral part of counseling, it is crucial that practitioners become competent in this area. A group of testing scholars—Moreland, Eyde, Robertson, Primoff, and Most (1995)—identified 12 competencies that are necessary for proper test use. These competencies can be coalesced into two major themes: (1) knowledge of the test and its limitations and (2) accepting responsibility for the competent use of the test. In some states, psychologists have attempted to restrict usage to only psychologists. In response to these efforts, the American Counseling Association (2003) published a policy statement asserting that professional counselors can be qualified to use tests given they are properly trained in the following seven areas:

1. *Skill in practice and knowledge of theory relevant to the testing context and type of counseling specialty.* Assessment and testing must be integrated into the context of the theory and knowledge of a specialty area, not as a separate act, role, or entity. In addition, professional counselors should be skilled in treatment practice with the population being served.
2. *A thorough understanding of testing theory, techniques of test construction, test reliability and validity.* Included in this knowledge base are methods of item selection, theories of human nature that underlie a given test, reliability, and validity. Knowledge of reliability includes, at a minimum: methods by which it is determined, such as domain sampling, test-retest, parallel forms, split-half, and inter-item consistency, the strengths and limitations of each of these methods; the standard error of measurement, which indicates how accurately a person's test score reflects their true score of the trait being measured; and true score theory, which defines a test score as an *estimate* of what is true. Knowledge of validity includes, at a minimum: types of validity, including content, criterion-referenced (both predictive and concurrent); and construct methods of assessing each type of validity including the use of correlation; and the meaning of significance of standard error of estimate.

3. *A working knowledge of sampling techniques, norms, and descriptive, correlational and predictive statistics.* Important topics in sampling include sample size, sampling techniques, and the relationship between sampling and test accuracy. A working knowledge of descriptive statistics includes, at a minimum: probability theory, measures of central tendency; multi-modal and skewed distributions, measures of variability, including variance and standard deviation; and standard scores, including deviation IQ's, z-scores, T-scores, percentile ranks, stanines/stens, normal curve equivalents, grade- and age-equivalents. Knowledge of correlation and prediction includes, at a minimum: the principle of least squares; the direction and magnitude of relationship between two sets of scores; deriving a regression equation; the relationship between regression and correlation; and the most common procedures and formulas used to calculate correlations.
4. *Ability to review, select, and administer tests appropriate for clients or students and the context of the counseling practice.* Professional counselors using tests should be able to describe the purpose and use of different types of tests, including the most widely used tests for their setting and purposes. Professional counselors use their understanding of sampling, norms, test construction, validity, and reliability to accurately assess the strengths, limitations, and appropriate applications of a test for the clients being served. Professional counselors using tests also should be aware of the potential for error when relying on computer printouts of test interpretation. For accuracy of interpretation, technological resources must be augmented by a counselor's firsthand knowledge of the client and the test-taking context.
5. *Skills in administration of tests and interpretation of test scores.* Competent test users implement appropriate and standardized administration procedures. This requirement enables professional counselors to provide consultation and training to others who assist with test administration and scoring. In addition to standardized procedures, test users provide testing environments that are comfortable and free of distraction. Skilled interpretation requires a strong working knowledge of the theory underlying the test, the test's purpose, statistical meaning of test scores, and norms used in test construction. Skilled interpretation also requires an understanding of the similarities and differences between the client or student and the norm samples used in test construction. Finally, it is essential that clear and accurate communication of test score meaning in oral or written form to clients, students, or appropriate others be provided.
6. *Knowledge of the impact of diversity on testing accuracy, including age, gender, ethnicity, race, disability, and linguistic differences.* Professional counselors using tests should be committed to fairness in every aspect of testing. Information gained and decisions made about the client or student are valid only to the degree that the test accurately and fairly assesses the client's or student's characteristics. Test selection and interpretation are done with an awareness of the degree to which items may be culturally biased or the norming sample not reflective or inclusive of the client's or student's diversity. Test users understand that age and physical disability differences may impact the client's ability to perceive and respond to test items. Test scores are interpreted in light of the cultural, ethnic, disability, or

linguistic factors that may impact an individual's score. These include visual, auditory, and mobility disabilities that may require appropriate accommodation in test administration and scoring. Test users understand that certain types of norms and test score interpretation may be inappropriate, depending on the nature and purpose of the testing.

7. *Knowledge and skill in the professionally responsible use of assessment and evaluation practice.* Professional counselors who use tests act in accordance with ACA's Code of Ethics and Standards of Practice (1997), Responsibilities of Users of Standardized Tests (RUST) (AAC, 2003), Code of Fair Testing Practices in Education (JCTP, 2002), Rights and Responsibilities of Test Takers: Guidelines and Expectations (JCTP, 2000), and Standards for Educational and Psychological Testing (AERA/APA/NCME, 1999). In addition, professional school counselors act in accordance with the American School Counselor Association's (ASCA's) Ethical Standards for School Counselors (ASCA, 1992). Test users should understand the legal and ethical principles and practices regarding test security, using copyrighted materials, and unsupervised use of assessment instruments that are not intended for self-administration. When using and supervising the use of tests, qualified test users demonstrate an acute understanding of the paramount importance of the well being of clients and the confidentiality of test scores. Test users seek ongoing educational and training opportunities to maintain competence and acquire new skills in assessment and evaluation (American Counseling Association, 2003, p.1-4).

Some of the specific themes related to being a responsible counselor regarding the use of assessments concern the need for multiple sources of convergent data, staying abreast of assessment issues, and consulting with professionals on interpretations. Gathering multiple sources of information is important because no assessment can perfectly measure complex psychological factors. Also, various circumstances can influence a client's performance during an assessment. For example, a client enters counseling and reports that she has been feeling fatigued, guilty, and depressed and she has had some suicidal thoughts. The counselor administers a depression inventory, and the results indicate a very low level of depression. If the counselor had made a therapeutic decision based solely on the results of the depression inventory, the client would have been ill-served. In this illustration, the client had been confused by the instrument's instructions and reversed the Likert scale that indicates the severity of the symptoms of depression. Thus, the results did not indicate she was depressed, when, in fact, she was depressed. In this case, the counselor explored why the results on the depression inventory did not match his clinical views and was able to uncover the scoring problem. Using multiple assessment strategies provides more comprehensive and clinically rich information, which typically increases a counselor's ability to help clients.

Another important issue concerning responsible test usage is counselors knowing the limits of their own assessment competency. To avoid harm to a client, counselors should never administer an assessment instrument without the necessary knowledge and training. Anastasi (1992) suggested that the major reason for the misuse of tests is inadequate or outdated knowledge about the statistical aspects of testing and about the psychological findings regarding the behavior that the assessment targets. Therefore, counselors must have knowledge about measurement concepts as well as an understanding of the psychological area being assessed and of the specific instrument being used.

This book provides an introduction to assessment and is geared toward counselors-in-training. It is designed to encourage counseling students to become well-educated assessment providers. Counselors must be able to evaluate assessment tools and to determine which instruments are appropriate for specific clients. The evaluation process continues even after appropriate instruments have been identified because counselors must also determine the best instruments for specific situations. In addition to evaluation skills, counselors need to know how to use instruments appropriately. Competent use of assessment tools involves determining what inferences can be made and understanding how to interpret results appropriately. The intent of this book is not only to provide selection and evaluation skills but also to provide information on the appropriate use of assessment tools and interventions in counseling. Thus, the book's focus is two-pronged: to provide a guide for evaluating and selecting assessment tools skillfully and to help the aspiring counselor use assessment instruments and interventions appropriately.

Types of Assessment Tools

To use assessment tools effectively in counseling, a practitioner needs to understand some of the basic types of assessment instruments. Assessment and testing are topics that often arise when counselors consult with other professionals (e.g., psychologists, social workers, and teachers). The field of mental health is moving toward a multidisciplinary team approach to treatment; hence, if counselors want to continue to be a part of this multidisciplinary team, they need to understand the nomenclature of assessment. Although there are many different ways to classify appraisal instruments, the following information provides an overview of some commonly used categories and terms.

Standardized vs. Nonstandardized

For an assessment device to be considered a standardized instrument, there must be fixed instructions for administering and scoring the instrument. In addition, the content needs to remain constant and to have been developed in accordance with professional standards. If the instrument is comparing an individual's performance with that of other individuals, the instrument must be administered to an appropriate and representative sample. A nonstandardized instrument has not met these guidelines and may not provide the systematic measure of behavior that standardized instruments provide.

Individual vs. Group

This distinction concerns the administration of the instrument. Some instruments can be given to groups, which is often convenient and takes less time than administering an instrument to one person at a time. With group administration, however, it is difficult to observe all the examinees and to note all of their behaviors while they take the instrument. A substantial amount of information can often be gained by administering an instrument individually and by observing a client's nonverbal behaviors. Some well-known psychological instruments are only administered individually in order to gather relevant clinical information.

Objective vs. Subjective

This categorization reflects the methods used to score the assessment tool. Many instruments are scored objectively; that is, there are predetermined methods for scoring the assessment, and the individual doing the scoring is not required to make any judgments. Subjective instruments, on the other hand, require the individual to make professional judgments in scoring the assessment. For example, many multiple-choice tests are objective instruments, with the scoring completed by noting whether the test-taker's response is correct or incorrect. Essay tests, however, are usually subjective instruments because the person grading these exams must make some judgments about the quality of the answers. Objectively scored instruments attempt to control for bias and inconsistencies in scoring. However, counselors are often interested in exploring clients' issues, which are not easily assessed by using only objective methods.

Speed vs. Power

This classification concerns the difficulty level of the items in an assessment. In power tests, the items in the examination vary in difficulty, with more credit given for more difficult items. A speed test simply examines the number of items completed in a specified time period. The determination of whether an assessment is a speed or a power test depends on the purpose of the assessment. If the aim of an assessment is to determine how quickly people can do a specific task, then a speed test is appropriate. If determining the mathematical abilities of an individual is the goal, then a power test is needed.

Verbal vs. Nonverbal

In recent years, counselors have become increasingly aware of the influences of language and culture on assessment. Instruments that require examinees to use verbal skills can be problematic for individuals whose primary language is not English. Imagine that you are being tested and you read the following instructions: "*Da prodes test ti moras zavoriti ovu knjigu i zafpati.*" Many people would fail this test because they would not be able to read the Bosnian instructions that say, "In order to pass this test, you must close this book and take a nap." (I know that some readers would be more than willing to oblige with these instructions now that they understand the translation.) Even when a test does not involve verbal skills, if the instructions are given orally or must be read, it is still considered a verbal instrument. Some people prefer the term *nonlanguage* instead of *nonverbal* to denote instruments that require no language on the part of either the examiner or examinee. Another term related to this topic is performance tests, which require the manipulation of objects with minimal verbal influences (e.g., putting a puzzle together, arranging blocks in a certain design). Sometimes there is not a clear distinction between a verbal and a nonverbal test. It is difficult to design instruments that have no language or verbal components. Hence, with some clients, the counselor may need to determine the degree to which language and verbal skills influence the results. In multicultural assessment, the practitioner needs to consider the degree to which both culture and language influence the results.

Cognitive vs. Affective

Cognitive instruments are those that assess cognition: perceiving, processing, concrete and abstract thinking, and remembering. Three types of cognitive tests predominate: intelligence or general ability tests, achievement tests, and aptitude tests. Intelligence tests are sometime called general ability tests because the term *general ability* does not have the same connotation as *intelligence*. Intelligence/general ability instruments typically measure a person's ability to think abstractly, solve problems, understand complex ideas, and learn new material—abilities involved in a wide spectrum of activities. Although intelligence is a complex phenomenon, it is essentially related to how "smart" the individual is (Sternberg, 1985). Achievement tests, which are measures of acquired knowledge or proficiency, measure the extent to which an individual has "achieved" in acquiring certain information or mastering certain skills. As an example, after individuals have gone through instruction or training, they are often assessed to determine how well they acquired the knowledge or skill. Classroom tests of a single academic subject are the most common form of achievement tests. Whereas achievement tests measure whether an individual has acquired some knowledge or skill, aptitude tests predict an individual's performance in the future. Achievement tests and aptitude tests can be similar in content, but their purposes are different. Aptitude tests do not measure past experiences; rather, they assess an individual's ability to perform in the future—to learn new material or skills.

Affective instruments assess interest, attitudes, values, motives, temperaments, and the noncognitive aspects of personality. Both informal and formal techniques have a dominant role in affective assessment. In the area of formal instruments, practitioners most frequently use one of two types of personality tests: structured instruments and projective techniques. Structured personality instruments include the Minnesota Multiphasic Personality Inventory-2 (MMPI-2), in which individuals respond to a set of established questions and select answers from the provided alternatives. With projective techniques, individuals respond to relatively ambiguous stimuli, such as inkblots, unfinished sentences, or pictures. The nonstructured nature of the projective techniques provides the examinee with more latitude in responding. It is theorized that these nonstructured responses are projections of the individual's latent traits. Although projective techniques are often more difficult for the examinee to fake, the examiner needs to be extensively trained to use these instruments appropriately.

History

To understand current assessment techniques and instruments, counselors need information about the history of assessment. The goal of this brief excursion into the development of assessment is to provide a context for understanding the current state of the field. Through knowledge of relevant issues and with an understanding of why and how some instruments were developed, counselors can begin the process of becoming informed, competent users of assessments.

Early Testing

Assessment is not a new phenomenon; testing has been around for many centuries (Anastasi, 1993; Bowman, 1989). There is some evidence that the Greeks might have used testing around 2,500 years ago. The Chinese used a civil services examination 2,000 years ago, and even then, there were discussions of the effects of social class, cheating, and examiner bias (Bowman, 1989). In general, however, the English biologist Francis Galton is credited with launching the testing movement. Galton did not set out to initiate testing, but in his study of human heredity during the late 1800s and early 1900s, he wanted a way to measure human characteristics of biologically related and unrelated individuals. Galton believed that he could use sensory discrimination tests to measure individual intelligence. He based this opinion on the premise that all information is conveyed through the senses, and, thus, the more perceptive a person is, the greater the amount of information that is accessible for intelligent judgments and actions. Galton's book *Hereditary Genius* was published in 1869. Galton also made a significant contribution in the area of statistics. The commonly used statistical technique of correlation came from his work in heredity and "co-relations."

Another psychologist who influenced early assessment was Wilhelm Wundt. Wundt, the man credited with founding the science of psychology, was also interested in measuring psychological constructs. Wundt's purpose was somewhat different from Galton's in that Wundt and his colleagues were more interested in identifying factors of intelligence that were common or innate to all human beings. Another prominent figure in the early testing movement was American psychologist James McKeen Cattell. Cattell was Wundt's student. Drawing from the work of both Galton and Wundt, Cattell expanded testing to include memory and other simple mental processes. Cattell was the first to use the term *mental test*, although his mental tests were quite simple in that they were not strongly related to estimates of school achievement or to other criteria now considered indicative of intelligence (Anastasi, 1993).

1900–1920

Just prior to the turn of the century, Binet and Henri published an article criticizing most available intelligence tests as being too sensory oriented. Binet was given the opportunity to develop his ideas when the French Minister of Public Instruction appointed him to a commission studying "educationally retarded" children. The result was the first version of the Binet-Simon scale, published in 1905. The instrument, which was individually administered to, was a simple instrument with only 30 items and a norming group of 50. The Binet-Simon scale was different from previous measures of intelligence in that it focused on assessing judgment, comprehension, and reasoning. The instrument was revised in 1908 to incorporate a ratio of mental age level to chronological age level. This was labeled the *intelligence quotient (IQ)*. This method of calculating IQ was used for many years, although, as will be discussed in later chapters, there are some problems associated with it. Binet's instrument was translated and adapted in several countries, including an adaptation by L. M. Terman at Stanford University. The revised test became known as the Stanford-Binet scale; however, the official title of Terman's 1916 publication is *The Measurement of Intelligence: An Explanation of and a Complete Guide for the Use of the Stanford Revision and Extension of the Binet-Simon Intelligence Scale.* Although other translations of Binet-Simon's scale were available at this time, Terman's normative sample and his methodical approach were credited with the success of the Stanford-Binet (Becker, 2003).

While individually administered intelligence tests were being developed, there was also some interest in group testing, particularly by military leaders in the United States during World War I. In 1917, the army contacted Robert Yerkes, who was then the president of the American Psychological Association, to have psychologists assist in developing a group intelligence test. The army hired psychologists and a group administered intelligence assessment was developed for use in selection and classification of personnel. The army used a multiple-choice format, which had only recently been introduced by Arthur Otis. These first group-administered intelligence tests were known as Army Alpha—used for routine testing—and Army Beta—, which was a nonlanguage instrument designed for use with illiterate or non-English speaking recruits. Although these instruments were never really used in World War I, shortly after the end of the war, the army released these two instruments for public use.

Another influential person of this time was Frank Parsons, who is often cited as being the father of guidance. Although Parsons did not develop any assessment, he did devise one of the first approaches to career counseling. In his three-step career counseling model, a counselor would (1) understand the person, (2) understand the world of work, and (3) match the person to the appropriate occupation in the world of work. Some career counselors have accomplished this first step of gaining an understanding of the person by incorporating some of the career assessments that have been developed since Parsons' time.

1920s and 1930s

Interestingly, the first intelligence tests were developed without a theoretical foundation, but in the 1920s and 1930s there was considerable theoretical attention to defining and explaining the construct of intelligence (Erford, Moore-Thomas, & Linde, 2007). Spearman (1927) proposed that intelligence consisted of two types of factors—one that pertained to general tasks and another that pertained to specific tasks. Thurstone (1938), on the other hand, proposed that there is no one general factor of intelligence; rather, there are seven primary mental abilities. This debate about whether intelligence is one general factor (g) or multiple factors continues and, even today, theoreticians have differing views of intelligence. During this time, there also was increased activity related to developing measures of intelligence. Terman and Merrill revised the 1916 version and the test was published using its current name, the Stanford-Binet. In 1939, another significant test, Wechsler-Bellevue Intelligence Scale, was published. The primary author was David Wechsler who continued to make significant contributions to intelligence testing until his death in 1981.

Interest in assessment was not restricted to intelligence testing alone. At the end of World War I, there was also an interest in identifying men who were not emotionally capable of serving in the armed forces. The army once again developed the prototype, but this time the group test, called the Woodworth's Personal Data Sheet, focused on personality assessment. Consistent with the Army Alpha and Army Beta, this self-report inventory was released for civilian use, where it spurred the development of other self-report personality inventories. In 1921, Rorschach described the technique of using inkblots as a tool for diagnostic investigation of the personality. Although his methods did not have a significant impact immediately, his writings had a major influence on clinical assessment later. Another projective test of personality (i.e., Thematic Apperception Test) was published in 1935. In this assessment, Murray and Morgan presented individuals with pictures and the examinees told stories about the pictures. The examiner would then evaluate the text in order to identify themes. A more detailed discussion of both of these projective assessments is included in Chapter 10.

As private industries began to see that tests could be used for selecting and classifying industrial personnel, special aptitude tests were developed, primarily for use in clerical and mechanical areas. There was also the development of vocational counseling instruments, such as the publication in 1927 of the Strong Interest Blank by E. K. Strong. Another individual active in the development of interest inventories for vocational counseling was G. Frederic Kuder, who first published the Kuder Preference Record—Vocational in 1932.

In 1923, the first standardized achievement battery, the Stanford Achievement Test, was published. This instrument was designed to provide measures of performance in different school subjects as opposed to testing in only a single subject. These achievement batteries also allowed educators to compare students' performances to other students from various parts of the country. In the mid-1800s, there was a move from oral achievement examinations to written essay testing. By the 1930s, there was considerable evidence concerning the difficulties of written essay examinations, particularly due to the lack of agreement among teachers in grading essay items. The desire for more objectivity in testing promoted the use of more objective items and the development of state, regional, and national achievement testing programs.

The rapid advancement in many areas of testing during the 1920s and 1930s led to a need for a resource to identify and evaluate testing instruments. The first edition of the *Mental Measurements Yearbook* was published in 1939 to fill that need. Oscar Buros established these yearbooks to provide information about instruments as well as to critique the properties of the instruments.

1940s and 1950s

Even though there were efforts to produce sound personality assessment tools, there was some dissatisfaction with many of these instruments because they were somewhat transparent and could easily be faked by an examinee. Therefore, projective techniques, such as the Rorschach, began to become more popular. With projective techniques, clients respond to a relatively unstructured task, and their responses are then evaluated. The increased use of projective techniques did not, however, hamper the development of self-report instruments. In the early 1940s, Hathaway and McKinley developed a prominent personality instrument, the Minnesota Multiphasic Personality Inventory (MMPI), which incorporated validity scales to assess the degree to which individuals portrayed themselves in an overly positive or negative way. The MMPI also contained items that were empirically selected and keyed to criterion rather than items that appeared to measure different aspects of personality.

Standardized achievement tests were also becoming well established in the public schools. Although single aptitude tests were already in existence, most of the multiple aptitude batteries appeared after 1940. Multiple aptitude batteries could indicate where an individual's strengths and limitations were. (E.g., Does an individual have higher verbal aptitude or higher numerical aptitude?) The development of multiple aptitude batteries came late compared with other assessment areas, which was directly related to the refinement of the statistical technique of factor analysis.

With the increased use of assessment instruments, problems associated with these instruments began to emerge. As criticisms of assessment rose, it became clear that there was a need for standards with respect to the development and use of instruments.

The American Psychological Association published the first edition of defined standards. In later years, three organizations—the American Educational Research Association (AERA), the American Psychological Association (APA), and the National Council on Measurement in Education (NCME)—collaborated on revised editions, titled *Standards for Educational and Psychological Testing*. These standards continue to be revised and serve as a significant resource in the evaluation and appropriate use of appraisal instruments.

As assessment became more established, it also became more sophisticated. Individuals began to see that centralized publication of tests would be convenient for consumers as well as, quite possibly, profitable for the publishers. For example, the testing functions of the College Entrance Examination Board (CEEB), the Carnegie Corporation, and the American Council on Education merged to form the Educational Testing Service. With the centralization of some publishing, electronic scoring became more cost-effective. Electronic scoring reduced scoring errors and allowed for more complicated scoring procedures.

1960s and 1970s

This period is marked by an examination and evaluation of testing and assessment. The proliferation of large-scale testing in the schools, along with the increased use of testing in employment and the military, led to widespread public concern. Numerous magazine articles and books questioned the use of psychological instruments and uncovered misuses of these instruments. Assessment instruments were particularly scrutinized for ethnic bias, fairness, and accuracy. This scrutiny revealed many limitations of existing instruments, particularly those concerning the use of some instruments with minority clients.

An interesting paradox occurred during the 1970s. Although there was substantial concern about the use of tests, there was also a grassroots movement related to minimum competency testing that encouraged more testing. This movement grew out of concern that high school students were graduating without sufficient skills. Because the public wanted to ensure that children reached a minimal level of competency before they graduated, many states enacted legislation requiring students to pass a minimum competency examination before they could be awarded a high school diploma (Lerner, 1981). In addition, legislation at the national level had a significant impact on testing. In 1974, the Family Educational Rights and Privacy Act was passed, mandating that parents and children older than 18 had the right to review their own school records. This legislation also specified topics that could not be assessed without parental permission.

As the country was beginning to take advantage of advances in technology, the field of assessment was also changing. Computers began to be used more, particularly for scoring. Near the end of the 1970s, the assessment field began to explore the interactive nature of computers and methods for using computers not only to score but also to administer and interpret assessment results.

1980s and 1990s

The use of computers in appraisal really blossomed in the 1980s. With the increased availability of personal computers, clients could take an assessment instrument on a computer and receive the results immediately. Computers could be programmed to adapt the order of items depending on a client's previous answer. For example, if a client got one item correct, then the next item could be more difficult; but if a client got the item wrong, the next item could be easier. There also was an increase in computer generated reports, where instead of a psychologist writing a report, the report was written by a computer.

Earlier criticisms of assessment techniques led to many instruments being revised. For example, the developers of the MMPI-2 attempted to eliminate many of the shortcomings of the MMPI. The most widely used instrument to assess children's intelligence, the Wechsler Intelligence Scale for Children—Revised (WISC-R), was revised to become the WISC-III. The adult version of the Wechsler scale (WAIS) was revised twice during this period. New instruments designed to be sensitive to cultural diversity were also developed (e.g., Kaufman Assessment Battery for Children). Issues related to cultural bias and sensitivity to multicultural influences that arose in the 1960s and 1970s continued to be researched and discussed. Many professional organizations began to realize that standards for multicultural counseling and assessment needed to be developed.

A major testing movement within the 1990s was authentic assessment, the purpose of which is to evaluate using a method consistent with the instructional area and to gather multiple indicators of performance. Authentic assessment has had a major influence on teachers' assessments of students' academic progress (Fisher & King, 1995). Teachers often use portfolio assessment, where multiple assignments are gathered together and evaluated. Rather than using only one multiple-choice test, teachers evaluate multiple essays, projects, and tests that are designed to represent the material being taught.

2000 to the Present

It is difficult to predict the future issues and trends that will evolve in assessment. Technology and the Internet are continuing to change the manner in which assessments are developed, administered, scored, and interpreted. It may be that assessment will not take place as much in the counselor's office; instead, many clients may take assessments via the Internet at home or other locations. There are also some drawbacks to technology's influence on assessment. Thousands of assessments are on the Internet; however, it is difficult for clients to determine what assessments have been researched and the degree to which validation evidence has been accumulated. Individuals might make important life decisions (e.g., whether to pay for an expensive training program) based on an instrument that has very low reliability.

Multicultural issues will continue to be a focus of research in the assessment area. Identifying methods of assessing individuals with different cultural backgrounds is complex, and it is hoped that the field will make strides in this area. A number of instruments have already been revised since 2000 with the goal of diminishing instrument bias.

Certainly the passage of the No Child Left Behind Act of 2001 has had a dramatic influence on achievement testing in the schools. The specifics of No Child Left Behind will be discussed in Chapter 14. In many ways, No Child Left Behind was passed to make schools more accountable. The theme of accountability is also evident for counselors interested in being mental health counselors. Indications are that counselors will need to be more accountable and provide effectiveness data. Hence, assessment knowledge is important for counselors working in diverse settings.

Summary

Often the terms *assessment* and *appraisal* have different meanings in the helping profession, depending on the situation and context. This book defines both terms as procedures, including formal and informal techniques, designed to gather information about clients. Assessment can involve formal tests, psychological inventories, checklists, scales, interviews, and observations. The degree to which counselors accurately assesses clients will influence the effectiveness of their counseling. Assessment is an integral part of the counseling process, and as such, counselors need to develop proficient assessment skills.

The history of assessment in counseling indicates that there has been an ebb and flow in assessment strategies. In the United States today, there is considerable interest in various areas of testing, and some environments, such as schools, have seen a significant increase in assessments. Given current social and political influences, it is even more important for counselors to understand issues in assessment. The development of assessment and appraisal skills involves knowledge of basic measurement techniques and methods for evaluating instruments. These skills also involve knowledge of the constructs (e.g., intelligence, personality) being measured and how to use the results in counseling. Assessment results can sometimes have a dramatic effect on a client; therefore, counselors should strive to ensure that appraisal results are used in a professional and ethical manner. In the past, psychologists have challenged whether counselors have the appropriate training and background to use assessment. If counselors want to continue to have a place in providing mental health services, then they need to be proficient in assessment. The following chapters are designed to provide counselors with an introduction to key issues in assessment with an emphasis on understanding basic concepts related to measurement.

CHAPTER 2

Basic Assessment Principles

Let's assume that you have just taken a test called the Counseling Aptitude Scale (CAS), and you received a score of 60 on this fictitious instrument. It is difficult to draw any conclusions based solely on this score of 60. For example, we don't know if the scores range from 0 to 60 or if the range is from 60 to 600. Even if the scores range from 0 to 60, a score of 60 would mean something different if everyone else taking the instrument had a score of 58 than it would if everyone else scored a 30. Any score on any instrument is difficult to interpret without additional information. The basic principles discussed in this chapter will assist counselors in understanding assessment scores and results and will help them begin to know how to interpret those scores to clients. Baker (2000) stated that "without basic knowledge of measurement principles, test users are navigating without compasses" (p. 278).

Measurement Scales

When counselors use assessments, they are attempting to ***measure*** some aspect of the client. Measurement typically involves the application of specific procedures for assigning numbers to objects. When an entity is measured, there are rules for how the measurement is performed. As an example, there is a rule related to the length of an inch—an inch is always the same distance regardless of the place or time that it is measured. In measuring any matter—a person's weight, the temperature outside, the number of lawyers in New York City, or the emotional stability of graduate students—the rules for measuring depend on the precision of the measurement scale being used.

There are four basic types of measurement scales: nominal, ordinal, interval, and ratio. Any measurement of a client (whether it is height or level of anxiety) involves one of these four types of measurement scales. Numbers at different levels or scales of measurement convey different types of information (Cohen & Swerdlik, 2005); therefore, counselors need to determine the type of measurement scale being used in an assessment in order to evaluate the instrument properly. Statistical tests are often used to analyze the psychometric qualities of an instrument. The type of measurement scale will influence the selection of appropriate statistical techniques. Therefore, one of the early steps in evaluating an instrument is to identify the measurement scale used and then determine if the statistical analyses are appropriate for that type of measurement scale.

The **nominal scale**, which is the most elementary of the measurement scales, involves classifying by name based on characteristics of the person or object being measured. In other words, the intent of the nominal scale is to name an object. If this scale is used, there is no indication of amount or magnitude. An example of a nominal scale is 1 = Democrats, 2 = Republicans, 3 = Libertarians, 4 = No party affiliation. When numbers are assigned to groups, it is not possible to perform many of the common statistical analyses. For example, the average for the above numbers for party affiliation is 2.5, which does not convey any real meaning. With a nominal scale, we can only get a count or a percentage of individuals who may fall into a specific category.

An **ordinal scale** provides a measure of magnitude and, thus, it often provides more information than does a nominal scale. An instrument with an ordinal scale makes it possible to determine which scores are smaller or larger than other scores. Ranking a group of children from best to worst behaved in the classroom is an example of an ordinal scale. The ordinal scale enables one to rank or order individuals or objects, but that is the extent of the precision. On the fictitious Counseling Aptitude Scale mentioned earlier, you received a score of 60, whereas Jason's score was 50 and Rebecca's was 90. Unless we know that there are equal intervals between points throughout the scale, all we can say is that Rebecca received the highest score, you were in the middle, and Jason had the lowest score of the group. With any kind of measurement, unless there are equal units (e.g., inches have equal units), the degree to which there is a difference between the scores cannot be precisely determined. It is often difficult to design instruments that measure psychological and educational aspects in equal intervals. Consider, for example, the difficulty in developing items for a depression scale in which the intervals would always be equal throughout the scoring of the instrument.

In an **interval scale**, the units are in equal intervals; thus, a difference of 5 points between 45 and 50 represents the same amount of change as the difference of 5 points between 85 and 90. An example of equal intervals is weight; if you gain 5 pounds, those pounds are always the same, whether you are going from 115 to 120 or from 225 to 230. In counseling, many instruments are treated as if there were interval data. For example, the difference between 85 and 100 on an intelligence test is supposedly the same as the difference between 100 and 115. Many of the statistical techniques used to evaluate assessment instruments also assume that there is an interval scale. There are instruments, however, that do not have an interval scale and that should not be evaluated using those statistical techniques. In evaluating instruments, counselors need to consider whether the scores can be classified on an interval scale because many of the statistical techniques discussed later in this book assume there is interval data. Sometimes a researcher will put together an instrument, for example using a Likert scale, where it is very difficult to achieve interval data (e.g., strongly disagree, disagree, agree, strongly agree). In this example, is the difference between strongly disagree and disagree equal to the difference between disagree and agree? The researcher may then use statistics that require interval data when that is not appropriate. We should be cautious in using an instrument developed in this manner.

A **ratio scale** has all the properties of an interval scale, but the former requires the existence of a meaningful zero. A good example of a meaningful zero is driving and miles per hour. When you are driving at zero miles per hour, you are stopped, and not moving is a meaningful zero. With intelligence tests, there is no definition of what a score of zero means. Therefore, the results from an intelligence test might be considered an interval scale but not a ratio scale. In measuring other entities, such as pulse or liquid ounces, there are meaningful zeros. Height is an example of a ratio scale because inches are equal units and a meaningful zero exists. With this type of scale, it is possible to compute ratios and make conclusions that something is twice as big as something else. For example, a person who is six feet tall is twice as tall as a person who is three feet tall. With interval scales, such as IQ, these types of conclusions cannot be made. Thus, we cannot say that someone whose IQ is 150 is twice as smart as someone whose IQ is 75.

As indicated earlier, the level of measurement influences the methods that can be used to evaluate the instrument. Therefore, counselors need to consider the scale of measurement when they begin to examine an instrument.

Norm-Referenced vs. Criterion-Referenced Instruments

To interpret a score on any instrument, practitioners first need to consider whether it is a norm-referenced or criterion-referenced instrument. In a **norm-referenced instrument,** an individual's score is compared with scores of other individuals who have taken the same instrument. The term ***norm*** refers to the group of individuals who took the instrument to which others' scores are then compared. A norming group can be quite large, such as a national sample of 2,000 adults who have taken a personality inventory. On the other hand, a norm could be your fellow classmates, such as when an instructor "grades on the curve." Simply stated, a norm-referenced instrument is one in which an individual's performance is compared with the performance of other individuals.

In a **criterion-referenced instrument,** the individual's score is compared with an established standard or criterion. Criterion-referenced instruments are sometimes called domain- or objective-referenced. With a criterion-referenced instrument, the interest is ***not*** on how the individual's performance compares with the performance of others, but rather on how the individual performs with respect to some standard or criterion. In criterion-referenced instruments, results are reported in terms of some specific domain. Therefore, to interpret a client's criterion-referenced test results, a counselor needs to understand the domain being measured, such as third-grade spelling words, multiplication of two-digit numbers, or knowledge of counseling theories. In criterion-referenced testing, the testing often pertains to whether a person has reached a certain *standard* of performance within that domain. For example, does Jerome get 70% of a sample of second-grade arithmetic problems correct? Does Lisa spell 90% of fifth-grade spelling words correctly? Many of the tests you have taken in your academic career have been criterion-referenced tests on which, for example, you needed to score 90% or better for an A, 80% or better for a B, 70% or better for a C, and so forth.

Sometimes with a criterion-referenced test there is a *mastery* component. In these cases, a predetermined cutoff score indicates whether the person has attained an established level of mastery. For example, a state's department of education may designate a certain test score that all high school students must achieve before they can graduate. Likewise, a teacher may test to find out if a student has mastered the multiplication table for the number 3 before allowing the student to learn the multiplication table for the number 4. Professional licensing examinations for counselors and psychologists are also examples of criterion-referenced tests that include a mastery component. To be licensed in many states, counselors must meet a pre-established score on a licensing examination that reflects a certain level of mastery. Individuals who do not attain that score are considered not to have mastered the body of knowledge necessary to perform as professional counselors.

There are several difficulties in developing sound criterion-referenced instruments. First, criterion-referenced tests are designed to measure a person's level of performance in a certain domain. Therefore, an instrument should adequately measure that domain. For example, to show mastery of a theories and techniques class in a counseling program, a criterion-referenced test for this class would need to adequately measure all the information in the domain of counseling theories and techniques. However, there is no universal agreement within the field about which theories are most important, nor is there complete agreement on which techniques are most effective. Therefore, it is difficult to determine what content should be included on a theories and techniques test. With higher-order knowledge areas, it is often quite difficult to define definitively the precise content domain and determine the degree to which topics within the content domain are particularly or less important. Anastasi and Urbina (1997) contended that criterion-referenced testing is best for assessing basic skills, such as reading and mathematics at the elementary level.

Another problem with criterion-referenced instruments is determining the criterion for mastery level. This issue centers on what exact score truly indicates that someone has mastered the content. For example, if the mastery level is preset at 90%, does it, in effect, mean that a person who receives 89% has not mastered the content? What about the person who scores below the mastery level because of a mistake in marking an answer? It is often difficult to determine the exact score that indicates whether someone has, indeed, mastered that content. The consequences of making mistakes in misidentification can often influence the setting of the mastery level. For example, in a professional licensing examination (e.g., in counseling), the consequences of misidentification can be quite serious if individuals are considered, by their performance on the instrument, to be competent when in fact they are not adequately prepared to counsel clients. To keep this from happening, the cutoff score might be set quite high to minimize the number of false positives. Although there are often numerous difficulties in developing sound criterion-referenced instruments, these instruments can be very useful in indicating an individual's level of performance in a certain content domain.

Interpreting Norm-Referenced Instruments

Let's return once again to our example of the Counseling Aptitude Scale (CAS) and your score of 60. In this example, this fictitious instrument is used to identify which individuals have the greatest potential for being superb counselors as compared with other individuals. Because we are comparing the scores of individuals, it is a norm-referenced interpretation. Often with norm-referenced instruments, we use statistics to help interpret the scores. If we examine the scores in Table 2.1, it would be difficult to simply look at the scores and to interpret your score of 60 compared with the scores of 39 other people. However, organizing the scores in a logical manner can facilitate the process of understanding the scores.

By converting the scores into a frequency distribution, as is reflected in Table 2.2 on the next page, we can better understand how your score of 60 compares with the others who also took the fictitious CAS. A frequency distribution is simply where the scores (X) are indicated on the first line and the frequency (f), or number, of people achieving that score is indicated beneath. A frequency distribution provides a visual display to help

TABLE 2.1
Raw scores on the Counseling Aptitude Scale

Names	CAS Scores	Names	CAS Scores
You	60	Tom	10
Alex	40	Angelina	50
Stacy	50	Max	40
Josh	50	Juan	50
Michael	70	Marilyn	20
Katlin	30	Satish	60
Morgan	60	Lisa	90
Ian	30	Omar	60
Christina	50	Matt	50
Hannah	80	Luisa	40
Marco	60	Rolando	90
Adam	50	Carmin	50
Rose	70	Yu-Ting	70
Kisha	50	Matt	50
Reggie	40	Logan	30
Kris	30	Regina	60
Bart	10	Colton	40
Rebecca	60	Punita	70
Scott	20	Javi	80
Shawn	60	Emily	40

TABLE 2.2 *Frequency distribution for the scores on the Counseling Aptitude Scale*

X	10	20	30	40	50	60	70	80	90
f	2	2	4	6	10	8	4	2	2

Note: X is for CAS scores, and *f* is for the frequency of individuals.

organize data so that it is easier to see how the scores are distributed. In the frequency distribution in Table 2.2, we can see that the number, or frequency, of people receiving scores of 10, 20, 80, and 90 is smaller than the number of people receiving scores of 40, 50, and 60.

Sometimes, actually graphing the frequency of scores can provide a better visual display of how a group of people scored on an instrument. A **frequency polygon** is often used in assessment because this graphic representation makes the data easier to understand. A frequency polygon is a graph that charts the scores on the *x*-axis (the horizontal) and the frequencies of the scores on the *y*-axis (the vertical). A point is placed by plotting the number of persons receiving each score across from the appropriate frequency. The successive points are then connected with a straight line. Figure 2.1 shows a frequency polygon for the CAS scores and reflects a graphic display of the information contained in the frequency distribution in Table 2.2. The frequency polygon in Figure 2.1 makes it easier to see that many more people had a score lower than your 60, although some individuals did have scores higher than yours. This frequency polygon also reflects that most of the people scored between 40 and 60, with the largest number of people receiving a score of 50.

Sometimes, we do not want to plot each individual score of an instrument because the range of scores is too large. For example, an instrument with a range of

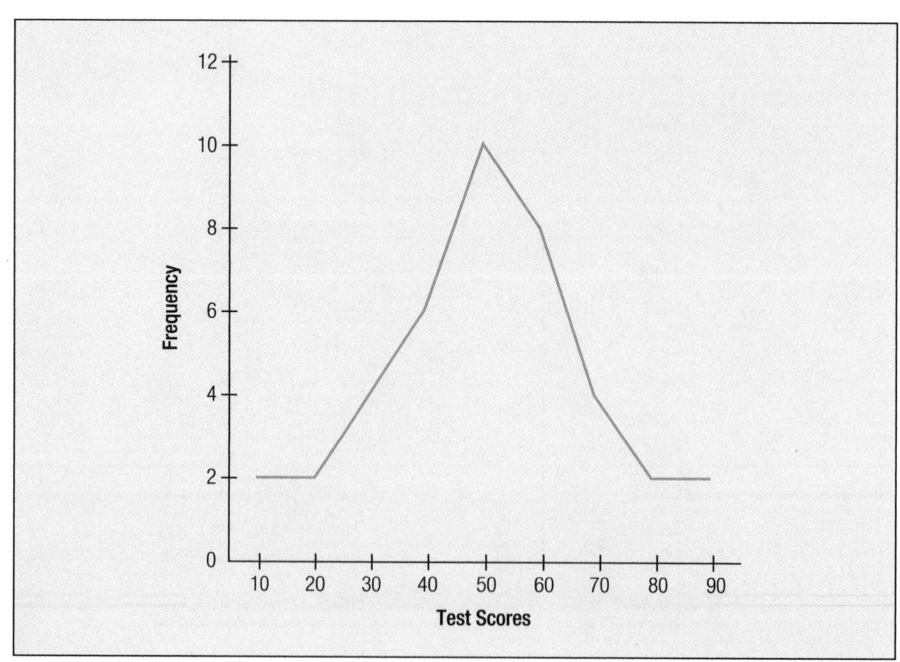

FIGURE 2.1 *Frequency polygon for Counseling Aptitude Scale scores*

scores from 1 to 200 would make a large frequency polygon if we plotted each possible score (1, 2, 3, . . ., 198, 199, 200). In this case, we may want to make the information more manageable by determining the frequency of people who fall within a certain interval of scores. Figure 2.2 contains a frequency polygon that groups the

FIGURE 2.2
Frequency polygon and histogram with interval scores

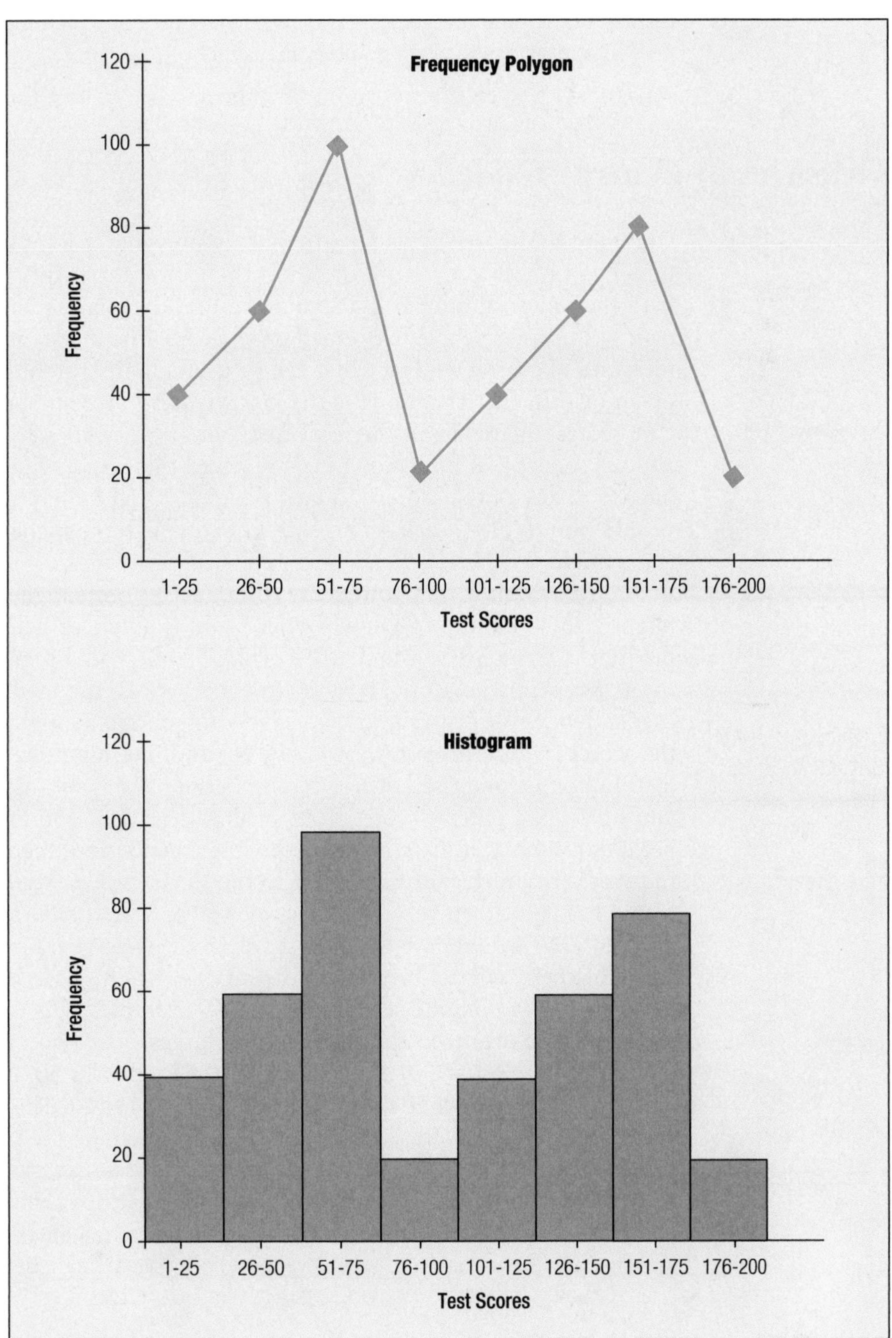

scores into convenient interval classes of 25 points each (e.g., 1–25, 26–50, 51–75, etc.). Figure 2.1 and Figure 2.2 are very similar except in 2.2 the scores are grouped into intervals. In a histogram, the height of the column over each class interval corresponds to the number of individuals who scored in that interval. As Figure 2.2 indicates, either a frequency polygon or a histogram can be used to provide a visual display of the same frequency of scores. The choice of which method to use depends on which provides the best graphic display.

Measures of Central Tendency

Graphing the scores by using a frequency polygon or a histogram can help you understand how your score of 60 on the Counseling Aptitude Scale compares with the scores of others. It also may be useful to have some indication of how *most* of the other people performed on the CAS. The mode, median, and mean are measures of central tendency that can be useful in interpreting individuals' results on an instrument. The mode is the ***most frequent*** score in a distribution. On the CAS scores, the mode, or the most frequent score, is 50, because both Tables 2.1 and 2.2 reflect that nine individuals received this score, which is the highest frequency of any of the scores. To find the mode, you merely count the number of people who received each score, and the score with the highest number of people is the mode.

You now know that your score of 60 is 10 points higher than the mode. It might also be helpful to know if your score is above or below the median. The median is the score at which 50% of the people had a score below it and 50% of the people had a score above it. In other words, the median is the score that evenly divides the scores into two halves. You determine the median by arranging the scores in order from lowest to highest and finding the middle number. If the distribution is comprised of an odd number of participants, then it is easy because you simply arrange the scores from smallest to largest and find the middle number. For example, if there are 25 score in a distribution, then you would arrange the scores in order and then count to the thirteenth score. The thirteenth score would be the median because 12 people (50%) would have a lower score and 12 people (50%) would have a higher score. In the CAS example, there are 40 scores and thus there will not be one middle number. In this case, you take the average between the two middle scores. In the CAS examples, this is easy because when the scores are arranged from smallest to largest, the two middle scores are 50 (and $50 + 50 \div 2 = 50$) and, therefore, the median is 50. As another example, let's say we have the following scores: 1, 1, 1, 3, 14, 16. The median would be 2 because that is the average between 1 and 3, which are the two middle scores in this distribution.

Although a mode of 1 and a median of 2 provides some useful information about the scores of 1, 1, 1, 3, 14, 16, these measures of central tendency do not really describe the variation in scores very well, because the higher scores of 14 and 16 are not really reflected in either the mode or the median. This is an example of why the mean is a useful measure of central tendency. The **mean** is the arithmetic average of the scores. The mean in the example of 1, 1, 1, 3, 14, 16 is 6, which provides a measure that represents the distribution of scores. In this book, which includes a few statistical formulas, the mean will always be notated by the letter *M* and an individual's score or some other data point by *X*. The Greek symbol Σ stands for sigma and means "to sum," and *N* represents the number of individuals in the group. In the formula for mean (M), we sum (Σ) the scores (*X*) and then divide by the number of individuals in the group (*N*) to get the mean or average (*M*). In the earlier example, we would sum the scores (1 + 1 + 1 + 3 + 14 + 16 = 36) and then divide 36 by the number of scores (*N* = 6), which is equal to 6. In case you are interested, the mean for the CAS scores listed in Table 2.1 is 50.50, whereas the median and the mode are both 50.

$$M = \frac{\Sigma X}{N}$$

Measures of Variability

Knowing the measures of central tendency assists you in understanding what your score of 60 on the Counseling Aptitude Scale means, because you now know that your score is larger than the mean, median, and mode. At this point, though, you cannot tell how much above the mean your score is in comparison with other people's scores. For example, it would suggest something very different if the 25 other people who took the Counseling Aptitude Scale all had scores of 60 as compared with the distribution of scores that was presented earlier (see Table 2.1). In assessments, it is important to examine how the scores vary so that we can determine if a person is high or low compared with others, and how much higher or lower a person's score is. For example, the scores of 1, 3, 6, 9, and 11 have a mean of 6, and the scores of 5, 6, 6, 6, and 7 also have a mean of 6. Even though the means are the same, the variations in scores affect how we would interpret a score of 7. Measures of variability provide useful benchmarks because they give us an indication of how the scores vary.

Range

Range provides a measure of the spread of scores and indicates the variability between the highest and the lowest scores. Range is calculated by simply subtracting the lowest score from the highest. On the Counseling Aptitude Scale, the highest score anyone received was 90, and the lowest was 10; therefore, the range is 80 (90 − 10 = 80). Range does provide an indication of how compact or wide the variation is, but it does not really assist us in interpreting your CAS score of 60 very well. Range is a simple and somewhat crude measure that can be significantly influenced by one extremely high or one very low score.

Variance and Standard Deviation

When interpreting scores to clients, counselors often use more precise measures to provide better information about how individuals vary from the mean. Variance and standard deviation fill this need by providing more precise measures that serve as indicators of how scores vary from the mean. In examining Table 2.3, we might be interested to know how these five scores (1, 2, 3, 4, 5), on the average, vary from the mean. In the second column, there is an indication of how each score varies from the mean of 3. If we wanted an average deviation from the mean, we could simply add these numbers together and divide by the number of scores. If we do that, however, what we get is 0. In fact, with any set of scores, given the way we calculate mean, we will always get 0. Therefore, to avoid this problem, we square the deviations, add these together, and divide by the number of scores. This number is **variance** or mean square deviation. In the case of Table 2.3, by adding the squared deviation in the third column and dividing the number of scores, the variance is 2. The problem with variance is that when we square the deviations, they are no longer in the same measurement unit as the original scores. Therefore, if we take the square root of the variance, it will take the deviation back to the original unit of measurement. The square root of variance is the **standard deviation,** which provides an indication of the average deviation from the mean in the original unit of measurement. In Table 2.3, the square root of 2 (variance) is 1.41, which is the standard deviation of those scores.

In the area of assessment, standard deviation is primarily used in two ways. First, standard deviation provides some indication of the variability of scores. The larger the standard deviation, the more the scores varied, or deviated, from the mean. Smaller standard deviations indicate that the scores are more closely grouped together around the mean. Based on the scores presented earlier, the standard deviation for the CAS is 19.10. A counselor cannot ascertain how much variation there is in scores based solely on the standard deviation; however, it is probably safe

TABLE 2.3
Illustrations of variance and standard deviation

Score (X)	Deviation ($X - M$)	Deviation² $(X - M)^2$
1	$1 - 3 = -2$	$-2^2 = 4$
2	$2 - 3 = -1$	$-1^2 = 1$
3	$3 - 3 = 0$	$0^2 = 0$
4	$4 - 3 = 1$	$1^2 = 1$
5	$5 - 3 = 2$	$2^2 = 4$
$\Sigma X = 15$	$\Sigma(X - M) = 0$	$\Sigma(X - M)^2 = 10$
$M = \frac{\Sigma X}{N}$		$s^2 = \frac{\Sigma(X - M)^2}{N}$ $s^2 = \frac{10}{5} = 2$
$M = \frac{15}{5} = 3$		$s = \sqrt{\frac{\Sigma(X - M)^2}{N}}$ $s = \sqrt{2} = 1.41$

to say that this standard deviation of 19.10 suggests that there is some variation in scores on the CAS.

The second way to use standard deviation involves interpreting individual scores. A standard deviation can provide an indication of whether a score is below the mean, close to the mean, or significantly higher than the mean. We can interpret your score of 60 on the CAS by saying that your score is quite close to one half a standard deviation above the mean (60 − 50.50 = 9.50), because one half a standard deviation for the CAS is 9.55 (19.10/2 = 9.55).

Normal Distributions

If the scores on an instrument fall into a normal distribution, or a normal curve, then standard deviation provides even more interpretive information. The distributions of a number of human traits (e.g., weight, height, intelligence, and some personality characteristics) approximate the normal curve. The normal curve has mathematical properties that make it very useful in the interpretation of norm-referenced instruments.

The normal curve is bell-shaped and symmetrical (see Figure 2.3). If the distribution of scores is normalized, there is a single peak in the center and the mean,

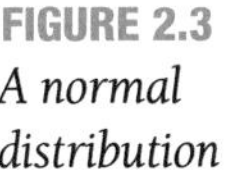

FIGURE 2.3
A normal distribution

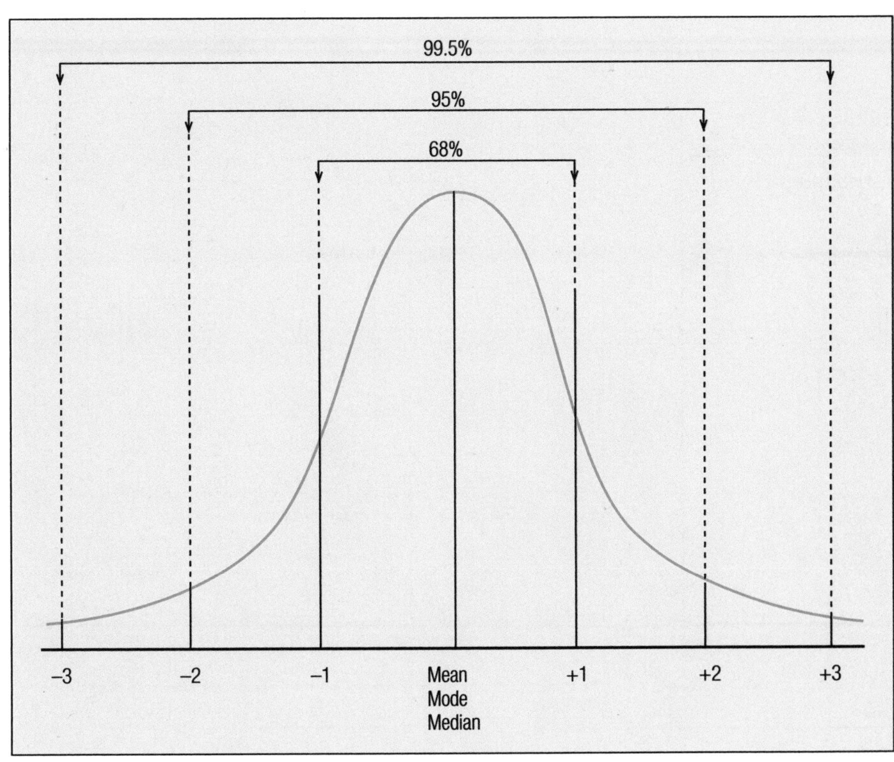

mode, and median are the same score. The normal curve reflects that the largest number of cases falls in the center range and that the number of cases decreases gradually in both directions. Specifically, 68% of the cases fall between 1 standard deviation below the mean and 1 standard deviation above the mean. Ninety-five percent of the cases fall between 2 standard deviations below the mean and 2 standard deviations above the mean, and 99.5% of the cases fall between 3 standard deviations below the mean and 3 standard deviations above the mean. The percentages of people falling within the different ranges of standard deviations are constant and have a normal distribution. In general, the larger the group, the greater the likelihood that the scores on that instrument will resemble a normal curve. If a counselor is using an assessment where the scores have a normal distribution, then a counselor interprets individuals' scores based on the characteristics of a normal distribution. For example, if an individual score is more than 3 standard deviations above the mean, we know that only a very small percentage of people score there, because 99.5% of the individuals score between 3 standard deviations below the mean and 3 standard deviations above the mean.

There are times, however, when the scores do not fall into a normal distribution, so using the normal curve to interpret scores would be inappropriate. Scores on an instrument can distribute in many ways other than a normal curve. They can be multimodal, which means the distribution has more than one peak. Distributions can also be skewed (see Figure 2.4), meaning that the distribution is not symmetrical and the majority of people either scored in the low range or the high range, as compared with a normal distribution in which the majority scored in the middle.

FIGURE 2.4 *Skewed distributions*

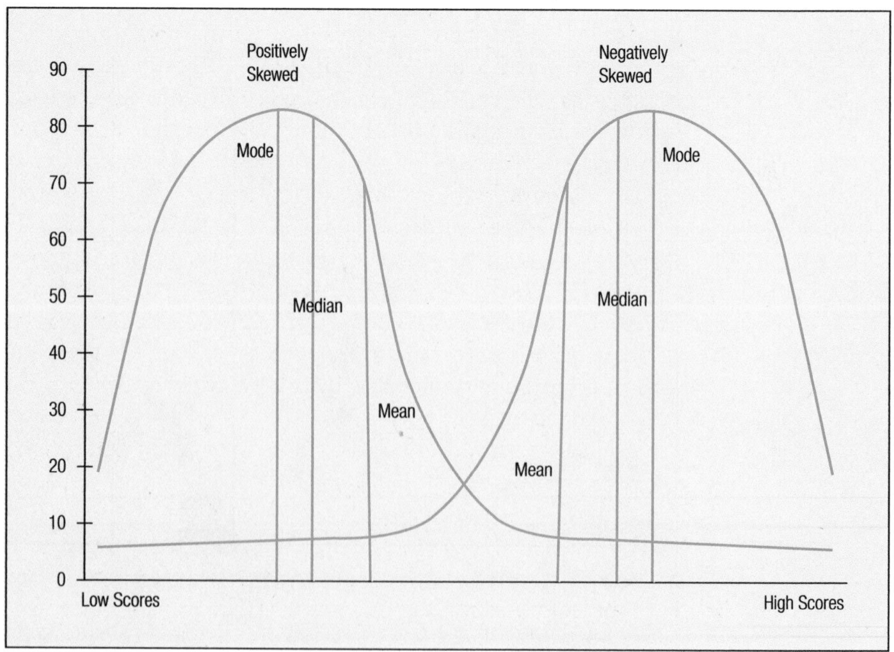

A positively skewed distribution is one in which the majority of scores are at the lower end of the range of scores. A negatively skewed distribution is the opposite, where the majority of scores are on the higher end of the distribution. The distribution of a criterion-referenced test, where most of the students had scores above 90%, would be an example of a negatively skewed distribution. Some students in an assessment course memorize the difference between positively and negatively skewed distributions simply by thinking that it is the opposite of what makes sense. You may use this technique for learning the difference, but there is a better explanation. If you look at Figure 2.4, you will notice that the mean is more positive as compared with the mode and median in the positively skewed distribution. The opposite occurs with the negatively skewed distribution, where the mean is more negative than either the mode or the median. Thus, a distribution is labeled either positive or negative, because the mean is skewed positively when the scores are mostly lower, and the mean is skewed negatively when the scores are mostly higher. Determining if the scores on an instrument are skewed is important, because professionals will sometimes interpret scores assuming there is a normal distribution when the distribution is actually skewed.

Types of Scores

Counselors often need to provide clients with interpretations of assessment results. For example, a school counselor interprets achievement test scores to students or parents, a mental health counselor interprets a personality inventory to a client, or a marriage and family counselor interprets a family functioning inventory to a family. Sometimes the manner in which test results are communicated to individuals can be quite confusing because clients have little exposure to terms such as *normal distribution, percentile,* or *stanine*. Therefore, counselors need to understand the different methods of scoring and become adept at communicating those results in ways that clients can understand.

The simplest of the scoring methods is the raw score, which is meaningless without any other interpretative data. We get raw scores by simply following the rules for scoring. Raw scores are those scores that have not been converted to another type of scoring (e.g., percentile, *T* score). As indicated earlier in this chapter, your raw score of 60 on the Counseling Aptitude Scale actually means nothing until we began to examine the distribution of scores, measures of central tendency, and measures of variability. When we examine these indicators, we typically have more information with which to interpret a score.

Sometimes, however, we want additional information concerning how an individual performed in comparison with the norming group, and this often is accomplished by converting the raw score to a percentile rank or percentile score. Percentile scores, or percentile ranks, indicate the percentage of people in the norming group who had a score *at* or *below* a given raw score. Percentiles should not be confused with the common scoring method of indicating the percentage of items answered correctly. Percentiles can be determined for any distribution of scores, not just for

TABLE 2.4 *Frequency distribution for the scores on the Counseling Aptitude Scale*

X	10	20	30	40	50	60	70	80	90
f	2	2	4	6	10	8	4	2	2
%	5	5	10	15	25	20	10	5	5
Percentile	5	10	20	35	60	80	90	95	99*

*The highest percentile is the 99th percentile.

normalized distributions. Table 2.4 reflects how percentiles can be calculated for the CAS scores. As you probably noticed, the first two lines of Table 2.4 are the same as the frequency distribution in Table 2.2. To find the percentile, we first have to determine how many people out of the group had each score, and then we calculate the percentage of people out of the total group who received that score. For example, for the score of 60, we can see that eight people received that score, and 8 divided by the total group of 40 is equal to 20%.

As stated earlier, percentiles are the ***percentage*** of people who received a score ***at*** or ***below*** a given raw score. Therefore, to get percentiles, we add the ***percentages*** of individuals who had a score ***at*** or ***below*** each of the raw scores. If we examine Table 2.4, we can see that the percentile for a score of 10 is the 5th percentile, because 5% of the people received this score (2/40 = .05) and no people had a score lower than this. We would interpret this score to a client by saying, "If a hundred people had taken this instrument, five people would have a score at or below yours." Let's look at your score (60) and see what your percentile would be. The percentage of people who received each of the scores is listed underneath the frequencies. Thus, to determine the percentile, we merely add the percentage of people at each score that are at or lower than 60 (5 + 5 + 10 + 15 + 25 + 20 = 80). In interpreting your score of 60, a counselor might say, "Eighty percent of the norming group had a score at or below yours." Another way of communicating this result is to say, "If a 100 people took the CAS, 80 of them would have a score at or below yours and 20 would have a higher score." In many ways, using percentiles may help you understand your score of 60 better than some of the other methods we have discussed so far.

Percentiles are used in many commonly used counseling instruments that have a normal distribution. Sometimes on such instruments as the Armed Services Vocational Aptitude Battery (ASVAB), the results are presented using a percentile band that is based on standard error of measurement (see Chapter 3). Percentile bands are useful because they can show a range of where clients could expect their scores to fall if they took the instrument multiple times.

Although percentiles are easy to understand and provide some useful information, there are drawbacks. Percentiles are not in equal units, particularly at the extremes of the distribution if the raw scores approximate a normal curve. Looking at the bottom of Figure 2.5, you will notice that there is a large difference between the 1st and 5th percentiles, whereas there is a very small difference between the 40th and 50th percentiles. With a normal distribution, scores will cluster near the median and mean, and there will be very few scores near the ends of the distribution. An example of the lack of equality in units can be seen from the distribution of CAS scores. As

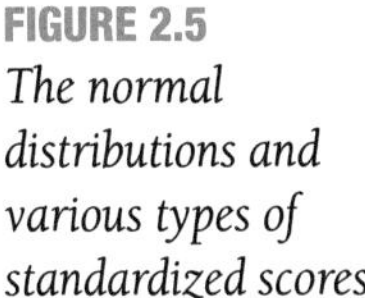

FIGURE 2.5
The normal distributions and various types of standardized scores

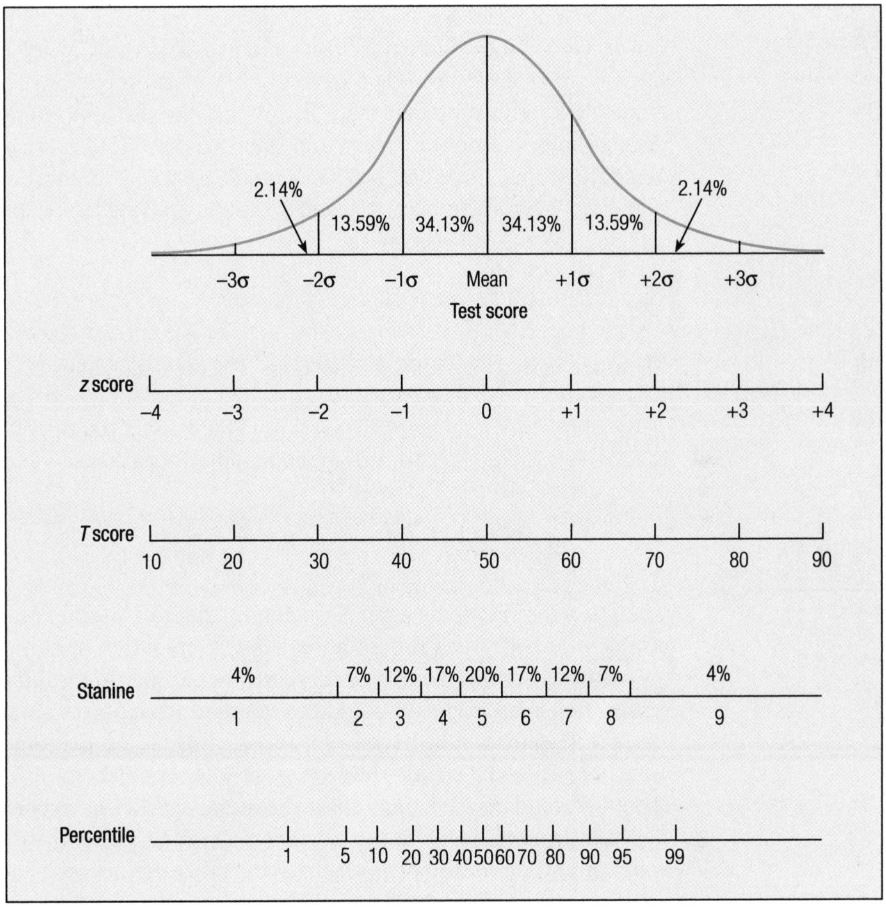

you will notice in Table 2.4, the difference in percentile scores between the raw scores of 80 and 90 is 4 (99 − 95 = 4). On the other hand, the difference in percentile scores between the raw scores of 40 and 50 is 25 (60 − 35 = 25). Consequently, the same 10-point difference in raw scores results in remarkable differences in percentile scores. Thus, percentile scores are helpful in providing information about each individual relative position in the normative sample, but they are not particularly useful in indicating the amount of difference between scores. In addition, percentiles are an ordinal scale and cannot be analyzed using statistics that require interval data.

Standard Scores

Standard scores address the limitation of unequal units of percentiles, while providing a "shorthand" method for understanding test results. Standard scores are different methods of converting raw scores so that there is always a set standard deviation and mean. Standard scores can be used with all types of instruments, including intelligence, personality, and career assessments. As a result, when we hear that a client has a z score of +1.00 or a T score of 60, we, as professional counselors, will automatically know where that score falls within the distribution without needing more detailed information (i.e., mean and standard deviation) on that specific instrument. Standard scores, therefore, provide a quick, easy way to know a client's relative position on an instrument because standard scores describe how many standard deviations a client's score is from the mean.

z Scores

There are various standard scores (e.g., T scores, deviation IQs), but all of them are based on z scores. To convert an individual raw score into a z score, we subtract the mean of the instrument from the client's raw score and divide by the standard deviation of the instrument. The formula for computing a z score is:

$$z = \frac{X - M}{s}$$

where z is the standard score, X is an individual's raw score, M is the mean of the instrument or test, and s is the standard deviation of that instrument. Because z scores are standard scores, there is always a set mean and a set standard deviation. With z scores, the mean is always 0 and the standard deviation is always 1. Table 2.5 illustrates the calculation of z scores for two individuals on the same instrument that has a mean of 75 and a standard deviation of 5. Abby's z score of 2.00 indicates that her score is 2 standard deviations ***above*** the mean, and Keith's z score of −.60 reflects that he is a little more than one half a standard deviation **below** the mean. With z scores, it is important for counselors to focus on whether the z score is positive or negative. A counselor would not want to communicate to a client that his or her score was above the mean when in actuality it was below the mean or vice versa.

If an instrument has a normal distribution, then z scores are considered to be normalized and can provide additional information. Therefore, counselors can then visualize the normal curve and identify where a particular z score would fall. For example, we can see that Abby's z score of 2.00 is 2 standard deviations above the mean,

TABLE 2.5
Calculations of z scores

***z* Score Formula**	**Sample Test**
$Z = \frac{X - M}{s}$	$M = 75$ $s = 5$
Abby's Score	**Keith's Score**
$X = 85$	$X = 72$
$Z = \frac{85 - 75}{5} = 2.00$	$Z = \frac{72 - 75}{5} = -.60$

and we can see that a large percentage of people, 98% to be exact, would have a score at or below Abby's. Keith's *z* score of −.60 is below the mean of 0, and a smaller number of people (27%) have a score at or below his. We can find the exact percentile score for each *z* score by using the conversion table in Appendix A, which lists the percentage of people who would fall at or below each *z* score.

T Scores

T scores, another standard score, have a fixed mean of 50 and a standard deviation of 10. A *z* score can be converted to a *T* score by multiplying the *z* score by 10 and adding or subtracting that number from 50. The *z* score is considered the base of standard scores because *z* scores are typically used when raw scores are converted to other standard scores. For examples, some test developers prefer to use *T* scores rather than *z* scores because they wanted to eliminate the decimals and positive and negative signs of *z* scores.

Normalized *T* scores have the same advantages as normalized *z* scores (see Figure 2.5). Although *T* scores are often normalized standard scores, it is important for counselors to check the manual of an instrument to ensure that this assumption is correct.

Some instrument developers will transform the data to normalize the distribution, which leads to an interesting dilemma concerning when it is legitimate to transform a nonnormal distribution into a normal distribution and when it is unacceptable to normalize a distribution. Anastasi and Urbina (1997) suggested that transforming a nonnormal distribution should be done only with very large samples and when the lack of normality is related to modest limitations of the instrument. Questions have been raised about some instruments and the transforming of the distribution when the construct is not normalized. As an example, some researchers have questioned whether marital satisfaction in the population really distributes normally; that is, are the levels of satisfaction for most couples around the mean, with very few people being very unhappy or very happy? Some instruments, such as the Marital Satisfaction Inventory—Revised, have been criticized for using transformed *T* scores on constructs that may not be normalized in the population.

Stanines

Another normalized standard score is the stanine scale; ***stanine*** is a contraction of ***stan***dard and ***nine***. Stanines, which range from 1 to 9 with a mean of 5 and a standard deviation of approximately 2, are different from other standard scores because they represent a range of percentile scores. Table 2.6 on the next page indicates the percentile scores and the percentage of people who fall within each stanine score. Raw scores are converted to stanines by having the lowest 4% of the individuals receive a stanine score of 1, the next 7% receive a stanine of 2, the next 12% receive a stanine of 3, and so on through the group.

A stanine has the advantage of being a single-digit number that many people find easy to use. The disadvantage is that stanines represent a range of scores, and sometimes people do not understand that one number represents various raw scores.

TABLE 2.6
Stanines

Stanine	Percentile Range	% of Individuals
1	1 to 4	4%
2	5 to 11	7%
3	12 to 23	12%
4	24 to 40	17%
5	41 to 59	20%
6	60 to 76	17%
7	77 to 88	12%
8	89 to 95	7%
9	96 to 99	4%

For example, if Josh scored at the 40th percentile and Maria scored at the 41st percentile, Josh's stanine score would be 4 and Maria's would be 5. On the other hand, if Sam scored at the 24th percentile, he would get the same score (i.e., 4th stanine) as Josh. Therefore, when information is needed for very important decisions in a client's life, practitioners usually should employ more precise measures than stanines.

Other Standard Scores

There are other standard scores, such as deviation IQs and CEEB scores, that mental health practitioners use. Deviation IQs are an extension of the ratio IQ, which was used in early intelligence tests. The earlier quotients were a ratio of mental age to chronological age times 100 (IQ = MA/CA × 100). If an individual's mental age were the same as her chronological age, her IQ score would be 100, a number that was considered the benchmark for normal performance. One of the difficulties with the ratio method of calculating IQ, however, is that it does not produce interval data. Furthermore, because different age groups have different standard deviations, it is difficult to remember all the different standard deviations. Therefore, deviation IQs have now replaced ratio IQs in intelligence tests. Deviation IQs are standard scores in which the deviations from the mean are converted into standard scores, which typically have a mean of 100 and a standard deviation of 15.

Another commonly used standard score is the College Entrance Examination Board (CEEB) score. In this standard score, the raw scores are converted into standard scores with a mean of 500 and a standard deviation of 100. Many people are familiar with this standard score, although they may not be familiar with the title "CEEB score," because instruments such as the Scholastic Assessment Test (SAT) and the Graduate Record Examination (GRE) use this standard score.

Age or grade equivalent scores. There are two common methods for calculating age or grade equivalent scores. One is through a procedure called ***item response theory*** (see Chapter 4) in which items are specifically developed to measure performance at certain developmental levels. The second method of calculating age norms or age equivalent norms is with a norm-referenced approach in which the focus is on comparing individuals with other individuals. Often, rather than comparing the individual with other age level performances, the process simply involves comparing the individuals with other individuals at that same age. The average performance score of 9-year-old children becomes the equivalent of a score of 9. Different age level equivalents are extrapolated depending on whether the individual is above or below the mean. Therefore, when this process is used to determine an age equivalent score, we should not interpret that a score of 12 reported for a 9-year-old student means that the child is functioning as an average 12-year-old. Rather, the 9-year-old student is being compared with other 9-year-old children and is performing at a considerably higher level than the average 9-year-old.

Grade equivalent norms, or grade equivalent scores, are based on the same reasoning as age norms. With grade norms, however, the average score for students in a particular grade is converted into the grade equivalent for that specific grade. Grade equivalent scores are widely used in the area of achievement testing, primarily because they are easy to communicate. It is often easier to say a child is performing at the sixth grade, second month (6.2) level than at the seventy-ninth percentile. Parents and others like grade equivalent scores because there is more of a context for interpreting those scores. For example, at a party, a parent can simply brag that little Jimmy is already reading at the fourth-grade level, and he is only in first grade. The problem with this is that Jimmy is probably not reading at the fourth-grade level; rather, his score indicates that he performed substantially higher than the average first grader. Moreover, a reading test for first graders may not even include any items that are truly fourth-grade reading items. Grade equivalent scores are typically extrapolated scores based on average performance of students at that grade level. Therefore, Jimmy's grade equivalent score does not indicate that Jimmy should be placed in a fourth-grade class for reading.

Professionals in the counseling field need to be aware of other problems with age norms and grade norms. A significant problem with extrapolated age and grade equivalent scores is that some professionals believe these scores reflect precise performance on an assessment, but that is not actually accurate. As a result of various problems with age or grade equivalent scores, Cronbach (1990) condemned the use of them.

The information that age and grade equivalent scores communicate is often ambiguous because there is no universal agreement on what constitutes age or grade achievement. For example, does eleventh-grade mathematics include trigonometry or a combination of algebra and geometry? Thus, one person's interpretation of a grade equivalent could be very different from another's interpretation.

A second problem with age and grade norms is that learning does not always occur in nice, equal developmental levels. Let's take the example of reading. Consider whether the difference in reading that typically occurs between first and second grades is equal to the change that takes place between seventh and eighth grades. Many people would contend that the change that takes place between first and second grades is far greater than the change between seventh and eighth grades; therefore, we do not have equal units of measurement in age or grade norms.

Another problem with age and grade equivalent scores is that instruments will vary in the scoring. One publisher's test could give a child a sixth grade, eighth month score (6.8), and another publisher's instrument could result in a score of 7.1. Although the two scores may be related to small differences between the instruments, consumers of the scores may have very different interpretations of scores that are really not all that discrepant. Another problem with age or grade equivalent scores is that teachers or administrators may expect all students to perform at or above their respective age or grade level. For example, teachers have been reprimanded because students have had scores below grade level.

These misconceptions fail to take into account that the instruments are norm-referenced; thus, the expectations are that 50% of the students will fall above the appropriate age or grade score and 50% will fall below this score. Therefore, in most classrooms, expecting all students to fall above the mean is unrealistic as well as inappropriate given norm-referenced testing.

Because age and grade equivalent scores are often misunderstood, counselors can be particularly helpful to parents or guardians by assisting them in understanding these scores. A case in point is Justin, a 10-year-old with academic and behavioral problems in school. Justin's parents entered counseling because they were having a major disagreement about whether Justin should repeat the fourth grade. At the beginning of the fourth grade, Justin's test scores showed that he had a reading grade equivalent of 3.4 (third grade, fourth month) and a language arts grade equivalent of 3.8. The father therefore anticipated that the counselor would automatically agree with him concerning the need for Justin to repeat the grade. The counselor explained to the parents that Justin was only slightly behind the average performance of fourth graders in language arts and a little more behind in reading. After working with the family for a few sessions and talking to Justin's teacher, the counselor realized that a number of complex issues were influencing Justin's academic and behavioral problems. Through counseling, the parents began to look at their parenting styles and found different methods they could use to assist Justin with his schoolwork. Although this case is an example of a situation in which the score is below grade level, parents also react to scores above grade level and want their child to be placed in a higher grade based on their child's grade equivalent test scores.

Evaluating the Norming Group

When using a norm-referenced instrument, it is not only important to consider what type of scoring is most appropriate (e.g., percentiles vs. *T* scores); it is also important to determine whether the norming group is suitable for the clients. You may wonder what the best type of norming group is; however, the answer to this question is dependent on a number of factors. The adequacy of a norming group depends on the clients being assessed, the purpose of the assessment, and the way in which that information is going to be used. Hence, there are *no* universal standards for what constitutes a good norming group; rather, the determination of an adequate norming group rests with the practitioner using the instrument. The *Standards for Educational and Psychological Testing* (AERA, APA, & NCME, 1999) clearly indicates that the norming group should be adequately described so that test users can evaluate whether it is appropriate for their uses.

One way to evaluate a norming group is to examine the methods used for selecting the group. In general, more credence is given to a sample that is drawn in a systematic method. In statistics, the word ***sample*** is often used to refer to the group that is actually being tested. This sample is drawn from the larger group of interest, or the ***population***. Returning to the Counseling Aptitude Scale example, the population would be the large group of all counseling students in the United States. It would be very difficult to have a norming group that included all of these counseling students; therefore, we might draw a sample of these students to represent this larger population.

One method of selecting a sample is to draw a ***simple random sample*** in which every individual in the population has an equal chance of being selected. Hence, if we wanted to use simple random sampling procedures with the CAS, we would have to give every counseling student in the United States an equal chance of being selected. Ensuring that every counseling student is entered into the pool from which the sample is drawn would be an extraordinarily difficult task.

A ***stratified sample*** is often used in the area of appraisal. In a stratified sample, individuals are selected for the norming group based on certain demographic characteristics. For example, instrument developers may want their norming group to match the percentage of African Americans, Hispanics, Native Americans, and Asian Americans in the nation. They would need to actively recruit a sufficient number of people for their norming group so that the proportions of individuals from these ethnic groups match the proportions found in the latest reports from the U.S. Census Bureau. Other demographic variables that commonly influence the gathering of stratified samples include gender, socioeconomic level, geographic location, amount of education, marital status, and religion. Sometimes an instrument will incorporate a ***stratified sampling technique*** for a specific purpose, such as selecting children with certain learning disabilities or including a specified proportion of both depressed and nondepressed adults. If a stratified sample is used, the counselor should evaluate not only the adequacy of the sample but also the methods used for recruiting the sample. For instance, there are some instruments for adults in which the developers have recruited primarily college students rather than a wider sample of adults.

Another sampling strategy commonly used in the assessment field is ***cluster sampling***, which involves using existing units rather than selecting individuals. By way of illustration, let's assume we are developing a measure of social skills for elementary age children. It would be unusually arduous to attempt a random sample and list all the elementary children even in one state. Therefore, the instrument developers might use a cluster sampling technique, where from a listing of all the elementary schools in a state, the instrument developer would randomly select a sample of elementary schools. The specific elementary students would not be randomly sampled; instead, larger units (i.e., elementary schools) would be randomly selected through cluster sampling.

When a counselor uses a norm-referenced instrument, the interpretation of the results is restricted based on the particular normative population from which the norm was derived. The size of the norming group should be sufficiently large to provide a solid comparison. To use an instrument appropriately, counselors need to know about the characteristics of the norming group. An instrument's manual should include precise descriptions of the population that was sampled. Most manuals now include detailed information on characteristics of the norming group, particularly in relation to gender, race or ethnicity, educational background, and socioeconomic status. Test developers are responsible for informing the test user if there are situations in which the norms are less appropriate for some groups or individuals than for others (AERA, APA, & NCME, 1999). The counselor or test user, however, has the ultimate responsibility for determining whether the norming group is appropriate for clients. If there are discrepancies between the norming group and the client, the counselor needs to carefully interpret the results and inform others of the need to use that information cautiously.

Summary

This chapter summarizes some of the basic methods by which instruments are categorized, scored, and interpreted. In examining an instrument, it is important to determine if it is norm-referenced or criterion-referenced. Norm-referenced instruments compare an individual's performance with other people's performance on the instrument. Alternatively, criterion-referenced instruments compare an individual's performance with an established standard or criterion. In regard to norm-referenced instruments, statistics assists us in organizing and interpreting the results. Frequency distributions are charts that summarize the frequencies of scores on an instrument. Frequency polygons and histograms graphically display the distribution of scores so that practitioners can easily identify trends. Measures of central tendency (i.e., mode, median, and mean) provide benchmarks of the middle or central scores. The mean or average score is often used to interpret appraisal results.

The measures of variability (i.e., range, variance, and standard deviation) indicate how scores vary and where an individual's score may fall in relation to the scores of others. Standard deviation is the most widely used measure of variability. Standard deviation has some important qualities if the distribution approximates the normal curve. With a normal distribution, 68% of the norming group will fall between 1 standard deviation above the mean and 1 standard deviation below the mean. With a normal distribution, the mean, mode, and median will all fall at the same point.

There are numerous methods for transforming raw scores in norm-referenced instruments. Percentiles provide an indication of what percentage of the norming group had a score at or below a client's. Standard scores, which convert raw scores so that there is always a set mean and standard deviation, express an individual's distance from the mean in terms of the standard deviation of the distribution. The most basic standard score is the z score, which has a mean of 0 and a standard deviation of 1. Counselors need to be careful when they use instruments that incorporate age equivalent or grade equivalent norms; they must know precisely how the results were calculated and how to interpret them appropriately. Furthermore, counselors need to fully examine the norming group of any instrument and understand the strengths and limitations of that group.

CHAPTER 3

Reliability

In Chapter 1, there was a discussion of the importance of examining an instrument's psychometric qualities to determine if it is appropriate for use. One psychometric indicator of the quality of an instrument is its **reliability**. According to the *Standards for Educational and Psychological Testing* (AERA, APA, & NCME, 1999), reliability refers to "the consistency of such measurements when the testing procedure is repeated on a population of individuals or groups" (p. 25). Of critical concern in assessment is the amount of *measurement error* in any instrument. In appraisal, counselors can typically assume that the traits or constructs being measured are, to some degree, stable and that fluctuations are due to errors in measurement. Reliability coefficients can be calculated to provide an indication of the amount of measurement error in an instrument. Counselors can then use these reliability coefficients in two ways. First, reliability coefficients can be useful in selecting instruments, because practitioners want to use instruments with the most consistency and the least amount of measurement error. Second, reliability coefficients can be used when interpreting the results of an assessment to a client, which involves the use of standard error of measurement (SEM). This chapter examines the theories behind reliability, how reliability coefficients are calculated, and how counselors can use these coefficients in their work with clients.

Classical Test Theory

Some people may have taken an assessment device (e.g., a test for a class) and believed that the test did not adequately measure their knowledge in the area. For instance, a person may have felt physically ill or may have had a disagreement with someone just before the test. It might also be that the test questions were vague or not particularly well written. Some people, however, have performed better on a test than they originally thought they would. This could be because they guessed right on a couple of questions or perhaps the instructor did not ask many questions about the content covered the day they missed class. Whatever the case, the test scores did not reflect the individual's actual knowledge, or, to state it in another way, there was some *error* involved in the test scores. In terms of reliability, classical test theory is built on the premise that any result from an appraisal device is a combination of an individual's true ability plus error (Crocker & Algina, 1986).

Although reliability is often considered an indicator of consistency, theoretically it is based on the degree to which there is error within the instrument. Classical test theory suggests that every score has two hypothetical components: a true score and an error component. Figure 3.1 presents this relationship with *Obs.* representing the observed score; *T*, the true score; and *E*, the error. In the field of assessment, no one has been able to develop a perfect instrument; so all instruments are a combination of a true measure and some degree of error. The pertinent question is: How much of any score is true, and how much is error? Figure 3.1 shows how, in theory, we progress from the simple concept of an observed score being equal to a true score plus

FIGURE 3.1 *Classical test theory and reliability*

- According to classical test theory, reliability is based on the concept that every observation (e.g., test score, instrument result, behavioral observation) is a combination of an individual's true score plus error:

$$Obs. = T + E$$

- Based on the above formula, theorists then proposed that the variance of the observation or score would be equal to the variance of the true score plus the variance of error:

$$s_O^2 = s_T^2 + s_E^2$$

- To make the above equation into something that can be used to determine reliability, we can divide the variance of observed on both sides of the equation:

$$\frac{s_O^2}{s_O^2} = \frac{s_T^2}{s_O^2} + \frac{s_E^2}{s_O^2}$$

- Because anything divided by itself is equal to 1, the equation then becomes

$$1 = \frac{s_T^2}{s_O^2} + \frac{s_E^2}{s_O^2}$$

- Theoretically, it is now possible to take the variance of error to the variance of observed off both sides of the equation:

$$1 - \frac{s_E^2}{s_O^2} = \frac{s_T^2}{s_O^2} + \frac{s_E^2}{s_O^2} - \frac{s_E^2}{s_O^2}$$

- Because anything minus itself is 0, the remaining equation is

$$1 - \frac{s_E^2}{s_O^2} = \frac{s_T^2}{s_O^2} = \text{reliability}$$

- Based on classical test theory, a measure of reliability provides an estimate of the amount of true variance to observed variance. Therefore, if an instrument's test manual indicates the instrument has a reliability coefficient of .80, this is interpreted, using classical test theory, as 80% of the variance is true to observed variance. In using the other side of the above equation, we can also see that 1 minus the error variance to observed variance equals reliability. Therefore, we can conclude that 20% of the variance is error variance (1 − .20 = .80).

error to reliability being a ratio of true variance to observed variance. Therefore, when counselors read an instrument's manual that includes a reliability coefficient, they often use classical test theory to interpret that coefficient. For example, a reliability coefficient of .75 would indicate that 75% of the variance is true to observed variance. As Figure 3.1 also indicates, 1 minus the ratio of error variance to observed variance is equal to reliability ($1.00 - x = .75$). Therefore, we can determine that the ratio of error variance to observed variance is .25 ($1.00 - .25 = .75$). Thus, we use a reliability coefficient to give us an *estimate* of how much of the variance is true variance and how much is error variance. However, this is only an estimate; current methods of calculating reliability are not sophisticated enough to indicate, in actuality, how much is true variance and how much is error variance. Thus, as we will see later in this chapter, there are different methods for calculating reliability; however, with all these different methods for calculating reliability coefficients, we often use classical test theory to interpret the reliability coefficients.

Reliability and Unsystematic Error

In theoretical terms, reliability is an estimate of the proportion of total variance that is true variance and the proportion that is error variance. Error variance, in this case, is only *unsystematic error*; it does not include systematic error. Reliability is calculated using the consistency of scores obtained by the same individuals, whereas variations in scores provide an estimate of error. Examining the difference between systematic and unsystematic error should clarify this distinction. *Systematic* means there is a system—methods are planned, orderly, and methodical. *Unsystematic* means the lack of a system—occurrences are presumed to be random. An example of systematic error is a test question that contains a typographical error and everyone who takes the test reads that same error. Reliability would not measure this error because it is systematic. Systematic errors are constant errors that do not fluctuate.

Unsystematic errors are those errors that are not consistent, such as a typographical error on just one person's test. Unsystematic errors can arise from a variety of sources. Sometimes there are situations in which an error occurs in the administration of an instrument. For example, a school counselor responsible for the administration of the Scholastic Assessment Test (SAT) at one school may not read the instructions correctly to students, while students at other schools receive the correct instructions. Illness, fatigue, and emotional factors can all affect an individual's performance on an assessment instrument. Scores may also be affected by such factors as the lack of sleep, lucky guesses, or test anxiety. There may be problems with the facilities during the administration of an instrument (e.g., the room may be too hot, cold, or noisy). The examinee's performance might be affected because he or she is starting to get sick and has a terrible headache, which may result in unsystematic error. The construction of the items on the instrument may be vague, and people may vary in how they interpret the items. With any instrument, it is important to know the degree to which unsystematic error is a problem, and reliability provides an estimate of the proportion of unsystematic error.

Correlation Coefficients

Reliability is frequently *calculated* based on the amount of consistency between two sets of scores (e.g., give a group an instrument once, wait a period of time, and then test them again to see if the scores change). Often when individuals want to examine consistency, they use the statistical technique of **correlation.** Correlation provides an indication of consistency by examining the relationship between scores. Figure 3.2 shows an example of a small class that took a test once and then took it again a week later. In this example, there is a perfect positive correlation (+1.00) because everyone in the class got the same score and the same rank the second time

FIGURE 3.2 *Scatterplots for positive and negative correlations*

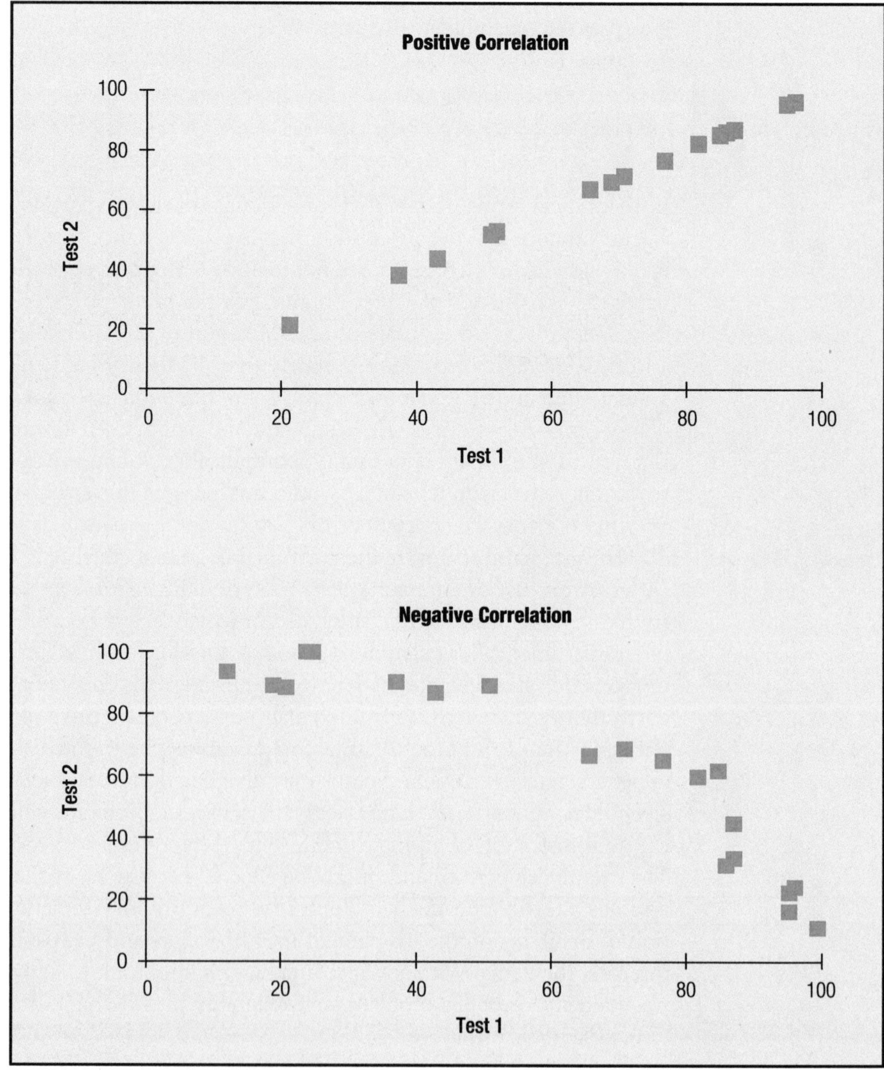

as they did in the first administration. The second scatter diagram in Figure 3.2 reveals a negative correlation—the scores on the x-axis increase, whereas the scores on the y-axis decrease. In some cases, we do not want a negative correlation. For example, with reliability, we would not want those who had the highest scores the first time they took the test to have the lowest scores the second time they took the test; nor would we want the reverse, where those who had the lowest scores at first have the highest scores the second time. There are occasions, however, when a negative correlation is expected. For example, if client hostility were to increase during the counseling process, we would expect the effectiveness of the counseling to decrease.

The statistical technique of correlation produces a **correlation coefficient**, which provides a numerical indicator of the *relationship* between the two sets of data. Remember that correlation is a statistic that is used not only to determine reliability, but it has multiple uses that involve examining the relationship between two sets of variables. Correlation coefficients can range from -1.00 to $+1.00$. The closer the coefficient is to 1.00 (either positive or negative), the stronger the relationship. On the other hand, the closer the coefficient is to .00, the smaller the relationship. A correlation coefficient of .00 indicates the lack of evidence of a relationship. Correlation coefficients can be computed in various ways, and it is the nature of the data that determines the appropriate method.

The most common method for calculating correlations is the *Pearson-Product Moment Correlation Coefficient,* which is essentially based on the simple concepts of a positive times a positive is a positive, a negative times a negative is a positive, and a positive times a negative is a negative; a big times a big is a big, and a small times a small is a small. Figure 3.3 on the next page shows how these concepts are used to calculate a correlation coefficient. The formula for the Pearson-Product Moment Correlation is

$$r = \frac{\Sigma z_1 z_2}{N}$$

In this equation, r represents the Pearson-Product Moment Correlation and characterizes the sum of the product of the z scores (take each person's z score on the first administration, multiply it by the z score on the second test, and then add these products together). In this equation, N represents the number of individuals. Converting each individual's scores into z scores provides an indication of whether they are above or below the mean. Remember that z scores above the mean are positive numbers and z scores below the mean are negative numbers. We would expect each test taker to be consistent; in other words, each would be either above the mean or below the mean on both administrations (a positive times a positive and a negative times a negative). Thus, if test takers were consistent in their performance, that would increase the product of the z scores and, thus, increase the correlation coefficient. On the other hand, if they are above the mean one time (a positive z score) and below the mean the second time (a negative z score), then a positive times a negative is a negative, which would decrease the correlation coefficient. The same applies to the size of the z scores because a higher z score (a big) times a higher z score (a big) will produce a larger number than a higher z score times a smaller z score. What is important to understand is that consistent scores contribute to a larger correlation

FIGURE 3.3
Calculating a Pearson-Product Moment Correlation

	First Administration		Second Administration	
	Raw Scores	***z* Scores**	**Raw Scores**	***z* Scores**
Joseph	62	−1.90	80	−.78
Hannah	78	−.38	78	−1.10
Geraldo	75	−.67	91	.94
Megan	84	.19	85	.00
Seth	88	.57	87	.31
Maria	92	.95	78	−1.10
Jason	95	1.24	96	1.73

$M = 82$ $\qquad$ $M = 85$

$s = \sqrt{\frac{774}{7}} = \sqrt{110.57} = 10.52$ $\qquad$ $s = \sqrt{\frac{284}{7}} = \sqrt{40.57} = 6.37$

Product of *z* scores

$-1.90 \times -.78 = 1.48$

$-.38 \times -1.10 = .42$

$-.67 \times .94 = -.63$

$.19 \times .00 = .00$

$.57 \times .31 = .18$

$.95 \times -1.10 = -1.05$

$1.24 \times 1.73 = 2.15$

2.55

$$r = \frac{\Sigma z_1 z_2}{N} = \frac{2.55}{7} = .36$$

coefficient (toward either a −1.00 or a +1.00), whereas inconsistent scores reduce the size of the correlation coefficient (toward .00).

There are easier methods for calculating a Pearson-Product Moment Correlation that do not require converting every raw score into a *z* score. The following formula is easier to calculate and will be less time consuming:

$$r = \frac{N\Sigma XY - (\Sigma X)(\Sigma Y)}{\sqrt{[N\Sigma X^2 - (\Sigma X)^2][N\Sigma Y^2 - (\Sigma Y)^2]}}$$

Even though this formula does not appear to take into consideration the consistency of raw scores, it actually does, because all the methods of calculating correlations take into account whether the two sets of data vary in the same manner. Sometimes with correlations, individuals want more than just an indicator of the relationship; they would like to know the percentage of common variances between the two sets of data. To find this percentage of shared variance between the two variables, we simply square the correlation coefficient. This statistic is called the **coefficient of determination** and is represented by r^2. Therefore, if a correlation coefficient is equal to .50, the amount

FIGURE 3.4
Venn diagram representing percentage of shared variance

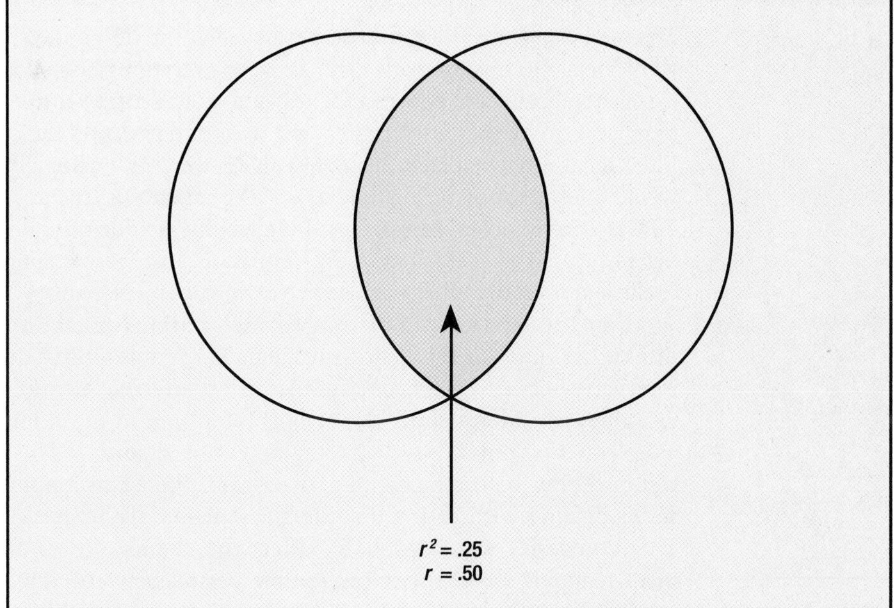

of shared variance is equal to .25 ($r^2 = .50^2$). The amount of shared variance is often represented in a Venn diagram (see Figure 3.4), which visually depicts the amount of overlap between the two variables. Hence, if there were a large degree of shared variance, there would be a large section where the two circles overlap; however, if r^2 were quite small, then the circles would hardly intersect.

Types of Reliability

The previous discussion of correlation is necessary for understanding how an estimate of reliability is actually calculated. As you will remember, reliability, in theory, provides us with an indication of the amount of true variance to observed variance. In everyday counseling, however, it is impossible to get a measure of "true" variance. Therefore, the statistical technique of correlation is often used to provide us with an estimate of reliability that is based on the concept of consistency (i.e., we would trust that a score is a "true" estimate if a person gets that same score consistently). The following discussion provides an overview of the typical methods for estimating the reliability of an instrument.

Test-Retest

A common method for estimating the reliability of an instrument is to give the identical instrument twice to the same group of individuals. With the **test-retest reliability** method, a reliability coefficient is calculated simply by correlating the performance on the first administration with the performance on the second administration. It is expected that the variation in scores between the first and second administrations would relate to unsystematic error because everything else should be the same. The correlation coefficient between the test and retest scores provides us with an estimate of reliability. We then use classical test theory to interpret the coefficient. Therefore, if the reliability coefficient using test-retest were .80, using classical test theory we would interpret it by saying that 80% of the variance is true to observed variance and 20% is error to observed variance. In reliability, we don't square the correlation coefficient or use the coefficient of determination. Instead, we simply use the reliability coefficient itself to evaluate the degree of measurement error.

Using test-retest as a method for determining reliability does present some difficulties. One of the major problems is the possibility that something could intervene between the first administration and the second administration. For example, consider a counselor who is interested in developing an instrument to assess clients' potential for having an eating disorder. This counselor gave the test once, but before he could give it again, there was a popular television miniseries dealing with eating disorders that many of the group members watched. This miniseries would probably affect the clients' scores on the retest. Instrument manuals should specify the time period between the first and second administrations in a test-retest situation. In general, reliability coefficients tend to decrease as the amount of time between the testing increases. Anastasi (1988) recommended that the time between the test and retest should rarely exceed six months. Sometimes a test-retest reliability coefficient will be called a *coefficient of stability* when there is a long period between the administrations of the instrument. In this case, the test-retest reliability provides an indication of the stability of the scores.

The test-retest method of estimating the reliability of an instrument is appropriate only if the following assumptions are met. First, the characteristic or trait that is being measured must be stable over time. If an instrument measured situational anxiety (not trait anxiety), we would anticipate much more fluctuation in scores, and the test-retest method would not be appropriate. Trait anxiety, however, is supposedly stable over time, so, in this case, test-retest would be an appropriate method for estimating reliability. The second assumption is that there should be no differential in practice effect. With many skills, people become more proficient as they practice, and the first administration of the test could serve as that practice. For example, in a psychomotor test where individuals are required to screw nuts and bolts together, individuals may improve with practice and score significantly higher on the retest. The third, and last, assumption is that there should be no differential in learning between the test and the retest. Exposure to education or psychological interventions between the testings can influence the performance on the second test. Sometimes learning can occur as a result of the first test. For example, sometimes people will simply remember the correct response to an item if the time between testings is fairly short. In addition, it is not uncommon for people to be bothered by a question and, after the test is over, seek the correct answer to that question. Some people may thus learn as a result of taking the first test. Therefore, there are instruments for which test-retest is appropriate to use and others for which test-retest is not appropriate. As consumers of assessment instruments, counselors need to decipher when the test-retest method is an appropriate technique for determining reliability of an instrument.

Alternate or Parallel Forms

Estimating reliability using **alternate** or **parallel forms** requires that there be *two* forms of an instrument. In this method, individuals are given one form of the instrument initially and then are assessed with a second alternate or parallel form of the instrument. The scores on the two instruments are then correlated, which results in an estimate of reliability. This method avoids the many difficulties of the test-retest method because it uses different forms of the instrument. Because the two forms eliminate the problems associated with individuals remembering responses, the forms can be given in immediate succession.

Care should be taken with alternate forms to ensure that the two forms are truly parallel. Ideally, the two forms of the instrument should be independently constructed to meet the same test specifications. For the instruments to be equivalent, there must be the same number of items, and the items must be in the same format. Content sampling becomes critical because both forms must adequately sample the content domain equally. Most content domains will vary in terms of difficulty, so instrument developers need to guard against one form being more difficult than the other. In the personality area, it is important to ensure that similar questions are addressing the same issue; even subtle wording changes can alter the context in which individuals answer questions. For example, some people would read the questions "Do you fight with your spouse?" and "Do you argue with your spouse?" as being equivalent. Others, however, may interpret *fight* as being physical and *argue* as being verbal. In the instrument's manual, there should be substantial evidence that instrument developers made substantial efforts to ensure the forms are truly equivalent.

Although the alternate-form method of estimating reliability offers many advantages, there are also some difficulties with using this method. Often in the area of counseling, it is difficult to develop even one sound instrument; the efforts required to develop two different but equivalent forms can be monumental. As a result, the alternate or parallel forms are a less prevalent method of estimating reliability. In addition, with alternate forms, the first instrument may have some influence on the administration of the second instrument (e.g., practice effect or learning) that will affect the reliability coefficient.

Internal Consistency Measures of Reliability

The following types of estimating reliability all use one administration and a single form of the instrument. Each method divides the instrument in different manners and correlates the scores from the different portions of the instrument. Thus, these forms of reliability examine the instrument "internally" to determine its consistency or lack of error.

Split-half reliability. In the **split-half reliability** method, the instrument is given once and then split in half to determine the reliability. The first step in this method involves dividing the instrument into equivalent halves. Splitting the instrument into the first half and the second half is often not appropriate because some tests become progressively more difficult. In addition, warming up and practice effect may influence performance on the first half, whereas fatigue and boredom may influence performance on the second half. Frequently, an instrument is divided in half by using the scores from the even items and the scores from the odd items. This odd-even splitting often minimizes some of the problems with equivalency, particularly if the items are arranged by order of difficulty. Other methods for dividing an instrument involve selecting items randomly or organizing the items on the instrument by content.

After the instrument has been divided into two halves, the second step involves correlating each individual's scores on the two halves. This is problematic, however, because a correlation coefficient is influenced by the number of observations involved in the calculation (i.e., in general, a larger number of observations will produce larger correlation coefficients and a smaller number of observations will produce smaller correlation coefficients). Therefore, when we split an instrument in half and correlate the halves, we are using half the original number of items in the calculation. For example, if an instrument involves 50 items, the split-half method provides an estimate of reliability based on 25 items. Because longer instruments usually have higher reliability coefficients than shorter instruments, split-half reliability coefficients will be smaller than those of other methods that use the original number of items. Research has shown that the **Spearman-Brown formula** provides a good estimate of what the reliability coefficient would be if the halves were increased to the original length of the instrument. Instrument developers often use the Spearman-Brown to correct split-half reliability estimates. The Spearman-Brown formula is

$$r_{ii} = \frac{2r_{hh}}{1 + r_{hh}}$$

where r_{ii} represents the Spearman-Brown correction of the split-half reliability coefficient and r_{hh} is the original split-half correlation coefficient. When comparing the reliabilities of different instruments, a split-half reliability coefficient should never be directly compared with a Spearman-Brown reliability coefficient, because it would be expected that the Spearman-Brown would always be higher. As an example, would you select the ABC Self-Esteem Inventory with a split-half reliability coefficient of .88 or the XYZ Self-Esteem Inventory with a Spearman-Brown reliability coefficient of .88? Because the Spearman-Brown is a correction of the split half, you should not assume that these two instruments are equally reliable. Therefore, you would be correct in selecting the ABC Self-Esteem Inventory because the split-half reliability coefficient of .88 would be increased if the Spearman-Brown formula were used.

Kuder-Richardson formulas (KR-20 and KR-21). The two **Kuder-Richardson formulas** also enable you to calculate reliability by examining the internal consistency of one administration of an instrument. The decision to use either Kuder-Richardson formula 20 (KR-20) or Kuder-Richardson formula 21 (KR-21) is based on the characteristics of the instrument, specifically whether the items are measuring a homogeneous or heterogeneous behavior domain. To see the difference between homogeneous and heterogeneous instruments, let's use the examples of instruments that measure family functioning. An example of a homogeneous instrument would be an instrument that measures family functioning and assesses only the *single* domain of family communication. On the other hand, with a heterogeneous instrument, multiple domains are examined, such as an instrument that measures family communication, family cohesion, family adaptability, and family conflict. The KR-20, which is purported to be an estimate of the average of all split-half reliabilities computed from all the possible ways of splitting the instruments into halves, is appropriate for instruments that are heterogeneous. The formula for computing a KR-20 is

$$r_{20} = \left(\frac{k}{k-1}\right)\frac{s_t^2 \, \Sigma pq}{s_t^2}$$

where r_{20} is the reliability coefficient of the instrument using the KR-20 formula, k is the number of items on the instrument, and s_t^2 is the standard deviation of the instrument squared, which is the variance of the instrument. The terms p and q may be new to you. We sum (Σ) the proportion of individuals getting *each* item correct (p) multiplied by the proportion of individuals getting each item incorrect (q). With the KR-20, one must calculate for each item the number of people who got it right and the number of people who got it wrong. Computers can be of assistance in calculating KR-20s because this method can be quite time-consuming.

The formula for the KR-21 is much simpler to compute, but it is appropriate only for an instrument that is homogeneous. The formula for the KR-21 is

$$r_{21} = \left(\frac{k}{k-1}\right)\left[1 - \frac{M(k-M)}{ks^2}\right]$$

where r_{21} is the reliability coefficient using the KR-21 formula, k is the number of items, M is the mean, and s is the standard deviation. Sometimes you may see an instrument manual in which the instrument developers report a KR-21 because it is easy to calculate when the developers should have used a KR-20. The KR-21 cannot be used if the items are not from the same domain or if the items differ in terms of difficulty level. In general, the Kuder-Richardson formulas tend to have lower reliability coefficients than the split-half method.

Coefficient alpha. In terms of internal consistency methods of estimating reliability, the discussion has so far concerned only examples where the scoring is dichotomous (e.g., right or wrong, true or false, like me or not like me). Some instruments, however, use scales that have a range, such as strongly agree, agree, neutral, disagree, and strongly disagree. On some personality tests, the answers to questions have different weightings. When the scoring is not dichotomous, then the appropriate method of estimating reliability is coefficient alpha or Cronbach's Alpha. Coefficient alpha (α) takes into consideration the variance of each item. (If you would like to calculate a Cronbach's Alpha, see Cronbach, 1951.) Coefficient alphas are usually low and conservative estimates of reliability.

Nontypical Situations

Typical methods of estimating reliability are not appropriate for some types of assessment tools. As consumers of appraisal instruments, counselors need to have an understanding of the assessment areas in which special consideration should be taken to determine the reliability of an instrument. One area in which typical methods of determining reliability are not appropriate is with speed tests, such as a psychomotor test where examinees are assessed to see how many nuts and bolts they screw together in a specified time period. A test-retest also may not be appropriate, because many individuals will become better at this task with practice. Also, splitting these timed tests in half or using other measures of internal consistency would probably result in nearly perfect reliability. For example, if an examinee got 22 nuts and bolts together in the allotted time, she would get 11 even "items" correct and 11 odd "items" correct, which would result in an overestimate of the instrument's reliability. Sometimes, to address this problem, instruments are split in half and people are given a certain time period to complete each half; in this case, the number of items in each timed period is correlated.

Another type of instruments in which typical methods for determining reliability may be problematic is with criterion-referenced instruments. As you will remember, criterion-referenced instruments compare an individual's performance with a standard or criterion. Criterion-referenced instruments are often used in achievement testing to determine whether a student has achieved a necessary level of performance. For example, a teacher may want to determine whether students have mastered multiplying one-digit numbers before allowing them to proceed with learning how to multiply two-digit numbers. Another criterion-referenced instrument could be one in which there is a cutoff score and all scores above that point would indicate that a client is considered to be depressed. With criterion-referenced instruments, we would expect that most of the scores would be close to the previously determined criterion or standard. In fact, in some situations, all of the examinees continue to receive instruction until the mastery score is achieved. For example, a teacher might require that all students show mastery of one-digit multiplication by getting 90% of the items on a test correct. Therefore, there is often little variability in criterion-referenced instruments. Remember the discussion of correlation and the phrase "a big times a big is a big, a small times a small is a small"? This phrase applies to criterion-referenced instruments because there will be only small variations from the criterion score; therefore, the correlation coefficients will be small due to the lack of variability. Typical methods of determining reliability use correlation, but these methods will frequently result in low reliability coefficients for criterion referenced instruments. Dimitrov (2007) contended that reliability evidence for criterion-referenced instruments is often provided by an indicator of *classification consistency*. In this case, the instrument may be given twice and a statistical analysis of consistency is conducted. If you are interested in examining the different methods of determining reliability for criterion-referenced instruments, the following resources may be helpful to you: Berk, 1984; and Subkoviak, 1984. In addition, it is difficult to determine estimates of reliability for those instruments that use item branching, where one's answer to one question will influence whether the next question is more difficult or, possibly, easier.

Instruments can also vary in the degree to which the scoring is more objective or subjective. As later chapters discuss, there are instruments in which the scoring involves clinical judgment, which requires some subjectivity in scoring. With subjectively scored instruments, we are not only interested in whether examinees score consistently, but we are also interested in examining any scoring differences among the examiners who score the same instrument. If the scoring of an instrument requires some professional judgments, then the instrument developers need to provide information on *interrater reliability*, which refers to how consistently different raters evaluate the answers to the items on the instrument. Although there are different methods for determining interrater reliability, the range is the same as for other reliability indices (.00 to 1.00). Interrater reliability becomes particularly important with portfolio assessments, simulation exercises, and performance assessments, which will be discussed in later chapters.

Evaluating Reliability Coefficients

The evaluation of an instrument's reliability should not be done in isolation. In instrument manuals, you will often find a range of reliability coefficients rather than just one coefficient. A counselor cannot just look at reliability coefficient(s) to determine whether there is adequate reliability. For instance, if you were to examine the reliability coefficient of .91, you might think that it was certainly acceptable. However, as will be discussed in a later overview of generalizability theory, reliability coefficients can convey quite different information. For example, a reliability coefficient could reflect various sources of error or possibly only one or two minimal sources of error. The manuals for most well-established instruments will include various reliability estimates for the user to evaluate. In evaluating reliability coefficients, a counselor should not assume that there are preferred approaches to estimating reliability. As the *Standards for Educational and Psychological Testing* (AERA, APA, & NCME, 1999) indicate, one should not infer that test-retest or alternate-form reliability estimates are always preferable to estimates of internal consistency, because the latter often approximate alternate-form coefficients. Furthermore, the appropriate procedures for estimating reliability will depend on the type of assessment and its purpose.

In order to determine whether an instrument has adequate reliability to use, we must first examine the purpose for using the instrument. If the results of an instrument could have a substantial impact on an individual's life, then we would want an instrument with very high reliability. In many school districts, for example, intelligence or general ability tests are part of the information used to determine whether a child can receive special educational services. It would be unfortunate if children did not receive the services they needed because of an unreliable test. As you will see in Chapter 7, some of the widely used intelligence instruments have overall reliability coefficients that are slightly higher than .91. However, many personality instruments do not have reliability coefficients in the .91 range. Therefore, in evaluating reliability, counselors must examine how they are going to use the instrument and be knowledgeable about the reliability coefficients of other instruments in that area.

In selecting an instrument, counselors also need to examine the characteristics of their clients and the reliability information applicable to that population. Sometimes an instrument will have acceptable overall reliability but will not be particularly reliable with certain subgroups (e.g., minority clients). As a general rule, instruments that assess younger children are less reliable than instruments for adults. Hence, a counselor could make a mistake by using an instrument that is not particularly reliable for the age group with whom he is working. The reliability coefficients for different ethnic groups or socioeconomic groups may also vary with instruments. Therefore, a counselor cannot rely on, for example, a brochure promoting the instrument; instead, she must examine the manual and evaluate all of the information concerning the reliability of the instrument.

Standard Error of Measurement

As previously stated, helping professionals should evaluate the reliabilities of different appraisal tools when selecting appropriate assessment interventions. Reliability, however, is useful to practitioners not only in selecting instruments; it can also be useful in interpreting clients' scores. Reliability is theoretically based on the concept of true score plus error. If a client took a test many times (e.g., 100 times), we would expect that one of those test scores would be the client's "true score." Hence, reliability is not something an instrument has but, rather, it is related to results and the degree of error in those results (AERA, APA, & NCME, 1999). Standard error of measurement provides an estimation of the range of scores that would be obtained if someone were to take an instrument over and over again. Therefore, with standard error of measurement, a counselor can provide the client with an expected range of where the client's true score would fall.

I once had a client who was struggling in his pre-med studies. This client was a junior with a grade point average of 2.88. He started counseling in an effort to learn better study skills because he was concerned that he would not be admitted to medical school with his grades. An assessment of his study skills revealed some minor problems; but, overall, he had developed many effective techniques for studying. During the counseling process, he learned that I was trained to do intelligence assessment, and he consistently requested that I test his abilities. I agreed to perform the assessment because the counseling was then focusing on whether he had the abilities to pursue a medical career while also making time for other activities. He was finding that he could achieve exemplary grades but was left very little time for any other activities. He had a family with small children, and he truly enjoyed civic activities. Standard error of measurement proved to be useful in interpreting the results of the intelligence assessment because SEM provides an estimated range of where a client's scores would fall if he took the test multiple times. For this client, it was expected that 68% of the time his IQ would fall between 110.8 and 117.20. Thus, he was certainly more intelligent than the average person but not in the range that is often considered superior. Providing the range of scores to this client was very helpful because he wanted an estimate of his highest ability. The results of this assessment were consistent with other information that indicated he would need to invest most of his energy in studying for his current classes to achieve the kind of grades that medical schools desire. He further concluded that if he were accepted to medical school, it would be enormously difficult and he would have little time for his other priorities.

As indicated earlier, standard error of measurement can provide a range of where people would expect their scores to fall if they took the instrument repeatedly. Standard error of measurement is based on the premise that when individuals take a test multiple times, the scores will fall into a normal distribution. Thus, when individuals take an instrument numerous times, they tend to score in a similar fashion to their original score, whereas dissimilar scores are far less prevalent. In Figure 3.5, the three bell-shaped curves indicate the expected range of scores for George, Michael, and Hillary if they took an instrument multiple times. Figure 3.6 is an enlargement of Figure 3.5, where we can examine just Michael's expected range. If Michael were to take an instrument multiple times, we would expect that 68% of the time his true scores would fall between 1 SEM below his original score and 1 SEM above his original score. In addition, we could expect that 95% of the time his true score would fall between 2 SEM below and 2 SEM above his score, and 99.5% of the time his true score would fall between 3 SEM below and 3 SEM above his score.

FIGURE 3.5
George, Michael, and Hillary's range of scores using standard error of measurement

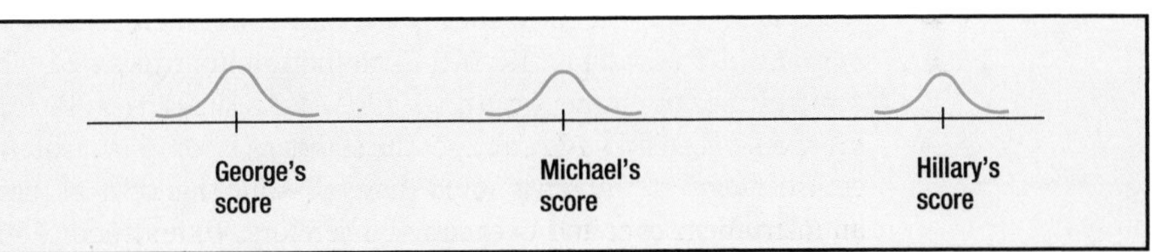

FIGURE 3.6
Ranges of Michael's scores using standard error of measurement

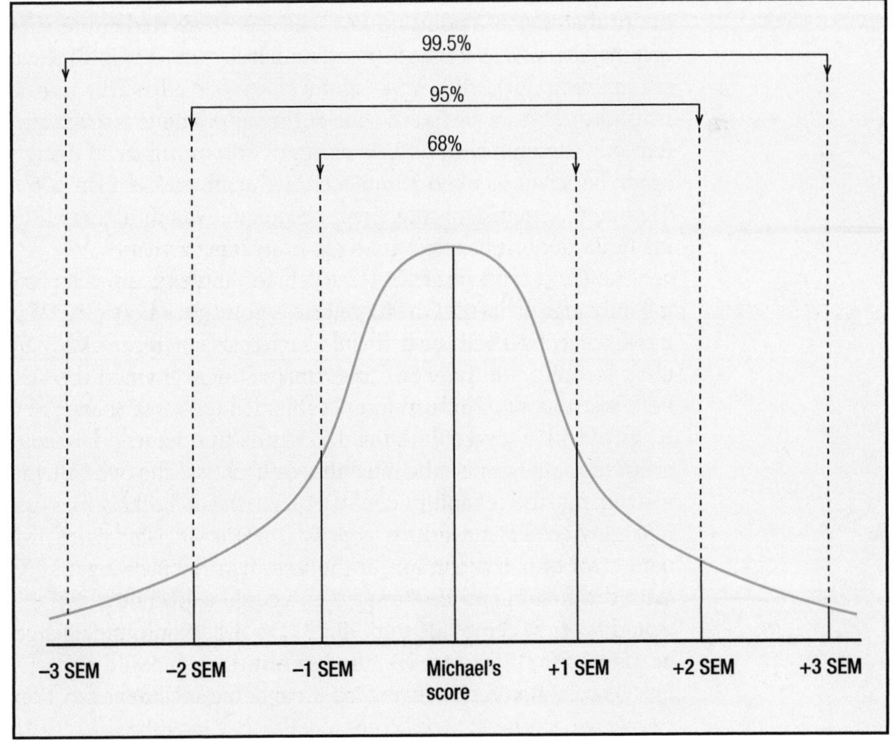

The formula for calculating the standard error of measurement is:

$$SEM = s\sqrt{1 - r}$$

where *s* represents the standard deviation of the instrument and *r* is the *reliability coefficient*. Many readers may be familiar with the Graduate Record Examination (GRE) general test—an instrument many graduate programs use in selecting and admitting students. The GRE has three sections, and an individual receives three scores: Verbal, Quantitative, and Analytical Writing. The score range for the GRE Verbal and GRE Quantitative is from 200 to 800. To understand how standard error of measurement can be used, let's use the example of Anne, who was disappointed in her score of 430 on the GRE Verbal. Often, the standard error of measurement is provided in the instrument's manual, so the counselor does not need to calculate it. In this case, however, we will calculate the standard error of measurement as an example. Although means and standard deviations for GRE scores vary, we will say that for this example the mean is 500 and the standard deviation is 100. The reliability coefficient for the GRE Verbal is .91 (Graduate Record Examination Board, 2007). Therefore, the standard error of measurement would be $100\sqrt{1.00 - .91} = 100\sqrt{.09} = 100(.30) = 30$. We would then add and subtract the standard error of measurement to Anne's score to get the range. A counselor could then tell Anne that 68% of the time she could expect her GRE-V score to fall between 400 (430 − 30) and 460 (430 + 30). If we wanted to expand this interpretation, we could use two standard errors of measurement (2 × 30 = 60). In this case, we would say that 95% of the time Anne's score would fall between 370 (430 − 60) and 490 (430 + 60). If we wanted to further increase the probability of including her true score, we would use three standard errors of measurement (3 × 30 = 90) and conclude that 99.5% of the time her score would fall between 340 (430 − 90) and 520 (430 + 90). This information might be very helpful to Anne if she were considering applying to a graduate program that admitted only students with GRE-V scores of 600 or higher. If Anne were to take the GRE again, her chances of obtaining a GRE-V score greater than 600 would be quite small. Therefore, a counselor might assist Anne in examining her GRE scores and considering other options or other graduate programs.

Standard error of measurement incorporates estimates of reliability in determining the range of scores. To illustrate this point, let's say there are two tests that measure intelligence, and both instruments have the same mean (100) and standard deviation (15). Joseph took these two instruments and obtained the same IQ score of 94 on both instruments. Because Joseph obtained the same score, we might expect that the range of where we would estimate Joseph's true score to fall would be similar, but this is not the case because the reliability estimates of the two instruments vary. In the first instrument, the reliability coefficient for the overall IQ measure is .90, whereas the reliability coefficient for the second IQ test is .71. Therefore, if we calculate the standard error of measurement for the first instrument, we get $15\sqrt{1.00 - .90} = 4.74$. With this first intelligence test, Joseph could expect that 68% of the time his IQ score would fall between 89.26 and 98.74. On the second intelligence test, the SEM would be $15\sqrt{1.00 - .71} = 8.08$. On this test, Joseph could expect that 68% of the time his IQ score would be between 85.92 and 102.08. As we see, the range, or score band, is notably larger for the second test because the instrument is less reliable. Standard error of measurement will always increase as reliability decreases.

Another matter to consider is that the standard error of measurement and reliability coefficients typically do not remain constant and will vary depending on the ability levels of the participants. For instance, the reliabilities of GRE scores have been found to vary across the span of scores (Graduate Record Examination Board, 2007). The *GRE Guide to the Use of Scores* includes conditional standard errors of measurement (CSEM) that reflect the variation in reliabilities of the scores. As an example, the CSEM for a score of 250 on the GRE-V is 21, but the CSEM for a score of 500 is 38. In using an instrument, it is important that the counselor determine if the instrument's reliability varies depending on ability level, age, or other factors.

An instrument's reliability can be expressed in terms of both the standard error of measurement and the reliability coefficient. The standard error of measurement is more appropriate for interpreting individual scores, and the reliability coefficient can be used to compare different instruments. Providing clients with a possible range of scores is a more proficient method of disseminating results than reporting only one score. Reporting a single score can be misleading because no instrument has perfect reliability. In the cognitive realm, a range of scores is a better indicator of a client's capabilities. People also vary in their personality and other affective dimensions, so using standard error of measurement can assist clients in understanding that variation. For example, a client may not be depressed on the day the results are interpreted and may dismiss information if the counselor provides only a single score indicating moderate depression. Presenting the results as a range takes into consideration the fluctuations in depression and increases the probability that the client will find the results useful. Counselors should be encouraged, whenever possible, to interpret assessment results by using a range of scores based on standard error of measurement. Because many instrument publishers are aware of the importance of reporting results using standard error of measurement, they are beginning to report results using score bands rather than single scores.

Although test scores have historically been used to evaluate and provide information about individuals, recently the use of group scores has increased (e.g., achievement scores for a school) to evaluate a program or a school's effectiveness.

The *Standards for Educational and Psychological Testing* (AERA, APA, & NCME, 1999) reflects that the error factors operating within the interpretation of group scores is different from those error factors influencing individual scores. The *Standards*, therefore, indicate that standard error of measurement should not be used for interpretation of group scores; instead, the more appropriate statistic is the standard error of the observed score means.

Standard Error of Difference

The purpose of some assessment situations is to compare certain aspects within the client. Often in counseling, for instance, a counselor wants to identify a client's strengths and limitations. Sometimes the focus concerns whether the individual

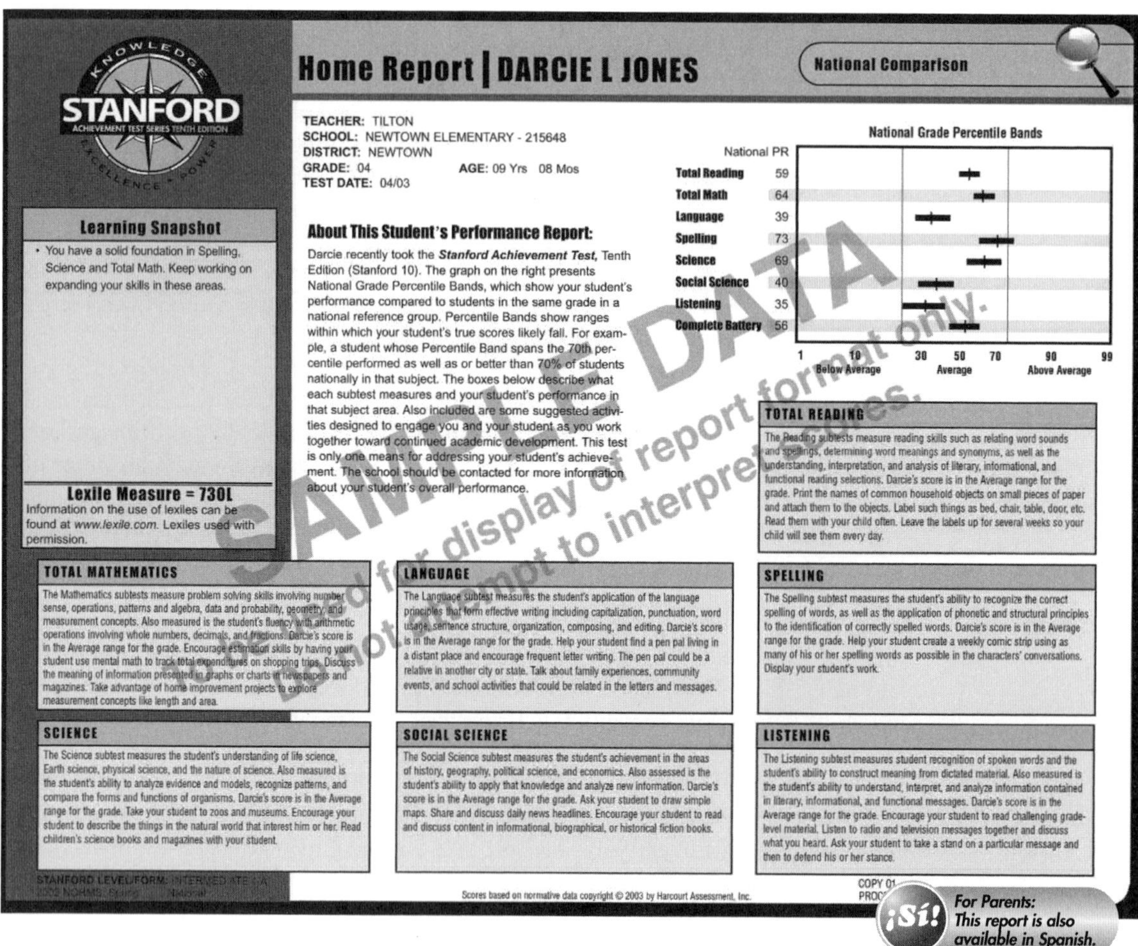

STANFORD ACHIEVEMENT TEST SERIES TENTH EDITION

KNOWLEDGE • EXCELLENCE • POWER

Home Report | DARCIE L JONES

National Comparison

TEACHER: TILTON
SCHOOL: NEWTOWN ELEMENTARY - 215648
DISTRICT: NEWTOWN
GRADE: 04 AGE: 09 Yrs 08 Mos
TEST DATE: 04/03

Learning Snapshot

- You have a solid foundation in Spelling, Science and Total Math. Keep working on expanding your skills in these areas.

Lexile Measure = 730L

Information on the use of lexiles can be found at *www.lexile.com*. Lexiles used with permission.

About This Student's Performance Report:

Darcie recently took the ***Stanford Achievement Test,*** Tenth Edition (Stanford 10). The graph on the right presents National Grade Percentile Bands, which show your student's performance compared to students in the same grade in a national reference group. Percentile Bands show ranges within which your student's true scores likely fall. For example, a student whose Percentile Band spans the 70th percentile performed as well as or better than 70% of students nationally in that subject. The boxes below describe what each subtest measures and your student's performance in that subject area. Also included are some suggested activities designed to engage you and your student as you work together toward continued academic development. This test is only one means for addressing your student's achievement. The school should be contacted for more information about your student's overall performance.

National Grade Percentile Bands

	National PR
Total Reading	59
Total Math	64
Language	39
Spelling	73
Science	69
Social Science	40
Listening	35
Complete Battery	56

TOTAL READING

The Reading subtests measure reading skills such as relating word sounds and spellings, determining word meanings and synonyms, as well as the understanding, interpretation, and analysis of literary, informational, and functional reading selections. Darcie's score is in the Average range for the grade. Print the names of common household objects on small pieces of paper and attach them to the objects. Label such things as bed, chair, table, door, etc. Read them with your child often. Leave the labels up for several weeks so your child will see them every day.

TOTAL MATHEMATICS

The Mathematics subtests measure problem solving skills involving number sense, operations, patterns and algebra, data and probability, geometry, and measurement concepts. Also measured is the student's fluency with arithmetic operations involving whole numbers, decimals, and fractions. Darcie's score is in the Average range for the grade. Encourage estimation skills by having your student use mental math to track total expenditures on shopping trips. Discuss the meaning of information presented in graphs or charts in newspapers and magazines. Take advantage of home improvement projects to explore measurement concepts like length and area.

LANGUAGE

The Language subtest measures the student's application of the language principles that form effective writing including capitalization, punctuation, word usage, sentence structure, organization, composing, and editing. Darcie's score is in the Average range for the grade. Help your student find a pen pal living in a distant place and encourage frequent letter writing. The pen pal could be a relative in another city or state. Talk about family experiences, community events, and school activities that could be related in the letters and messages.

SPELLING

The Spelling subtest measures the student's ability to recognize the correct spelling of words, as well as the application of phonetic and structural principles to the identification of correctly spelled words. Darcie's score is in the Average range for the grade. Help your student create a weekly comic strip using as many of his or her spelling words as possible in the characters' conversations. Display your student's work.

SCIENCE

The Science subtest measures the student's understanding of life science, Earth science, physical science, and the nature of science. Also measured is the student's ability to analyze evidence and models, recognize patterns, and compare the forms and functions of organisms. Darcie's score is in the Average range for the grade. Take your student to zoos and museums. Encourage your student to describe the things in the natural world that interest him or her. Read children's science books and magazines with your student.

SOCIAL SCIENCE

The Social Science subtest measures the student's achievement in the areas of history, geography, political science, and economics. Also assessed is the student's ability to apply that knowledge and analyze new information. Darcie's score is in the Average range for the grade. Ask your student to draw simple maps. Share and discuss daily news headlines. Encourage your student to read and discuss content in informational, biographical, or historical fiction books.

LISTENING

The Listening subtest measures student recognition of spoken words and the student's ability to construct meaning from dictated material. Also measured is the student's ability to understand, interpret, and analyze information contained in literary, informational, and functional messages. Darcie's score is in the Average range for the grade. Encourage your student to read challenging grade-level material. Listen to radio and television messages together and discuss what you heard. Ask your student to take a stand on a particular message and then to defend his or her stance.

STANFORD LEVEL/FORM:

Scores based on normative data copyright © 2003 by Harcourt Assessment, Inc.

COPY 01

¡Sí! For Parents: This report is also available in Spanish.

FIGURE 3.7

Illustration of score bands from the Stanford Achievement Test

Differential Aptitude Tests; Fifth Edition with Career Interest Inventory. Copyright © 1990 by NCS Pearson, Inc. Reproduced with permission.

has more aptitude in the verbal area as compared with the numerical area. On an achievement test, parents may want to know if their child's score in reading is significantly lower than in other academic areas. Examining differences in factors within a client also applies to personality assessment. Figure 3.7 illustrates percentile bands provided in the scoring profile of the Stanford Achievement Test. In this profile, the band around the percentile score represents a range from 1 SEM below the percentile score to 1 SEM above. With this profile, the counselor can examine strengths and limitations in terms of academic achievement. In examining Figure 3.7, you will notice that some of the percentile bands overlap, whereas there is no overlap among other percentile bands. If the bands overlap, you should *not* conclude that these scores are different. Differences can be attributed to areas where there is no overlap between the bands. With some instruments, the standard errors of measurement are not visually presented, so a counselor will need to compute the point difference to determine if scores are truly different. In examining differences between two scores, counselors need to take into account the errors of measurement from *both* scores. Examining the standard error of measurement from just one score will not be sufficient to determine the amount of difference actually needed to indicate a meaningful distinction. The **standard error of difference** enables counselors to calculate the exact amount of difference needed between scores. Standard error of difference takes into consideration the standard errors of measurement of both of the scores, as indicated in the following formula:

$$SE_{diff} = \sqrt{SEM_1^2 + SEM_2^2}$$

In this formula, SE_{diff} is the standard error of differences, SEM_1^2 is the standard error of measurement for the first score squared, and SEM_2^2 is the standard error of measurement for the second score squared.

Alternative Theoretical Models

Thus far, the examination of reliability has only addressed the "true score" model or the classical model. Although these models continue to be influential, a discussion of reliability should also include an exploration of alternative models. In **generalizability theory** or **domain sampling theory**, the counselor is interested in the dependability, or "generalizability" of the scores. With a true score approach, the focus is on identifying the portion of the score that is due to true score variance as compared with error variance. In generalizability or domain sampling, however, the focus is on estimating the extent to which specific sources of variation under defined conditions contribute to the score on the instrument. According to Cronbach (Cronbach, 1990; Cronbach, Gleser, Rajaratnam, & Nanda, 1972), the same instrument given under the exact same conditions should, theoretically, result in the exact same score. With generalizability theory, the focus is on the degree to which scores can be generalized across alternative forms, test administrators, number of items, and other facets of assessment. Therefore, when reliability information is gathered, there needs to be a description of the "universe." Instead of using the term *true score*, the term in generalizability theory is *universe score*, which represents the average of taking the instrument multiple times in the same universe (e.g., same purpose and same conditions). When counselors use a single score and assume it represents a universe of scores, they are generalizing from that score. Cronbach preferred the word *generalize* to *reliability* because the former implies the act of generalizing to a specific purpose rather than an all-inclusive evaluation of the instrument.

Thus, generalizability theory requires multiple reliability coefficients or *coefficients of generalizability*. This theory encourages the study of variations in test scores with the intent of identifying sources of variation. For example, researchers would attempt to identify the portions of the variance that are due to practice effect, examinees' levels of motivation, administrators' styles, and room temperature. Generalizability theory directs us to consider that reliability is not a stagnant notion; instead, reliability varies depending on the purpose, setting, conditions, and use of the instrument. The interest is still in determining the degree to which the instrument is free from error. In fact, using this theoretical approach, a researcher would attempt to identify sources of error and, when it is appropriate, to generalize from the assessment results.

Vaacha-Haase (1998) developed a meta-analytic method to explore variability in reliability estimates called **reliability generalization.** Similar to other meta-analytic procedures, reliability generalization involves combining reliability estimates across studies, which allows researchers to characterize and explore variance in score reliability. Vaacha-Haase's technique has spurred a number of reliability generalization studies of instruments. A few examples of reliability generalization are: for the Dyadic Adjustment Scale (Graham, Liu, & Jeziorski, 2006), the Myers-Briggs Type Indicator (Capraro & Capraro, 2002), the Minnesota Multiphasic Personality Inventory (Vaacha-Haase, Kogan, Tani, & Woodall, 2001) and the Learning Styles Inventory (Henson & Hwang, 2002).

Another alternative to classical test theory is Item Response Theory (IRT), which is discussed in Chapter 4. In item response theory, the focus is on calibrating each item and examining which items an individual answers correctly. Because the focus is on each item, typical measures of score consistency are not applicable. Hypothetically, the standard error of measurement in an IRT-based assessment is the standard deviation of a distribution of measurement errors that occurs when a given population is assessed (AERA, APA, & NCME, 1999). IRT is complex and involves examining the characteristic curve of each item; thus, the evaluation of precision or error within the instrument is also quite complex and statistically sophisticated.

In conclusion, the field of measurement is continuing to refine methods and approaches to reliability. These advances are critical to counselors because these researchers are advancing methods for assisting counselors in considering whether client scores are reliable. Although classical test theory is still influential, counselors should keep abreast of changes in the field of measurement and refinements related to reliability.

Summary

Reliability concerns the degree to which scores on an instrument are consistent and the degree to which those score may be influenced by error. Using classical test theory, we interpret a reliability coefficient as the ratio of true variance to observed variance. A reliability coefficient of .87 indicates that 87% of the variance is true variance. It is impossible, however, to measure true variance; thus, individuals often calculate reliability using measures of consistency. Some of the common methods for estimating reliability include test-retest, alternate or parallel forms, and measures of internal consistency (e.g., split-half, coefficient alpha). Reliability coefficients range from 0 to 1.00, with coefficients closer to 1.00 indicating higher reliability. One of the critical steps in selecting psychometrically sound instruments involves the evaluation of instruments' reliability. Evaluating reliability is not a simple task, and counselors need to consider various factors when examining the information on reliability of different instruments.

Reliability is not only useful in evaluating instruments, but it is also helpful in interpreting clients' scores and results. Standard error of measurement is another representation of an instrument's reliability, and provides a band or range of where a counselor can expect a client's "true score" to fall. Depending on the confidence level that is needed, a counselor can use standard error of measurement to predict where a score might fall 68%, 95%, or 99.5% of the time. Many professionals in the assessment field encourage counselors to interpret results using a band or range of scores based on standard error of measurement. Professionals should use standard error of difference, however, to determine whether the scores on an assessment battery are actually different.

In conclusion, reliability needs to be considered before it is possible to evaluate an instrument's validity. Validity indicates what scores or results from taking an assessment means. If scores from an instrument have a high degree of error, then those scores cannot have much practical value. Therefore, it is important to remember that reliability is the precursor to validity.

CHAPTER 4

Validity and Item Analysis

Validity

Validity concerns what an instrument measures and how well it does that task. The *Standards for Educational and Psychological Testing* (AERA, APA, & NCME, 1999) states: "[V]alidity refers to the degree to which evidence and theory support the interpretations of test scores entailed by proposed uses of tests" (p. 9). Validity is not something that an instrument "has" or "does not have"; rather, validation information informs a counselor when it is appropriate to use an instrument and what can be inferred from the results. Validity is an overall evaluation of the evidence and a determination of the degree to which evidence supports specific uses and interpretations. The interpretation of what the scores or results mean is derived from the validity evidence. For example, an instrument's title might indicate that it measures marital satisfaction; however, if we were to examine the validity information for that instrument, we might find that it is only good at predicting the number of arguments a couple has. Some people might contend that the number of arguments a couple has is not a valid indicator of marital satisfaction because some couples who are deeply dissatisfied may not even talk to each other, let alone argue. It is important that helping professionals have the skills to evaluate the validity of both formal and informal instruments. In fact, the *Standards for Educational and Psychological Standards* (AERA, APA, & NCME, 1999) clearly states that validity is *most fundamental* in developing and evaluating assessments.

The validation of an instrument is a gradual accumulation of evidence that provides an indication of whether or not an instrument does indeed measure what it is intended to measure. For many instruments, validity information is provided in the instrument's manual. It is not the instrument that is validated; rather, it is the *uses* of the instrument that are validated. In later chapters, we will examine instruments that are valid for certain purposes, but the validation information is not supportive of certain other usages of some instruments. Validation is a process where research is conducted to determine if the instrument's results represent the intended purpose and whether the scores or results are relevant to the proposed use (AERA, APA, & NCME, 1999). Therefore, before using an instrument, a counselor must evaluate the validation evidence and determine if there is enough support for using that instrument in that specific manner.

Reliability is a prerequisite to validity. If an instrument has too much unsystematic error, then the instrument cannot measure anything consistently. The reverse can also be true, however, when an instrument is reliable but not valid. For example, an instrument may measure something consistently, but it may not be measuring what it is designed to measure. Therefore, although reliability is necessary for an instrument to be sound, high reliability does not guarantee that the instrument is a good measure. In selecting assessment tools, a counselor should first examine the reliability and see if the instrument measures consistently. The counselor should then move to *what* the instrument measures and *how well* it measures what it was designed to assess.

In the field of assessment, there has been a movement away from the three traditional categories of validity (i.e., content-related, criterion-related, and construct-related evidence). Historically, **content-related validity** concerned the degree to which the evidence indicated that the items, questions, or tasks adequately represent the intended behavior domain. For example, content validity traditionally involved examining the content or items, such as does a test of third grade spelling contain typical words that educators would expect third graders to know how to spell. **Criterion-related validity** concerned the extent to which an instrument was systematically related to an outcome criterion. With criterion-related validity, we were interested in the degree to which an instrument was a good predictor of a certain criterion. An example of criterion-related validity is whether the Scholastic Assessment Test (SAT) predicted academic performance in college. The third historical type of validation evidence is **construct validity**, which concerns the extent to which the instrument may measure a theoretical or hypothetical construct or trait. As the *Standards for Educational and Psychological Testing* (AERA, APA, & NCME, 1999) indicates, construct validation evidence involved a gradual accumulation of evidence such as the interrelation of the test with other variables, the structure of the assessment, and analysis of the responses to the items. In the most recent *Standards for Educational and Psychological Testing* (AERA, APA, & NCME, 1999) all educational and psychological tests are measuring a construct, hence, validation evidence is always related to what was previously categorized as construct validity, and the term *validation evidence* more accurately represents the concepts. Although readers should be aware of the three historical types of validity (i.e., content-related, criterion-related, and construct), many experts in measurement now argue that construct-related validation evidence is what is pertinent with any assessment used by counselors.

The gathering of construct validity information is analogous to the techniques used in the scientific method where the starting point is the instrument and theories about the trait or construct. Predictions are made related to the instrument based on theory or previous research. These predictions are empirically tested, and the results of those empirical tests are either supportive of the validity of the instrument or not. This process is continually repeated, and the accumulation of evidence is evaluated to determine an instrument's construct validity. Counselors need to review the accumulation of information and determine the appropriate uses of the instrument.

This view of validation as a unitary concept is shared by a number of leaders in the assessment field, such as Messick (1995), who contended that dividing validity into three types only fragments the concept. Messick argued that a comprehensive view of validity integrates consideration of content, criteria, and consequences into a construct framework in which the practitioner then evaluates the empirical evidence to determine if it supports the rational hypotheses and the utility of the instrument. Messick suggested that validity is best viewed as a comprehensive view of construct validity. Messick further argued that a more comprehensive view of validity should take into account both score *meaning* and the *social values* in test interpretation and test use. Therefore, in evaluating the empirical evidence, the counselor needs to consider both score meaning and the consequences of the measurement.

Table 4.1 includes different methods for acquiring validation evidence according to the *Standards for Educational and Psychological Testing* (AERA, APA, & NCME, 1999). It should be noted that validation is a shared responsibility among the developers and the practitioner. The instrument's developer is responsible for providing relevant research and evidence related to using the instruments and the counselor is responsible for determining whether sufficient evidence supports using it in assessing a certain client or clients. The type of instrument and how the instrument is going to be used will influence the methods used to gather validation evidence. In some circumstances, the evidence related to items or content of the instrument may be particularly pertinent. In other circumstances, a counselor would be more interested in evidence concerning whether the instrument predicts certain behaviors (e.g., does the instrument predict clients who are likely to attempt suicide). These different types of validation evidence should not be considered as distinct types of validity because validation requires examining the bulk of evidence and determining whether the assessment is appropriate for certain uses. Furthermore, frequently other researchers and not just the instrument developer conduct research that adds to the validation evidence.

TABLE 4.1
Validation evidence from the Standards for Educational and Psychological Testing

- **Evidence Based on Test Content** Concerns analyzing the evidence of the relationship between the instrument's content and the construct it is intended to measure.
- **Evidence Based on Response Processes** Includes theoretical and empirical investigations of individual's cognitive, affective, or behavioral response processes. (This evidence concerns whether the examinee is responding in a manner consistent with the intent of the assessment.)
- **Evidence Based on Internal Structure** Involves analyzing the internal structure of the instrument to determine whether it conforms to the intended construction of the instrument. For example, factor analyses could be performed to examine whether the interrelationship of items corresponds to the appropriate subscales of an instrument.
- **Evidence Based on Relations to Other Variables** Entails examining the relationship between the assessment scores and other pertinent variables. For example, investigating whether an assessment of self-esteem correlates with other measures of self-esteem.
- **Evidence Based on Consequences of Testing** Concerns the evidence about the intended and unintended consequences of the use of this instrument. For example, studies of whether an employment test results in different hiring rates for different groups of people.

Evidence Based on Instrument Content

Although the *Standards for Educational and Psychological Testing* (AERA, APA, & NCME, 1999) uses the term *test* (see Table 4.1), I am going to use the term *instrument* in discussing methods related to gathering validation evidence. Evidence based on instrument (or test) content is related to the traditional term *content validity*. Often practitioners need to examine the evidence related to the development of items, questions, or tasks to consider whether the content of the instrument seems to adequately represent the intended construct. As an example, let's pretend (although it may not be merely a fantasy for some readers) that you are going to take a test soon covering basic principles of assessment, or Section I of this book. You may carefully study the content in each of the five chapters and feel quite prepared to take the test. You take the test, however, and find that all of the questions address concepts solely related to reliability! You could then argue that there was a problem with the content of the test because, with all the questions coming from one chapter, the content domain (basic appraisal concepts) was not adequately sampled or represented. In providing validation evidence related to the content of an instrument, the developers should discuss how they analyzed the construct and how they selected the items or questions that measured the construct.

With evidence related to the content of an instrument, the central focus is often on how the instrument's content was determined. Documenting the procedures used in instrument development often provides evidence of content validation. Common instrument development procedures are sensitive to content validation issues. Instrument developers should first begin by identifying the behavior domain they wish to assess. At first glance, this seems to be an easy step, but in actuality, it is often one of the more difficult ones. In counseling, there are often different theoretical perspectives concerning the areas we wish to assess (e.g., self-esteem, personality, career interests), and there is no universal agreement on the definitions of these constructs. Let's use an example of developing an instrument to measure client change that may occur because of counseling. Consistent with other counseling topics, there are various views on what constitutes client change and how to measure it. Hence, if we are attempting to construct a measure of client change, we would first need to define and conceptually clarify this concept. After initially clarifying the concept, we would then draw up *test specifications*. Test specifications provide the organizational framework for the development of the instrument. A common first step in test specification is to identify the goals or the content areas to be covered. In the example of client change assessment, we need to bear in mind that client change is a very broad area. Therefore, the instrument developers would need to consider whether to measure behavioral change, affective change, or cognitive change. The process of identifying goals and content is helpful because it requires us to clearly articulate the intended purpose(s) of the instrument. The instrument's manual should include a rationale for each intended use of the instrument and provide theoretical and empirical information relevant to those intended usages.

The next step in test specification is to precisely state the objectives or processes to be measured. For example, in client change, who will assess the change (e.g., client report, counselor report, or someone else)? Once the objectives have been established, they need to be analyzed, and the relative importance of each objective needs to be considered. We would probably want to include more items related to objectives that are of greater importance. Before writing any of the items, the test specification process also involves determining the level of difficulty or level of abstraction of the items. For example, in the assessment designed to measure client change, we would need to determine whether the instrument was going to be for children or adults, the level of complexity of the items, and the appropriate reading level. Any instrument manuals should describe in detail the procedures used in developing the instrument before any items were written. Developers create a more refined and better quality instrument if significant work is exerted before the items are written.

Another method of providing evidence of content-related validity is by having experts review the instrument. Experts can be scholars in the instrument's content area or, perhaps, practitioners working in the field. Experts will typically analyze the degree to which the instrument's content reflects the domain, whether the weighting of the instrument is appropriate, and the degree to which the content is assessed in a nonbiased manner. In general, these critiques generally will lead to revisions of the instrument. The manual should provide the number of experts used, a description of the experts, and an explanation of why these individuals were selected. If experts' judgments were used, then the manual should describe what was done to respond to these judgments.

Content-related validation evidence should not be confused with *face validity*, which means what it says—on the surface, the instrument looks good. Face validity is not truly an indicator of validity and should not be considered as one. An instrument can look valid but may not measure what it is intended to assess. Remember that an instrument is not valid or invalid, rather the validation evidence informs the clinician of the appropriate uses of that assessment. Therefore, a helping professional cannot simply examine an instrument's questions or items and decide to use that assessment tool. Rather, counselors need to evaluate the content validation evidence provided in the instrument's manual and determine if there is sufficient evidence to use it. Although content validation evidence is always important, there are situations in which it is particularly vital. An example is with achievement tests, where we are interested in how much an individual has learned. We cannot expect someone to learn something unless he has had exposure to that information. Therefore, there needs to be a direct correspondence between the information presented and the contents of the assessment. In fact, you may have had the experience in your academic career where you took an achievement test in a class, and there was little connection between what was taught and what you were tested on. In this case, the content of the test did not reflect the information taught and you could conclude that there was a problem with content validity.

Evidence Based on the Response Processes

As researchers have learned more about information processing, this knowledge has been applied to instrument development. The goal of this type of validation evidence concerns whether individuals either perform or respond in a manner that corresponds to the construct being measured. For example, if an assessment is attempting to measure vocational interest, then the instrument developers might examine whether people are answering the items based on what they like to do rather than what they can do. An example of how researchers might examine this is to have individuals "think aloud" while taking the interest inventory. The test takers' verbalizations of their thoughts while taking the interest inventory would be recorded, and researchers then analyze the manner in which the test takers processed the inventory to see if they were considering their interests while taking the assessment.

Another example of gathering validation evidence based on response processes is to question examinees about their performance strategies or responses to items. As an example, if it is an assessment of mathematical reasoning, the examinees would be queried about their strategies for solving each problem to see if they used the intended mathematical concepts. Sometimes it is interesting to examine if there are subgroup differences (e.g., race or ethnicity) regarding the processing of information. It may be that a distractor within an item confuses individuals from certain groups when they try to apply the intended mathematical concepts, but does not distract members from other groups. By examining the response process used by different groups, the test developers can rewrite the item so that it is processed in the same manner by individuals from diverse groups.

Particularly in the area of achievement, there have been significant advancements concerning models or theories of cognition and learning. Based on these models and theories, there can be computer simulated performances on assessment items and then researchers can compare the performance of children or adults to the model-based answers produced by computer (National Research Council, 2001). Hence, if individuals' responses match the computer's theory-developed answer, then there is some evidence that individuals are using the intended theory. Validation evidence based on response processes can often provide keen insight about an instrument and instrument manuals are increasingly including this type of evidence.

Evidence Based on Internal Structure

The *Standards for Educational and Psychological Testing* (AERA, APA, & NCME, 1999) suggests that analyses of the internal structure of an instrument can also contribute to the validation evidence. An instrument may be designed to measure one clearly defined construct or it may have subtests or scales within the instrument. In analyzing the validation evidence, it is often useful to examine whether the items in one subscale are related to other items on that subscale, a task which involves examining the internal structure of the instrument. For example, the NEO Personality Inventory—Revised (NEO PI-R) is designed to measure five factors of personality: neuroticism, extraversion, openness to experience, agreeableness, and conscientiousness (Costa & McCrae, 1992). When using the NEO PI-R, a counselor should examine whether the items that measure neuroticism are related because it would be disconcerting if several of the items designed to measure neuroticism were more closely related to items on the agreeableness subscale as compared to items on the neuroticism subscale.

Factor analysis is often used to examine the internal structure of instruments because factor analysis is a statistical technique used to analyze the interrelationships of a set or sets of data. There are a variety of reasons for using factor analysis in gathering validation evidence, including exploring patterns of interrelationships among variables (Agresi & Finlay, 1997). Hence, results of a factor analysis often provide information on the pattern of interrelationships among items and a clinician can see if those interrelationships correspond to the appropriate subscales. In examining the internal structure of the instrument, factor analysis can also identify items that may be redundant (i.e., very highly related to each) so that instrument developers may present results in a manual to explain their process for reducing the number of items in a subscale or in an instrument. Also, as will be discussed in Chapter 15, researchers study the internal structure of instruments with different groups, such as men and women or individuals from different racial or ethnic backgrounds. It sometimes happens that results from factor analyses indicate that the internal structure for an instrument corresponds to the intended design of the instrument for one group but the internal structure of an instrument might be quite different for another group.

Evidence Based on Relations to Other Variables

Another commonly used method for gathering validation evidence is to analyze the instrument's relationship with other variables. For example, an instrument developer may want to show that an instrument designed to measure depression is associated with other indicators of depression (e.g., feeling blue, lack of interests). When the validation evidence concerns examining the relationship of the instruments with other variables, clinicians need to consider the quality of the other variables. An instrument may be highly related to another variable, but if the other variable is not anything meaningful, then that greatly reduces the likelihood that you would want to use that instrument with clients. In examining the validation evidence, counselors want to see that the instrument is related to other variables that are *relevant* and *pertinent* to client issues or that add to our knowledge about using that instrument.

A statistical tool often used in providing validation evidence related to an instrument's relationship with other variables is the **correlational method.** As discussed in Chapter 3, the statistical technique of correlation is used to explore the relationship between two variables. Counselors often want to examine the degree to which an instrument is related to other pertinent variables or a *criterion*. Because the focus is on the degree to which there is a relationship, it is logical to use correlation to provide an indication of the magnitude of that relationship. There are several steps in gathering validation evidence using correlation. First, select an appropriate group to use in the validation study. Second, administer the instrument. Depending on how the instrument is going to be used, sometimes the criterion data is gathered immediately or with instruments that predict future behavior—there may be a time lapse before the criterion information is gathered (e.g., waiting until the group finishes college to gather academic performance information). Once the criterion information is collected, the final step is to correlate the performance on the instrument with the criterion information. The result of that calculation is often labeled a **validity coefficient.**

Validity coefficients can be helpful to counseling practitioners in two ways. Counselors can compare the validity coefficients from different instruments and select the instrument that has the highest relationship between the instrument and the relevant variables or criteria. Although this sounds quite easy, in practice it can sometimes be complex because there are correlations with a number of different variables. The second way that validity coefficients can be useful in practice is by allowing the counselor to examine the amount of shared variance between the instrument and pertinent variables. As you will remember from the discussion of correlation in Chapter 3, a correlation coefficient can be squared, resulting in a *coefficient of determination*, which provides an indication of the amount of shared variance between the two variables. Thus, by squaring the validity coefficient, we get the percentage of variance between the assessment instrument and the other relevant variables. In many discussions of validity coefficients, a question arises about the magnitude of the coefficient and how large a validity coefficient should be. Kaplan and Saccuzzo (2005) indicated that validity coefficients are rarely larger than .60 and that they often fall in the .30 to .40 range. Anastasi and Urbina (1997) suggested that validity coefficients should at least be statistically significant, which means we can conclude that the coefficient had a low probability of occurring by chance.

As I indicated earlier, the constructs of interest in counseling (e.g., depression, academic achievement, work values) are complex and, therefore, evidence of validity cannot be confirmed with one correlation coefficient. Consequently, when examining an instrument's manual, counselors will often find that the validation of an instrument has been explored by seeing if it relates to other variables that are consistent with its use and seeing if the instrument has a low relationship with incompatible constructs. Examining an instrument's relationships with similar constructs and purportedly different variables is called convergent and discriminant evidence. **Convergent evidence** means an instrument is related to other variables to which it should theoretically be positively related. For example, if an instrument is designed to measure depression and correlates highly with another instrument that measures depression, then there is convergent evidence. **Discriminant evidence**, on the other hand, exists when the instrument is not correlated with variables from which it should differ. For example, there is evidence of discriminant validity when an instrument designed to measure depression is not significantly correlated with an instrument that measures trait anxiety. According to Anastasi and Urbina (1997), discriminant validation information is particularly important in terms of evaluating the validity of personality instruments, in which irrelevant variables may influence scores in assorted ways.

Campbell and Fiske (1959) suggested using a **multitrait-multimethod matrix** in order to explore construct-related validity. This procedure involves correlating an instrument with traits that are both theoretically related to the instrument and traits that should be unrelated to the construct being measured. This process also involves correlating the instruments with other instruments that use the same and different assessment methods (e.g., self-reports, projective techniques, behavioral ratings). The result of these various correlations is a matrix that enables professionals to evaluate the relationship between the instrument and measures of (1) the same traits using the same testing method, (2) different traits using the same testing method, (3) the same traits using different testing methods, and (4) different traits using different testing methods. Support for the construct validity of an instrument would be indicated when the correlations are higher between the same trait using different assessment methods as compared with different traits using the same methods or with different traits using different methods.

It should be remembered that correlation coefficients provide only an indication of the relationship between the instrument and another variable. Therefore, if the intent is to *predict* behaviors based on the instrument's results, then researchers need to use additional techniques to see if the instrument can be used for prediction.

Prediction or instrument-criterion relationships. Sometimes we want an instrument that predicts future behavior and, therefore, the validation evidence should focus on the degree to which the instrument does predict relevant behaviors. In assessment, when an instrument was developed to predict or identify, then traditionally users would examine the criterion-related validity. Examples of instruments for which practitioners examine the evidence related to an instrument's ability to predict (what was historically labeled criterion-related validity) are the Scholastic Assessment Test (SAT) and the Armed Services Vocational Aptitude Battery (ASVAB). The SAT predicts academic performance in college, and the ASVAB is designed to predict performance in training and job performance in both civilian and military settings.

Historically there are two types of criterion-related validity: concurrent validity and predictive validity, with the difference being the period of time between taking the instrument and gathering the criterion information. In concurrent validation, there is no time lag between when the instrument is given and when the criterion information is gathered. Prediction is used with concurrent validity in a broad sense because it is predicting behavior based on the current context. This type of criterion-related validity is used when we want to make an immediate prediction, such as with diagnosis. On the other hand, with predictive validity, there is a lag between when the instrument is administered and the time the criterion information is gathered. For example, if we wanted to develop an instrument that would identify couples who will stay married for more than 10 years, we would administer the test right before a couple was married and then wait 10 years to gather the criterion evidence, which would be whether the couple was still married.

In considering variables that an assessment is designed to predict (i.e., the criterion), we should be particularly interested in precisely what the criterion is and its psychometric qualities. A good criterion is truly a variable of interest. As an example, there would be problems if I were developing an instrument to measure hopefulness and used as my criterion whether I simply thought the person looked hopeful. The criterion should be *reliable* and relatively free from unsystematic error. If there is a large degree of error in the criterion, then there is a very good possibility that the instrument will be unable to predict anything useful. Using an assessment without a reliable criterion is like trying to predict to a target that is always moving. We also want the other variable to be *free from bias*. As an illustration, if an instrument were developed to predict a firefighter's effectiveness, the criterion should be an assessment of job performance. It would be a problem if the criterion variable was supervisors' evaluation of job performance, and the supervisors used in this validation study happened to be biased against female firefighters. Finally, we want the other variable to be *immune from criterion contamination*. Criterion contamination occurs when knowledge of the instrument influences the gathering of criterion information. For example, criterion contamination may occur if those determining a *DSM-IV-TR* diagnosis had prior knowledge of a participant's performance on an instrument designed to diagnose. A practitioner could easily be influenced by the information from the instrument and might tend to assign a diagnostic label that was consistent with the instrument. In this example, the correlation between the instrument and the diagnostic categories would appear artificially high. Thus, the criterion, in this case, is "contaminated" by the prior knowledge of the individual's performance on the diagnostic instrument.

In providing validation evidence related to an instrument's abilities to predict behavior, researchers often use regression-related statistical techniques or expectancy tables.

Regression The statistical technique of **regression** is another commonly used method for gathering validation evidence. Regression, which is closely related to correlation, is commonly used to determine the usefulness of a variable, or a *set* of variables, in predicting another important or meaningful variable. In appraisal, we are usually specifically interested in whether the instrument predicts some other specific behavior (the criterion variable). For example, does an instrument designed to measure potential suicidal behaviors actually predict suicidal behaviors? Regression is based on the premise that a straight line, called the *regression line*, can describe the relationship between the instrument's scores and the criterion. In Figure 4.1, the scores on an instrument are plotted in relation to the scores on the criterion. The line that best fits the points is the regression line. Once a regression line, or line of best fit, is established, it is possible to use it to predict performance on the criterion based on scores on the instrument.

To illustrate the concepts of regression, imagine you are interested in an instrument that predicts people's abilities to be "fun" (please note that this is only an illustration). In this example, you are comparing three instruments to use for the

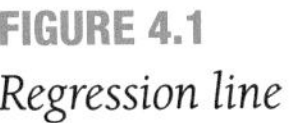
FIGURE 4.1
Regression line

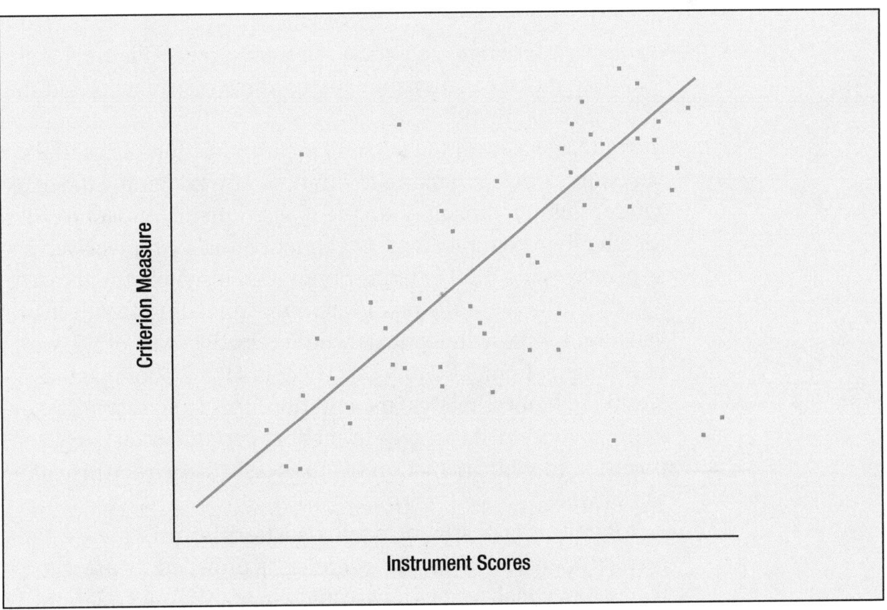

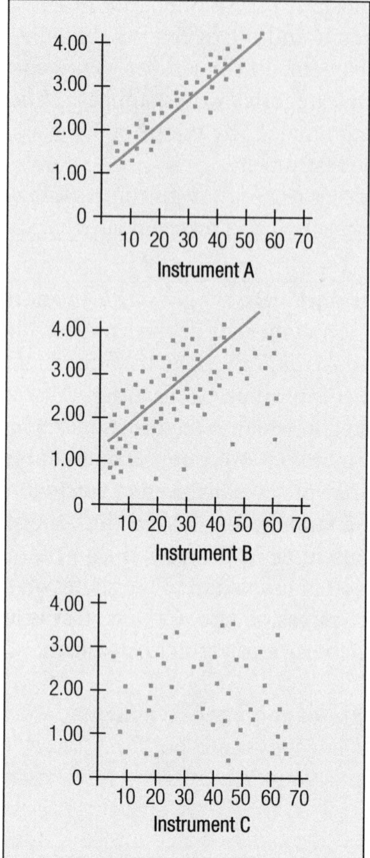

FIGURE 4.2 *Scatterplots between scores on three instruments and the criteria for these instruments*

screening of friends, neighbors, and coworkers. Figure 4.2 shows three scatterplots that describe the relationship among three instruments and the criterion. In all three of these cases, an individual took one of the three instruments and then friends of that individual evaluated the person's ability to be fun. Thus, the criterion, which is plotted on the *y*-axis, is a rating of "funness." By examining the diagrams in Figure 4.2, we can see that Instrument A is a pretty good predictor because all scores are located near the line. For example, most of the individuals who received a score of 50 were rated as being around 3.00 in terms of funness. Instrument B, however, is not quite as good a predictor because the points are more spread out. With Instrument B, there is wide variation for those individuals who received a score of 50, with the evaluation of funness ranging from 2.00 to 4.00. There is such a poor relationship between Instrument C and the funness ratings (the criterion) that a regression line or a line of best fit could not be determined. To help in making certain social decisions, you may want more precision in your prediction of "funness" than either Instrument B or Instrument C can provide.

Rarely in assessment does a scatterplot provide evidence of an instrument's predictive ability; rather, the evidence is provided by using the statistical technique of regression, which tells us if we can use a **regression equation**. This equation describes the linear relationship between the predictor variable and the criterion variable. The regression equation is

$$Y' = a + bX$$

where Y' is the predicted score; a is the *y-intercept*, or the *intercept constant;* b represents the *slope*, which is the rate of change in Y as a function of changes in X; and X is the individual's score on the instrument. The slope is usually called the *regression coefficient* or the *regression weight.* Thus, in an instrument's manual, the instrument developers will provide information on whether the instrument can significantly predict the criterion. (I.e., can the data be fitted into a significant regression equation?) While on the subject of regression, note that there is also *multiple regression*, in which there are multiple predictor variables. As an example of multiple regression, suppose that two predictor variables, a pre-college test (e.g., SAT or ACT) and high school grades, are used to predict academic achievement in college. In multiple regression, the equation is extended to include the additional variables that have different weightings. ($Y' = a + b_1X_1 + b_2X_2 + b_3X_3 + \cdots + b_nX_n$). In using multiple regression, it is possible to determine which variables are the best predictors as well as how much variance is explained when additional variables are added to the equation. Hence, it is possible to analyze whether high school grades or a pre-college test is a better predictor of college performance and the amount of variance that these variables explain, both in combination and separately.

Just as no instrument can have perfect reliability, no instrument can have perfect criterion-related validity. As discussed in Chapter 3, we take the lack of perfect reliability into consideration and provide scores in a range using standard error of measurement. The same logic applies with predicting to a criterion, where the lack of a perfect relationship between the instrument and the criterion is taken into consideration in the interpretation of the criterion scores by using **standard error of estimate.** Standard error of estimate indicates the margin of expected error in an individual's predicted criterion score as a result of imperfect validity. The formula for standard error of estimate (SE_{est}) is similar to the formula for standard error of measurement except that the focus of standard error of estimate is on the validity coefficient:

$$SE_{est} = s_y\sqrt{1 - r_{xy}^2}$$

In this equation, s_y is the standard deviation of the criterion and r_{xy} is the validity coefficient (correlation between the scores on the instrument and the criterion), which is squared (r_{xy}^2). Although standard error of estimate can be used for predicting an individual's performance on the criterion, it is more commonly used to look at error around a cutoff point. A developer of an instrument designed to predict suicidal behaviors would want to use standard error of estimate when determining the score at which counselors should be concerned about their clients. As with standard error of measurement, standard error of estimate provides a range of scores; however, with standard error of estimate, the range is on the criterion.

Decision Theory Another method that examines the relationship between an instrument and a criterion or predictor variable is *group separation* or *expectancy tables*. This approach is sometimes referred to as **decision theory** because instruments are often used in decision making, and this approach evaluates the accuracy of the decision making. Group separation concerns whether the scores of the instrument correctly differentiate. For example, do people who score high on the test get the high grades, as predicted? Decision theory attempts to assist in the selection and placement process by taking available information and putting it into a mathematical form (see Cronbach & Gleser, 1965). In terms of aiding the decision-making process, we want to know how often the instrument is right (a *hit*) and how often the instrument is wrong (a *miss*). For example, to what extent does the instrument accurately predict those who will succeed in college versus those who will not succeed? An **expectancy table** is the table that is developed to examine whether an instrument differentiates between the groups. An expectancy table can be used in two ways. First, an expectancy table can help in making decisions, such as admissions or hiring decisions. Second, it can provide clients with information on the probabilities of succeeding in college or an occupation given their scores on the instrument.

Let's return again to the fictitious Counseling Aptitude Scale (CAS). As you will remember, the CAS is supposed to predict who will be effective counselors and who will not. If we were the developers of this instrument, we could use an expectancy table to see (1) if the CAS does predict effective counseling and (2) if we could use the CAS to determine cutoff scores for admission to counseling programs. After we develop the expectancy table, we could then use it to provide potential students with an indication of how successful they might be as counselors. To develop an expectancy table, we must first find a criterion to use in validating the instrument.

Hypothetically, the Counseling Aptitude Scale will predict counseling effectiveness. Because this is a difficult concept to measure, we might want to use performance in a graduate program in counseling as a criterion. (I know some will argue that performance in a graduate program is not a very good measure of people's effectiveness in actual counseling, but let's just go ahead with this as an example.) After we have established the criterion of grade point average (GPA) in a counseling program, we next have to gather data. To do so, we would take a group of students who had been admitted to a counseling program, and, before they began classes, we would give them the Counseling Aptitude Scale. We would then sit back and let these students proceed with their counseling program. After the students graduated, we would gather GPA information to construct our expectancy table. Figure 4.3 shows an imaginary expectancy table for the CAS scores and the GPAs of 60 students. We would examine the first table to determine if the CAS can differentiate between those students who did well in a graduate counseling program and those who did not perform well.

In examining this table, we can see that those who did well on the CAS tended to have higher GPAs than those who did poorly on it. We would then examine this table to determine how many times the instrument "hit" (was an accurate predictor) and how many times it "missed" (was not an accurate predictor). Examining the hits and misses not only helps to evaluate the criterion-related validity of the CAS; it can also aid us in determining cutoff scores for use in future admissions decisions.

FIGURE 4.3
Expectancy tables for the Counseling Aptitude Scale

	1–20	21–40	41–60	61–80	81–100
A			7	5	2
B	1	2	10	3	
C	4	10	3		
D	3	8			
F	2				

	1–20	21–40	41–60	61–80	81–100
A			7	5	2
B	1	2	10	3	
C	4	10	3		
D	3	8			
F	2				

	1–20	21–40	41–60	61 -80	81–100
A	False negatives		7	5	2
B	1	2	10	3	
C	4	10	3		
D	3	8	False positives		
F	2				

Often in graduate school, a student must earn a grade point average of B or above to continue in a program. Therefore, in the second table in Figure 4.3, a squiggly line has been drawn under the B row to indicate which students earned a B or better. As you can see from the second table, 30 students had GPAs above B (1 with scores of 1–20, 2 with scores of 21–40, 17 with scores of 41–60, 8 with scores of 61–80, and 2 scores of 81–100). If we set the cutoff score at 21 and above (signified by the single line), then we would have 38 hits and 22 misses. The 22 misses would include the one person who received a score between 1 and 20 but achieved a GPA of B even though that wasn't predicted, as well as the 18 who scored between 21 and 40 but had grades of either C or D and the 3 people who scored between 41 and 60 who received a C. What we now need to do is to determine the hits and misses if the cutoff score is set at 41 and above (signified by the dark line) and 61 and above (signified by the line with dashes). If we set the cutoff score at 41, there are 54 hits and only 6 misses. On the other hand, if we set the cutoff score at 61, there would be 40 hits and 20 misses. Therefore, if the decision were based solely on the most hits and the least misses, then the cutoff score of 41 seems best.

In addition to identifying hits and misses, expectancy tables can provide information about **false positives** and **false negatives.** A false positive occurs when the instrument predicts that individuals have "it" (the criterion) when in fact they do not. Thus, if we examine the third table in Figure 4.3, we can see three false positives—the three individuals who had scores at or above the 41-point cutoff but who received a C average in graduate school. A false negative occurs when the instrument predicts that test takers do not have it when in fact they do. Figure 4.3 shows three false negatives—individuals who had a score of less than 41 but earned a B average in graduate school. Hence, the assessment predicted these students would not do well, but the prediction was a false negative because the students actually had a B average.

The assessment situation influences whether individuals should try to minimize the false positives or the false negatives in setting cutoff scores. For example, if an instrument were used to select individuals for a very expensive training program, we might want to minimize the number of false positives. The purpose would be to select only people who would be successful and to not spend the money to train people who wouldn't. On the other hand, a false negative can also be quite costly. For example, a false negative on an instrument designed to assess suicide potential means the instrument would not identify someone as being at risk for committing suicide when, in fact, he or she is at risk. In this case, a false negative could mean the loss of life. Sometimes expectancy tables are used to identify the false positives or false negatives and then identify other characteristics of those individuals (e.g., personal characteristics, background characteristics) that may contribute to the misclassification. Using the last table in Figure 4.3, we might find it interesting to gather more information about the three individuals who scored between 41 and 60 but who did not achieve a B average in graduate school. There may be characteristics about these individuals that could help in screening those who appear to have counseling potential based on their CAS scores but who do not do well in their graduate counseling program.

Expectancy tables are commonly used for selection and placement purposes. They can also be used in counseling to provide probability information to individuals (e.g., What is the probability of achieving an A average given a Counseling Aptitude Scale score of 35?). The probability information is calculated by determining the percentage of people who fall in certain criterion categories. In looking at Figure 4.3, for example, we see that the probability of achieving an A average with a CAS score of 35 is zero because no one who received a score of 21–40 achieved an A average. There is, however, a 10% chance that a person receiving a score of 35 could achieve a B average because 2 of the 20 people who scored between 21 and 40 received a B average. The probability of receiving an A average with a CAS score of 90 is 100% because all of the people who scored between 81 and 100 achieved an A average.

Other factors need to be considered when using expectancy tables to determine cutoff scores for selection or placement purposes. One factor concerns the degree to which the process is *selective.* In many ways, a cutoff score is easier to determine if the process is very selective. The opposite is also true—the selection process is simplified if the intent is to select most individuals and only weed out a few who are extremely low. Another factor that influences the decision-making process is *base rate*, which refers to the extent to which the characteristic or attribute exists in the population. The third factor that influences the decision-making process is the way in which the scores *distribute*. The selection process is considerably more difficult when scores are grouped closely together than when there is more variability in scoring.

Validity generalization. In the *Standards for Educational and Psychological Testing* (APA, AERA, & NCME, 1999), the last subcategory related to validation evidence based on relations with other variable is *validity generalization*. Validity generalization was initially debated in employment testing and concerned the degree to which test validation research could be generalized to new situations. In general, findings from one study are not conclusive and there is a need for replication. When there are numerous studies related to an instrument, then there are methods for analyzing the data to determine if the relationship among the instrument and criterion are related to statistical artifacts or research methodologies or if the relationship is quite robust and can be generalized. The statistical procedure used to examine whether an instrument's validity can be generalized is *meta-analysis*. In meta-analysis, researchers combine the results of many studies and examine the influences of different research factors to determine whether a particular instrument has a significant relationship with a criterion.

Generalizing the validation evidence requires that a large number of studies have been conducted with the instrument. Furthermore, the researchers must employ complex meta-analytic procedures that allow for the examination of consistent patterns of relationships between the instrument and criteria. After this type of complex meta-analytic research is completed, researchers examine the findings to determine if the results warrant a generalization of the previous validation evidence to other uses of the instrument. An example of validity generalization is related to research conducted by Hunter and Schmidt (1983) and their colleagues regarding general ability or intelligence scores and job performance. Their research is discussed in Chapter 7.

Evidence-based consequences of testing. Another topic related to validity evidence that the *Standards for Educational and Psychological Testing* (AERA, APA, & NCME, 1999) clarifies is the concept that practitioners have a responsibility to examine the evidence related to the consequences of testing when considering using an instrument. Examples of social consequences of assessment are group differences in test scores on instruments used for employment selection and promotion and group differences in the placement rate of children in special education programs. Validity is a unifying concept in which the counselors simultaneously examine the evidence considering use, interpretation, and social implications. Considering both validation evidence and issues of social policy becomes particularly important in cases when there are differing consequences related to test usage among different groups (AERA, APA & NCME, 1999). Practitioners should evaluate the evidence to determine if there is a compelling argument that justifies the test use and the appropriate interpretation. This concept of considering social implications is particularly relevant to counselors who have the ethical responsibility to consider what is in the client's best interest when they are counseling clients.

In some situations, it is suggested that testing will result in some defined benefits, such as increased student motivation. The *Standards for Educational and Psychological Testing* (AERA, APA, & NCME, 1999) suggests that these benefits should not be automatically accepted and in evaluating the validation evidence, clinicians need to examine the research related to the positive or negative consequences of such testing. As argued earlier, counselors are responsible for conducting assessments that are in the best interest of the client and, therefore, it is a counselor's responsibility to investigate the evidence or lack of evidence regarding the benefits or deleterious effects of testing.

Conclusion on validation evidence. In conclusion, the validity of an instrument is indicated by the gradual accumulation of evidence; consequently, there is usually not a clear-cut decision on whether an instrument has construct validity or not. It must be remembered, however, that validation evidence provides the basis for our interpretation of the results. To interpret the results of an instrument appropriately, a counselor must evaluate the validity information and determine what can be inferred from the results. Cronbach (1990) suggested that validation should be seen as a persuasive argument in which we are convinced by the preponderance of evidence on the appropriate use of an instrument. An instrument with strong construct validity will attempt to resolve critical uncertainties and explore plausible rival hypotheses. Many times the evaluation of the validation evidence need not be done by the counselor in isolation, because many instruments have been critiqued by knowledgeable scholars in publications such as the *Mental Measurements Yearbooks* and *Test Critiques*.

The emphasis in this chapter has been, to a degree, on formal assessment tools; yet, the concepts associated with validity apply to *all* types of client assessment. For example, counselors need to consider the concepts of validity when they do an intake interview with a client. In interviewing a client, a counselor needs to consider the content of the interview and the evidence that the interview questions address the appropriate behavior domain. Furthermore, counselors often make predictions about clients' behaviors and they should examine what informal assessments they are basing those predictions on and whether there is an accumulation of evidence that supports those hypotheses. Construct validity, which many leaders in the assessment field believe is synonymous with validity, is also pertinent because client traits or constructs frequently are an integral part of assessment. Research tend to support the contention that practitioners who rely only on intuition and experience are biased in their decisions (Dawes, 1994). Therefore, it may be helpful for practitioners to focus on the concept of construct validity in their informal assessment of clients. Counselors who purposefully analyze an accumulation of evidence will probably make more valid assessments of their clients.

Item Analysis

This chapter includes information on both validity and item analysis. **Item analysis** focuses on examining and evaluating each item within an assessment. Whereas validity evidence concerns the entire instrument, item analysis examines the qualities of each item. Item analysis is often used when instruments are being developed or revised because it provides information that can be used to revise or edit problematic items or eliminate faulty items. Some of the simpler methods of item analysis can easily be used to evaluate items in classroom tests, questionnaires, or other informal instruments. There are also some extremely complex methods for analyzing items and this discussion will include a brief overview of the typical methods used to analyze items.

Item Difficulty

When examining ability or achievement tests, counselors are often interested in the difficulty level of the test items. The difficulty level of an item should indicate whether an item is too easy or, possibly, too difficult. Item difficulty, which is an index that reflects the proportion of people getting an item correct, is calculated by dividing the number of individuals who answered the question correctly by the total number of people who answered the question:

$$p = \frac{\textit{number who answer correctly}}{\textit{total number of individuals}}$$

An item difficulty index can range from .00 (meaning no one got the item correct) to 1.00 (meaning everyone got the item correct). Item difficulty does not really indicate difficulty; rather, because it provides the proportion of individuals who got the item correct, it shows how easy the item is. Let's use an example of an item on a counseling assessment test where 15 of the students in a class of 25 got the first item on the test correct. In this case, we would say the item difficulty (p) is .60:

$$p = \frac{15}{25} = .60$$

There are no clear guidelines for evaluating an item difficulty index and the desired index difficulty level depends on the context of the assessment. In the previous example, we would need more information to interpret the index of .60 (interpretation of this item difficulty index might also depend on whether an individual is in the group who got the item correct or the group who got it wrong!). If the intent is to have items that differentiate among individuals, then a difficulty level of around .50 is considered optimum. Some assessment experts have suggested that in multiple-choice items, the probability of guessing needs to be considered in determining the optimum difficulty level (Cohen & Swerdlik, 2004; Kaplan & Saccuzzo, 2005). In other contexts, however, an instructor might be pleased with an item difficulty level of 1.00, which would indicate that everyone in the class was able to comprehend the material and answer the item correctly. Therefore, the determination of the desired item difficulty level depends on the purpose of the assessment, the group taking the instrument, and the format of the item. Evaluating an item difficulty index can frequently provide useful information to an instructor. For example, an easy item might have a low index because students find it confusing; whereas, a difficult item may have a comparatively high item difficulty because the item may be written in a manner that students can figure out the correct response without knowing the content.

Item Discrimination

Item discrimination, or item discriminability, provides an indication of the degree to which an item correctly differentiates among the examinees on the behavior domain of interest. For example, have you ever taken a test and felt as if an item didn't discriminate between those individuals who studied hard and knew the material and those individuals who didn't? Not only is item discrimination applicable to achievement or ability tests; it can also indicate if items discriminate in other assessment areas, such as personality and interest inventories. For instance, we may want to know if individuals who have been diagnosed as being depressed answered an item one way and if individuals who do not report depressive symptoms answer the same question another way. There are several methods for evaluating an item's ability to discriminate.

One of the most common methods for calculating an item discrimination index is called the *extreme group method.* First, examinees are divided into two groups based on high and low scores on the instrument (the instrument could be a class test, a depression inventory, or an assertiveness scale). The item discrimination index is then calculated by subtracting the proportion of examinees in the lower group (lower %) from the proportion of examinees in the upper group (upper %) who got the item correct or who endorsed the item in the expected manner:

$$d = \text{upper } \% - \text{lower } \%$$

Item discrimination indices that are calculated with this method can range from +1.00 (all of the upper group got it right and none of the lower group got it right) to –1.00 (none of the upper group got it right and all of the lower group got it right). An item discrimination index with a negative number is a nightmare for test developers (particularly for instructors with vengeful students in the upper group who find out the item did not discriminate between those who studied and those who did not). Like item difficulty, interpretation of an item discrimination index depends on the instrument, the purpose it was used for, and the group taking the instrument.

The determination of the upper group and the lower group with item discrimination depends on the distribution of scores. Kelley (1939) showed that if there is a normal distribution, then optimal dispersion is accomplished by using the upper 27% for the upper group and the lower 27% for the lower group. Anastasi and Urbina (1997) suggested that with small groups, such as the typical classroom of around 30 students, the exact percentages to select each group need not be precisely defined but should be in the general range of 25–33%.

Another method for determining item discrimination is through the *correlational method.* These correlational approaches report the relationship between the performance on the item and a criterion. Often the criterion is performance on the overall test. The point biserial method and the phi coefficient are two commonly used correlational techniques. A thorough explanation of these techniques would be too lengthy for this discussion, but interested readers are directed to Crocker and Algina (1986). The result of these methods is a correlation coefficient that ranges from +1.00 to –1.00, with the positive and larger coefficients reflecting items that are better discriminators.

Item Response Theory

Before moving on to other topics, it is important to briefly address item response theory (IRT). Embretson and Hershberger (1999) argued that item response theory is one of the most important recent developments in psychological assessment and that practitioners need knowledge about these approaches to assessment. **Item response theory**, or **latent trait theory**, builds on the concepts of item analysis. The basis for item response theory is different from classical test theory, where the focus is on arriving at one true score and our attempts to control error in the instrument. In classical test theory, the items on the instrument are a sample of the larger set of items that represents the domain and we get an indication of the individual's performance based on the combined items. In item response theory, the focus is on each *item* and establishing items that actually measure a particular ability or the respondent's level of a latent trait. Item response theory rests on the assumption that the performance of an examinee on a test item can be predicted by a set of factors called traits, latent traits, or abilities. Using an item response theory approach, we get an indication of an individual's performance based not on the total score but, rather, on the *precise items* the person answers correctly. As an example, with a traditional approach, we might say a score above 70 indicates that the student is reading at the sixth-grade level. With an item response approach, however, the student would need to answer items 5, 7, 13, 19, 20, 21, and 24 correctly to achieve a score indicating a sixth-grade reading level. The goal with this approach is to develop items that assess sixth-grade reading (not fifth- or seventh-grade reading). Item response theory involves the scaling of items, a procedure that requires quite sophisticated mathematical analyses. A thorough discussion of item response theory is not appropriate for this book; interested readers are directed to Hambleton, Swaminathan, and Rogers (1991), van der Linden and Hambleton (1997) and Wilson (2005).

In IRT, there are two fundamental assumptions: *unidimensionality* and *local independence* (Henard, 2000). Unidimensionality means that the theoretical view is that each item will be constructed so that it measures only one ability or latent trait. This is difficult to meet in reality because of factors such as test anxiety and reading ability on tests of personality. Sometimes developers of assessments based on item response theory will use the term *dominant* factor, which acknowledges other factors may be slightly involved. The second assumption, local independence, requires an examinees' response on each item to be unrelated to responses on other items. Because the focus is on each item, it is assumed that the answer on one item does not influence an answer on another item. In IRT, the only factor that would influence item response is the latent trait (Henard, 2000).

Item response theory suggests that the relationship between examinees' item performance and the underlying trait being measured can be described by a monotonically increasing function called an *item characteristic function* or an *item characteristic curve* (Hambleton et al., 1991). To construct an item characteristic curve, an instrument developer starts by constructing an item that he believes will measure the ability of interest. The developer then gives the item to an appropriate group or groups and then plots the results for each item using an item characteristic curve. With an item characteristic curve, the instrument developer plots a measure of trait or ability (e.g., age or grade level) on the horizontal axis and the probabilities of getting the item correct on the vertical axis. He obtains the probabilities by determining the proportion of persons at different levels who passed an item. Figure 4.4 shows a simplified example of plots of item characteristic curves. In this figure, the measure for the trait or ability is chronological age and the proportions of 6-year-olds, 7-year-olds, 8-year-olds, and 9-year-olds who answered the questions correctly are the probabilities. With a "good" item, we would expect the probability of getting the answer correct to increase as the underlying trait (e.g., age) increases. The probability of a 7-year-old getting item "a" right is very high (over 90%), while the probability of getting item "b" right is around 50%. The item curves are plotted from mathematical functions derived from the actual data.

Another strength of an IRT approach is it enables researchers to conduct rigorous tests of measurement across experimental groups (e.g., depressed versus non-depressed individuals). IRT approaches also have cross-cultural applications, where researchers compare the item characteristic curves of various ethnic/racial groups.

There are different IRT models, and the mathematical functions to plot the item characteristic curves vary. An elementary approach in an IRT model would involve examining item difficulty (a one parameter model). Figure 4.4 shows item characteristic curves that are plotted based on item difficulty and the percentage of individuals who got the item correct. Good items result in a somewhat slanted *S* shape. With this one parameter model, the point on the ability axis where there is a 50% (.50) probability of getting the item correct is typically considered the pivotal point.

FIGURE 4.4 *Hypothetical item characteristic curves*

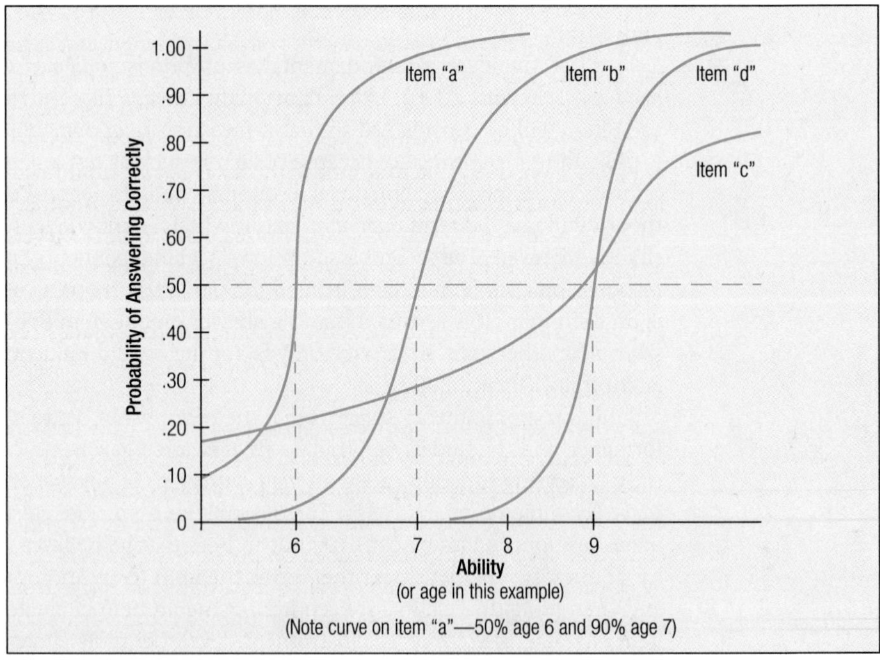

Item response theory is based on the concept that each item has nuisances or error variables that escape standardization (van der Linden & Hambleton, 1997). Therefore, we need to control the error for each item, which can be done mathematically (similar in concept to analysis of covariance [ANCOVA], where we statistically control a variable). More complex IRT models consider more parameters than just item difficulty. For example, a parameter that is often included is the slope of the curve, which provides an indication of how well the item discriminates. Steeper slopes indicate the item is a good discriminator, whereas flat slopes reflect that an item does discriminate very well. In Figure 4.4, item "c" does not discriminate as well as the other items. What is sometimes called the location is the place where the probability of getting a correct response is .50. An item that 50% of the fourth graders got right would be considered a fourth-grade item. In Figure 4.4, item "a" would be a 6-year-old item, item "b" would be 7-year-old item, and items "c" and "d" would be 9-year-old items. Many models also consider the basal level, which is an estimate of the probability that a person at the low end of the trait or ability scale will answer correctly. Also, many models of item response theory take into consideration the liability of guessing. The combination of parameters produces item characteristic curves that are evaluated to determine the suitability of the item. Consistent with the simpler model, the slanted *S* curve is desired in the item characteristic curves of the more complex models.

Instruments developed with an item response approach are not evaluated the same way as those developed with classical test theory approach. An item response approach to instrument development will theoretically result in an instrument that is not dependent on a norming group. Therefore, the methods for determining standard error of measurement are also different. With IRT, the standard error of measurement differs across scores (Embretson, 1996). Furthermore, IRT can be particularly useful in developing comparable test scores across multiple forms of an instrument because items with similar item characteristic curves can be selected for each different form of the instrument, thus allowing for interchangeable test forms.

There are numerous approaches to using item response theory in instrument development, and the methods continue to become more sophisticated (van der Linden & Hambleton, 1997). Item response theory is having an influence on large-scale testing programs, particularly in the area of achievement. Another application concerns building item banks that include items scaled to different levels. Publishers have assembled some item banks for fractions, decimals, and long division (Cronbach, 1990). These sophisticated item banks can provide useful information in terms of identifying individuals' academic strengths and limitations. Because of the extensive analysis and calibration of the items, item response theory can be particularly useful in the development of criterion-referenced tests. It is also having an effect on computer-administered adaptive testing in which performance on certain items influences the future items presented to the examinee. For example, if students cannot multiply a one-digit number by a one-digit number, it makes little sense to give them numerous questions about multiplying two-digit numbers by two-digit numbers. Thus, the computer sorts the questions based on previous responses. Item response theory can be particularly useful in achievement and ability adaptive testing, because the calibrated items can be used to quickly pinpoint an individual's ability level and identify possible gaps in knowledge. Item response theory is also serving as the theoretical base for measures of personality and psychopathology. The approach is the same as achievement. We can find an example of using the item response theory approach to analyze an instrument in Beevers, Strong, Meyer, Pilkonis, and Miller (2007), who examine the Dysfunctional Attitude Scale.

Summary

Validity concerns whether an assessment measures what it is designed to measure. An instrument is not validated; rather, it is the uses of the instrument that are validated. Validation evidence informs counselors on what they can infer from the results. A counselor is responsible for examining the accumulation of validation evidence and for determining how the instrument can be used and what can be inferred from the results. The field of measurement is moving away from the three traditional types of validity to an overall, integrated view of validation evidence. Therefore, the three sources of evidence should not be viewed as separate and distinct types but, rather, as ways of accumulating evidence that contributes to overall evaluation of the appropriate uses and interpretations of the assessment. Content validation evidence concerns the content of the instrument and the degree to which the content corresponds to the behavior domain. Criterion-related validation evidence is related to how well the instrument predicts to a defined criterion. There are two types of criterion-related validity: concurrent and predictive. With concurrent, there is no time lapse between the taking of the instrument and the prediction, whereas with predictive, there is a time lapse. The third type of validity is construct validity, which applies to instruments that measure theoretical constructs or traits. Construct validation evidence requires the gradual accumulation of evidence and can include both content- and criterion-related validity. Many different techniques can be used in the process of gathering construct-related evidence. Counselors evaluating the validity of an instrument should examine what the preponderance of evidence indicates about whether that instrument can be used in a specific manner.

Items in well-constructed instruments are also analyzed. Two of the most common methods of item analysis involve determining the item difficulty and the item discrimination indices. Item response theory, which involves developing items that are calibrated to measure abilities or traits, is also having a substantial influence on instrument development.

CHAPTER 5

Selecting, Administering, Scoring, and Communicating Assessment Results

Before moving on to the second and third sections of this book that address specific assessment areas and issues related to assessment in counseling, it is important to address the specific topics of selection, administration, scoring, and communicating assessment results. Particularly in terms of the use of formal instruments, problems related to assessment can often be traced to clinicians' confusion or misjudgments in one of these areas. This discussion of selecting, administering, scoring, and communicating results may seem to reinforce the idea that assessment is a separate and distinct process for counseling. My philosophy, however, is that counselors are continually assessing clients throughout the counseling process and that clinicians need to be mindful of the appropriate use and interpretation of both informal and formal assessment techniques.

Preliminary Identification of Assessment Instruments or Strategies

A practitioner who selects and uses a faulty assessment tool in counseling could adversely affect a client's life. The most glaring example would be to mishandle an assessment of suicidal ideation. Therefore, the selection of an assessment tool or strategy is an important clinical decision. In some counseling situations, the selection of assessment strategies is neglected due to heavy caseloads or comfort with existing methods. Yet, assessment is the foundation of the counseling process because it provides much of the information used to determine the therapeutic goals and interventions. Therefore, the selection of assessment methods needs to involve careful consideration and evaluation of strategies and approaches. The following steps may be helpful in selecting an assessment instrument or strategy: (1) determine what information is needed, (2) analyze strategies for obtaining information, (3) search assessment resources, (4) evaluate assessment strategies, and (5) select an assessment instrument or strategy.

Determine What Information Is Needed

The first step in the process is to determine what information would be useful. An assessment tool is helpful only if it provides useful information. Therefore, before counselors can determine what assessment strategies to further consider and evaluate, they first need to determine what information is truly needed. Doing so can involve identifying the information needed for a specific client or determining what general information clinicians in an organization may need about their clients. Sometimes counselors skip this first step and implement an assessment approach without considering whether the process will yield useful information. As reflected in Appendix B, the *Code of Fair Testing Practices in Education* (Joint Committee on Testing Practice, 2004) clearly reflects that the first responsibility for test users is to "Define the purpose for testing, the content and skills to be tested, and the intended test takers. Select and use the most appropriate test based on a thorough review of available information" (p. 5). According to Anastasi and Urbina (1997), the use of formal assessment is most productive when it answers a client's question and is seamlessly integrated into the counseling process. Sometimes when counselors are considering assessment strategies and client information that would be useful, they do not consider information that may already be accessible. For example, school counselors often have access to substantial information in students' educational records and mental health counselors frequently have clients complete some forms before an initial session. Hence, sometimes information can be accessed in advance and the assessment process can focus on strategies for eliciting particularly pertinent client information. It should also be stressed that gathering assessment information is not applicable just at the beginning of counseling and counselors often need to determine assessment strategies at various points throughout the counseling process.

Analyze Strategies for Obtaining Information

Once clinicians have identified the pertinent client information, the second step is to determine the best strategies for obtaining that information. A primary decision for a counselor is whether information can best be gathered through *formal* or *informal* techniques. Frequently, both formal and informal assessment tools provide an optimum situation, because the strengths of one method complement the other, and together they provide an in-depth analysis of clients. Counselors also need to consider which assessment method would be most suited to a client or clients (e.g., paper-and-pencil self-report, behavioral checklist, computer assessment). Often counselors will become comfortable with certain assessment strategies (e.g., interviewing) and not consider other strategies that may correspond to client characteristics. Analyzing client attributes before selecting an assessment strategy may increase both the quality and quantity of the information selected. Furthermore, counselors also need to consider their own professional limitations and the types of instruments they can ethically administer and interpret.

Search Assessment Resources

Once the pertinent information and the most effective strategies for gathering that information are identified, the next step is to peruse existing instruments or assessment strategies. Duckworth (1990) suggested that, whenever possible, the client should be involved in the selection of instruments. This does not mean that counselors should provide a detailed lecture, using psychometric information, on choices of instruments. Instead, counselors should engage clients in a brief discussion of possible avenues to consider.

It is impossible for any practitioner to be familiar with the thousands of published and unpublished assessment tools in the counseling realm. In addition, it is not always easy to identify possible instruments to use. Because no one source describes every formal and informal assessment tool that has ever been developed or used, practitioners often need to use a variety of sources and technologies to develop a list of possible tools. Counselors should regularly examine assessment resources because new instruments are continually being developed that may provide better information. In addition, many instruments are continually revised and a counselor would not want to use an older version of an instrument when a more recent and improved version is available. Although it may be tempting to use the Internet and some of the more popular search engines (e.g., Google) to identify assessment resources, this approach has some problems. I recently used Google to identify career interest inventories and it identified 19,400,000 websites. Even though I do find the examination of new interest inventories quite fascinating, even I am not going to visit and thoroughly evaluate all 19,400,000 sites! Furthermore, based on the information provided in some of the websites, it is somewhat difficult to differentiate between legitimate, psychometrically sound interest inventories and ones with little evidence regarding the instrument's psychometric qualities. Chapter 16 will more thoroughly explore issue related to the Internet and assessment, but some alternative resources for identifying possible assessments that are a little more professionally oriented than those found simply using a search engine are discussed in the next section.

Assessment search resources. A number of resources can assist counselors in searching for different assessment instruments. One of the most important assessment resources is the *Mental Measurements Yearbooks* (MMY). This series of yearbooks contains critiques of many of the commercially available psychological, educational, and career instruments.

Oscar K. Buros published the first yearbook in 1938 and continued to spearhead the publication of subsequent yearbooks until his death in 1978. Each yearbook extends information in the previous yearbooks by reviewing instruments published or revised during a specific time period. The *Seventeenth Mental Measurements Yearbook* is currently in production and should be completed before the publication of this book. The Buros Institute of Mental Measure can be accessed on-line at http://www.unl.edu/buros/bimm/index.html. Most academic libraries have book forms of the *Mental Measurement Yearbooks* and test reviews can be retrieved either on-line or through a library. By using the Buros Institute home page, clinicians can use "Test Reviews On-line" in which counselors can search a large database of commercial assessments. For example, typing in the term *anxiety* recently brought up a lengthy list of assessments that measure anxiety. By clicking on an instrument's name, a counselor can then get specific information on the instruments, including title, author, purpose, acronym, publisher, publisher's address, and in which edition of the *Mental Measurements Yearbook* the assessment was reviewed. It is also possible to order the review (for a fee) directly from the website. These reviews and critiques are written by authorities in the assessment field and provide an overview of each instrument's strengths and limitations. Another resource published by the Buros Institute is *Tests in Print*, which is useful in identifying tests by content area. The current version, *Tests in Print VII* (Murphy, Plake, & Spies, 2006), summarizes information on most commercially available tests published in English. *Tests in Print* can also be accessed on-line at http://www.unl.edu/buros/bimm/index.html. The instruments listed in *Tests in Print* are also cross-referenced with the *Mental Measurements Yearbooks.*

Another good resource for identifying possible instruments is Educational Testing Service (ETS) Test Link, which also can be accessed on-line. Test Link includes the Test Collection at ETS, which includes information on more than 25,000 tests and other measurement devices. The ETS Test link website indicates they are planning to offer an annual online subscription to the Tests on Demand collection for libraries. The plan allows students whose institutions subscribe to download assessments and have royalty-free permission to reproduce the tests for research purposes.

A prominent publisher for assessment resources is PRO-ED, which publishes *Test Critiques.* Similar to the *MMY*, more recent assessments are discussed in the later volumes of *Test Critiques.* PRO-ED also published *Tests: A Comprehensive Reference for Assessments in Psychology, Education, and Business* (Maddox, 2003), which provides descriptive information, including purpose, costs, available data, and scoring on approximately 2,000 instruments in the areas of psychology, education, and business.

Some counselors may be interested in identifying unpublished instruments to use in counseling or research. A useful resource is the *Directory of Unpublished Experimental Mental Measures* (Goldman & Mitchell, 2002), which identifies and describes noncommercial and more experimental measures in the fields of psychology, sociology, and education. The most recent volume (Volume 9) includes tests published from 2001 to 2005 in 36 of the top journals. Similar to other testing resources, earlier editions of this resource have information on older assessments. Although critiques are not provided in this resource, it does provide descriptions of noncommercial assessments.

Evaluate Assessment Strategies

After identifying possible assessment strategies, the next step is to evaluate those strategies in order to select the most effective methods or instruments. One of the first steps in determining if an instrument is appropriate to use is to ascertain if the instrument's purpose corresponds to the counselor's needs. If an instrument does not measure the behavior or construct of interest, then there is no need to further investigate the psychometric characteristics of that instrument. As mentioned earlier, an instrument is worthwhile only if it provides pertinent information that is needed in the counseling process. Sometimes, determining an instrument's purpose involves sifting through the information provided in the manual. Occasionally, the purpose stated in the manual may be a little different from what the name of the instrument implies. Furthermore, it is important to determine if the design of the instrument corresponds to the intended purpose. Some instruments fail to achieve their intended purpose because of problems in construction. An instrument's manual should provide a description of the instrument's purpose as well as a detailed explanation of how the instrument measures the behaviors related to that purpose.

Instrument development. Counselors need to closely scrutinize the procedures that instrument developers used in constructing the instrument. Most instruments have a theoretical or empirical base that influences the overall development. If detailed information about the development of an instrument is not provided, counselors should be concerned, and its psychometric properties should be carefully evaluated. For many instruments, the development of the actual items plays a central role in instrument construction. For example, if an instrument is based on item response theory, the development and analysis of each item is critical to the interpretation of results. Evidence of careful construction of items, as well as of detailed item analysis, adds credence to the instrument's value. Counselors should also read the items and consider if they are appropriate for the client(s). Furthermore, if counselors will use the instrument with clients from different ethnic groups, then they should examine whether *differential item functioning* has been conducted to control for group differences (see Chapter 15).

Appropriate selection of norming group or criterion. Depending on the type of instrument, either the norming group in a norm-referenced instrument or the criterion in a criterion-referenced instrument will need to be evaluated. In a norm-referenced instrument, an analysis of the makeup of the norming group is critical. First, counselors must determine if the norming group is appropriate for their clients. For example, if a counselor is working with adults who did not complete high school, then an instrument that used college students as the norming sample for adults would probably not be appropriate. Counselors should also evaluate the suitability of the norming sample in terms of age, gender, ethnic makeup, socioeconomic representation, educational level, and geographic location. A norming group's ethnic makeup is of particular importance and should be carefully considered. The size of the norming sample is another consideration in evaluating a norm-referenced instrument. Although there are no clear guidelines for determining the appropriate size of a norming group, large samples drawn in a systematic manner tend to garner more confidence.

The evaluation of the criterion in a criterion-referenced instrument involves analyzing the procedures the developers used to determine the criterion. As you will recall, criterion-referenced instruments measure whether an individual has attained a certain level or standard (the criterion). With a criterion-referenced instrument, the evaluation of the criterion is the most important step. In response to federal legislation and other influences in our society, there is currently substantial interest in setting standards or determining the criteria for passing achievement tests. Publishers of some achievement tests will include information pertinent to setting a criterion for passing that may include standards from professional organizations, reviews by leading researchers, and studies of curriculum. The manual should supply sufficient documentation to convince the reader that the determination of the criterion was based on suitable information and careful analysis.

Reliability. Evaluating an instrument's reliability evidence is an important step in determining whether to use it. When I am teaching an assessment course, counseling students sometimes ask, "How high should a reliability coefficient be to indicate adequate reliability?" My answer is, "It depends." There are no clear guidelines in determining what constitutes an acceptable reliability. The type of instrument affects how the reliability coefficients are evaluated. In the second section of this book, the reliability coefficients of some commonly used instruments are provided in order to furnish a reference. Reliability can be estimated in different ways, and in some instruments' manuals, counselors will find a range of coefficients that were calculated using different methods. In comparing instruments, counselors should take into consideration the methods used for determining the coefficients, because some methods of determining reliability tend to have lower estimates than others. Standard error of measurement is also often provided in the manuals of well-developed instruments. Another trend to consider when evaluating an instrument's reliability is that reliability coefficients tend to be lower with younger participants. Therefore, you can expect lower coefficients with preschoolers than with adults.

Validity. Evaluating the validity of an instrument involves studying the validation evidence. In examining the validation information, counselors should not expect a definitive conclusion, such as the instrument either has validity or does not have validity. Rather, the evaluation of validity involves determining the degree to which there is support for particular *uses* of the instrument. The analysis of validity concerns whether there is a preponderance of evidence to support the use of an instrument in a specific manner or context. The manual should include ample evidence that the instrument is valid for the desired purpose. If there is not ample evidence, the instrument should be used very cautiously or not at all.

Bias. In the past 25 years, there has been substantial concern about test bias and multicultural assessment. An instrument's authors should provide evidence that the instrument was evaluated for possible bias. Chapter 15 provides an overview of how instruments are typically examined to detect possible bias. Because some instruments may be inappropriate for certain populations, the manuals should address those limitations. If a manual recommends that an instrument not be used with certain clients, then alternate assessment strategies should be explored.

Interpretation and scoring materials. If an instrument has adequate psychometric qualities, counselors will want to examine the materials that were designed to assist in the interpretation of the results. The manual or additional resources should provide the necessary information for interpreting the results. Many instruments have a variety of scoring options and interpretative reports.

In examining the interpretative materials, counselors also need to consider how they are going to use the information in counseling and what would be the most effective way to share the information with the client. Some instruments have interpretative booklets, which can be given to clients to assist in the counseling process. These booklets should never replace the counselor explaining the results, but these types of resources can sometimes be helpful.

Another consideration when choosing an instrument is how it is scored. Today, many instruments are computer scored, which may require access to an appropriate computer and other equipment (e.g., a scanner). An organization's resources often affect which instruments and scoring services can be considered for use.

User qualifications. In selecting an instrument, practitioners should also consider their own competencies and training. Counselors can select instruments only from the pool of instruments that they can ethically use. Moreover, counselors must become competent in using a specific instrument before giving it to a client. Instruments vary in the amount of training and experience that is necessary. Some instruments can be used with knowledge gained from studying the manual, whereas other instruments require supervised instruction on the appropriate use of those devices. One attempt that some publishers make to address the variations in needed training is a grading system that classifies instruments based on certain user qualifications. The following list provides an example of the levels used by a publisher.

> *Level A:* Typically these instruments can be adequately administered, scored, and interpreted solely by using the manual. The orientation to these instruments is usually left up to the institution or organization in which the individual works. Test publishers often will not send these materials out unless the individual is employed in a legitimate or recognized organization or institution, or the individual has verification of licensure or certification recognized by the publisher. Examples of instruments at this level are achievement tests and the *Self-Directed Search* (SDS).
>
> *Level B:* These instruments and aids require technical knowledge in instrument development, psychometric characteristics, and appropriate test use. To qualify for Level B, the test user must have a master's level degree in psychology or education, or the equivalent with relevant training in assessment. Alternatively, the individual must have verification of licensure or certification recognized by the publisher. Examples of instruments at this level are the *Myers-Briggs Type Indicator, Suicidal Ideation Questionnaire, NEO PI-R,* and the *Strong Interest Inventory.*
>
> *Level C:* These instruments and aids require substantial knowledge about the construct being measured and about the specific instrument being used. Often the publisher will require a Ph.D. in psychology or education, with specific coursework related to the instrument. Examples of instruments at this level are the *WISC-IV*, the *Stanford-Binet*, the *Rorschach*, and the *Rotter Incomplete Sentence Blank* (2nd ed.).

Although these levels are used by some publishers, a counselor needs to check the category system used by each publisher because there are variations. For example, Pearson Assessments—which publishes the MMPI-2—has Level 1, Level 2, and Level 3.

The *ACA Code of Ethics* (American Counseling Association, 2005a) indicates that counselors need to recognize their level of competence and perform only those testing and assessment services for which they have been trained (see Appendix C). These standards also indicate that the ultimate responsibility for appropriate use of an instrument rests with the practitioner. Therefore, if an organization wants counselors to use instruments for which they are not properly trained, the counselors have an ethical responsibility to refrain from using those assessments. There can be legal ramifications (e.g., losing a professional license or being sued for malpractice) for practitioners who use instruments that they are not qualified to use.

One of the arguments related to restricting testing and assessment only to psychologists is that unqualified users are using psychological instruments. Qualified and competent use requires more than having the necessary training—the practitioner must also be knowledgeable about the specific instrument being used. The discussion of instruments in the following chapters of this book does not provide enough information to serve as training for using an instrument. Sufficient knowledge of an instrument is gained *only* through the thorough examination of the manual and the accompanying materials. In some cases, a practitioner also must have supervised training on the use of a particular assessment before being allowed to use it. The counselor must know the limitations of an instrument and for what purposes the instrument is valid.

Practical issues. When selecting an assessment, there are often a number of practical issues to keep in mind. In many settings, the cost of the instrument plays a role in the decision process. Certainly, a counselor should consider whether the instrument provides information that is sufficiently useful to warrant the costs. Some instruments are quite expensive; however, if used appropriately, they can be enormously helpful to clients. Another consideration is time and whether the time investment is worth it. Some clients may be reluctant to spend hours taking numerous assessment tools, or some parents may object if instructional time is used for assessment. If, however, the clients understand the benefits of the assessment, they may be less concerned about the amount of time involved.

In conclusion, the selection of an assessment instrument is an important task. Assessment tools have been used inappropriately in the past, and sometimes this was because professionals did not devote sufficient time to selecting an appropriate tool for a specific client. A selection decision should not be made without thoroughly examining an instrument and its manual. Figure 5.1 provides some questions to consider when evaluating assessment instruments in counseling.

FIGURE 5.1
Example of a form to evaluate assessment instruments

1. Is the purpose of the instrument clearly stated in the manual?	Yes ______ No ______
2. Does the purpose of the instrument meet my clinical needs?	Yes ______ No ______
3. Do I have the professional skill and background necessary to competently administer and interpret this instrument?	Yes ______ No ______
4. Given the logistics of my organization, can the instrument be administered in an appropriate manner?	Yes ______ No ______
5. Is there evidence that the authors developed clear goals and objectives (i.e., instrument specifications) for the instrument before the instrument was developed?	Yes ______ No ______
6. Was care taken in constructing and evaluating all of the items?	Yes ______ No ______
7. Did they perform adequate item analysis of all items?	Yes ______ No ______
8. Did they evaluate the items for possible bias?	Yes ______ No ______
9. For norm-referenced instruments, does the norming group seem appropriate for my client(s)?	Yes ______ No ______
10. For norm-referenced instruments, does the size of the norming group appear sufficient?	Yes ______ No ______
11. For norm-referenced instruments, does the norm group appear to represent the pertinent population in terms of the appropriate characteristics?	Yes ______ No ______
12. For criterion-referenced instruments, is the criterion clearly stated?	Yes ______ No ______
13. For criterion-referenced instruments, was the criterion selected appropriately?	Yes ______ No ______
14. For criterion-referenced instruments, is there compelling evidence that the level of expected performance is appropriate?	Yes ______ No ______
15. Has the reliability of the instrument been explored sufficiently?	Yes ______ No ______
16. Is there reliability information for different groups and are the coefficients acceptable for these different groups?	Yes ______ No ______
17. Does the instrument appear to have acceptable reliability for my uses?	Yes ______ No ______
18. Does the manual provide the standard error of measurements for all the appropriate scales and subscales?	Yes ______ No ______
19. Does the manual provide validity information?	Yes ______ No ______
20. Is there sufficient validation evidence for me to feel comfortable in using this instrument for the specific purpose I need?	Yes ______ No ______
21. Does the validity evidence indicate I should be careful in using this instrument with certain clients or in certain situations?	Yes ______ No ______
22. Can the instrument be scored in a manner that fits the situation?	Yes ______ No ______
23. Is there sufficient information and resources for me to feel I can adequately interpret the results of this instrument to each client?	Yes ______ No ______
24. Are there appropriate materials to help the client understand the results?	Yes ______ No ______
25. Can the organization afford to use this instrument?	Yes ______ No ______
26. Do the benefits of this assessment outweigh the costs and time commitments?	Yes ______ No ______

Administering Assessment Instruments

Many counselors, particularly those in school settings, are responsible for administering certain assessment instruments. This is an important task because assessment results can be invalidated by careless administration. As the *Standards for Educational and Psychological Testing* (AERA, APA, & NCME, 1999) indicates, the usefulness and interpretability of test scores *require* that a test be administered according to the developer's instructions. Thus, the major focus of this section is on *knowing the administration materials and being prepared!*

It is important for professionals to have read the administration materials before the time of administration. With many instruments, pretesting procedures must be completed in a required manner. For example, the administration procedures might require that the room be set up in a specific way to minimize the opportunity for examinees to see others' answer sheets. Other procedures might include specific registration procedures in which the examinee must provide two forms of identification to sit for the examination. Thus, preparedness for the administration of an instrument should start well before the actual administration.

Administrators also need to be aware if there are precise instructions for administering the assessment. Many instruments have detailed instructions on how the instrument is administered, often including a specific script that is read to the examinee(s). In addition, they also need to be familiar with testing materials and equipment, and sometimes there are even specific rules about whether the test booklets or the answer sheets are disseminated first. For some school counselors, the administration of state-wide achievement tests has become quite specific and there are strict rules related to overseeing the testing process. Adherence to a time schedule is often part of the administration responsibilities. For example, a careless mistake in timing on the SAT could significantly affect students' scholarship awards and admission into certain colleges. The *Standards for Educational and Psychological Testing* (AERA, APA, & NCME, 1999) indicates that any modifications to standardized test administration procedures need to be documented. Some standardized instruments will provide a form on which the test administrator can report any problems or unusual circumstances that occurred during the administration.

An individual administering an assessment instrument also needs to know the boundaries of what is acceptable. For example, instruments vary in terms of what is considered an appropriate relationship and the degree of rapport the administrator is to have with the examinee(s). Some instruments require a certain degree of reserve, whereas other instruments encourage the administrator to be quite warm and encouraging. Examples of knowledge about what is acceptable include knowing what to do if people have to go to the restroom, procedures if the administrator suspects cheating, or testing protocol if an examinee comes in 30 minutes late. An example of a recent administration problem I witnessed occurred during a scholastic aptitude test, when some administrators allowed students to use calculators and other test administrators did not. The importance of knowing the administrative procedures cannot be emphasized enough. Following the procedures provided in Figure 5.2 may assist counselors who are administering an assessment for the first time. In summary, the key to effectively administering any assessment is knowledge of the procedures and preparing for possible problems.

FIGURE 5.2
Sample checklist for instrument or test administration

Pretesting Procedures

_______ Ensure that all testing materials are kept in a secure place
_______ Read instrument manual to familiarize yourself with all administrative procedures
_______ Check possible testing facilities for size, seating, lighting, and ventilation
_______ Schedule testing facilities
_______ Check to ensure there are no conflicts with arranged testing time(s) and facilities
_______ Send out any pretesting materials that need to be sent
_______ Review testing materials to ensure that all needed materials are available
_______ Arrange for any posting of signs to direct examinees to testing location
_______ Thoroughly study exact procedures for administering the instrument
_______ Read and practice the directions for administering the test
_______ Check stopwatch or other device if time limits are involved
_______ Prepare for questions that might be asked

Immediately Preceding Testing

_______ Make sure that facilities and seating arrangements are appropriate
_______ Organize any registration processes
_______ Organize testing materials

Administration of Instrument

_______ Perform any registration duties in the specified manner
_______ Distribute appropriate materials in the specified manner
_______ Administer instrument using the prescribed methods
_______ Adhere to specified time limits
_______ Note any behavioral observation of the client if individually administered
_______ Note any irregularities

After Completion of Testing

_______ Gather testing materials in the specified manner
_______ Follow specific directions for either scoring the instrument or sending the materials to be scored

Scoring

Many instruments are scored either by hand or by computer. Some instruments are self-scored, meaning the client is able to score the instruments, typically by adding columns together or counting responses. An example of an instrument that can be self-scored is the *Self-Directed Search* (Holland, Fritzsche, & Powell, 1994) on which clients simply count the number of items that correspond to Holland's (1997) six personality types. The manual, however, warns that scoring errors do occur and that the counselor should take steps to minimize any errors. For example, some practitioners will double-check clients' scoring, whereas others will simply have clients recheck their addition.

Although hand scoring is becoming less prevalent, some clinical situations may involve hand scoring of an assessment. Even if the scoring is quite easy, there are times when it is therapeutically inappropriate to have the client score the instrument. In addition, with many instruments, hand scoring typically involves placing a template over the answer sheet and counting the answers that correspond to various scales. If hand scoring is used, counselors need to ensure that this often tedious process is completed with attention to detail and accuracy.

Computer scoring, when compared with hand scoring, is often more accurate, rapid, and thorough. Computers are not biased and will not unintentionally consider factors such as race or gender in scoring. In addition, computers can be programmed to complete complex scoring procedures that would take humans weeks to perform. Furthermore, computers can be programmed not only to score but also to interpret the results. Computer scoring, however, is not always error free. Humans program the computers to perform the scoring, and errors in programming can result in problems. To ensure accurate scoring, the *Standards for Educational and Psychological Testing* (AERA, APA, & NCME, 1999) calls for test-scoring services to document the procedures they use when scoring. In addition, it calls for scoring services to monitor their scorings and correct any errors that might occur. This mandate, however, does not guarantee that all computerized scoring programs are sound, because individuals who lack sufficient training could write a program that improperly scores and interprets instruments. Before using a computerized scoring service, practitioners should investigate the integrity of that service and the steps that were taken to develop the scoring program. Another problem with computer scoring and interpreting relates to the ease with which assessment results can be generated. Because of this, some organizations might be tempted to skimp on staff training on an assessment device, or they might allow assessments to be conducted without appropriate professional oversight.

Not all assessments are scored by computers and some instruments require clinician judgment as a part of the scoring process. For example, with some individual intelligence or general ability tests, the examiner needs to make some professional judgments in scoring and interpretation. The manuals for these instruments attempt to reduce the ambiguity in these judgments by providing explicit scoring instructions. In the personality area, many of the projective techniques involve professional judgments. For many projective techniques, there are systematic methods for scoring the client's responses. Another area in which scoring is more unstructured is with performance or authentic assessment.

The terms **performance assessment** and **authentic assessment** are often used interchangeably, but there is a slight distinction between the two (Oosterhof, 2000).

Both performance and authentic assessments are typically associated with testing that goes beyond paper-and-pencil tests to assessment that more closely approximates the skill being measured. All authentic assessments are performance assessments, but the reverse is not always true. Authentic assessments involve the performance of "real," or authentic, applications rather than proxies, or estimators, of actual learning. Authentic and performance assessments are typically associated with achievement testing. Performance assessment, however, has its roots in industrial and organizational psychology (Bray, 1982), where individuals were given activities such as the "in-basket technique." With these types of assessments, multiple-choice items are typically avoided; instead, performance on open-ended tasks is evaluated. Because many of the same strengths and limitations in scoring apply to both performance and authentic assessments, this portion of the book will simply use the term *performance assessments* with the intent of also encompassing authentic assessment.

One of the goals of these types of assessments is to see if knowledge can be applied. For example, instead of giving a multiple-choice test on the rules of grammar, a performance test would involve writing a grammatically correct business letter. Another example of performance assessment is observing a student complete a lab experiment. Performance assessments seek to assess complex learning and processes by assessing both the product and the process. Thus, they involve observation and professional judgments about how the individual performed the tasks (e.g., the process of performing a lab experiment) and the product produced (e.g., the results of experiment). Performance assessments can sometimes assess the more abstract learning skills that traditional multiple-choice tests cannot adequately measure. There are, however, many difficulties associated with scoring these assessments.

The reason authentic and performance assessment is discussed here concerns issues of scoring. Objectivity in scoring becomes more difficult with the open-ended methods that are typically used in performance assessment. Sometimes the criteria for evaluating these measures are not adequately defined, and, thus, other factors can influence the judgments that are made. Particularly when process rather than product is being assessed, evaluators may fail to observe some important behaviors or will attend to behaviors that are unrelated to the skills being assessed. Because subjectivity is often part of performance assessment, examiners need to attend to multicultural issues in scoring. Evaluators' biases can sometimes seep into their observations and evaluations. The use of checklists and rating scales can increase both the reliability and validity of the scoring of a performance assessment (Oosterhof, 2000). Performance assessment requires a well-thought-out scoring plan or rubric.

Scoring a performance assessment is admittedly more complex than grading a multiple-choice examination. Research related to methods for ensuring sound measurement (Airasian, 2000; Oosterhof, 2000) has found that the procedures for scoring a performance assessment will be enhanced if:

- The assessment has a specific focus.
- The scoring plan is based on qualities that can be directly observed.
- The scoring is designed to reflect the intended target.
- The setting for the assessment is appropriate.
- Observers use checklists or rating scales.
- The scoring procedures have been field-tested before they are used.

The previous discussion focused on the scoring of performance assessment, with many of the issues pertaining to scoring instruments that are not multiple choice.

When scoring involves subjectivity, practitioners need to find methods for ensuring objective assessment. These guidelines also apply to nonacademic assessment, in which objectivity is also needed. Hence, practitioners should consider these guidelines with many of the subjective assessment strategies they use with clients.

Communicating Results

Once an instrument is scored, counselors often have the responsibility for interpreting the results based on the validation evidence and communicating the assessment results to clients, parents, or other individuals. Communicating the results to clients is often one of the most important aspects of the assessment process. Although counselors are trained in communication skills, the interpretation of assessment results requires specialized knowledge and competencies. The communication of results is an important process because if this information is not communicated effectively, clients or others may misperceive the assessment results. For example, a common problem is confusing the percentile with the percentage correct. I once had a client who was initially upset with her performance at the 50th percentile. When she saw her score on the mathematical section of an aptitude test, she began to weep and said that she had never been good in math. As I explained that her performance was in the average range, she looked puzzled and questioned my interpretation. As the discussion progressed, I began to see that she believed the score indicated she had gotten 50% of the items correct even though I was using terms such as the *50th percentile*. Once the misunderstanding was corrected, the client was pleased with her performance and seemed to feel more efficacious about her mathematical skills.

The communication of testing or assessment results should not be perceived as a discrete activity but should be interwoven into the counseling. The reason for using any informal or formal assessment is to answer questions that either the counselor or the client has. Thus, reporting results should be directly connected to the counseling's focus. Counselors need to be knowledgeable about the instrument and the client's specific results so that the focus during the interpretation of results can be on the client's questions and reactions rather than on what the scores mean.

Research Related to Communication of Results

Surprisingly, there is little research related to how practitioners can best communicate results to clients. Much of the research related to the benefits of clients receiving test information is in the area of career counseling. A number of studies conducted before 1985 related to test interpretation and communicating results from career assessments (Whiston, 2002a). In a meta-analysis that included career assessment studies, Oliver and Spokane (1988) found an effect size of .62 for individual test interpretation and an effect size of .76 for group test interpretation. This means that those who received the test interpretation were more than two thirds of a standard deviation higher on the outcome measures used than those who did not receive the interpretations. Concerning assessment in personal counseling, Goodyear (1990) also noted the lack of research, but concluded tentatively that those who receive test interpretations, regardless of the format, do experience greater gains in counseling than those who do not receive an interpretation. Related to working with couples, Worthington et al. (1995) found that married couples gained more from assessment feedback as compared with those who only completed the questionnaire.

In the area of personality assessment, some researchers have found that sharing personality assessment information can be therapeutic. Researchers (Finn & Tonsager, 1992; Newman & Greenway, 1997) have found that providing MMPI-2 feedback increases clients' self-esteem and reduces levels of distress. In particular, they found clients reported better outcomes when counselors communicated MMPI-2 results using a collaborative model. In Finn and Tonsager's (1997) model of collaborative therapeutic assessment (TA), clients are provided with assessment feedback that most closely aligns with their self conceptualizations and then presented with information that is progressively more discrepant from their conceptualizations of self. Ackerman, Hilsenroth, Baity, and Blagys (2000) found that clients whose initial sessions involved Finn and Tonsager's model of collaborative therapeutic assessment were more likely to begin therapy than those who received the more traditional information gathering approach. Furthermore, the results indicated that this method of providing results was highly correlated with a good therapeutic relationship later in the counseling process. On the other hand, Hanson and Claiborn (2006) found mixed results related to encouraging client involvement in the interpretation of a personality assessment as compared to other methods of interpreting the assessment results.

In addition, Jones and Gelso (1988) found that individuals perceived interpretations that were tentative as being more helpful than interpretations that were more absolute. These individuals also expressed more willingness to see a counselor who used a tentative interpretation approach over one whose approach was more absolute.

Counselors sometimes want to know whether it is better to interpret results individually or in groups. Interestingly, the research is inconclusive in this area. However, when given a preference, clients *prefer* to receive results individually. Furthermore, clients report more satisfaction, clarity, and helpfulness when the interpretation is performed individually as compared with other formats, such as groups (Goodyear, 1990). Benziman and Toder (1993) examined whether children in mental health settings would prefer to receive assessment feedback from the examiner or therapist as compared with receiving the information from their parents. In this study, the children voiced a strong preference for receiving assessment results from their parents.

Although clients may prefer individual interpretation, some organizations may need to consider group interpretation because of the cost. Krivasty and Magoon (1976) found that individual interpretation was six times more expensive than group interpretation. Some counselors (e.g., school counselors) may want to consider combining modes of interpretation, such as providing group interpretation for general interpretive information and then following up with individual sessions to discuss specific results.

There is limited research related to client characteristics and evaluation of assessment processes and procedures. One result that seems logical is that more intelligent clients tend to remember test results better as compared with less intelligent clients. In addition, researchers are beginning to explore the relationship between personality and interpretation of assessment results. Lenz, Reardon, and Sampson (1993) investigated the effect of selected client characteristics (i.e., gender, personality, level of identity, and degree of differentiation) on clients' evaluation of SIGI-Plus, which is a computerized career guidance system. Surprisingly, only personality had a significant influence on the clients' ratings of the system. The researchers found that as scores on the Social and Enterprising scales increased, individuals' rating of the system's contribution to their self and occupational knowledge decreased. In addition, Kivlighan and Shapiro (1987) found that Investigative and Realistic individuals were more likely than other personality types to benefit from a test feedback intervention.

The following provides some general guidelines to consider when communicating.

Guidelines for Communicating Results to Clients

- Before any type of interpretation or communication of results to a client can be done, the counselor needs to be knowledgeable about the information contained in the manual. Validity information is the basis for the interpretation because this information informs practitioners on appropriate uses and interpretations. Furthermore, most manuals will explain the instrument's limitations as well as areas in which clinicians should proceed with caution.
- Hanson and Claiborn (1998) suggested that, in preparing clients to receive test feedback, counselors should take time to "optimize" the power of the test (e.g., "This test is useful in particular ways, within particular limits"), rather than allowing the client to "maximize" it (e.g., "This test speaks the truth").
- Interpreting assessment results is part of the counseling process, and, thus, typical counseling variables (e.g., counseling relationship, interaction between client and counselor) need to be considered. To communicate assessment results adequately, counselors need to use effective general counseling skills.
- Counselors need to develop multiple methods of explaining the results.
- Sometimes the communication of results involves terms such as *standard deviation, normal curve,* and *stanines,* which may not be familiar to many individuals. Preparing to explain the results in multiple ways is necessary, because some clients will not understand their results if the counselor uses only standard psychometric terms. When appropriate, counselors should include visual aids because some people understand better by seeing the results rather than by hearing a report.
- Whenever possible, the interpretation should involve descriptive terms rather than numerical scores. For example, if a client's score is at the 83rd percentile, a counselor could explain this as, "If a hundred people took this instrument, 83 of them would have a score at or below your score." It is better to provide a range of scores rather than just one score. The description of the results should be tied to the reason for the assessment. As an example, if a counselor gave a personality inventory to a couple, the counselor would need to explain the rationale for taking the personality inventory and how the results can be useful.
- The assessment results should not be presented as infallible predictions. When probability information is available, counselors should explain the results in terms of probabilities rather than certainties. There is, however, considerable research indicating that people attribute very different meanings to many of the probabilistic words—such as *unlikely, possible, probable,* and *very likely*—commonly used in appraisal (Lichtenberg & Hummel, 1998). These findings indicate that counselors

vary widely in their interpretations of probabilistic statements in interpretative reports. Lichtenberg and Hummel suggested that counselors should use numerical descriptors (e.g., there is a 95% chance) rather than verbal ones (e.g., there is a high probability) to convey more precise information.

- Although the results should contain detailed information, Jones and Gelso (1988) found that individuals perceived interpretations that were tentative as being more helpful than interpretations that were more absolute.
- The results should be discussed in context with other client information. Interpretation should never be done in isolation; rather, the interpretative process should explore how the assessment information conforms to other pertinent information. A competent interpretation involves not only analyzing the assessment results but also integrating diverse client information into a comprehensive understanding. Assessment results can be viewed as pieces of a puzzle, with other puzzle pieces being used to understand the total picture.
- When describing results, therapists should involve clients in the interpretation.
- Clients need to be involved in the process so that they can address questions about whether the results make sense or if the results fit with other information.
- Counselors should monitor client reaction to the information, which can best be accomplished by having the client provide feedback throughout the process.
- Asking the client for reactions early in the assessment process lays the foundation for an interactional interpretation.
- Any limitations of the assessment should be discussed in nontechnical terms. Some clients will be confused by comments such as, "The reliability coefficients are low." An explanation of the limitations needs to be geared toward the client's level of assessment sophistication. If there are questions related to the instrument's results in terms of the gender, racial background, or other characteristics of the client, then this also needs to be explained.
- The counselor should encourage the client to ask questions during the process.
- Occasionally, clients believe they will appear foolish to their counselors, so they may be reluctant to ask questions. To determine whether clients understand the assessment information, counselors can use incomplete sentences with the client filling in the information or completing the sentence. Counselors must ensure that clients do not leave confused or ill informed about the results.
- At the end of the conversation, it is often helpful to summarize the results, reiterating and stressing important points. This summarization process provides a second opportunity for the client to question inconsistent results.

Guidelines for Communicating Results to Parents

The guidelines in the preceding list also apply to communicating assessment results to parents; however, some specific issues do arise when interpreting results with parents. Parents frequently receive achievement test information, but they may have little background in testing. In addition, schools sometimes send assessment results

TABLE 5.1
Questions parents commonly ask counselors

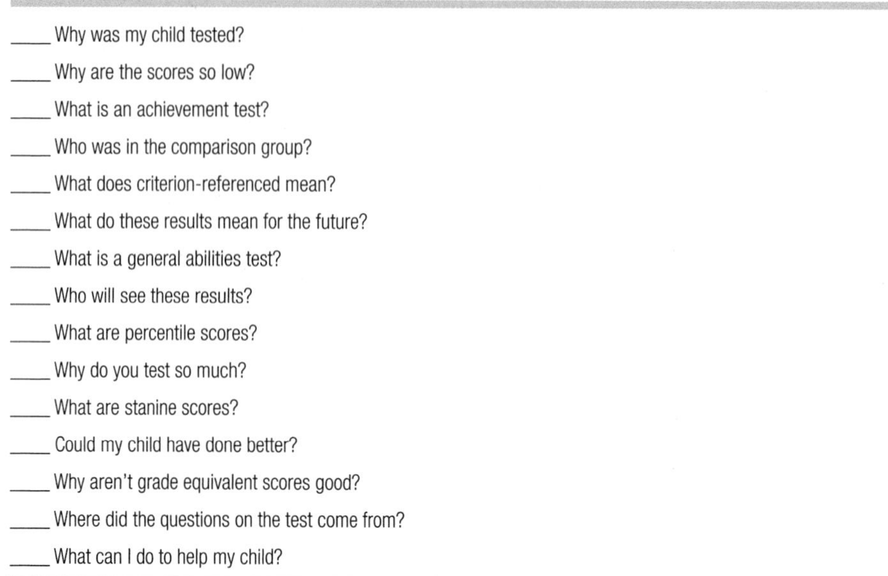

____ Why was my child tested?
____ Why are the scores so low?
____ What is an achievement test?
____ Who was in the comparison group?
____ What does criterion-referenced mean?
____ What do these results mean for the future?
____ What is a general abilities test?
____ Who will see these results?
____ What are percentile scores?
____ Why do you test so much?
____ What are stanine scores?
____ Could my child have done better?
____ Why aren't grade equivalent scores good?
____ Where did the questions on the test come from?
____ What can I do to help my child?

home even though the materials may not adequately explain the results. When interpreting the results, parents often seek help from a school counselor. Any counselor, school or otherwise, who works with a family should be prepared to interpret achievement and aptitude testing results. Table 5.1 contains a list of common questions that all counselors should be prepared to answer. Occasionally, a parent may ask questions about standardized tests to "break the ice" with a counselor with the goal of discussing other issues. Therefore, when results are being interpreted, counselors should provide parents with opportunities to extend the discussion to other clinical topics.

Increasingly, counselors are members of multidisciplinary teams that collaborate in the delivery of mental health services. As a part of a team, counselors may be responsible for counseling parents after a child has been diagnosed with a disorder. Examples of the more typical diagnoses a child may receive from a school psychologist or community practitioner are Mental Retardation, Motor Skills Disorders, Communication Disorders, Autistic Disorder, Asperser's Disorder, Attention Deficit/Hyperactivity Disorder (ADHD), Oppositional Defiant Disorder (ODD), and Conduct Disorder. In these cases, parents usually have received an explanation of the testing that was performed, but they are often overwhelmed with the amount of information presented. During their work with parents on coping and parenting issues, counselors must have an understanding of the testing used and the symptoms of the disorder. If counselors are not part of the multidisciplinary team and do not have access to the testing results, they can gain access to the information by having parents sign an informed consent form to release the information to them.

Parents often struggle with the news that their child has a disorder; a counselor can be instrumental in helping them adjust to the situation. Many parents in such a situation have experienced numerous difficulties and frustrations and need to interact with an individual who can empathize with their situation. A family's reaction to the diagnosis of a disability tends to go through five stages: impact, denial, grief, focusing outward, and closure (Fortier & Wanlass, 1984). To progress through the stages, a family often needs help in understanding the child's condition. This may involve discussing the assessment report more than once. It is particularly important that the counselor be prepared to discuss the results by using a variety of techniques. The counselor may also help the parents focus on the child's abilities and not just on his or her disabilities—the entire family can benefit from understanding that the disability is only one aspect of a child's life. Sattler (2001) also encouraged clinicians to emphasize the active role that parents and their child can play in coping with the disability. The counselor should attempt to frame the family's response into an active, coping approach rather than a succumbing, victim framework.

Focusing on coping methods does not mean that the counselor should ignore the negative emotions a family is feeling. It is often very difficult for parents to hear that their child is, for example, mentally retarded or autistic. Both the parents and the child often experience feelings of guilt and think that they somehow caused the problems identified in the testing. Frequently, there are also feelings of sorrow and loss. Even parents who have been aware of developmental delays and other problems for a period of time tend to experience feelings of loss when confronted with the actual results of testing. In general, these feelings are associated with the loss of the "perfect child" that most parents fantasize about at some point. Counselors, therefore, need to provide a therapeutic environment in which issues related to loss, anger, and frustration can be openly addressed.

In addressing negative reactions to the assessment results, the counselor needs to monitor the parents' responses so that the child does not internalize their negative reactions. Sometimes, a child will interpret the parents' disappointment in the testing result as disappointment in the child. The child may also be concerned about rejection by peers. Often when psychodiagnostic evaluation is completed, educational interventions are implemented (e.g., the child goes to a resource room or receives other special education services). The child may fear the reactions of other children as they become aware of the situation. Hence, this may be a time when the child is particularly vulnerable and, at the same time, is unsure of his or her parents' level of affection.

Psychological Reports

Many times assessment results are communicated in written form, which is typically called a **psychological report** or psychoeducational report. This is particularly the case when psychologists, using a battery of tests, conduct a psychological evaluation. For example, a neuropsychologist may have conducted a battery of tests to assess an individual after a traumatic brain injury, or a school psychologist may have given a child a set of tests to determine if there is a learning disability. In most traditional positions, counselors will not be writing these extensive psychological reports but will use these reports in their work with clients. For instance, a counselor could be assigned to assist the individual with the traumatic brain injury cope with his injuries. To provide effective counseling, this counselor would need to be able to understand the neuropsychologist's psychological report. Likewise, school counselors often work closely with school psychologists and, thus, must be able to understand the psychological reports. Although there may be occasions when a counselor is called upon to write a psychological report, the focus of the following section is more on counselors evaluating others' reports and applying the information in counseling interventions. A psychological report completed by a skillful clinician can provide an abundance of clinical information. However, psychological reports can vary in quality; therefore, counselors need to be able to evaluate the quality of the report before implementing interventions based its content. (A detailed discussion on the writing of psychological reports is beyond the scope of this book; counselors who need these skills are directed to Ownby (1997) and Sattler (2001).)

The purpose of psychological reports is often to disseminate assessment information to other professionals rather than to clients. For example, a report written by a school psychologist may focus on intelligence and achievement testing, with the interpretation directed toward teachers and how to improve their instruction. Many times, the psychological report is not geared exclusively toward the client, and the content may be difficult for some clients to understand because the information is technical in nature and often focuses on diagnostic and clinical decisions. A well-written report will not merely report test results but will also incorporate a wide array of relevant information. Thus, in evaluating psychological reports, counselors should expect a comprehensive overview of the client and an interpretation of the assessment results in a contextual manner. A psychological report should be carefully crafted with attention to detail. The caliber of the report can be initially evaluated by examining typographical errors, use of vague jargon, careless mistakes, and lack of detail.

Common Areas in a Psychological Report A counselor can expect a psychological report to contain certain information. Table 5.2 lists the typical sections included in a psychological report. Because there are no established guidelines for writing a report, not all reports will follow this outline. A quality report, however, will include all of these major areas. Many reports will have a heading, such as PSYCHOLOGICAL REPORT: FOR PROFESSIONAL USE ONLY. This heading clearly identifies the document and stresses that the document is for professional use only.

TABLE 5.2
Typical sections in a psychological report

Identifying information
Reason for referral
Background information
Behavioral observation
Assessment results and interpretation
Recommendations
Summary
Signature

Identifying Information This section of the report provides some demographic information on the client. It is often done in outline format and includes the following information:

Client's name
Date of examination
Date of birth
Chronological age
Date of report
Grade (if applicable)
Examiner's name
Tests administered

Other possible information includes the individual's gender, the teacher's name, or the parents' names. All of this is important information and is necessary introductory information to the reader of the report.

Reason for Referral The second section of a psychological report typically addresses the reason for the referral for testing. Some practitioners will use the label "Reason for Counseling" in order to broaden the focus. It should be noted that the term *psychological report* is typically associated with the reporting of assessment information. The information customarily included in this section is the name and position of the referral source (e.g., teacher); the reason for the referral; and a brief summary of the symptoms, behaviors, or circumstances that led to the referral. The reason for the referral often guides the practitioner in the selection of instruments or procedures. In evaluating a psychological report, the practitioner should find a direct connection between the instruments or procedures used and the reasons for the referral.

Background Information This section is critical for many readers because it provides a context in which to interpret the assessment results. The background information portion of the report should provide the reader with an overview of relevant information regarding the client. This section should also provide sufficient detail about the client's past so that the reader can understand the current issues and concerns. The information in this section may come from interviews with the client; interviews with other family members (e.g., parents if the client is a minor); or past educational, counseling, or health records. The focus of the background review will vary depending on the reasons for the assessment, but it should include significant past events related to the assessment purpose. Educational history is often relevant, as well as the current family situation. Notable physical and mental health events in the client's life should be discussed. If other assessments have been performed, there should be a summary of those assessment results and the progress made since the prior evaluations. For adult clients, this section should include a description of the current employment situation and any other past or present work-related information germane to the assessment.

Behavioral Observations Practitioners unfamiliar with standard protocol may not include this important section of a psychological report. However, a well-written psychological report will describe what is observed during the assessment process. This information is critical to interpreting the results, for it addresses issues such as motivation, anxiety, concentration, and self-efficacy. The behavioral observations are reports of the client's behaviors while taking the instruments. The behavioral observation section will usually include a brief description of physical appearance, client comments and reactions to the process, responses to different assessment activities, unusual mannerisms or behaviors, variations in activities, and changes in voice tone and facial expressions. If inferences are made about the client's behavior, then those inferences should be accompanied by descriptions of behaviors supporting the conclusions. For example, a report might include statements such as, "The client appeared somewhat tense and chewed her fingernails. She also reported that she was feeling anxious about the testing."

Assessment Results and Interpretations This is the heart of the psychological report and will be the longest section. Sattler (2001) suggested that this section be entitled "Assessment Results and Clinical Implications," which directs attention to using the results to assist the examinee. Topics included in this section are the assessment findings, the meaning of the results, and the clinical and diagnostic impressions. In the discussion of the assessment findings, the precise scores on every scale and subscale may not need to be presented. The focus should be on the pertinent findings and *interpreting* rather than simply reporting the findings. The report should include sufficient detail so that a reader unfamiliar with the specifics of the instrument can understand the meaning of the results. Names of the instruments and descriptions of the scores and scales will help the reader understand the results. The interpretation of the results will often include an exploration of the client's strengths and limitations. Furthermore, there should be a discussion of both consistent and inconsistent scores and results. The reader will also expect to find an explanation or possible hypotheses about any notable results. The psychometric qualities of the instrument are not directly reported in the report, but the interpretation needs to incorporate any psychometric limitations. For example, limited validation evidence should be stressed. When a diagnosis is presented in a report, there should be sufficient evidence to support that diagnosis. Consistent findings from different sources provide the sort of documentation expected for a diagnosis. The report should be organized in an easy-to-follow manner. Many practitioners organize their reports in a domain-by-domain framework. A summary is not needed at the end of the results and interpretation section because one will be provided later in the report.

In evaluating a psychological report, a counselor should consider the quality of information and how the report is written. First, the writing needs to be specific and concrete rather than vague and ambiguous. A reader with little background in assessment should be able to understand the report. A vague statement such as "Pat has low self-esteem" is problematic because it is not clear what is meant by "low," nor is it clear what is meant by "self-esteem." Although the report should be clearly written, it should not include declarative statements about people. For example, a report should not say, "Michael is an extrovert." Michael may only be portraying himself to be extroverted because he thinks that is more socially acceptable. Instead, a report writer should report, "Michael's answers on the Myers-Briggs Type Indicator *indicated* that Michael's preference is toward the extroverted function, which reflects a preference for . . . ." The focus should be on what the scores reflect or indicate, not on some specific label. A clinician cannot say Mary's IQ is 102 because the next time she takes an intelligence test her IQ may be 104. It would be more appropriate to present the results as, "Mary's scores on the [insert test name] reflect that her IQ is around 102." A better strategy would be to use standard error of measurement and say, "Mary's performance on the [insert test name] indicates that 68% of the time Mary's IQ could be expected to fall between 99 and 102."

Recommendations The recommendations section extends the material presented in the report into future actions that will be beneficial to the client. The rationale for the recommendations should have been made in the previous sections of the psychological report. The recommendations should be realistic, with consideration of the client's resources and situation. There also needs to be sufficient detail so that the recommendations can be easily implemented. Many times this requires the clinician to have information about community resources.

Summary The summary is a succinct summarization of the entire report, with a focus on the results and interpretation. The summary is usually only one or two paragraphs, but it contains the major aspects of the report. As one of my teachers once said, "Write the summary as if that will be the only thing anyone reads." The summary provides an opportunity to reiterate and emphasize important results. Sometimes the summary and recommendations will be combined into one ending section.

Signature The report writer's name, degree, and professional title or capacity should be typed at the end of the report. The writer then signs her or his name above the typewritten name.

In conclusion, a thorough psychological report written by a well-trained clinician can provide a wealth of information that can be used in treatment planning. Most credible reports will identify both strengths and limitations of the client and will include pertinent recommendations. A quality report will not only provide the assessment results but will also integrate other information to produce a thorough report. Counselors who write psychological reports should ensure that their writing is clear and concise and that it accurately describes and interprets the client's assessment results. More often, counselors will be consumers of psychological reports and will need to analyze the report to determine the quality of the information.

Summary

This chapter examined instrument selection, administration, scoring, and communication of results. Selecting and using an inappropriate instrument can have a negative impact on clients. An instrument should not be used with a client until the counselor has thoroughly evaluated it, including the instrument's purpose, the procedures used in constructing the instrument, the appropriateness of the norming group or criterion, the reliability, and the validation evidence. Instruments should also be evaluated for potential bias, particularly in multicultural counseling situations. The practitioner's qualifications should also be considered in determining whether to use an instrument. It is unethical for counselors to use an instrument for which they have not received the proper training. Some publishers use a three-level qualification system (e.g., Level A, Level B, and Level C). The ultimate responsibility for ethical use of an instrument, however, rests with the test user.

Part of using an instrument appropriately is ensuring that the instrument was properly administered. Counselors often shoulder this responsibility, even in settings such as schools where achievement tests are actually administered by classroom teachers. The key to ethical instrument administration is understanding and following the administrative instructions. Most manuals provide instructions detailing the manner in which an instrument should be administered. Counselors need to follow these guidelines and prepare for potential difficulties. Foresight and planning can often circumvent potential problems in instrument administration.

Accurate scoring must be ensured to guard against erroneous findings. For many instruments, computer scoring is becoming more prevalent than hand scoring. Some instruments involve intricate scoring procedures and can only be computer scored. With certain types of instruments, scoring involves professional judgments by the person scoring the results. An assessment area that has been of increasing interest is performance and authentic assessment. Although subjectivity can be problematic in these types of assessment, there are procedures that can enhance the scoring process.

Research findings reflect that clients who receive test interpretations, regardless of the format, experience greater gains in counseling than those who do not receive an interpretation. Communicating the results to clients is often one of the most important aspects of the assessment process. However, there is surprisingly little research related to the most effective methods for communicating assessment results. In general, it is more effective to integrate the communication of assessment results into the counseling process. Clients prefer to have results interpreted to them individually, but group interpretations also appear to be effective and are significantly cheaper.

Assessment results must be interpreted in context, and part of this process involves examining whether the results are consistent with other information about the client. In addition, to facilitate understanding, the practitioner should be prepared to explain the results by using multiple methods. Clinicians may also need to explain results to parents to assist them in understanding the results and in making informed decisions about their children. Sometimes, the assessment information that counselors are interpreting to clients is from psychological reports written by other professionals (e.g., school psychologists). Counselors need to be able to distinguish quality reports from those that are carelessly or haphazardly compiled. A sloppily written report may be indicative of imprecision and carelessness in the entire assessment process. Occasionally, counselors may be required to write psychological reports; they should seek training on report writing and on appropriate documentation and interpretation of assessment results.

SECTION II

Overview of Assessment Areas

CHAPTER 6

Initial Assessment in Counseling

You have just been hired as a counselor for a community mental health center. Your first client is Cal, a 56-year-old African American male. The center does not have a structured intake procedure and leaves the process up to the clinician. Because you have never conducted an initial intake interview at this location, you are unsure of how to maximize your initial time with Cal. This community mental health center has a reputation for working with substance abuse clients. Therefore, you think you should explore substance use with Cal, although you are not sure how to ask appropriate questions that will get honest appraisals of substance use. Furthermore, you do not want to miss any significant issues or important problems. Your supervisor has indicated there are some brief assessments in a file drawer that you can use if you think it might be helpful. Because the session is only scheduled for 50 minutes, you will need to use your time wisely.

How a counselor begins the counseling process has been found to be critical to the eventual effectiveness of the counseling. Many clients do not return for a second session and this may be related to counselors' skills in identifying client issues and building positive expectations about the counseling process based on that assessment. Researchers have found that clients' expectations about counseling before they enter have very little influence on eventual outcome; however, the expectations that clients build during those initial sessions have a significant influence on outcome (Clarkin & Levy, 2004). Building positive expectations, however, needs to be based on accurate assessment of client concerns. Some of us have had the experience of going to a medical doctor and feeling like the physician is not really attending to our reporting of our symptoms. This analogy applies to counseling because clients want a clinician who can assist them with their specific issues. Also, building a therapeutic relationship starts early in the counseling process. Beutler et al. (2004) found that it is the quality of the therapeutic relationship in the early sessions of psychotherapy, rather than later in the process, that significantly predicts long-term positive results. Hence, from the beginning counselors should consider the initial session as being critical to the effectiveness of the overall process. In addition, counseling tends to be more efficacious when the counselor is able to quickly conceptualize the relevant issues.

Clients often come to counseling with scattered information regarding current issues, problems, and circumstances. Sometimes the presenting concerns are somewhat vague and ill defined. The concerns are often presented in statements such as, "I am not getting along with my husband," "The kid won't listen," "I keep making the same dumb mistakes," "I can't stand my job anymore," "I just can't get motivated to do anything," or "My son never does his homework, and he lies." Counselors need to become skilled in taking these vague concerns and identifying relevant issues and problems. Cormier and Nurius (2003) suggested that problems are rarely related to one factor, are usually multidimensional, and typically occur in a social context. Therefore, counselors need finely tuned initial assessment skills to identify the complex interaction of factors related to the client's problems.

Initial Intake Interview

Counselors often use interviewing skills to begin the counseling process and obtain relevant clinical information. Initial, or intake, interviews usually gather information about the range and scope of the concerns, pertinent details about the current situation, and background information relevant to the current problems. Nelson (1983) found that this type of interview was one of the most commonly used assessment strategies. Despite research findings that the interview is the most popular assessment strategy used, it is not always easy to conduct one effectively. Research evidence indicates that guidelines and training are needed for counselors to obtain accurate, valid information from an interview (Duley, Cancelli, Kratochwill, Bergan, & Meredith, 1983).

In Hill and O'Brien's (2004) model of helping or counseling, the first stage of the process is *exploration*. In this stage, the counselor seeks to establish rapport, develop a therapeutic relationship with the clients, encourage clients to tell their stories, help clients explore their thoughts and feelings, facilitate the arousal of client emotion, and learn about clients from their own perspective. An effective initial interview is a balance between gathering information and building a therapeutic relationship. In Hill and O'Brien's model, the first stage of exploration lays the foundation for the second stage, *insight*, which leads to the final stage of the client taking *action*. The initial assessment and information gathering need not have a detrimental effect on the relationship, because a skilled clinician can gather pertinent information while beginning to establish a working alliance. Therefore, this discussion first addresses information customarily gathered in an initial interview and then proceeds with an overview of therapeutic skills for conducting that interview.

Information Gathered in the Initial Interview

The information gathered in an initial counseling interview varies somewhat depending on the setting (e.g., school or agency) and the services delivered by the organization. The initial interview often provides information that influences the treatment phase of counseling and clinical decision making such as: What are the client's major issues? Can counseling be effective with this person? and What is the best treatment approach or modality? To gather sufficient information to make sound clinical decisions, the initial interview needs to address demographic information, client background information, medical information, the client's presenting concern, and other relevant information concerning difficulties the client is experiencing.

Demographic Information

Typically in mental health settings, demographic information is gathered through the intake paperwork of an agency. For school counselors, much of the demographic information already exists in the student's educational file. It is important, however, to ensure that the demographic information is current and correct. Accurate telephone numbers and emergency numbers can be critical in crisis situations. In addition, pertinent demographic information needs to be gathered to make clinical decisions. For example, it could be important for the practitioner to have information on the client's marital status, race or ethnicity, employment status, and occupation. Also, for cases in which clinicians need to report suspected child abuse, information on all individuals living in a household and where the children attend school could prove to be important.

Client Background Information

To facilitate counselors' understanding of the client, they typically need to gather background information. Some clinicians call this gathering of background information a **psychosocial interview**. Gathering background information is not a detailed exploration of the client's past but rather an overview of the client's background, particularly as it relates to the presenting problem. Table 6.1 on the next page includes the common areas that are addressed in gathering background information. Counselors should explain to the client their reasons for gathering this background information. All of this information does not need to be collected in every intake interview. For example, in some mental health centers it may be more efficient to gather some of this information by using an easy-to-complete form. In some settings (e.g., schools) or for specific issues (e.g., career counseling), the counselor may not need to gather extensive information about the client's background. Nevertheless, to develop an effective treatment strategy, counselors will need to gather or have access to background information that is germane to the client's issues and the types of services provided by the counseling facility.

Health and Medical History

As part of gathering a client's background information, clinicians must have knowledge about the client's medical conditions so that they can holistically understand the

TABLE 6.1
Client background information

1. **Identifying Information**
   Client name, address, phone number, age, gender, marital status, occupation, workplace or school, work telephone numbers, name of another person to contact in case of an emergency
2. **Purpose of Counseling/Presenting Problem**
   Presenting concern and detailed information on the problem/concern
3. **Physical Appearance**
   Clothing, grooming, height, weight
4. **Present Level of Functioning in Work/School, Relationships, and Leisure**
   Analysis of present level of functioning in work, relationships, and leisure activities; degree that presenting concern affects activities
5. **Medical History and Current Status**
   Present health, current health complaints, health history, treatments received for current complaints, date of last physical examination, current medications, other drugs (either OTC or "street drugs"), sleep patterns, appetite level or changes, exercise patterns
6. **Past Counseling Experiences or Psychiatric History**
   Type of treatment, concerns addressed, length of treatment, types of outcome, positive results, unhelpful results, medications prescribed for emotional/psychological problems
7. **Family Information**
   Current marital status, number and ages of children living at home, other people living at home, any violence or physical abuse, family-of-origin makeup, significant influences of family-of-origin on present problems, family history of psychiatric problems, family history of substance abuse
8. **Social/Developmental History**
   Significant developmental events that may influence the present, any irregularities in development, current social situation, religious affiliation and values
9. **Educational/Occupational History**
   Occupational background, educational background, reasons for terminating previous jobs, military background, overall satisfaction with current job, stresses related to occupation
10. **Cultural Influences**
    Race and/or ethnicity, socioeconomic status, sexual orientation, acculturation, experiences of discrimination, perceived internal and external barriers

client. This exploration of health issues should include an analysis of current health issues, including a listing of current medications. Because counselors want to ensure that there is no physiological base to the client's concerns, it is often wise to refer a client to a physician for a physical examination. Even if a client has had a recent physical, it is important to gather medical information and explore the possible side effects of any medications the client is taking. Certainly, with many clients, a thorough assessment needs to include an analysis of drug and alcohol use. Under the umbrella of health issues, counselors should also gather information on past psychiatric illnesses and treatments.

Client's Presenting Concern(s)

Many clients enter counseling because of specific issues that are causing them difficulties. It is important for the counselor to understand the issues or problems that may have motivated the client to counseling. Outcome research results indicate there is a connection between attending to a client's presenting concerns and an effective outcome. This process involves more than noting the presenting concern. It also includes gathering information on when the issue started as well as surrounding events that may be relevant. The counselor should also explore the frequency of the problem, the degree to which the problem is affecting the client's daily functioning, and methods the client has used to attempt to deal with the problem in the past.

Other Relevant Information

In discussing an initial interview, it is difficult to address all of the necessary information that counselors should seek because counselors work in diverse settings and with a variety of clients. Hence, the content of an initial interview will vary and counselors may need to gather additional information that will augment what has already been covered in this chapter. In considering other information, clinicians need to focus on gathering *relevant* information. Counselors are human and have their own interests, which may influence their approach to an initial interview. For example, I am very interested in issues related to individuals' work and often I find it interesting to hear about individuals' employment history and their analysis of how they ended up in their current occupation. For some clients, focusing on work issues is relevant; however, for other clients it is not. Therefore, clinicians need to consider whether the information they are gathering is relevant in defining the client's problems.

Defining the Client's Problem

Once the clinician has gathered information about the presenting concern and about the client's background, the initial interview should focus on defining the client's problem or problems. Problem assessment plays a critical role in counseling, because it is crucial that the counselor have a clear understanding of the presenting issues and concerns. Mohr (1995) found that one of the major reasons counseling can result in a negative outcome is that clinicians underestimate the severity of the client's problems. Many clients seek counseling for multiple issues rather than one specific problem. Therefore, it is important that counselors investigate the range of issues. Once the counselor has identified the dominant concerns or problems, the counselor should then explore each issue in detail. The following are topics to address in the examination of significant problems.

1. *Explore each significant problem from multiple perspectives.* Counselors should attempt to view the problem or concern from diverse vantage points. They can accomplish this by having the client describe the problem in terms of affective, behavioral, cognitive, and relational perspectives. If a counselor is working with a family, then having each member describe the problem contributes to a multidimensional perspective. If a counselor is working with a single client, then asking the client how others may describe the problem can promote a better understanding of the problem.
2. *Gather specific information on each major problem.* The counselor should encourage the client to describe the problem(s) in detail. Included in this description

should be information on when the problem began, the history of the problem, what events were occurring when the problem arose, and what factors or people contributed to the situation. Information on the antecedents and consequences of the problem can be particularly helpful later when selecting treatment interventions.

3. *Assess each problem's intensity.* Counselors need to assess the degree to which the problem or issues are affecting the client. The problem's severity and the frequency or duration of problematic behaviors should be explored. One example of doing this is to have clients rate the severity of the problem on a scale from 1 to 10, which can provide an indication of the degree of negative impact. In certain situations, such as anxiety attacks, the counselor may have the client chart or record the when and where the problematic behaviors occur.
4. *Assess the degree to which the client believes each problem is changeable.* When assessing client problems, it is important to explore the degree to which the client believes the problems are malleable or immutable. Assessment in this area will be helpful later in determining interventions and possible homework assignments.
5. *Identify methods the client has previously used to solve the problem.* Counselors need to explore methods the client has already used to address the problem. Doing so provides insight into the client and avoids duplicating efforts that have already been attempted.

Once the counselor has assessed each significant problem the client is experiencing, the next step is to prioritize them. If the counselor addresses all of the problems at once, the counseling process will likely be stymied. Prioritizing the problems is considered part of the assessment process and can serve as a transition into the treatment phase. Determining which problems to address first in counseling depends on the situation, the client, and the counseling relationship.

Assessing the Change Process

Within the counseling field, there is increasing acknowledgment that not all individuals enter counseling at the same place in regards to changing. As an example, Bandura (1977) and Mahoney (2000) encouraged clinicians and researchers to explore the fundamental principles and processes of change. The transtheoretical model (Prochaska, DiClemente, & Norcross, 1992) is considered one of the most influential models of behavior change (Morera et al., 1998). According to this model, counselors select interventions based on the client's stage in the change process. By studying people in counseling and self-changers, Prochaska et al. (1992) identified five stages of change, described in the following text. Much of Prochaska's research has been related to modifying addictions, but these same stages have been found to pertain to clients with diverse problems.

Prochaska and associates (Prochaska, 2000; Prochaska & DiClemente, 1992; Prochaska & Norcross, 2001) found that because people progress through five stages as they change, counseling will be more effective if the interventions are geared toward the individual's stage in the change process. In fact, Prochaska, Velicer, Fava, Rossi, and Tsoh (2001) found that by proactively gearing the interventions to the assessed stage of change, 80% of their clients remained in therapy as compared to the typical rate of only 50%. *Precontemplation* is the first stage in the change process. At this stage, the individual has no intention of changing behavior in the foreseeable future. Many clients may be unaware or underaware that there is even a problem. They often enter counseling because they are coerced or pressured by others. They may attempt to demonstrate change because of the pressure, but they will quickly return to old behaviors when the pressure is off.

The second stage is *contemplation*, in which individuals become aware that a problem exists and begin to consider the problem. At this stage, however, they have not made a commitment to take action. The contemplation stage is characterized by serious consideration of the problem, with clients beginning to weigh the pros and cons of seeking solutions. In *preparation*, clients begin to make small alterations in behavior, with the intention of taking action within the next month. For example, clients will cut down on cigarettes or drink only on the weekends. Their actions may be small, but they intend to take stronger action in the near future.

In the *action* stage, individuals modify their behavior, experiences, or environment to address their problems. The action stage involves overt behaviors and the devotion of considerable time and energy to the change process. Counselors often mistakenly equate this stage with actual change and ignore the requisite process that the client needs to go through to implement change.

The last stage in the transtheoretical model of change is *maintenance*. Here the individual works to prevent relapse and to consolidate the gains achieved in the action stage. This is not a static stage; rather, maintenance is the continuation of the changed behavior. In general, maintenance lasts for at least six months, during which time the client focuses on methods for stabilizing and continuing the change.

Assessing a client's stage and level of change is not a traditional part of the intake interview. It does, however, dovetail nicely with the developmental perspective of counseling and the contention that the counselor's role is to facilitate positive change. Assessment of the client's stage in the change process is usually accomplished through interviewing the client. Responses to questions related to the client's presenting concerns and background typically reflect the stage in the change process. There is also an instrument, the Stages of Change Questionnaire (McConnaughy, DiClemente, Prochaska, & Velicer, 1989; McConnaughy, Prochaska, & Velicer, 1983) that can be used with clients to assess their stage within the change process. Once an understanding of the client's current stages has been obtained, the clinician can then draw from over 25 years of research on processes of change that work best in each stage to facilitate progress (Prochaska, Prochaska, & Johnson, 2006).

In conclusion, with regard to the content of the initial interview, a counselor should consider the major types of information they want to elicit from a client before beginning the initial interview. Initial interviews often provide the foundation for further assessment and, therefore, should cover a spectrum of topics. Typical information gathered in these interviews concerns demographic information, client background information, medical information, presenting concern, and sufficient information to define the problem. The goal of interviewing is to gain valid information. However, to elicit information from a client, the counselor must establish an atmosphere in which the client feels comfortable in divulging personal information. Thus, conducting sound initial assessments usually requires excellent interviewing skills and the effective implementation of interviewing techniques.

Interviewing Skills and Techniques

A sound interview is accomplished by gathering information in a therapeutic manner. Therefore, counselors need to attend to both the content of the initial interview and to the processes they use in gathering that information. Because typical content has been covered already in this chapter, I want now to focus on the process of interviewing and the skills and techniques involved in the initial interview. The initial interview is the first contact with the client, and first impressions do have an influence on counseling outcome. Counselors should consider the degree to which they appear to be credible to the client in terms of being seen as trustworthy, expert, and attractive. LaCrosse (1980) found that initial client perceptions of counselors' expertness accounted for 31% of the variance in favorable therapeutic outcomes. Clients who perceive their counselors as being trustworthy, expert, and attractive helpers have better outcomes in counseling than clients who do not have these perceptions of their counselors (Heppner & Claiborn, 1989).

Numerous people have written about the importance of using effective communication skills in initial interviews (Cormier & Nurius, 2003; Okun & Kantrowitz, 2007). Communication skills are needed to communicate to the clients that they are being heard and understood in their responses to the interview questions. Open-ended questions are often used in interviewing because they are less likely to lead or unduly influence the client. In closed-ended questions, there is a set of "closed" responses from which the client can select an answer, such as answering either "yes" or "no" to questions such as "Did you come to counseling because you are feeling depressed?" Open-ended questions require a more elaborate answer that the client has to construct. Examples of open-ended questions are "What brought you to counseling?" "Can you describe for me the problems that you are having now?" "What situations are not going as well as you would like them to go?" With interviews that do not have a structured format, counselors may use other communication skills to draw out the client. Commonly used techniques are paraphrasing, clarifying, reflecting, interpreting, and summarizing (Okun & Kantrowitz, 2007). Furthermore, the counselor's vocabulary should be adjusted to correspond to the client's educational and social background.

A counselor's verbal and nonverbal behaviors impact the effectiveness of the initial interview. The climate the counselor builds during the interviewing process influences the degree to which clients are willing to disclose personal information. Asking questions is not the counselor's only verbal behavior during the initial session; restatement and reflection of feeling can both solicit additional information and facilitate a therapeutic environment. Table 6.2 includes some general guidelines for conducting initial counseling interviews. It should be remembered that clients respond differently to various therapeutic styles and there is not one correct manner of conducting an initial interview.

TABLE 6.2 *Common guidelines for conducting an initial interview*

- Assure the client of confidentiality (clearly state any exceptions, such as child abuse or harm to self or others).
- Word questions in an open-ended format rather than a closed format.
- Avoid leading questions.
- Ask questions in a courteous and accepting manner.
- Listen attentively.
- Consider the client's cultural and ethnic background.
- Adjust your approach to the individual client (some clients are more comfortable with a more formal process; others prefer a more warm and friendly approach).
- Avoid "chatting" about unimportant topics.
- Encourage clients to openly express feelings, thoughts, and behaviors.
- Avoid psychological jargon.
- Use voice tones that are warm and inviting, yet professional.
- Allow sufficient time, and do not rush clients to finish complex questions.
- If clients drift from pertinent topics, gently direct them back to the appropriate topics.
- Vary your posture to avoid appearing static.

Interviewing Children

The previous suggestions on interviewing, such as establishing rapport, gearing the vocabulary toward the client's educational level, and asking questions in a warm professional manner, apply to children as well. Children, however, are sometimes more difficult to interview, so the counselor needs to adjust the initial interview to the child's developmental level. Starting with statements such as "I am going to talk with you for a little while to see if the two of us can figure out some ways to make your life better" or "Your mom told me some problems were going on, but I would like to hear what you think is going on" may help children understand the purpose of the initial interview.

It may also be helpful for counselors to provide an explanation of why they are asking questions at this stage in the counseling. For example, "I really want to understand, so I am going to ask you some questions to help me understand." Children, in particular, need to understand the purpose for the interview and counseling, because they have had little exposure even to media representations of counseling. Many children see a counselor as an adult in a punitive role and will have difficulty trusting the counselor. Therefore, when attempting to identify problems with a child, it is important for counselors to define the limits of confidentiality.

Merrell (2007) contended that to interview children effectively, the interviewer must have knowledge of some basic developmental issues and be able to structure the interview so that it is developmentally appropriate. For children in early childhood, Merrell recommended (1) using a combination of open and closed questions; (2) not attempting to maintain total control of the interview; (3) reducing the complexity of the questions; (4) using toys, props, and manipulatives; and (5) establishing familiarity and rapport. Even though children are able to think more complexly as they move into middle childhood, Merrell suggested that the counselor (1) avoid abstract question; (2) rely on familiar activities and settings; (3) not maintain constant eye contact; (4) provide contextual clues (e.g., pictures, examples); and (5) use physical props in context. In adolescence, children typically have the ability to reason abstractly and problem solve systematically so that the interview can be less concrete. With adolescents, Merrell recommended that the interviewer (1) consider the degree of emotional liability and stress, (2) avoid making judgments based solely on adult norms, and (3) show respect.

If, during a counseling session, a child becomes involved in disruptive play, begins crying, or misbehaves in some way, Greenspan and Greenspan (1981) recommended not stopping the behavior too quickly. They suggested that observing this behavior rather than stopping it may be insightful and that disciplining too quickly may negatively affect the interviewing process. On the other hand, counselors do not have to sit and watch children destroy their offices. Simple statements such as "Can I ask you not to do that?" "We don't allow behavior like that in the center," or "Let's talk for just 10 minutes, and then we will do something else" can be helpful. Periods of silence or times when the conversation halts are more common in interviewing children than with adults. Silence may be an indication that the child is thinking about what to say or is reflecting on a situation or problem. If the silence becomes extreme, then the counselor might intervene with a question such as "These questions seem difficult for you to answer. Can you tell me about that?" or "You seem a little quiet. What are thinking about right now?" In assessing children and their problems, counselors need to be more patient and skillful during the assessment than they are with adults.

Structured and Unstructured Initial Interviews

One of the decisions a counselor needs to make about the initial session is whether to use a structured or an unstructured interview. Sometimes this decision will be made for the counselor, because some agencies require that a structured interview be performed with each new client. In a **structured interview,** counselors ask an established set of questions in the same manner and sequence for each client. In an **unstructured interview,** counselors may have an idea about possible items to address but gear the interview in a unique manner, depending on the client's needs. A **semistructured interview** is a combination of the structured and the unstructured interview formats; certain questions are always asked, but there is room for exploration and additional queries. There are advantages and disadvantages to all three methods of interviewing.

The major advantage of the structured interview is that it is more reliable (Aiken & Groth-Marnat, 2005). Reliability concerns the proportion of error, which counselors want to minimize. Furthermore, as Chapter 4 addressed, reliability is a prerequisite to validity. Thus, a structured interview may possibly be more valid than an unstructured interview, though this is not guaranteed. Some practitioners believe that structured interviews have a negative impact on the counseling relationship because the client may feel interrogated. This is not necessarily true, because the interviewer's style has a significant influence on the counseling relationship and the degree of comfort the client feels in disclosing information. The soundness of a structured interview is intimately linked to the questions included in the interview and to the counselor's ability to elicit crucial information. It is difficult to assemble a structured interview that responds to the array of problems and situations faced by clients. Therefore, with structured interviews, it is important for counselors to include a question at the end to encourage the client to disclose any important information that may not have been addressed.

The advantage of unstructured interviews is that they can be easily adapted to respond to the unique needs of the client. Unstructured interviews, however, are less reliable and more prone to error than structured interviews. In my supervision of counseling students, I have seen unstructured interviews in which the initial interviews focused entirely on a relatively minor issue and the counselors neglected to gather adequate information. In unstructured interviews, gathering information tends to take longer as compared with well-developed structured interviews. The decision to use either a structured or an unstructured interview should be based on the interview's purpose. For example, if the purpose of the initial interview is to screen clients to determine if they are appropriate for a clinic, then a structured interview that reduces the amount of error is probably better. If, on the other hand, the purpose is to better understand the specifics of an individual client, then an unstructured interview may allow for more individualized exploration. The unstructured interview requires much more skill on the part of the interviewer than does the structured interview.

The following dialogue is an example of an unstructured initial interview with Emily, a 16-year-old female client who has entered counseling at her mother's insistence.

Counselor: Hello, Emily. I understand from your paperwork that your mom wants you to be in counseling, but I would like to know from you what you think is going on.

Emily: Oh, I don't know. My mom is really controlling and wants me to be perfect. She is the one who should be in counseling.

Counselor: What kinds of things do you do that upset your mom?

Emily: She gets upset about my grades. She wants me to be "clone-child" and get all As.

Counselor: What are your grades? Tell me about your last report card.

Emily: Well, they weren't as good as they used to be; but still, I only had two Fs.

Counselor: What were your grades in the past?

Emily: Oh, I used to get really good grades, like mostly As, and my mom keeps harping that I should still be getting those kind of grades again.

Counselor: When was the last time you got grades that didn't upset your mom?

Emily: Oh, I don't know. I was still on the honor roll when I was first in high school, but I haven't been for, maybe, a year.

Counselor: Has anything changed for you?

Emily: What do you mean?

Counselor: Is it a different school? Are you taking different classes? Are your friends different? Do you feel different about school?

Emily: I do feel differently about school—I just hate to go.
Counselor: Tell me more about this hating to go.
Emily: I just hate going to school. The kids there are so into themselves and who's in their group that they never even talk to anyone else. The teachers just want to make your life hard and point out what you did wrong. I just never want to go in the mornings.
Counselor: So you hate to go . . .
Emily: I hate it when I'm there, and I'm not learning anything worthwhile. I learn more when I stay home and read or watch TV. I don't really need to go to school, and it's better when I just stay home.
Counselor: Do you stay home from school sometimes?
Emily: Well sometimes.
Counselor: How often, on average, do you stay home?
Emily: A couple of times a week.
Counselor: In the past two weeks, how many times have you missed school?
Emily: Lots.
Counselor: I'm not sure what that means. I'm not going to give you a lecture, so tell me how many days you went to school in the past two weeks.
Emily: Twice.
Counselor: When you don't go to school, what do you do? Tell me about a typical day.
Emily: Are you going to tell my parents?
Counselor: No, unless you're doing something to hurt yourself or others.
Emily: Well, I just stay home. My parents already sorta know because the school has contacted them and everything. I get up in the morning and act like I'm going to school, but my parents usually leave for work before I need to leave for school. I just wait until they leave and stay at home. My mom has kinda gotten wise to this lately and has been going into work late. On those days, I go sit in the shed behind our house and wait until she leaves. Then I go back into the house and watch TV. I'm not hurting anybody, so I don't know what all the fuss is about.
Counselor: Tell me about how you feel when you're home and how you feel when you're at school—I want to understand this better.
Emily: When I am at school, I just feel yucky. No one talks to me; I don't have anyone to eat lunch with. The kids just look through me, or there's this group in my first period class that makes these stupid remarks when I do come to class. At home, I don't have to put up with that, I can just be myself and watch TV. I mean, sometimes, I'd like to be at school and be popular and everything, but it's so hard. I don't have any friends. The friends I used to have don't want me in their group—they made that very clear. It's just easier to stay home because being at school is terrible.
Counselor: I'm getting this feeling that being at school is quite painful for you. On a scale of 1 to 10, with 1 being you are feeling very happy and comfortable and 10 being the most awful pain, what number on the scale would represent your feelings while at school?

Emily: About an 8 most of the time that I'm there. It's most difficult when I first get there in the mornings and at lunchtime.

Counselor: Not that I'm saying your parents understand it very well, but if I asked them about this problem of you not going to school, what would they say?

Emily: They would say I'm lazy and that I'm being childish. They tell me to make some new friends.

Counselor: I imagine you've tried to make new friends; tell me about some of the ways you've tried.

Emily: I try to go up and talk to people, but I'm not very good at it. I want to make friends. I'm just really shy, and it's hard for me. When I start to talk to people, I sound stupid, so I stop.

Counselor: I know it's difficult to make new friends, and some people find it easier than others. On the other hand, I think we can work together and find some ways that you can be comfortable with to make some friends. It sounds like the lack of friends is what keeps you from going to school—am I hearing that correctly?

Emily: Yes, you're hearing it right. If I had some friends, especially to eat lunch with, then I could go to school.

Counselor: How about we meet together for three sessions for the next three weeks and see where we are and if we're making progress on making friends. Could you do that?

Emily: I could do that.

Strengths and Limitations of Interviewing

As mentioned earlier, in terms of reliability, structured interviews are more reliable than unstructured ones. The quality of the questions asked influences the validity of an interview and what information can be inferred from the client's responses. Counselors should also consider the validation evidence and the inferences they make about a client based on the initial interview. The information gathered in an interview must be carefully analyzed. In addition, counselors should consider other evidence that may substantiate or challenge the clinical judgments being made. The strength of any type of interview is its ability to directly question the client about issues, problems, and personal information. The limitations of interviews usually relate to the lack of validation evidence and the influences of counselor subjectivity. As Dawes (1994) demonstrated, clinicians tend to be biased in decision making. Therefore, clinicians need to ensure that they gather and analyze the information gained from interviews by using objective and sound methods.

All clients will not respond in the same manner to a clinical interview. Certainly, gender and culture should be considered in determining whether to use this assessment strategy. Some cultures do not encourage immediate self-disclosure to someone outside of the family. Clients may have difficulty relating to questions and formulating a response. A counselor could perceive this difficulty as resistance when it may be more a matter of unfamiliarity and discomfort. Interviews are a good method for gathering initial information; however, they are not the only method. Counselors may consider supplementing their intake interviews with other information, such as checklists or rating scales, to provide information not addressed in the interview. Furthermore, the information from checklists or rating scales may complement the interview and aid the counselor in identifying the more pressing and significant issues.

Other Strategies That Can Be Used in Initial Assessment

The counseling process frequently begins with the counselor gathering information about clients and their concerns. Most practitioners start this process by talking with clients and using a structured, semistructured, or unstructured interview. Some counselors, however, supplement the interview with other assessment tools. These tools may include informal assessment instruments (e.g., checklists or rating scales) that are incorporated into the initial paperwork. Other assessment devices may be more formal instruments that provide information on symptoms and issues.

Checklists

A checklist can be a relatively simple and cost-effective method for gathering initial information from clients. Usually in a checklist, individuals are instructed to mark the words or phrases in the list that apply to them. Checklists can be filled out by the client or by an observer (typically a parent or teacher). When multiple individuals complete the same checklist on a client, a counselor can acquire a rich body of therapeutic information from diverse perspectives. For example, clinicians working with children can expand on in-session observations by having children's parents and teachers complete a brief checklist.

Standardized Checklists

Counselors can construct their own checklists or use a number of existing standardized checklists. Some of the existing standardized checklists focus on clients reporting their current symptoms. *The Symptom Checklist-90—Revised* (SCL-90-R; Derogatis, 1994) and the *Brief Symptoms Inventory* (BSI; Derogatis, 1993) are two popular instruments that often are used at intake in many mental health settings. These instruments are related and are very similar; the main difference is that the SCL-90-R contains 90 symptoms, whereas the BSI contains 53. In these checklists, the client simply responds to the listed symptoms using a 5-point scale of distress, ranging from 0 (not at all) to 4 (extremely). The SCL-90-R takes about 15 minutes to complete; the BSI is less time consuming.

There are two methods for using these two symptom inventories as valuable initial screening tools. First, a clinician can simply scan the results of these instruments and examine which symptoms are distressing to the client. Included in these measures are items such as thoughts of ending their life, feelings of worthlessness, feeling afraid in open spaces, and feeling that most people cannot be trusted. Alternatively, the SCL-90-R and the BSI can be scored by providing measures on the following nine scales: somatization, obsessive-compulsive, interpersonal sensitivity, depression, anxiety, hostility, phobic anxiety, paranoid ideation, and psychoticism. There are also three composite scores that can be particularly helpful to counselors in determining whether to refer a client for psychiatric evaluation: the Global Severity Index, the Positive Symptom Total, and the Positive Symptom Distress Index. Client responses can be compared with nonpatient adults, nonpatient adolescents, psychiatric outpatients, and psychiatric inpatients. The internal consistency measures and test-retest coefficients for the SCL-90-R and the BSI are quite high over short time periods. Derogatis (1993) recommended that the results of either the SCL-90-R or the BSI are good for no more than seven days. Derogatis (2000) also developed an 18-item symptom inventory called the Brief Symptom Inventory-18 (BSI-18) for settings that want a quick assessment or short instrument, and the total score is designed to provide a Global Severity Index. In addition, the BSI-18 contains six items that assess the three subscales of Somatization, Depression, and Anxiety. There are many other commercially available checklists that can be used with adults.

A number of checklists have been developed for use with children and adolescents. A widely used set of checklists for children is the *Achenbach System of Empirically Based Assessment*, which has three versions (Preschool, School-Age, and Young Adults). With these instruments, clinicians can gather information from multiple sources (parent, teacher, and child or adolescent). Although these instruments are labeled checklists, in many ways they are more similar to a rating scale. One of the more commonly used assessments from this set is the Child Behavior Checklist/6–18 (CBCL/6–18), which is appropriate for children ages 6 to 18 and is completed by the parents or guardians. The version completed by the teacher is the Teacher Report Form/6–18, and the version completed by the child or adolescent is the Youth Self-Report/11–18 (YSR). Boys and girls are scored separately and there are T scores and percentiles for Total Competence, three Competence scales (Activities, Social, and School), eight Syndrome scales, and six DSM-Oriented scales. The Syndrome scales are Anxious/Depressed, Withdrawn/Depressed, Somatic Complaints, Social Problems, Thought Problems, Attention Problems, Rule-Breaking Behavior, and Aggressive Behavior. There are also three broad scores related to Internalizing, Externalizing, and Total Problems. It is also possible to get scale scores that are *DSM*-oriented. Flanagan (2005) complimented the developers of these scales on the refinement of these instruments from an earlier version and was particularly positive about the authors' efforts to obtain a nationally representative sample.

Informal checklist. Some counseling centers and agencies have developed informal checklists to be used in their facilities. (For an example of one of these brief checklists, see Table 6.3 on the next page.) Some of these agencies have performed studies on the reliability and validity of these instruments, but many have not. If there is no psychometric information available for a checklist, then the practitioner should proceed with caution. Although it is possible to gather some preliminary information from these informal checklists, counselors need to be cautious in using these results

TABLE 6.3
Example of an informal checklist

Personal Checklist

Please check the concerns that apply to you.

____ Depression	____ Emotional/physical/sexual abuse	____ Career issues
____ Anxiety	____ Binge eating	____ Academic concerns
____ Stress	____ Self-induced vomiting	____ Financial pressures
____ Anger control	____ Relationship problems	____ Multicultural issues
____ Panic attacks	____ Family conflict	____ Sleep disturbance
____ Fears/phobias	____ Conflict with friends	____ Physical complaints
____ Grief/loss	____ Conflict with people at work	____ Obsessive thinking
____ Suicidal thoughts	____ Lack of relationship	____ Alcohol/drug concerns
____ Unwanted sexual experience	____ Indecisiveness	____ Lack of assertiveness
____ Sexuality issue	____ Low self-esteem	____ Trauma/assault/accident
____ Other (please specify): ____________		

without reliability and validity information. The results of informal checklists that do not have psychometric information can be viewed only as possible problems; a counselor's clinical decisions should never rest on this information alone. In using informal checklists, clinicians should also be aware that some clients have a tendency to check numerous items whereas others check very few. Therefore, a client who has checked numerous problems should not necessarily be viewed as being more disturbed than a client who checked only a few.

Rating Scales

A rating scale is slightly more sophisticated than a checklist, because it asks the client or an observer to provide some indication of the amount or degree of the problem, attitude, or personality trait being measured. Sometimes rating scales contain a numerical scale, with numbers assigned to different categories. For example, clients may be asked to rate their level of anxiety from 1 (not at all anxious) to 5 (extremely anxious). Another common rating scale is the semantic-differential, in which individuals choose between two bipolar terms (see Table 6.4 for an example).

When counselors interpret ratings, they should keep in mind a number of findings related to these measures. In general, people tend to respond in the middle of the ratings, which is called *central tendency error*. Individuals are less likely to rate themselves, or others, at either the low or the high extremes. Another finding pertains to *leniency error*, which concerns an individual's reluctance to assign unfavorable ratings. People are more likely to endorse the positive as compared with the negative. Finally, in terms of an individual's ratings of someone else, there is often a *halo effect*. Research indicates that people are influenced by first impressions, and these impressions influence subsequent ratings. Thus, there can be either a positive halo or a negative halo effect.

TABLE 6.4
Example of an informal rating scale

Personal Rating Scale

Please place an X on the point that most accurately reflects how you typically feel.

Calm	___ ___ ___ ___ ___	Nervous	Courageous	___ ___ ___ ___ ___	Afraid
Superior	___ ___ ___ ___ ___	Inferior	Optimistic	___ ___ ___ ___ ___	Pessimistic
Sad	___ ___ ___ ___ ___	Happy	Independent	___ ___ ___ ___ ___	Dependent
Indecisive	___ ___ ___ ___ ___	Decisive	Abusive	___ ___ ___ ___ ___	Victimized
Outgoing	___ ___ ___ ___ ___	Shy	Adventurous	___ ___ ___ ___ ___	Timid
Strong	___ ___ ___ ___ ___	Weak	Confident	___ ___ ___ ___ ___	Anxious
Fearful	___ ___ ___ ___ ___	Confident	Irrational	___ ___ ___ ___ ___	Rational
Compulsive	___ ___ ___ ___ ___	Lackadaisical	Energetic	___ ___ ___ ___ ___	Lethargic
Patient	___ ___ ___ ___ ___	Impatient	Confused	___ ___ ___ ___ ___	Insightful
Trusting	___ ___ ___ ___ ___	Suspicious	Honest	___ ___ ___ ___ ___	Shrewd
Aggressive	___ ___ ___ ___ ___	Submissive	Moral	___ ___ ___ ___ ___	Wicked
Relaxed	___ ___ ___ ___ ___	Tense	Impulsive	___ ___ ___ ___ ___	Cautious
Hostile	___ ___ ___ ___ ___	Gentle	Competitive	___ ___ ___ ___ ___	Cooperative
Sluggish	___ ___ ___ ___ ___	Active	Hopeless	___ ___ ___ ___ ___	Elated
Sick	___ ___ ___ ___ ___	Well	Even-paced	___ ___ ___ ___ ___	Erratic

Informal rating scales can be incorporated into the initial assessment of clients. For example, clients could be asked to rate on a 5- or a 7-point scale the severity of the presenting problem, the degree to which the problem is affecting their daily functioning, their commitment to addressing the problem, and the likelihood that the problem will change. These informal rating scales can be asked verbally or incorporated into an intake form. There are also standardized rating scales, such as the *Conners' Rating Scales-Revised* (Conners, 1996). The Conners' Rating Scales-Revised are instruments designed for screening children ages 3 through 17, with the instrument being completed by the parent, teacher, or adolescent. The three versions of the scale (for parent, teacher, and adolescent) include both long and short forms. This rating scale includes a number of scales (e.g., oppositional, anxious/shy, social problems). Furthermore, this instrument is often used in the diagnosis of Attention Deficit/Hyperactivity Disorder because it includes a scale for ADHD (i.e., the Conners' ADHD Index).

Other Screening Inventories

A number of other initial screening instruments are neither checklists nor rating scales. An example of one these instruments is the *Problem Oriented Screening Instrument for Teenagers* (POSIT), which was developed in the Adolescent Assessment/Referral System, a program initiated by the National Institute on Drug Abuse (NIDA; Rahdert, 1997). The project's aim is to identify an assessment and treatment referral system for troubled youths 12 through 19 years of age. The purpose of the POSIT is to screen for potential problem areas that should be assessed more thoroughly before selecting appropriate treatment options. The POSIT, which comprises 139 yes/no items, assesses 10 functional areas. The results indicate whether a problem may exist in one or more of the 10 areas. Currently, the POSIT and a personal history questionnaire are used to determine if further problem assessment is necessary.

In conclusion, a number of both formal and informal instruments can supplement the initial client information gathered in an intake interview. Some counselors incorporate these techniques routinely, whereas others periodically use checklists, rating scales, or other types of inventories, depending on the situation. Counselors can improve their effectiveness by using multiple methods for gathering information. No one source of information, such as a test, should be the sole basis of any decision. Multiple sources of information will provide a more comprehensive overview of clients and their problems. Sometimes, in the process of gathering information, a counselor will determine there is a need to assess the client more thoroughly on a specific problem. For example, during the initial intake interview, the counselor may see signs of depression and want to gather information specific to depression. Thus far, we have discussed general initial assessment, but counselors also need to consider methods for assessing specific client problems.

Assessing Specific Problems in the Initial Sessions

Certain problems should be given special consideration during counseling's initial stages because if these specific issues are overlooked, there could be negative results, even the death of a client. A significant example is suicide, for if a counselor does not assess a client's suicide potential, a client might attempt suicide when treatment might have prevented this attempt. Depression is significantly related to suicide and is a second factor that counselors should consider during the initial stage of counseling. A third area that counselors should assess in the initial intake is substance abuse because of the psychological and physiological effects of psychoactive substances. Although clinicians will want to consider many other specific problem areas in the initial assessment stage, these three are discussed in detail because of the potentially serious ramifications of misdiagnoses.

Assessment of Suicide Potential

In the initial session, a counselor needs to evaluate each client's potential for suicide. Neglecting to identify a client with suicidal ideation could result in an avoidable death. The probability of working with a potentially suicidal client is high. According to the National Institute of Mental Health (NIMH, 2006), suicide is the eleventh leading cause of death in the United States. The American Association of Suicidology (2006) reported that in 2004 in the United States, an average of 88.6 individuals committed suicide each day. Rogers, Guelulette, Abbey-Hines, Carney, and Werth (2001) found that 71% of counselors had worked with individuals who had attempted suicide, and 28% of these practitioners had a client who had committed suicide. Predicting which clients might commit suicide is very difficult because individuals' moods often vary greatly from day to day and even from hour to hour. A counselor may work with a client who appears to be at minimal risk; however, a few hours later something may happen to significantly alter the risk of suicide (e.g., the client's spouse asks for a divorce).

Having information on the demographic factors that research shows are related to suicide can assist counselors in screening clients for potential suicide. In general, men are more likely than women to commit suicide, although some studies show women are more likely to attempt suicide (NIMH, 2003). These results, however, do not indicate that a woman's disclosure of suicidal thoughts is any less serious than a man's disclosure. White men account for 73% of all suicides, with the highest rate being for white men over the age of 85. Adolescent suicide has increased 300% in the past 20 years (NIMH, 2003), with suicide now being the third leading cause of death among individuals 15 to 24 years old. Although suicide is somewhat rare for children before puberty, it does exist. For children ages 5 to 14, suicide is the seventh leading cause of death. Marital status has also been found to be associated with suicide risk; those who are single, divorced, or widowed are at greater risk than those who are married. Individuals responsible for children under the age of 18 have also been found to be at lower risk than individuals without those responsibilities.

There are also clinical aspects to consider when evaluating clients for the potential of committing suicide. Major depression and alcoholism account for between 57% and 86% of all suicides, with the majority of these deaths being related to depression (Clark & Fawcett, 1992). The relationship between depression and suicide is so significant that all depressed clients should be regularly evaluated for possible suicidal ideation. One of the important signs to look for in suicide assessment is a sense of hopelessness or helplessness. For most suicidal clients, the situation seems hopeless, and the only way to end the pain is through death. In addition, those who have previously attempted suicide are likely to try again. For children, adolescents, and adults, a recent loss, divorce, or separation increases the chances of attempting suicide. Other personality factors that are related to suicide include impulsivity, inability to express emotions, perfectionism and super responsibility, sensitivity, pessimism, and dependency (Stelmachers, 1995). A client with a history of a psychiatric disorder is also at greater risk than one who has never suffered from a disorder. About 10% of individuals with schizophrenia tend to commit suicide, often in the first few years of the illness (Morrison, 2007). Some research indicates that 30% to 40% of suicides are completed by individuals with a personality disorder, particularly individuals with borderline or antisocial personality disorders (Sanchez, 2001).

In determining the risk of suicide, Sanchez (2001) also suggested that the counselor assess whether there are some "protective factors," which have been found to reduce the risk of attempting suicide. For example, being married or in a significant relationship seems to serve as a protective factor. In addition, people who have children under the age of 18 are less likely to attempt suicide. Having a general purpose for living and a support system also seem to be important protective factors. Other positive factors to consider are whether the individual is employed or involved in a structured program (e.g., going to school).

Counselors need to be proficient in detecting suicidal thoughts and assessing the intensity of those thoughts. Counselors must assess this information accurately to determine if clients are in immediate danger of harming themselves. If the client is deemed to be in immediate danger, then the practitioner must have procedures for responding quickly to this potentially deadly situation. Stelmachers (1995) recommended that clinicians concentrate on the following seven areas when assessing the risk of suicide.

1. *Verbal communication.* A client who verbalizes the thought of suicide is providing a clearly identifiable signal for the counselor to investigate the situation's lethality. Counselors need to listen closely, because some clients are very subtle in their disclosures. For example, a client may say in a casual manner, "Sometimes I just want to end it all." Themes of escape, reducing tension, punishing, or self-mutilation can be signs of possible suicidal ideation. Sometimes beginning-level counselors feel uncomfortable asking clients if they are going to commit suicide. A less abrupt approach is to ask clients if they have ever considered harming themselves. Even jokes about suicide should be pursued. A counselor should never be lulled into a false sense of security if a client denies having any suicidal thoughts.
2. *Plan.* If there is any indication of possible suicidal thoughts, the next step for the counselor is to assess if there is an actual suicide plan. The counselor's concern for the client should increase if a plan exists, particularly if the plan is specific, concrete, and detailed. However, impulsive clients who may not yet have developed a plan may still commit suicide if their situation deteriorates.
3. *Method.* The counselor should investigate whether a client has selected a specific method of self-harm or suicide. In analyzing the method, the counselor should evaluate the availability and the lethality of the method. McIntosh (1992) found that firearms accounted for more than half of suicidal deaths, followed by hanging, strangulation, and suffocation; taking poisons often did not result in death. A counselor needs to determine the degree to which there is a risk and the feasibility of the suicidal plan. The counselor should also explore if the method includes provisions to avoid being rescued (or the opposite, if the plan facilitates being rescued).
4. *Preparation.* Another area to explore in suicide assessment involves whether the client has started the preparation process. For example, some clients will have secured the gun or pills already or even have written the suicide note. Sometimes the preparation process will be subtle, with the client giving away possessions or getting finances in order. The level of danger is proportionally related to the amount of preparation already completed.
5. *Stressors.* Another area to assess is past, present, and future stressors. A client may not be in immediate danger but may quickly become suicidal if certain circumstances occur. Stressors commonly associated with suicide are loss (particularly loss of a significant relationship), physical illness, and unemployment. For some clients, anniversaries or other special days are difficult and may exacerbate the sense of loss and depression. Identifying the potential stressors will also be

helpful in the continual monitoring of suicide potential. If counselors identify potential stressors, then they can respond more proactively when the stressors begin to build.

6. *Mental State.* The assessment of the client's mental state is important in determining both the immediate and long-term risks for suicide. As discussed earlier, certain psychological factors, such as depression, are clearly associated with attempting suicide. Clients who report being despondent, impotent, angry, guilty, distraught, and/or tormented should be continually monitored. Sudden improvement in a client should not always be viewed as a positive development. Some clients, while in the process of becoming more actively suicidal, will have uplifted spirits because they have finally found a solution to ending their pain. In the assessment of mental state, the practitioner should also assess the client's use of alcohol and drugs, because these psychoactive substances can affect impulsivity and other emotions, thereby increasing the suicidal risk. Another consideration is possible homicidal behaviors, which are occasionally combined with suicidal behaviors.
7. *Hopelessness.* Most suicidal clients exhibit a degree of hopelessness. Study after study has documented the prevalence of this affective state with suicidal individuals (Stelmachers, 1995). Suicidal clients often see death as the only method for relieving their pain. The degree of hopelessness should be explored with clients who verbalize some suicidal thoughts. In addition, the level of hopelessness is a gauge for determining the risk for clients who do not report any suicidal thoughts.

The following is an example of an initial session that explores the possibility of suicidal ideation. In this case, Mary is a 39-year-old woman whose husband has recently moved out of their home. Mary works as an accountant for a large accounting firm. Her husband told her three weeks before that he had met with a lawyer to initiate divorce proceedings and that he wants to have shared custody of their 11-year-old son, Sean.

Counselor: Can you tell me what brought you in to counseling?

Mary: My husband left me three weeks ago, and I'm having trouble coping with that. Although I had gotten angry with him for working so much, I never thought he would leave me. We've been together for 15 years, and the thought of not being together is just so difficult for me. It is so painful not to be with him.

Counselor: Tell me more about the pain.

Mary: It's almost like a physical pain. I feel empty and hurt and there are times that I can't stop crying. I can't describe the pain and the emptiness. I just hurt so much and I can't find any way to stop the pain. I sometimes throw up because I'm in so much pain. I spend hours crying in the bathroom and I can't get myself to stop. I cannot imagine a life without him. I have begged him to come back but he tells me that he can't stay married to me. When I call him, he hangs up on me and says he can't take any more. I feel so helpless and I can't get him to listen. I never felt so terrible . . . I can't think about anything else.

Counselor: You seem very hurt by his decision to leave?

Mary: Very hurt doesn't quite describe it. I have never felt so hurt and rejected. I feel like nothing matters except for Sean. I try to do things like cook dinner for Sean, but it's very hard. I'm so depressed and I can't find the energy to even cook dinner. The future looks so bleak . . . I don't want to think about living without him. I don't see a way to feel anything but pain. I wish I could find a way to end the emptiness and pain.

Counselor: Sometime when people are in as much pain as you are in, they'll do anything to stop the pain, including committing suicide. Have you ever thought about suicide as a way to stop the pain?

Mary: Although I don't want to admit it, I have thought about killing myself because I think that's the only way I could stop this pain.

Counselor: I understand the desire to stop the pain. When you thought about stopping the pain, what have you thought about?

Mary: I just think about how nice it would be not to hurt so much and that feeling nothing would be so much better than how I feel now.

Counselor: When was the last time you felt like this?

Mary: Last night. I always try to cry in the bathroom so that Sean won't see how I upset I am and I thought I'd like to climb in the shower and slit my wrist.

Counselor: Is that the first time you felt like killing yourself?

Mary: No, I guess I've thought about climbing in the shower a couple of times.

Counselor: It sounds like you've thought about killing yourself in shower but have you thought about other ways you might kill yourself?

Mary: Not really. It's during my spells when I can't stop crying that I think about ending it. I know it sounds crazy, but the shower wouldn't leave such a mess.

Counselor: Have you thought about how you'd cut your wrists?

Mary: I've thought that I would need to buy those old-fashioned razor blades.

Counselor: Have you bought those?

Mary: No, I can't do that to Sean. I wouldn't want Sean to suffer and it would hurt him.

Counselor: Mary, I know you are in a lot of pain and I worry that you might hurt yourself to try and stop that pain. Are there other ways than slitting your wrist that you have thought about to kill yourself?

Mary: No. I won't have a gun in the house and I don't have any pills. I am embarrassed that I told you about the shower.

Counselor: You don't need to be embarrassed because I understand the desire to stop the pain. I am, however, very worried about you and about you hurting yourself.

Mary: Because of Sean, I won't do anything. I don't want to saddle him with the pain of having his mother commit suicide. I just want the pain to abate for just a little while.

Counselor: I think we can work together and that the pain will get better, but that will take you coming to counseling. Right now I need some reassurances that you won't hurt yourself. I probably should inform the authorities to keep you from killing yourself. What kind of assurances can you give me that you won't hurt yourself?

Mary: To be honest, I can promise you that I won't kill myself.

Counselor: I need something more. I'm going to go get a paper that we both will sign, which is a contract between you and me, where you promise not to kill yourself. I am also going to give you a phone number of a suicide hotline that I want you to call if you have an episode where you start to think about getting in the shower to hurt yourself. Also you need to promise me that you won't buy any razor blades or anything else that you might use to hurt yourself.

Mary: I can promise all of that.

Formal instruments have been constructed to assess the risk of suicide. Most clinicians, however, do not use these instruments in isolation; instead they use both interviewing and observation in conjunction with a formal instrument. Figure 6.1 provides a nice mnemonic for counselors to use in the assessment of suicidal ideation. It should be remembered that a counselor does not assess suicide risk just once. A suicide assessment is time-limited and pertains only to the risks at that time and under those current conditions. Therefore, counselors need to continually reevaluate the suicide potential of clients because circumstances often change and the risk of suicide can increase or decrease depending changes within the client's life.

Suicide potential instruments. The *Suicide Probability Scale* (Cull & Gill, 1992) is a 36-item instrument that provides an overall measure of suicide risk. The scale includes subscales that assess hopelessness, suicidal ideation, negative self-evaluation, and hostility. An advantage of this instrument is that it includes separate norms for normal individuals, psychiatric patients, and lethal suicide attempters (those who have attempted suicide using a method that could have been lethal).

Aaron Beck, the noted cognitive therapist, has constructed two scales related to suicide potential. The *Beck Scale for Suicide Ideation* (Beck & Steer, 1991) can be used

FIGURE 6.1 *SAMHSA's mnemonic for red-flags for suicidal behavior*

IS PATH WARM

Ideation: Threatened or communicated

Substance abuse: Excessive or increased

Purposeless: No reasons for living

Anxiety: Agitation/insomnia

Trapped: Feeling there is no way out

Hopelessness

Withdrawing: From friends, family, society

Anger (uncontrolled): Rage, seeking revenge

Recklessness: Risky acts, unthinking

Mood changes (dramatic)

to identify and screen clients who will acknowledge suicidal thoughts. This scale uses five screening items, which reduce the amount of time spent completing the scale for clients who are not reporting any suicidal ideation. The manual recommends that this instrument not be used alone but in combination with other assessment tools. Another of Beck's instruments, the *Beck Hopelessness Scale* (Beck & Steer, 1993), relates to measures of suicidal intent and ideation. This instrument also has norms available for suicidal clients. Another noted contributor in the area of assessment, William Reynolds (1988), who developed the *Suicidal Ideation Questionnaire*, which has two forms, one for grades 10 through 12 and a second (SIQ-JR) for grades 7 through 9. Reynolds (1991) also developed the *Adult Suicidal Ideation Questionnaire*.

Validating instruments that assess the potential to commit suicide is somewhat problematic. It would not be ethical to give a sample of potentially suicidal individuals an instrument and then simply sit back and collect data on which ones actually committed suicide. Hence, a counselor using one of these instruments needs to examine the validation information to determine what the instrument measures (e.g., suicidal ideation, correlation with depression measures, attempted suicide). None of the instruments designed to specifically identify suicide potential is sufficiently refined to use in isolation. To screen for suicide, the counselor needs both astute observational and interviewing skills, combined with trained clinical decision making. Some practitioners will also use other instruments—such as measures of depression, personality, or symptom checklists—in the global assessment of suicide potential. A counselor should consult with another professional if there are any concerns related to the assessment of suicide risk. Oftentimes with a suicidal client, a counselor may need to ensure that the client receives a psychiatric evaluation.

Assessment of Depression

Because of depression's direct connection to suicide, it is important for counselors to begin assessing for depression early in the counseling process. Because of its frequency and detrimental effects on individuals, Morrison (2007) advised mental health clinicians to assess level of depression with every client. Depression is characterized by feelings of sadness, ranging from the common "blues" to severe depression.

To properly assess whether a client is depressed, a counselor needs familiarity with the common characteristics of depressed clients. With some clients, the symptoms of depression are easily recognized. With other clients, there may be "masked" depression, with the individual concealing the dysphoric mood or denying the depressed feelings. In cases of masked depression, practitioners need to detect the subtle signs of depression and explore the issue further if initial suspicions of depression are confirmed.

According to McNamara (1992), the symptoms of depression usually include a dysphoric mood, often accompanied by feelings of anxiety, guilt, and resentment. Depression is characterized by difficulties with concentration, decision making, and problem solving. Depressed clients tend to be pessimistic and have negative attitudes toward themselves, others, and the world. Behavioral and physical symptoms are also usually present, particularly if the depression is more serious. Social withdrawal is another symptom, and depressed individuals are often prone to crying, lethargy, and loss of interest in activities that were previously pleasurable. In terms of physical symptoms, fatigue is almost always present, sometimes accompanied by a loss of appetite and an inability to sleep. The reverse may also be true, with appetite and amount of sleep required substantially increased. Headaches, muscle aches, and decreased libido are other indicators of possible depression. In some cases, there may be a reduction in speech and a slowing of body movements. Included in the clinician's assessment of depression is whether the client should be referred for a psychiatric evaluation and possible medication.

The assessment of depression includes determining both the severity of the depression and the type of depression. Chapter 12, which addresses diagnosis, discusses different types of depression. Practitioners must be skilled in differentiating among the types of depression and assessing the risk of suicide. Sometimes clinicians will employ one of the following standardized instruments to assess the severity of the depression.

Beck depression inventory-II. Ponterotto, Pace, and Kavan (1989) identified 73 different measures of depression that researchers or mental health practitioners use. Of these different measures, the *Beck Depression Inventory* (BDI) was the most commonly used. In fact, the BDI was used 10 times more often than the second most popular instrument. The latest version of this instrument is the *Beck Depression Inventory II* (BDI-II; Beck, Steer, & Brown, 1996). The BDI was revised to align with the *Diagnostic and Statistical Manual of Mental Disorders—Fourth Edition* (DSM-IV) criteria for depression. Like its predecessor, the BDI-II contains only 21 items and usually takes clients about five minutes to complete. With each item, there are four choices that increase in level of severity. Therefore, the BDI-II results provide an index of the severity of depression. With college students, Steer and Clark (1997) found an overall coefficient alpha for the BDI-II of .92 and support for the construct validity of the instrument. Dozois, Dobson, and Ahnberg (1998) found that the factor structure of the BDI-II is stronger than that of the BDI. Furthermore, Beck recently published the *Beck Youth Inventories*, one of which is the *Beck Depression Inventory for Youth.*

Other depression instruments. Other standardized instruments that could also be used in the assessment of depression. For children and adolescents, there are the *Children's Depression Inventory-2003 Update* (Kovacs, 1992); the *Children's Depression Rating Scale-Revised* (Poznanski & Mokros, 1996); the *Reynolds Adolescent Depression Scale-2nd Edition* (Reynolds, 2002); and the *Reynolds Child Depression Scale* (Reynolds, 1989). For adults, another instrument (besides the BDI-II) is the *Hamilton Depression Inventory* (Reynolds & Kobak, 1995). The *Revised Hamilton Rating Scale for Depression* (Warren, 1994) also assesses the client's level of depression; however, the clinician rather than the client completes this instrument. In conclusion, a substantial number of depression assessments have been developed and the practitioner has some options in selecting an assessment of depression.

Assessment of Substance Abuse

According to Adesso, Cisler, Larus, and Hayes (2004), the assessment of substance use is a relevant task for clinicians regardless of the population with whom or the setting in which the therapist works. On the other hand, Greene and Banken (1995) contended that clinicians frequently fail to recognize clients' symptoms as reflecting substance abuse or dependence. A recent survey of employed adults found that more than 8.2% (more than 9 million) employed adults reported using illicit drugs in the past month and 8.8% (more than 10 million) reported heavy alcohol use in the previous month. Among unemployed adults, a staggering 18.6% reported illicit drug use and 13.6% indicated heavy alcohol use (Substance Abuse and Mental Health Services Administration, 2007). In the United States, Grant et al. (2004) found the highest prevalence of alcohol dependence among 18- to 20-year-olds who began drinking in early adolescents. Adesso et al. (2004) cited studies that indicated that in most mental health settings between 29% and 50% of the individuals seeking services will also have a substance use disorder. Problematic use of a substance(s) is a unitary disorder and there are distinctions between such problems as abuse and dependence. Chapter 12 will briefly discusses the criteria for diagnosing various substance related disorders.

Adesso et al. (2004) contended that assessing substance use is not conducted solely during the initial session. They suggested that assessment is necessary through all of the following steps if during the screening period the counselor detects a possibility of a substance use problem:

1. Screening
2. Brief problem assessment
3. Diagnosis
4. Comprehensive pretreatment problem assessment
5. Treatment-related factors
6. Outcome assessment

Adesso et al. (2004) articulated these different levels and provided a list of formal assessments that can be used at each level. For clinicians or agencies that provide substance-related counseling, this comprehensive listing of formal assessment may be particularly informative.

Given the number of clients who have a substance-related issue, it is important that counselors assess substance use early in the counseling process. A counselor who does not explore the possibility of substance abuse could easily proceed with addressing only issues that are essentially a result of the client's substance abuse. One method for exploring the possibility of substance abuse is simply to ask the client. Oetting and Beauvais (1990) found that self reports were reasonably reliable. There are, however, some problems with validity, because some clients are reluctant to disclose the use of certain substances or the amount of use. Nevertheless, counselors should explore with every client what drugs they are taking and the amount of alcohol they typically consume. In terms of medications, use of prescription, over-the-counter, *and* street drugs should all be explored for several reasons. First, heavy use of any of these types of drugs can be problematic. A second reason for exploring all types of drugs is that even some commonly used over-the-counter medications have side effects. Sometimes a client's symptoms (e.g., being tired all the time) result from the medication; therefore, counselors need to consult the *Physician's Desk Reference* in order to be knowledgeable about the side effects of any drug the client is taking. Table 6.5 includes some

TABLE 6.5
Examples of questions related to substance use

1. Do you take any medications, over-the-counter drugs, or other drugs such as street drugs? If medication or over-the-counter drugs are used, for what and how much? If street drug, what and how much?
2. Do you drink alcohol? If yes, how many drinks in a typical week?
3. How often do you get drunk or high in a typical week?
4. When did you start drinking or taking the drug(s)?
5. Has anyone ever mentioned that this is a problem? Who? Why do you think they see it as a problem?
6. Where and with whom do you usually drink or use drugs?
7. Has drinking or taking drugs ever caused you any problems (e.g., problems with family, employers, friends, or the law)?
8. Have you ever tried to quit? What happened? Were there any withdrawal symptoms?
9. Is your drinking or drug use causing you any financial difficulties?
10. Do you ever mix drugs or mix drugs and alcohol? Do you ever substitute one substance with another substance (e.g., do you ever use amphetamines instead of cocaine)?

examples of questions to ask clients, particularly if they indicate that they are drinking or taking drugs.

In assessing substance use, counselors need to focus on assessing which substances are used and the amount taken. Other areas that should be included in assessment of substance abuse are the social and interpersonal aspects, because this information will be helpful in the treatment phase. Treatment will vary depending on whether the client is drinking or using alone or with friends. Another goal is to identify the internal and external triggers that precede the use of the substance. For counselors working with adolescents, it is important that clinicians understand the risk and protective factors related to substance abuse. Counselors interested in this area are directed to the Substance Abuse and Mental Health Services Administration (SAMHSA) website (http://guide.helpingamericasyouth.gov/).

Standardized instruments in substance abuse. A number of standardized instruments are designed specifically to assess substance abuse. One instrument is the *Substance Abuse Subtle Screening Inventory* 3 (SASSI-3; Miller, 1997). The SASSI Institute purported that the SASSI-3 has a 93% rate of accuracy in identifying individuals with substance-related disorders. There is also the SASSI-A2 (Miller, 2001), a screening instrument for adolescents who may have a substance use disorder.

Another assessment tool that is often used in medical settings is the CAGE, which is an interviewing technique. The CAGE (Mayfield, McLeod, & Hall, 1974) is a mnemonic device for the following four questions:

1. Have you ever felt you need to *cut down* on your drinking?
2. Have people *annoyed* you by criticizing your drinking?
3. Have you ever felt bad or *guilty* about drinking?
4. Have you ever had a drink first thing in the morning to steady your nerves or get rid of a hangover (*eye opener*)?

If the answers to these questions indicate a problem, then the clinician should gather more detailed information about the client's drinking.

Sometimes, however, clients will deny that drinking or drug use is a problem. One technique to help clients admit a drinking or drug use problem is to have them self-monitor and record all drinking and drug use. Some clients will be surprised by the amount recorded. Another technique, sometimes referred to as the "acid test," is to ask clients to control or limit their drinking. For example, a client is asked to have no more than three drinks at any one occasion for three months. This technique provides an indication of whether the drinking can be controlled.

In the assessment of substance abuse, counselors must also assess whether they can provide the appropriate services for a client. Some clients will need to be referred to specialists in the area of substance abuse or to an outpatient or inpatient facility specializing in substance abuse.

Mental Status Examination

Although not a formal psychometric instrument, counselors in many hospitals and mental health settings need to be able to conduct and write the results of a **mental status examination** (MSE; Polanski & Hinkle, 2000). The mental status examination is used to describe a client's level of functioning and self-presentation and is generally conducted during the initial session or intake interview. The MSE is not necessarily a separate and distinct portion of the interview, although it is often integrated into the initial counseling process. Morrison (2007) concluded that the mental status examination is simply a statement of how a person looks, feels, and behaves at the moment of the initial examination. The information gathered in an MSE is often used for diagnostic purposes and to organize client information. The MSE is frequently organized around the following categories: (1) appearance, attitude, and activity; (2) mood and affect; (3) speech and language; (4) thought process, thought content, and perception; (5) cognition; and (6) insight and judgment (Trzepacz & Baker, 1993).

Although there are some variations among the precise categories of information included in a mental status examination, most procedures start with the clinician noting the client's general *appearance*, including such physical attributes as grooming, dress, cleanliness, and any notable abnormalities. Polanski and Hinkle (2000) suggested that counselors also include a notation on attitude and physical activity in this first category. In terms of *attitude*, counselors should note a client's presenting attitude and approach to the interview, including such descriptors as *cooperative, hostile, guarded, tense,* or *regressed.* Because the level and type of physical *activity* can indicate neurological problems, substance abuse, anxiety, or hyperactivity, Polanski and Hinkle also suggested including documentation on the level and quality of a client's physical or motor movements. A mental status examination report may also include pertinent physical movements or manifestations (e.g., crying, laughing, pacing, grunting) that are either inappropriate or incongruent with the context.

A client's *mood and affect* is typically the second category on which a clinician remarks in an MSE. Morrison (2007) suggested that clinicians consider three qualities when discussing mood: its type, lability, and appropriateness. According to Trzepacz and Baker (1993), most moods can be partially captured by the descriptors of euthymic (normal), dysphoric, euphoric, angry, anxious, and apathetic. When reporting on mood, it is often useful for counselors to include the client's own words. Lability concerns the degree to which moods seem to change in a given time frame. Some clients present with a high degree of lability and their moods change frequently during an initial interview; whereas, other clients exhibit a more consistent mood through the first interview. In addition, some moods are appropriate (e.g., depression after the death of a spouse) and other clients may exhibit moods that may not coincide to their circumstances. In a mental status examination a clinician usually describes the client's mood in a few sentences.

As the third category, Polanski and Hinkle (2000) recommended that clinicians include analysis of *speech and language* in a mental status examination. Morrison (2007) labeled this section "flow of speech." In particular, a counselor should note derailments in speech, loose associations, flights of ideas, tangential speech, poverty of speech, or pressured speech. As will be discussed in Chapter 12, characteristics of the client's speech can be very helpful in determining a diagnosis.

The fourth major category included in a mental status examination includes *thought process, thought content, and perception*. Analysis of thought process and content is important not only in diagnosing psychotic disorders but it can also be useful in diagnosing mania, depression, dementia, drug intoxications, and some personality disorders. Once again, counselors should note unusual thought processes or content in an MSE. Also like mood, the clinician should consider whether the thought content is consistent with the client's current circumstances (Morrison, 2007).

Cognition is typically the fifth category assessed in the MSE. Cognition refers to intellectual functioning and the ability to think logically and rationally. Morrison (2007) suggested that clinicians also consider the intellectual resources that the client may be able to use in further treatment. Unlike other portions of the MSE, this section can frequently involve a formal instrument, with the most common being the Mini-Mental State Exam (Folstein, Folstein, & McHugh, 1975).

Finally, Polanski and Hinkle (2000) indicated that counselors should include an analysis of *insight and judgment*. In this case, insight refers to clients' awareness of their own personality and behaviors that may be contributing to their current difficulties.

In managed care situations and other mental health situations, clinicians are often required to write an MSE report or an abbreviated summary of the client's presenting issues and background. Polanski and Hinkle (2000) suggested that this report include pertinent psychosocial background information in addition to the six categories listed previously. The focus of the report should be on describing the client's behavior during the initial session or intake procedure and the order of the content is not typically prescribed. Often in managed care situations, the MSE report must include information that supports the diagnosis. (Detailed information on diagnosis is covered in Chapter 12.) The following is an example of an MSE report.

> Michael is a 33-year-old Caucasian male employed as a research analyst for a department within his state government. Michael came to counseling because his supervisor has insisted that he seek help because he has missed a number of workdays in the past three months and is substantially behind on a number of projects. Michael appeared appropriately dressed for work in a professional office, but his clothes were wrinkled, and he indicated he had not had

time to shower in the past three days. Michael reports that his supervisor believes Michael's problems at work may be related to his drinking and occasional drug use. Michael reports that he sometimes drinks to excess on weekends and snorts cocaine about once a week. His speech seemed somewhat pressured, and he often skipped from topic to topic and had difficulty staying focused on many of the topics. He also complained of "cotton mouth." Michael appeared to be of above-average intelligence and seemed logical and rational in his cognitions. No gross or fine motor impairments were noted, but there appeared to be some occasional tremors in both hands. He reports he is under a physician's care but is not taking any prescribed medications. Although he expressed some "anxiety" about the possibility of losing his job, his mood often appeared euphoric. He consistently laughed, smiled, and appeared jovial, even when discussing difficult issues. He seemed to avoid questions related to the amount of his drinking and drug use and "couldn't remember" if he had used cocaine in the past week. Insight into the degree to which substance use may play into his difficulties seemed limited.

Summary

The initial information-gathering process in counseling usually involves the counselor interviewing the client. The skill with which the counselor performs this initial assessment has an influence on the overall effectiveness of the counseling. Because interviewing is one of the most frequently used counseling assessment tools, counselors should consider the reliability and validity of their own interviews. Within the initial, or intake, interview, it is important that counselors not only identify the most pressing problems but also explore these issues from diverse perspectives. Gathering detailed information about the presenting concerns provides a sound foundation for the selection of interventions and treatment approaches. In gathering client information, structured, semistructured, and unstructured interviews each have strengths and limitations, and the choice of which to use depends on the setting and the primary purposes of the clinical interviews.

Some counselors incorporate formal and informal assessment measures into the initial paperwork completed by the client. Checklists and rating scales can be efficient methods for gathering information. Commonly used instruments are the Symptom Checklist-90—Revised or the shorter version of this instrument, the *Brief Symptoms Inventory*. These measures of symptoms can also be used throughout the counseling process to monitor changes in symptoms (e.g., feeling anxious) as a result of the counseling. With some of the checklists and rating scales for children, a parent or guardian completes the forms rather than the child. In addition to using standardized instruments, counselors can develop their own informal checklists and rating scales; however, these should be used with extreme caution.

The counselor's initial assessment of a client also needs to consider specific issues, such as potential suicide, depression, or substance abuse. Assessment of these potential problem areas should involve a multifaceted approach. Because of the lethal aspects of suicide, counselors should routinely include an investigation of suicidality in their counseling. An assessment of suicidal risk should include an investigation of possible intent, whether there are plans and a specific method, the progress made in instituting the plan, and an evaluation of the client's mental state, particularly the degree of hopelessness.

The evaluation of suicide potential should not be a single step but rather a continual monitoring and evaluating of the potential risk. Because depression is a common disorder, counselors need to be aware of the subtle signs of depression so that they can assess the severity of the depression. Substance use is another area counselors need to include in their initial assessment. Counselors should systematically explore the use of both drugs and alcohol with clients because this is a prevalent problem. The assessment of substance abuse needs to include inquiry into the amount of the substance(s) used, whether the use can be controlled, and the consequences of the use.

In some settings, a counselor may be required to write a summary of a mental status examination. A mental status examination is typically not a "formalized" assessment, although some settings may have a structured interview and then the clinician writes the mental status examination after completing the interview. As part of conducting a mental status examination, practitioners sometimes will briefly assess the client's level of intellectual functioning by using the Mini Mental Status Exam (Folstein et al., 1975).

CHAPTER 7

Intelligence and General Ability Testing

As a school counselor in an elementary school, you receive a voice-mail message from the mother of Justin, a fourth grader at your school. Justin has recently been tested for the school's academically accelerated, or "gifted," program, and his mother is upset because Justin was determined not eligible for the program. In your school district, a student must have an intelligence quotient (IQ) of 130 to be in this accelerated program. Justin's mother wants information on the intelligence test used, and she questions the test's legitimacy because she says she knows her son and is convinced that he is highly intelligent. Justin's mother is quite upset that her son was not accepted into the accelerated program with an IQ score of 123, and his mother questions whether 7 points really reflect a significant difference in intellectual capabilities. As you prepare to return this parent's phone call, you begin to investigate the intelligence test used by the school psychologist in your district. Furthermore, you begin to think about what it means to be highly intelligent and how we actually assess intellectual abilities. In addition, you begin to contemplate what an IQ score of 130 actually represents and if it is significantly different from a score of 123.

As indicated in the discussion of Justin, intelligence or general ability tests often are used to determine if a student is placed in an accelerated program in a school. In addition, these same assessments are used in making decisions about the most appropriate instructional approaches for students with cognitive difficulties. Very few counselors will be involved in the administration of individual intelligence tests in their careers; however, many counselors will be involved in activities that require knowledge of intelligence testing. A school counselor is often a regular member of the committee that compiles Individual Educational Plans (IEPs) for students with special educational needs. Mental health counselors frequently work with individuals who have learning disabilities or other cognitive impairments that were diagnosed with intelligence testing. Parents may seek the help of a marriage and family counselor when family friction results from a child not achieving in school at a level reflective of the child's intellectual level. A rehabilitation counselor may work with a client who has recently experienced a traumatic brain injury. In all of these cases, knowledge of intelligence testing will assist counselors in better serving their clients.

Although terms such as *intelligence* and *IQ* are a common part of everyday language, there is a lack of consensus within the profession concerning the specifics on definition and structure of intelligence. In the United States, Sternberg, Conway, Ketron, and Bernstein (1981) found that both laypeople and experts had some common ideas about intelligence that included some kind of problem solving, a factor related to verbal ability, and some kind of social competence. Some professionals in the field of assessment prefer the term *general ability* because of the negative connotations associated with intelligence testing. The debate about the meaning of intelligence and intelligence test scores is somewhat emotionally charged. According to Neisser et al. (1996), political agendas, rather than scientific knowledge, often fuel the debate related to intelligence testing. To facilitate an understanding of intelligence testing, this chapter briefly reviews several different perspectives on the nature of intelligence. This overview of models lays a foundation for the discussion of specific intelligence or general ability tests. Both individually administered and group tests are included in the discussion. This chapter concludes with a summary of research related to pertinent issues in intelligence or general ability testing.

Models of Intelligence

Psychometric Approach to the Study

Since the beginning of the twentieth century, a major influence on the study of individual differences in intelligence has been the *psychometric* (or differential) *approach*. Psychometric theories of intelligence are based on the premise that intelligence can be described in terms of *mental factors* (Bjorklund, 2005), which are general mental skills that influence mental performance in a variety of situations. The term *factor* is used in this approach because many theorists have based their assertions on the statistical technique of factor analysis. From this theoretical perspective, researchers need to identify one or more factors of intelligence, and then develop intelligence tests to measure differences on those identified factors. Theorists, however, are not in total agreement on the number or types of factors that constitute intelligence.

At one extreme in terms of the number of factors in intelligence is Spearman's (1927) model. Spearman was one of the first theorists to discuss factors. He postulated a two-factor theory of intelligence. He contended that everyone has the first factor—a *general ability factor* (*g*) that influences a person's performance on all intellectual tasks. Spearman contended that the second type of factors was specific factors that influence performance in specific areas. According to Spearman, these specific factors were all to some degree correlated with *g*, and that, in essence, intelligence is a rather homogeneous construct. To put it very simply, smart people are smart, and unintelligent people are not smart. This homogeneous view of intelligence has had considerable influence on peoples' views of intelligence.

At the other end of the continuum concerning the number of factors in intelligence is Guilford's (1988) structure-of-intelligence theory, which includes 180 unique intellectual factors organized around three dimensions. Figure 7.1 illustrates this complex model in which the first dimension is *mental operations* and contains six forms. These mental operations can involve five *content areas*, which is the second dimension. Finally, there are six possible *products*, the third dimension, that interact with the combinations of operations and content areas.

Between the extremes of Spearman and Guilford is another early theorist, Thurstone, who also had considerable influence on others' views of intelligence. Thurstone (1938) originally proposed a model of seven *primary mental abilities* rather than one solitary

FIGURE 7.1
Guilford's Structure-of-Intelligence model
From Educational and Psychological Measurement, Vol. 48, p. 1-4. Reprinted by permission of Sage Publications.

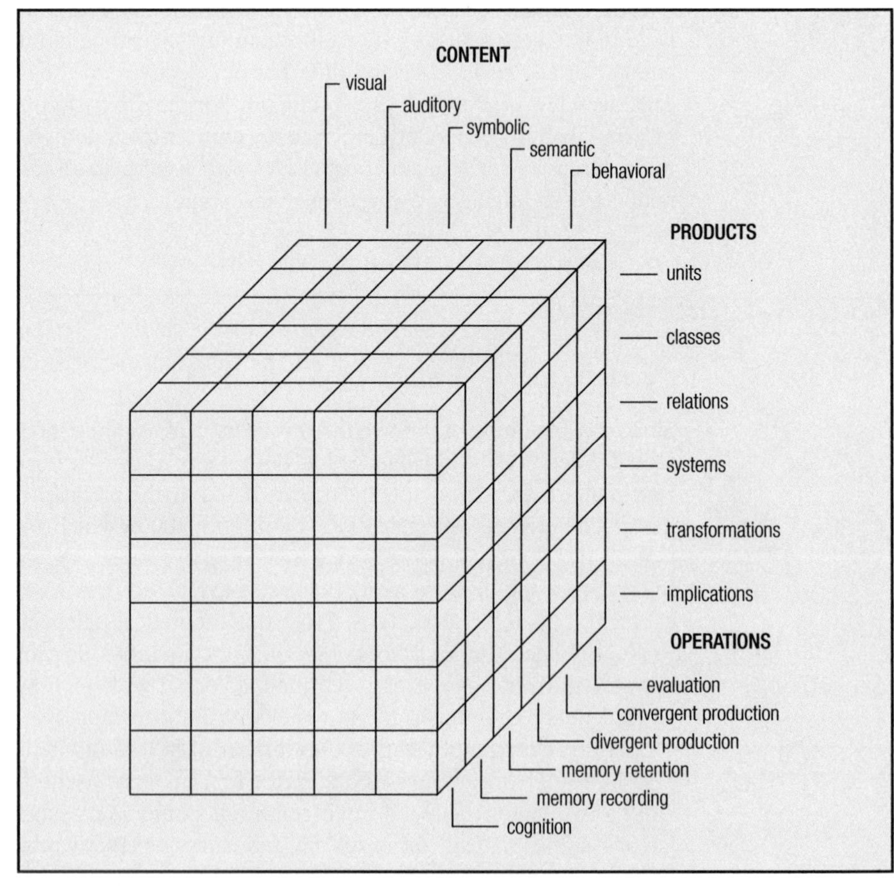

factor. In several studies, Thurstone demonstrated that seven common factors collectively accounted for most of the individual differences associated with intelligence. These seven primary mental abilities were:

1. Verbal comprehension
2. Word fluency
3. Number facility
4. Perceptual speed
5. Memory
6. Space
7. Reasoning

Thurstone's original theory did not include a general ability factor (*g*), but he did propose that the different factors were somewhat related to each other.

Other factor theorists primarily used a hierarchical approach. For example, Vernon (1950) contended that at the top of the hierarchy was g that influenced all other factors. According to Vernon, there were two second order factors: verbal and educational aptitudes (v:ed) and spatial, mechanical, and practical aptitudes (k:m). Finally, other abilities branched down from these levels to these two second order factors into third, fourth, and other order factors.

Cattell-Horn-Carroll Model

Although some consider the Cattell-Horn-Carroll model of cognitive abilities to be one of the more influential contemporary theories (Evans, Floyd, McGrew, & Leforgee, 2002), this is not a theory that three theoreticians collaborated on, but rather, a theory that has evolved from the work of three individuals. Cattell (1971, 1979) was a theorist who suggested that g was composed of two second-order factors. In Cattell's model, the second-order factors are *fluid abilities* (Gf) and *crystallized abilities* (Gc). Cattell proposed that fluid abilities are biologically determined and affect all fields of relational perception. Because fluid abilities are considered relatively culture-free, they are often reflected in memory span and spatial thinking tests. Crystallized abilities, on the other hand, include acquired skills and knowledge that are influenced more by cultural, social, and educational experiences. Tests of verbal comprehension and social relations tap crystallized abilities. Horn and Cattell (1966) and Horn (1985) expanded Catell's Gf-Gc model by adding several other intelligences. Carroll (1997) used an analogy based on geology in which intelligence is a hierarchical structure. The top stratum is g or general intelligence; the second stratum that underlies the first stratum is made up of eight abilities and processes; and the third stratum below each of the second stratum abilities is comprised of more specific factors that relate to and support the eight second stratum factors. McGrew (1997) proposed that the similarity between the Cattell-Horn model and the Carroll model reflected a single model, which he labeled the Cattell-Horn-Carroll Theory of Cognitive Abilities. McGrew and Flanagan (1998) further refined and the theory, focusing on 10 broad-stratum abilities that provide the foundation for the Woodcock-Johnson III (see Chapter 8).

More similarities exist among the psychometric approaches to intelligence than might at first appear. Toward the end of their careers, Spearman and Thurstone became more similar in their views. Spearman acknowledged that separate group factors (e.g., verbal abilities, mathematical reasoning) exist, and Thurstone concluded that correlation exists among his primary factors, suggesting the possibility of one general factor. Overall, most psychometricians agree that there is both one general ability factor (*g*) *plus* a number of lower-level factors that reflect more specific skills. Differences among the theorists primarily relate to the extent to which intelligence can be described by g and the content of the lower-level factors (Bjorklund, 2005).

Developmental progressions. Rather than focusing solely on the structure of intelligence, developmental theorists have suggested that intelligence can be better understood by examining how intelligence develops. The most well-known developmental theorists is probably Jean Piaget (1972). Unlike the psychometricians, Piaget had little interest in how individuals might differ in intellectual abilities, because he was interested in children's development. Others have adapted Piaget's concepts to the analysis of individual differences and to measuring intelligence. One of the ways in which Piagetian approaches have influenced the measuring of intellectual functioning is through the examination of individual differences in development.

Piaget suggested that intelligence involves a developmental progression, with individuals moving sequentially through the stages of the *sensorimotor, preoperational, concrete,* and *formal operations* periods. Children move through these successively higher stages of intellectual development through the use of two intellectual functions. One of these is *assimilation*, which is the process by which a child incorporates a stimulus into an existing cognitive structure or schema. The second process is *accommodation*, a process by which the child creates a new schema or significantly alters an existing schema based on new information. According to Piaget, cognitive development does not occur only through maturation; learning and the environment also influence the process. Piaget's tasks can be modified to serve as measures of individual differences; however, the tasks have not directly influenced the major standardized tests of intelligence.

Another developmental theorist whose work is having an increasing influence on the field of education is the Russian psychologist Vygotsky. His theories are complex and currently are having a significant influence on instruction but, currently, little affect on intelligence testing.

Some researchers have recently been interested in biological development, particularly the study of the brain as the basis for measuring intelligence (Neisser et al., 1996). With the increasing sophistication in brain imaging technology, it soon may be possible to understand more about the influence of biological development and specific characteristics of brain functioning.

Related to biology is Ceci's (1990, 1993) bioecological theory, which is a recent theory that also incorporates a developmental perspective in the conceptualization of intelligence. Ceci believes that biological factors have a major influence on intelligence; however, he contends that there is no single, underlying factor (g), nor is human intelligence highly heritable. Ceci, along with others, sees intelligence as being multifaceted, with individuals varying in the domain-general abilities. These theorists posit that there are no intelligent people, there are only people who are intelligent in certain domains. *Context* is central to Ceci's theory, for he argued that intellectual abilities are highly influenced by the context in which they are performed. For example, one of his studies showed that children learned better when the context was a video game versus a laboratory. The context in which people learn affects the knowledge base they possess, an idea that is central to Ceci's theory. Thus, Ceci argued, an individual's intelligence might not be reflected in the methods currently used to assess intelligence. He further contended that intelligence is reflected in knowledge acquisition and in the ability to process, integrate, and elaborate on the knowledge in a complex manner.

Information processing. Rather than studying the structures or development of intelligence, information-processing models focus on how individuals process information. Hence, the focus is not on *what* we process (factors of intelligence) but on *how* we process. One information-processing approach that has had an influence on intelligence testing is the work of Luria (1966). Luria proposed that intellect could best be described by two methods of processing information: simultaneous processing and sequential processing. **Simultaneous processing** involves the mental ability to integrate input all at once. To solve simultaneous processing items correctly, an individual must mentally integrate fragments of information to "see" the whole. **Sequential processing** involves a different set of processing skills that requires the individual to arrange stimuli in sequential or serial order to solve a problem. The Kaufman Assessment Battery for Children-Second Edition (KABC-II, Kaufman & Kaufman, 2004) was influenced by Luria's theory.

Another information-processing theory that has recently received some attention is Sternberg's (1985, 1988) triarchic theory. This theory of intelligence is quite extensive and incorporates three subtheories: (1) the internal world of the individual or the mental processes that underlie intelligence, (2) the experiential subtheory, and (3) the individual's contextual or external world. The information-processing portion of the theory is part of the first subtheory. According to Sternberg, an individual's ability to process information depends on the use of three components: the metacomponents, the performance components, and the knowledge-acquisition components. The *metacomponents* are the higher-order executive processes that are used to plan what to do, monitor it while it is being done, and then evaluate it after it is completed. Consider, for example, the interaction between planning abilities and intellectual capabilities. Sternberg argued that more intelligent people focus on critical issues that need to be solved, while less intelligent people attend to less important situations. The metacomponents influence the selected *performance components* (e.g., encoding, mental comparisons, retrieval of information). Once again, individuals vary in their abilities to use these performance skills. According to Sternberg, intelligence is related to selecting the appropriate strategies for processing diverse information. The third component, *knowledge acquisition*, involves individuals selectively encoding, combining, and comparing information to add to their knowledge base. Thus, Sternberg argued, differences in intelligence are a reflection of differences in people's abilities to process information at the metacomponent, performance, and knowledge-acquisition levels.

The second subtheory within Sternberg's triarchic theory concerns the relationship between experience and intelligence. This subtheory relates to an individual's ability to process information within existing experience. According to Sternberg, intelligence is best measured when the task is rather novel or when the task is in the process of becoming automatized. In Sternberg's view, the ability to deal with novelty is a good measure of intelligence. In essence, people who are more intelligent are able to react more quickly and process new information more efficiently than people who are less intelligent. Another of Sternberg's contentions is that the ability to automatize is also an indicator of intellect. If a person is effective at automatizing information, then that individual will have more resources available for dealing with novelty.

The third subtheory within Sternberg's theory concerns the contextual or external world of the individual. Sternberg argued that intelligence is contextually bound. For example, having an uncanny knowledge of elephants' migratory patterns is not highly valued in many settings in Western society. Thus, people will vary in their abilities to select, adapt to, and shape environments, which are also, according to Sternberg, marks of intelligence. Although Sternberg's theory has not yet had a direct influence on intelligence instruments, his contention that intelligence tests only measure a selective portion of the complex construct of intelligence is having an influence on the understanding of what intelligence is. Most of us probably know someone who would not do particularly well on the instruments discussed later in this chapter, even though that person may be "street smart" or "have an uncanny ability to size up the situation." Sternberg is a leader in promoting the expansion of methods to view and measure intelligence.

Other Theories

Another theorist who advocated for expanding our views of intelligence is Gardner (1993). Gardner's theory of multiple intelligences avers that any set of adult competencies that is valued in a culture merits consideration as a potential intelligence. As the name of his theory implies, he argued that there are *multiple* intelligences rather than a single entity. Gardner's theory is different from others, such as Thurstone, in that he proposes nine relatively independent frames of mind: (1) linguistic, (2) logical-mathematical, (3) musical, (4) spatial, (5) bodily-kinesthetic, (6) interpersonal, (7) intrapersonal, (8) naturalist, and (9) existential. Gardner suggested that current psychometric tests only measure linguistic, logical, and some aspects of spatial intelligence, while ignoring the other intelligences. He argued that measures need to value intellectual capacities in a wide range of domains and that the methods should be appropriate for each domain (e.g., for spatial ability, testing an individual's ability to navigate in a new city). There are some difficulties with adapting Gardner's ideas in assessment, but his theory has attracted considerable attention in the assessment area.

In conclusion, the different theoretical approaches have influenced the assessment of intelligence. The psychometric approach has had the most direct influence on the instruments commonly in use today. The newer theories, however, provide some important insight into the complexities of intelligence and may influence future methods of assessment. Defining and conceptualizing intelligence is often perplexing, which means the measuring of intelligence is also plagued by many of these same issues.

Individual Intelligence Testing

As stated earlier, counselors are typically not responsible for the administration, scoring, and interpretation of individual intelligence tests. In order to administer an individual intelligence test, a professional must have completed certain coursework and received specific training and supervision on the use of that instrument. This chapter does not provide the necessary information to become proficient in the administration and interpretation of these instruments. Rather, the intent of this chapter is to give an overview of commonly used tests so that counselors can use the results in counseling contexts or when participating in multidisciplinary teams involving intelligence assessment. This overview includes a brief description of the most widely used instruments.

Wechsler Scales

David Wechsler had extraordinary influence on the testing of intelligence. He developed a series of three intelligence instruments that are similar in approach but designed for different age groups. The *Wechsler Preschool and Primary Scale of Intelligence III* (WPPSI-III, Wechsler, 2002) is designed for children ages 2 years, 6 months through 7 years, 3 months old; the *Wechsler Intelligence Scale for Children—Fourth Edition* (WISC-IV, Wechsler, 2003) is for children ages 6 years, 0 months through 16 years, 11 months old; and the *Wechsler Adult Intelligence Scale—Third Edition* (WAIS-III, Wechsler, 1997a) is for individuals 16 through 89 years old. In addition to these three major assessments, there are also the *Wechsler Abbreviated Scale of Intelligence* (WASI) and the *Wechsler Intelligence Scale for Children—Fourth Edition Integrated* (WISC-IV Integrated). The Wechsler scales are commonly cited in research, and numerous reports on test usage indicate that the Wechsler instruments are the most frequently used intelligence tests (Archer, Maruish, Imhof, & Piotrowski, 1991; Archer & Newsom, 2000). Furthermore, even if we examine all types of tests (e.g., personality), research results indicate that counselors frequently use the Wechsler scales. Elmore, Ekstrom, Diamond, and Whittaker (1993) found the WISC-R to be the most widely used assessment instrument among school counselors. Likewise, Bubenzer, Zimpfer, and Mahrle (1990) found the WAIS-R to be the third most widely used instrument and the WISC-R the fifth most widely used instrument by community mental health counselors. Therefore, counselors should be familiar with these instruments and with their strengths and limitations.

The earlier versions of the WPPSI-III, the WISC-IV, and the WAIS-III included measures of Full Scale IQ (FSIQ), Verbal IQ (VIQ), and Performance IQ (PIQ). This, however, appears to be changing as the most recent revision of these assessments, the WISC-IV, has a measure of FSIQ and four index scores: Verbal Comprehension Index (VCI), the Perceptual Reasoning Index (PRI), the Working Memory Index (WMI), and the Processing Speed Index (PSI). The WAIS-III retains the FSIQ, VIQ, and PIQ, but also has four index scores (see Table 7.1 on the next page). With the WPPSI-III, a supplemental subtest can be added to produce a Processing Speed Quotient. The WAIS-IV, which will be released in 2008, will use the four index scores.

With the WPPSI-III, WISC-IV, and WAIS-III, the FSIQ is the global and aggregate measure of cognitive abilities and has a mean of 100 and a standard deviation of 15. The

TABLE 7.1
Indexes and subtests for the WPPSI-III, WISC-IV, and WAIS-III

WPPSI-III	WISC-IV	WAIS-III
Verbal IQ	***Verbal Comprehension Index***	***Verbal Scale***
Information	Similarities	Similarities
Vocabulary	Vocabulary	Vocabulary
Word Reasoning	Comprehension	Comprehension*
Comprehension*	Information*	Information
Similarities*	Word Reasoning*	Digit Span
Picture Naming**		Letter-Number Sequencing**
Receptive Vocabulary**		
Performance IQ	***Perceptual Reasoning Index***	***Performance Scale***
Block Design	Block Design	Block Design
Matrix Reasoning	Matrix Reasoning	Matrix Reasoning
Picture Concepts	Picture Concepts	Picture Completion
Object Assembly*	Picture Completion*	Digit Symbol-Coding
Picture Completion*		Picture Arrangement*
Coding**		Object Assembly
Symbol Search**		Symbol Search**
		Mazes
	Working Memory Index	
	Digit Span	
	Letter-Number Sequencing	
	Arithmetic*	
	Processing Speed Index	
	Coding	
	Symbol Search	
	Cancellation*	

*supplemental subtest
**expanded

other indexes or composite scores also have a mean of 100 and a standard deviation of 15. Due to the similarities of all the Wechsler intelligence instruments, the following information on the *Wechsler Intelligence Scale for Children—Fourth Edition* (WISC-IV, Wechsler, 2003) should also acquaint readers with some aspects of the WPPSI-III and many aspects of the WAIS-III (see Figure 7.2). For the WISC-IV, the four index scores are the

- *Verbal Comprehension Index* measures verbal attention, concentration, and processing speed and involves the subtests of Similarities, Vocabulary, and Comprehension.
- *Perceptual Reasoning Index* assesses fluid reasoning abilities, perceptual organization, and motor skills and includes the subtests of Block Design, Picture Concepts, and Matrix Reasoning.

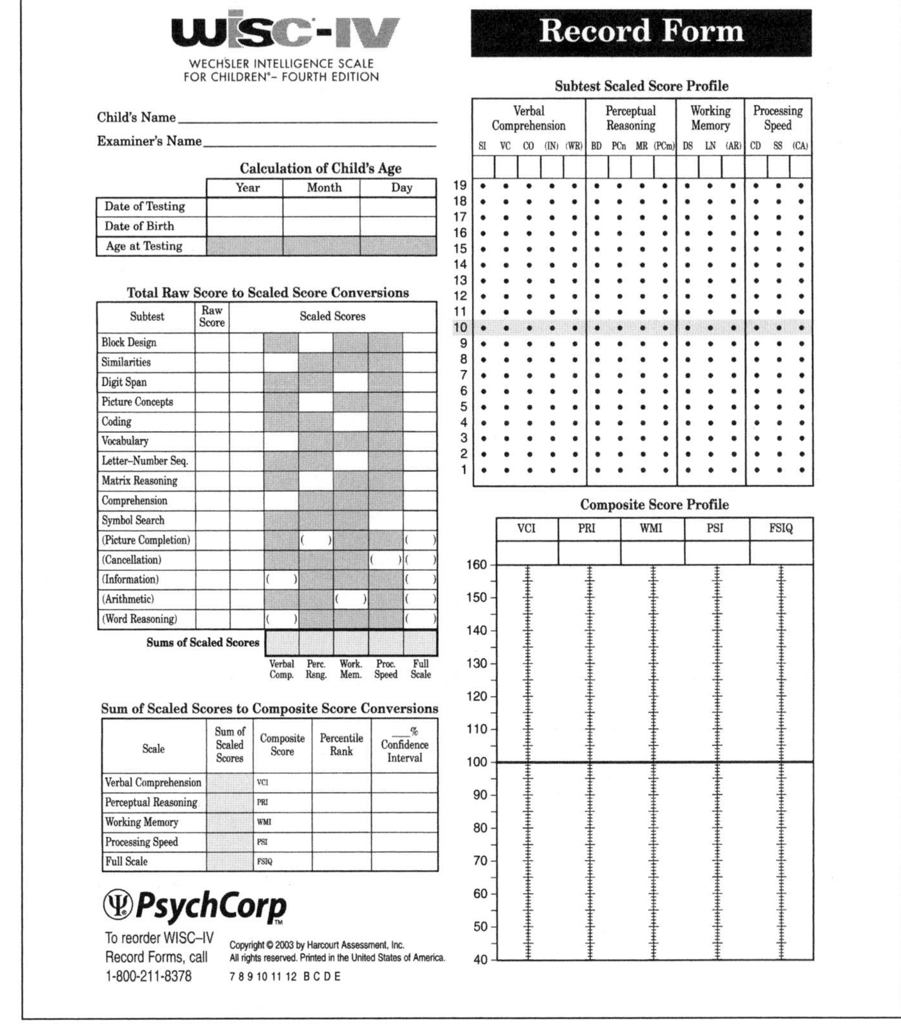

WISC-IV

WECHSLER INTELLIGENCE SCALE FOR CHILDREN®– FOURTH EDITION

Child's Name ______________________

Examiner's Name ______________________

Calculation of Child's Age

	Year	Month	Day
Date of Testing			
Date of Birth			
Age at Testing			

Total Raw Score to Scaled Score Conversions

Subtest	Raw Score	Scaled Scores				
Block Design						
Similarities						
Digit Span						
Picture Concepts						
Coding						
Vocabulary						
Letter–Number Seq.						
Matrix Reasoning						
Comprehension						
Symbol Search						
(Picture Completion)			( )			( )
(Cancellation)					( )	( )
(Information)		( )				( )
(Arithmetic)				( )		( )
(Word Reasoning)		( )				( )
Sums of Scaled Scores						
		Verbal Comp.	Perc. Rsng.	Work. Mem.	Proc. Speed	Full Scale

Sum of Scaled Scores to Composite Score Conversions

Scale	Sum of Scaled Scores	Composite Score	Percentile Rank	___% Confidence Interval
Verbal Comprehension		VCI		
Perceptual Reasoning		PRI		
Working Memory		WMI		
Processing Speed		PSI		
Full Scale		FSIQ		

PsychCorp™

To reorder WISC–IV Record Forms, call 1-800-211-8378

7 8 9 10 11 12 B C D E

Record Form

Subtest Scaled Score Profile

Verbal Comprehension					Perceptual Reasoning				Working Memory			Processing Speed		
SI	VC	CO	(IN)	(WR)	BD	PCn	MR	(PCm)	DS	LN	(AR)	CD	SS	(CA)

19 18 17 16 15 14 13 12 11 10 9 8 7 6 5 4 3 2 1

Composite Score Profile

VCI	PRI	WMI	PSI	FSIQ

160 150 140 130 120 110 100 90 80 70 60 50 40

FIGURE 7.2
Record Form for the Wechsler Intelligence Scale for Children-Fourth Edition

Wechsler Intelligence Scale for Children® - Fourth Edition. Copyright © 2003 by NCS Pearson, Inc. Reproduced with permission. All rights reserved. Wechsler Intelligence Scale for Children and WISC is a trademark, in the US and/or other countries, of Pearson Education, Inc. or its affiliate(s).

- *Working Memory Index* measures a person's information-processing capacity and the active use of incoming information. The subtests involved are Digit Span and Letter-Number Sequencing.
- *Processing Speed Index* concerns mental and motor speed and the ability to organize, plan, and implement appropriate strategies. This index involves the subtests of Coding and Symbol Search.

The WISC-IV developers contended that these four discrete domains are important because working memory and processing speed, which relate to learning acquisition, can be distinguished from verbal comprehension tasks and perceptual organization tasks. This breakdown becomes particularly important when diagnosing attention deficit/hyperactivity disorder (ADHD), learning disabilities, and other cognitive deficiencies. Although the WAIS-III has the traditional measures of Verbal IQ (VIQ), and Performance IQ (PIQ), MacCluskie, Welfel, and Toman (2002) recommended closely examining the four index scores. The WAIS-IV is currently being developed and is expected to measure the four indexes contained in the WISC-IV and not have the verbal and performance dichotomy.

The scoring of the Wechsler subscales is somewhat complex because different points are awarded depending on the quality of the responses. Items in each subtest are arranged hierarchically, beginning with the easier items and ending with the more difficult items. Similar to the Stanford-Binet, the administrator uses a reverse sequencing procedure in determining the *basal level*, which involves moving to easier items if a certain number of items are missed at the beginning of the subtest, and then proceeding through the testing until a *ceiling level* is reached (i.e., a certain number of items are consecutively missed). Throughout the administration of the scales, the examiner also gathers anecdotal information, such as task-approach skills, level of concentration, and motivation. A qualified examiner can extract rich and important information from the performance on these intelligence tests as well as from observing the individual during the testing.

Tables 7.2, 7.3, 7.4, and 7.5 provide brief overviews of the subtests that comprise the index scores (i.e., Verbal Comprehension, Perceptual Reasoning, Working Memory, and Processing Speed) of the WISC-IV. The interpretation of the WISC-IV is complex and that is why specific training and supervised practice in using the Wechsler assessments is needed in order to use them. The examiner's manual provides various ways to compare and contrast an individual's performance at the Index level and in

TABLE 7.2
Brief description of the Verbal Comprehension subtests on the WISC-IV

- *Similarities.* On this subtest, the individual must identify similarity between two verbal concepts, each represented by a single word. The lower level test items measure learned association, but as the items increase in complexity, the test becomes a measure of higher-order skills. This subtest assesses the ability to analyze relationships, concept formation, and the level of logical and abstract reasoning.
- *Vocabulary.* On the Vocabulary subtest, the individual must provide the definition of a given word. This subtest has the strongest relationship with general ability of any of the subtests. Vocabulary assesses word knowledge, language development, fund of knowledge, and learning ability. The open-ended format often provides information of clinical significance in terms of both academic background and other psychological factors, such as ability to retain and produce material learned in diverse settings. It is most predictive of academic aptitude.
- *Comprehension.* For this subtest, the individual is asked open-ended questions for which he or she must provide an oral response. The questions typically involve providing a rationale for commonly accepted social norms, rules, or laws, but can also involve explaining a proverb or explaining what the individual would do in a given situation. This subtest measures judgment more than it does previous academic learning. It also measures verbal comprehension, verbal expression, and long-term memory. The Comprehension subtest provides an indication of awareness of social convention and is considered a clinically rich subtest.
- *Information.* This is a supplemental subtest within the Verbal Comprehension Index that taps an individual's level of general knowledge. The subtest requires the examinee to answer factual questions (e.g., "In what direction does the sun rise?"). The subtest involves crystallized intelligence and provides an indication of knowledge base, verbal expressive skills, and long-term memory. Educational and cultural background have more of an influence of performance on the Information subtest than on some of the other subtests.
- *Word Reasoning.* The Word Reasoning subtest is also a supplemental subtest in Verbal Comprehension. Individuals are asked to identify the common concepts described in a series of clues. It has been shown to measure verbal comprehension, domain knowledge, reasoning abilities, and the ability to integrate and synthesize information.

TABLE 7.3
Brief description of the Perceptual Reasoning Index subtests on the WISC-IV

- *Block Design.* Materials for the Block Design include nine identical blocks; each has two sides all red, two sides that are all white and two sides that are half red/half white. The individual must use these blocks to copy certain designs. Block Design is usually considered the best indicator of nonverbal intelligence. The subtest taps nonverbal concept formation, visual perception, and organization. Furthermore, the subtest analyzes the degree to which visual input is integrated with motor functions and simultaneous processing.
- *Picture Concepts.* The examinee is presented with two or three rows of pictures and must select one picture from each row, showing the objects that have common characteristics. It is designed to measure fluid reasoning and the ability to use abstract categorical reasoning.
- *Matrix Reasoning.* In this subtest, the individual examines a matrix from which a section is missing and then identifies from a group of pictures which one is the missing section, either by its number or by pointing to the appropriate selection. Matrix-related tasks have often been considered good measures of fluid reasoning and general intellectual ability.
- *Picture Completion.* Picture Completion is a supplemental subtest in the WISC-IV. The individual is shown a picture in which an important part is missing (e.g., the cord on a telephone). He or she must identify the missing detail. To eliminate verbal influences, respondents can point to the missing part. Picture Completion measures visual perception, alertness, visual memory, concentration, and attention to detail.

TABLE 7.4
Brief description of the Working Memory Index subtests on the WISC-IV

- *Digit Span.* There are two parts of this subtest, with the first portion involving the examinee repeating a series of numbers in the same order that the examiner says them. In the second portion, the examiner says a sequence of numbers and the examinee responds by saying the numbers in reverse order. The subset assesses auditory short-term memory and process. It also measures attention, concentration, and rote learning.
- *Letter-Number Sequencing.* In this subtest, the examiner reads a string of numbers and letters, and the examinee first repeats the numbers in ascending order and then provides the letters in alphabetical order. This subtest provides an indication of auditory discrimination, memory, attention, and sequencing abilities.
- *Arithmetic.* The Arithmetic subtest is a supplemental test on the WISC-IV. It requires the individual to answer mathematical questions that are presented orally. At the lower levels, the examinee can simply count to find the answer. The majority of the items are "word problems" and must be solved without calculators or paper and pencil. The subtest measures reasoning, concentration, alertness, and short-term auditory memory and mastery of basic mathematics calculation facts.

TABLE 7.5
Brief description of the Processing Speed Index subtests on the WISC-IV

- *Coding.* This subtest is titled Digit Symbol Coding on the WAIS-III. In Coding, the individual copies symbols that have been paired with simple geometric shapes or with numbers. The examinee needs visual perception skills, basic motor skills for copying, and short-term memory skills to complete the task efficiently. The subtest also measures degree of persistence and speed of performance.
- *Symbol Search.* The examinee is presented with a series of paired groups of symbols, with each pair containing a "target" group and a "search" group. The examinee quickly indicates whether either of the pair of symbols in the target group appears in the search group. There are two forms depending on the child's age. The subtest measures visual-motor processing speed and visual acuity.
- *Cancellation.* Cancellation is a supplemental subtest. Examinees scan both structure and random arrangements of pictures and mark target pictures. It was developed to measure processing speed, visual selective attention, and vigilance.

using the individual subtests. Individual variations in subtest and index results provide insights into the learning strengths and limitation of many students.

The norming sample for the WISC-IV was 2,200 children ages 6 years, 0 months to 16 years, 11 months old (6:0–16:11). In addition, samples of children from specific groups were included in the standardization process. There are 11 age groups (e.g., 6:0–6:11, 7:0–7:11, 8:0–8:11, etc.), with 200 children in each. The norming group has an equal number of males and females, and the sample was drawn to represent U.S. population in terms of racial/ethnic makeup. Furthermore, parent education level and geographic location were taken into account in establishing the national norms. According to Mallor (2005) the reliability estimates for the FSIQ are impressive, with coefficient greater than or equal to .96 for every age group. Except for the Processing Speed Index, the reliability coefficients for the index scores are above .90. Standard errors of measurements for the Full Scale IQ, all index scores, and subtest scores are provided in the technical manual. The technical manual also contains substantial information related to the WISC-IV scores and correlations with other relevant measures and results of both exploratory and confirmatory factor analyses.

An extension of the WISC-IV is the WISC-IV Integrated (Wechsler et al., 2004) that focuses on identifying processing problems and involves the administration of a selection of 16 process subtests in addition to the administration of the WISC-IV. The WISC-IV Integrated is not an updated version of the WISC-IV, but it is designed to expand on the information gathered in the WISC-IV particularly as it relates to identifying information processing strengths and limitations. The process subtests expand on the WISC-IV subtests and a knowledgeable psychologist can provide more detailed information about a child's cognitive processes. It should be interesting to see if school psychologists will move toward using the WISC-IV Integrated in their assessment of children and adolescents who may have learning disabilities.

With baby boomers getting older, there is also increased interest in older adults' neurological disorders and there is increased use of the WAIS-III in assessing neurological disorders (e.g., Alzheimer's, Parkinson's). The WAIS-III was revised in conjunction with the *Wechsler Memory Scale III* (Wechsler, 1997b); these two instruments share similar research methodologies, normative samples, and validation procedures. These instruments share a technical manual and are designed to provide a proficient examiner a method of comparing intellectual ability and memory functioning. The pairing of intellectual ability and memory functioning is becoming increasingly important in many areas of assessment (e.g., with geriatric populations). In their reviews of the WAIS-III, both Hess (2001) and Rogers (2001) concluded that the WAIS-III is an improvement over the earlier edition and is built on a substantial history of research and instrument development.

In conclusion, the Wechsler instruments are the most widely used individually administered intelligence tests. A skilled psychologist can derive an abundance of useful information from the administration of the WPPSI-III, WISC-IV, or WAIS-III. Although most interpretations of the results will focus on cognitive abilities, some psychologists are able to use these testing results to identify personality factors and learning styles. Spanish versions of the Wechsler scales are also available and have been researched and validated.

Stanford-Binet Intelligence Scale

One of the oldest and most widely used intelligence assessments is the *Stanford-Binet*, which is now in its fifth edition (Roid, 2003). The Stanford-Binet evolved from the Binet-Simon, which was first published in 1905 and contained only 30 items. The Binet-Simon was revised in both 1908 and 1911. The first version of the Stanford-Binet was published in 1916 under the leadership of Terman at Stanford University. This version of the instrument was the first to include an intelligence quotient (IQ), derived from the ratio of mental age to chronological age. Major revisions of the Stanford-Binet were performed in 1937, 1960, 1972, and 1986. The fourth edition abandoned the ratio IQ in favor of a deviation

IQ. The fifth edition of the Stanford-Binet (SB5) was built on this extensive historical experience and the substantial research that has been conducted related to earlier versions of the Stanford-Binet. In addition, some of the procedures were revised in order to address criticisms of earlier editions, particularly related to measuring the nonverbal aspects of intelligence and to making the assessment more engaging for diverse groups.

The current version of the Stanford-Binet was constructed for use with individuals 2 through 85 years old. According to Becker (2003), the SB5 contains an equal balance of verbal and nonverbal content. Norm-referenced scores are determined for Verbal IQ (VIQ), Nonverbal IQ (NVIQ), and Full Scale IQ (FSIQ). There are five factors for both the verbal and nonverbal areas. These are:

1. *Fluid Reasoning* concerns an examinee's abilities to solve verbal and nonverbal problems using inductive and deductive reasoning.
2. *Knowledge* assesses an examinee's accumulated fund of general information acquired at home, school, work, or through life experiences.
3. *Quantitative Reasoning* measures facility with numbers and numerical problem solving, whether with word problems or figural relationships (emphasis is on problem-solving more than mathematical knowledge).
4. *Visual-Spatial Processing* involves an examinee's abilities to see patterns, relationships, spatial orientation, and the gestalt among diverse aspects of visual displays.
5. *Working Memory* measures short-term memory processing of verbal and visual information, with an emphasis on "transformation" or "sorting out" of diverse information.

Similar to the Wechsler instruments, the Stanford-Binet's three intelligence score composites (i.e., FSIQ, VIQ, and NVIQ) have a mean of 100 and a standard deviation of 15. Previous editions of the Stanford-Binet had a mean of 100 and a standard deviation of 16 (see Figure 7.3). Within the Nonverbal Domain there are five Scaled Scores (e.g., Nonverbal Fluid Reasoning, Nonverbal Knowledge) and within the Verbal Domain there are five Scaled Scores (e.g., Verbal Fluid Reasoning, Verbal Knowledge) that have a means of 10 and standard deviations of 3. The Scaled Scores for each domain are combined to produce five composite factor scores (i.e., FR, KN, AR, VS, and WM) that also have means of 100 and standard deviations of 15 (see Figure 7.3).

The SB5 contains items and content from the fourth edition of the Stanford-Binet; however, the administration procedures are somewhat different. The administration of the SB5 starts with administering the Nonverbal Reasoning Routing Subtest (Object Series/Matrices) and then moving to the Verbal Knowledge Routing Subtest (Vocabulary). Once the routing tests have been administered, the administrator begins testing in the Nonverbal Domain until a ceiling has been reached for Nonverbal Knowledge, Nonverbal Quantitative Reasoning, Nonverbal Visual-Spatial Processing, and Nonverbal Working Memory. Once the ceiling levels are established in the nonverbal area, the administrator then begins to assess the Verbal Domain by completing the activities related to Verbal Fluid Reasoning, Verbal Quantitative Reasoning, Verbal Visual Spatial Processing, and Verbal Working Memory.

The standardization sample for the current version of the Stanford-Binet was more than 4,800 individuals. The reliability estimates, using a measure of internal consistency for the Full Scale IQ, is .98. Because the SB5 was only recently published,

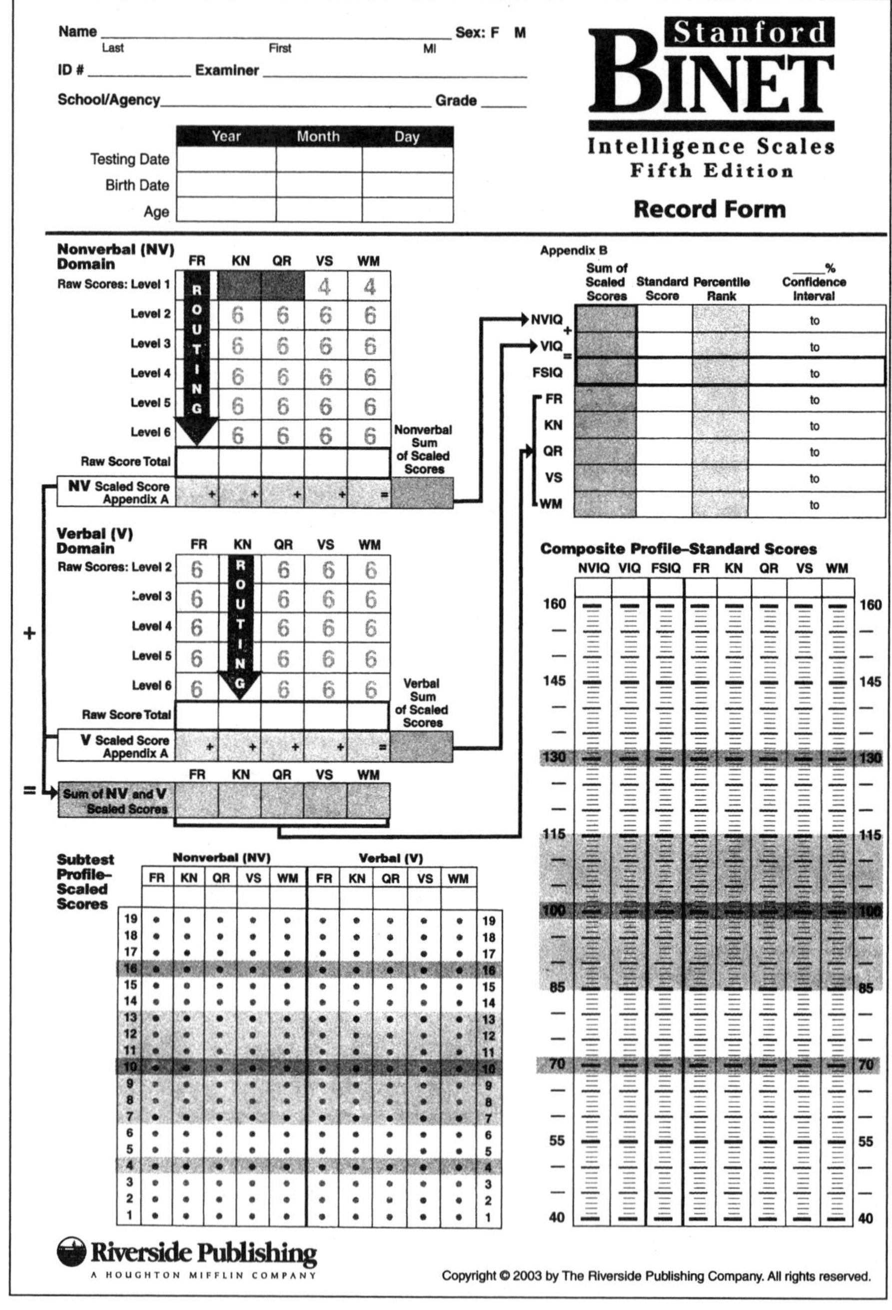

Name ______________________ Last First MI Sex: F M

ID # __________ Examiner ______________________

School/Agency ______________________ Grade ______

Stanford BINET Intelligence Scales Fifth Edition

Record Form

	Year	Month	Day
Testing Date			
Birth Date			
Age			

Nonverbal (NV) Domain

	FR	KN	QR	VS	WM
Raw Scores: Level 1	ROUTING			4	4
Level 2		6	6	6	6
Level 3		6	6	6	6
Level 4		6	6	6	6
Level 5		6	6	6	6
Level 6		6	6	6	6
Raw Score Total					
NV Scaled Score Appendix A	+	+	+	+	= Nonverbal Sum of Scaled Scores

Verbal (V) Domain

	FR	KN	QR	VS	WM
Raw Scores: Level 2	6	ROUTING	6	6	6
Level 3	6		6	6	6
Level 4	6		6	6	6
Level 5	6		6	6	6
Level 6	6		6	6	6
Raw Score Total					
V Scaled Score Appendix A	+	+	+	+	= Verbal Sum of Scaled Scores

	FR	KN	QR	VS	WM
Sum of NV and V Scaled Scores					

Appendix B

	Sum of Scaled Scores	Standard Score	Percentile Rank	___% Confidence Interval
NVIQ				to
VIQ				to
FSIQ				to
FR				to
KN				to
QR				to
VS				to
WM				to

Composite Profile–Standard Scores

NVIQ VIQ FSIQ FR KN QR VS WM

160 — — 145 — — 130 — — 115 — — 100 — — 85 — — 70 — — 55 — 40

Subtest Profile–Scaled Scores

Nonverbal (NV): FR KN QR VS WM — Verbal (V): FR KN QR VS WM

19 18 17 16 15 14 13 12 11 10 9 8 7 6 5 4 3 2 1

Riverside Publishing

A HOUGHTON MIFFLIN COMPANY

FIGURE 7.3
Stanford-Binet Intelligence Scale, Fifth Edition

Copyright © 2003 by The Riverside Publishing Company. "Stanford-Binet Intelligence Scale, 5th edition Record Form Figure 7.4 page 152" from the Stanford-Binet Intelligence Scales, Fifth Edition (SB5) reproduced with permission of the publisher. All rights reserved.

reviews of its psychometric qualities were not available at the time of this book's publication. However, because the Stanford-Binet is a commonly used instrument that historically has been influential, research related to its qualities will be available soon.

Kaufman Instruments

Another prominent name in the field of intellectual assessment is Kaufman. Alan and Nadeen Kaufman are a husband-and-wife team of psychologists with extensive experience in test development. In the 1980s, they published the *Kaufman Assessment Battery for Children* (K-ABC, Kaufman & Kaufman, 1983a, 1983b), which reflected many advances in intelligence testing, but also was the focus of some controversy. They next published the *Kaufman Adolescent and Adult Intelligence Test* (KAIT, Kaufman & Kaufman, 1993). Recently, the *Kaufman Assessment Battery for Children, Second Edition* (KABC-II, Kaufman & Kaufman, 2004) was published, which is grounded in Luria's processing model and the Cattell-Horn-Carroll model. The Kaufman instruments are not as widely used as the Wechsler instruments and, therefore, are not covered in the same degree of detail.

The Kaufman Assessment Battery for Children, Second Edition was designed to assess children ages 3 to 18. Both the KABC and the KABC-II were designed with the intention of fairly assessing children from diverse backgrounds and minimizing ethnic group differences in performance. The KABC-II yields four or five scales depending on whether the examiner is using the Cattell-Horn-Carroll (CHC) or the Luria approach. From a CHC perspective, the KABC-II yields measures of Short-Term Memory, Visual Processing, Long-term Storage and Retrieval, Fluid Reasoning, and Crystallized Abilities. A composite of these five scales is the Fluid-Crystallized Index. From a Luria perspective, the scales are named Sequential Processing, Simultaneous Processing, Learning Ability, and Planning Ability. The global score from the Luria approach is titled Mental Processing Index. Kaufman and Kaufman (2004) recommended that examiners use the CHC approach unless the examinee is likely to have deficiencies in crystallized abilities due to nonstandard learning experiences. Baden and Ouzts (2005), however, contended that the KABC-II does not measure intended constructs consistent with Luria's theory and that marketing it as utilizing both theories is misleading.

The KABC-II has 18 subtests; however, an examiner would not use all 18 with one child. The selection of subtests is based on the child's age and which of the theoretical approaches is used for scoring. The KABC-II was standardized with a sample of 3,025 and the make-up of the sample was reflective of the demographics of the 2001 U.S. Census. The reliability coefficients, particularly test-retest, vary somewhat depending on the theoretical approach, but for the major components from both approaches, the range is from .77 to .92. The validation evidence is complex, but both Baden and Ouzts (2005) and Thorndike (2005) question the degree to which the instrument measures Luria's theory.

The *Kaufman Adolescent and Adult Intelligence Test* (KAIT, Kaufman & Kaufman, 1993) is designed for individuals 11 to 85 years old. The Core Battery can be given in 60 minutes, whereas the Expanded Battery, which has a neurological focus, can be administered in 90 minutes. The KAIT includes three intelligence scales: Fluid (Gf), Crystallized (Gc), and Composite Intelligence. It has six subtests, three that assess fluid intelligence and three that assess crystallized intelligence. Flanagan (1995) criticized the KAIT for having a dichotomous view of fluid and crystallized intelligence that is neither supported by current theorists in the area nor by research. The instrument appears to be well standardized, with a national sample of 2,000. The reliability information provided is acceptable. Although the manual provides extensive validity information, there is some concern about the KAIT, particularly related to the instrument's ability to assess fluid intelligence (Flanagan, 1995).

Additional Individual Instruments

A few other individually administered intelligence tests are used sufficiently to merit a brief overview. The *Differential Ability Scales-Second Edition* (DAS-II, Elliot, 2006) is based on the British Ability Scales, which has been used in England since 1983. The DAS-II has been standardized in the United States, and, in 2008 the publishers are planning to produce a version specifically for Australia. As the name implies, the focus of the DAS is on identifying specific abilities. It is designed to provide insight, particularly to school psychologists, into how a child processes information. The diagnostic subtests measure abilities such as verbal and visual memory, immediate and delayed recall, visual recognition and matching, processing and naming speed, phonological processing, and understanding numerical concepts.

Another frequently used instrument is the *Slosson Intelligence Test-Revised, Third Edition* (SIT-R3, Nicholson & Hibpshman, 1990). The SIT-R3 provides a relatively quick assessment of cognitive abilities for children and adults. It takes approximately 15 to 20 minutes to administer and score (Erford, Klein, & McNinch, 2007). It consists of 187 items that are given orally; the examinee's language skills will influence performance. The norms for the SIT-R3 were recalibrated in 1998. This shorter assessment is not quite as reliable as the longer, individually administered intelligence assessments. On the positive side, the SIT-R3 is highly correlated with the Verbal Scale and Full Scale IQ scores of the Wechsler instruments.

As discussed later in this chapter, there has been criticism of intelligence tests being culturally biased. In response to this criticism, some individually administered intelligence tests have been developed that focus on trying to diminish the effects of cultural biases and the influences of language proficiency on intelligence. For example, the *Raven's Standard Progressive Matrices* (Raven, Court, & Raven, 1983) contains matrices that have a logical pattern or design with a missing part. The examinee selects the appropriate item that completes the pattern. Hence, progressive matrices are nonverbal; however, some researchers contend that culture also influences these skills. Another attempt to reduce cultural bias is the *Peabody Picture Vocabulary Test—III* (Dunn & Dunn, 1997), which measures receptive vocabulary knowledge. There are both English and Spanish versions. In both versions, the individual is given a word and asked to simply point to the corresponding picture. The *Test of Nonverbal Intelligence 3* (TONI-3, Brown, Sherbenou, & Johnsen, 1997) is another example of a language-free measure of intelligence in which the instructions are pantomimed and the examinee points to the answers.

Conclusion

In conclusion, the information gained from individually administered intelligence tests can be helpful to counselors. The amount of useful information depends on the expertise of the individual administering and interpreting the results. Counselors need to become proficient consumers of psychological reports that include intelligence assessment.

This involves having sufficient information about the instruments used to be able to evaluate the psychologist's report. For example, a counselor who receives a psychological report for a Hispanic 9-year-old boy with limited English proficiency needs to understand the cultural influences on the intelligence test used. Instrument manuals, critiques and reviews of instruments, journal articles, and books can all aid the counselor in becoming an informed professional in the area of individual intelligence assessment.

Group Intelligence Testing

Group intelligence tests are used more frequently than individual tests, particularly in school settings. These tests are often given in conjunction with group achievement tests in schools; thus, their use is often connected with evaluating student performance. In some school settings, group intelligence tests serve as initial screening tools to identify those children who should receive additional testing to identify a possible learning disability or developmental delay. Another use of group intelligence tests concerns evaluating entire schools. For example, school boards, administrators, or legislators may want to evaluate a school's performance, so they examine the differences between ability levels (as measured by group intelligence test results) with academic performance (as measured by group achievement test results). The following example of Alicia provides another example of how to use group intelligence test information in counseling.

> Alicia is an 11-year-old fifth grader. Her parents sought counseling for her because she was doing "poorly" in school. The parents reported that Alicia was getting mostly Cs and an occasional B. The parents were both professionals with graduate degrees. They reported that Alicia was not performing up to her abilities, and they wanted the counselor to identify methods to help motivate her. Alicia, on the other hand, told the counselor that she was trying hard to do well in school. The counselor asked about homework, once again receiving discrepant information from Alicia and her parents. Alicia contended that she worked diligently for hours on homework, whereas her parents reported that she dawdled the hours away. The counselor secured a release of information from the parents to talk with Alicia's teacher and review Alicia's school records.
>
> Children in Alicia's school took an annual standardized group achievement test that also included a measure of intelligence or general ability. The counselor found that Alicia consistently scored slightly below average in terms of intellectual abilities compared with both national and local norms. In fact, the results consistently indicated that Alicia's IQ was in the 40th to 44th percentile range, even though instruments from different publishers had been used in this school district. Alicia's teacher concurred with the results of the group intelligence tests and voiced that she believed Alicia was probably overachieving rather than underachieving.

Group intelligence or ability tests can provide certain information, but they also have certain limitations. With individually administered intelligence tests, it is possible to observe behaviors that often reflect the level of motivation. In a group setting, however, it is impossible to document the behaviors of the entire group, and sometimes individuals are not motivated to perform at their highest level. Many of us have heard of children who, when taking group-administered tests, bubbled the answer sheets into attractive patterns rather than reading the questions! Furthermore, group intelligence tests require more reading than individually administered tests and are, therefore, more problematic for individuals with limited reading skills. Counselors also need to consider a client's culture, background, and language proficiencies when interpreting the results from group intelligence tests. Consistent with good assessment practices, the results of any instrument should never be interpreted in isolation, and this practice is particularly germane to group intelligence tests because they are not as sophisticated and detailed as individually administered intelligence tests.

The *Cognitive Abilities Test* (CogAT), a revision and extension of the Lorge-Thorndike Intelligence Test, is designed to assess the pattern and level of children's reasoning abilities. There are different levels of the instrument appropriate for kindergarten through grade 12. The current form of the instrument, Form 6, provides separate scores for verbal, quantitative, and nonverbal reasoning; a composite score can also be provided. The stated intent of the CogAt is to assess the level and pattern of cognitive development of students. The time allotted to take the CogAT is between 30 and 50 minutes, depending on the child's grade level. For schools interested in administering combined ability and achievement testing, the CogAT is concurrently normed with the Iowa Tests. When given with one of the Iowa Tests, the CogAT provides schools with predictive achievement scores, which can aid in identifying students who may display a discrepancy between expected achievement level and performance. The CogAT Web site (http://www.riverpub.com/products/cogAt) contains an interesting Interactive Results Manager, a web-based reporting application for teachers and administrator that analyzes assessment data from CogAT and the Iowa Test. The Resource Manager can disaggregate results (e.g., race/ethnicity and students with disabilities) to respond to requirements of the No Child Left Behind Act.

Another frequently used group intelligence test is the *Otis-Lennon School Ability Test,* Eighth Edition (OLSAT-8). The OLSAT-8 is also for students in kindergarten through grade 12 and has recently been re-normed. This test measures cognitive abilities related to a student's ability to learn and succeed in school. Although previous editions used the term "mental ability," the current version does not use that nomenclature. The scores provided are Total, Verbal, and Nonverbal, in addition to five cluster scores (Verbal Comprehension, Verbal Reasoning, Pictorial Reasoning, Figural Reasoning, and Quantitative Reasoning). The maximum time requirement for the OLSAT-8 is 75 minutes. The OLSAT-8 was standardized with the *Stanford Achievement Test, Tenth Edition* (Stanford-10). Both the OLSAT-8 and the CogAt have a mean of 100 and standard deviation of 16.

In View is a test of cognitive skills developed and concurrently standardized with the TerraNova, The Second Edition (see Chapter 8). This group test of intelligence, which can be used with students in grades 2 through 12, employs problems of sequences, analogies, verbal reasoning-words, verbal reasoning-content, and quantitative reasoning. In addition, it provides a score on the Cognitive Index designed to indicate a measure of overall academic aptitude.

The *Naglieri Nonverbal Ability Test* (Naglieri, 1997) is a group-administered, brief measure of ability designed to be sensitive to cultural and socioeconomic differences in children. The matrix style of the items requires children to select the shape or design that is consistent with the provided matrix. The Naglieri Nonverbal Ability Test—Multilevel Form (NNAT-MF) was conjointly standardized with the *Stanford Achievement Test, Ninth Edition* (Stanford-9). Stinnett (2001) supported the use of the NNAT-MF if there is a need for a brief measure of general nonverbal intellectual abilities; however, counselors must remember that the matrix format is somewhat narrow in its approach to assessing intelligence. In addition, there is a version of the Naglierei Nonverbal Ability Test that can be administered individually.

The *Multidimensional Aptitude Battery II* (MAB-II, Jackson, 1998) is another group intelligence test, although it is not designed for use in schools. Instead, the MAB-II was designed as a convenient alternative to the WAIS-R. The MAB-II is for either adolescents or adults and can be given either individually or in groups. Like the Wechsler instruments, this test provides a FSIQ, a VIQ, and a PIQ. There are five verbal and five performance subtests, with each subtest having a time limit of seven minutes.

Another group intelligence test that is primarily used in industrial settings is the *Wonderlic Personnel Test* (WPT, Wonderlic Personnel Test, Inc., 1998), also known as the Wonderlic Personnel Test and Scholastic Level Exam. Typically, most ability tests involve both speed and power; however, the WPT (a 50-item test with a 12-minute time limit) is weighted more toward speed. There are paper-and-pencil, PC, and online versions of the WPT, which allow individuals to take the instrument multiple times.

Issues in Intelligence Testing

Controversy and debate about intelligence testing are certainly not new phenomena. For example, both Jensen's (1969) oft-cited article and Hernstein and Murray's (1994) *The Bell Curve: Intelligence and Class Structure in American Life* have received enormous media attention and have ignited significant debates about the nature of intelligence and the meaning of intelligence test scores. It is important for counselors to understand some of the issues related to the construct of intelligence and the controversies surrounding the assessment of intelligence or general ability. Hence, the third section of this chapter will examine some of the issues related to intelligence testing and summarize the research findings related to these topics.

Is Intelligence Stable?

One of the major questions about intelligence test scores concerns whether they remain stable as individuals develop and age, or do scores change over time, depending on the variable influences the individual experiences in life? Infants and preschool children have the least stable intelligence test scores, a fact reflected in the lower reliability coefficients of the instruments for these younger children. The answer to whether intelligence is stable from childhood through old age depends on what research is examined.

Early research in this area indicated that intelligence tended to gradually decline after the age of 20, with the decline becoming more apparent for individuals in their 50s through their 70s. There is a commonly held notion that as we age, our memory, speed of processing, and mental agility decrease. You have probably heard people cite their age as the reason for forgetting some detail. The findings of these early studies, however, have not been supported by more sophisticated research methodologies.

Early research on intellectual stability involved *cross-sectional studies*, in which people at different age levels were tested and their intelligence scores compared.

What these early findings did not take into account, however, were the cultural differences that affected the scores of different generations of individuals. For example, in these cross-sectional studies, many of the older individuals did not have the same educational experiences as the younger individuals. The assessment field is in general agreement that these early results indicating decreases in intellectual function were the result of cultural differences among the different generations (Anastasi & Urbina, 1997). Later researchers were able to complete *longitudinal studies*, in which the same people were tested repeatedly at different ages in their lives. Some of the more prominent longitudinal studies (e.g., Bayley & Oden, 1955; Tuddenham, Blumenkrantz, & Wilken, 1968) indicated that intelligence gradually increases from childhood into middle age and then levels off.

Probably the best indicators of the stability of intelligence come from those studies that employed both cross-sectional and longitudinal designs, following the same individuals over time, as well as comparing 30-year-olds in 1950 with 30-year-olds in 1980 (Schaie, 1996). These well-designed studies indicated intelligence is fairly steady throughout adulthood, with slight declines occurring approximately after the age of 65. The intellectual declines that do occur tend to be in the area of fluid, as compared with crystallized, intelligence (Kaufman, 1990). As Verhaeghen (2003) indicated, there is little decline over the lifespan on tests that measure experience and knowledge, but there is decline on tests that require speed of processing and mental manipulation. The degree to which there may be decline in intelligence, however, appears to be related to a complex interaction of variables, such as physical health, mental activities performed in the later years, and the degree to which education is continued throughout the lifespan.

What Do Intelligence Test Scores Predict?

Earlier, this chapter presented different views concerning what constitutes intelligence and different methods for measuring intelligence. The conclusion is that there is no generally agreed upon definition of intelligence, nor is there consensus on the most appropriate methods for assessing this somewhat elusive construct. Yet, intelligence tests continue to be used in our society; therefore, it is important for counselors to understand the research findings related to what these tests actually measure. The following discussion does not address findings related to any specific instrument; rather it looks at general trends in intelligence testing.

Intelligence tests appear to be related to academic performance. The correlation between intelligence and school performance is consistently near .50 (Neisser et al., 1996). Although this is often considered a substantial coefficient, it is important to remember that only 25% of the variance is explained by the relationship between intelligence and school performance. Therefore, success in school is related to many other factors (e.g., socioeconomic factors, motivation) in addition to intelligence. However, children with higher intelligence test scores are shown to be less likely to drop out of school as compared with children with lower scores.

The relationship between IQ scores and occupational success and income is not as simple to determine. The degree to which intelligence scores are related to occupational prestige, and to a lesser degree to income, is partly due to the connection between education and intelligence. Higher-prestige occupations, such as doctor or

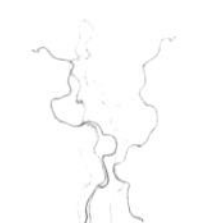

lawyer, typically require more than a college education. Admissions scores for college (e.g., SAT) and post-degree work (e.g., GRE) are highly correlated with intelligence tests. Although Hernstein and Murray (1994) contended that intelligence scores predict occupational attainment, a task force appointed by the American Psychological Association (Neisser et al., 1996) did not reach the same conclusion. At most, the latter authors concluded that intelligence accounts for about one-fourth of the social status variance and one-sixth of the income variance. This relationship further decreased when the parents' socioeconomic status was taken into consideration.

Concerning the relationship between IQ scores and occupational success, the research conducted by Hunter and Schmidt (e.g., Hunter, 1986; Hunter & Schmidt, 1983) is often cited because they studied the effects of abilities and aptitudes on job performance. The findings, which Hunter and Schmidt termed **validity generalization**, are primarily related to aptitude testing and the *General Aptitude Test Battery* (GATB), a vocational aptitude test developed by the U.S. Department of Labor. The GATB does include a measure that some professionals contend is synonymous with intelligence; thus, Hunter and Schmidt's findings do have some relevance in regard to the predictive ability of intelligence tests.

Hunter and Schmidt, and their associates, were primarily interested in studying which variables predicted successful personnel selection. In studying the effectiveness of tests in employment selection, they focused on the GATB because numerous validation studies had been conducted. Other researchers contended that the GATB was fine at predicting performance in some occupations but not good at predicting performance in other occupations. By examining the variations in validity coefficients of job performance tests, which primarily involved the GATB and performance in various occupations, they found that differences in validity coefficients were mainly due to measurement and sampling error (Pearlman, Schmidt, & Hunter, 1980; Schmidt & Hunter, 1977; Schmidt, Hunter, & Caplan, 1981). In a large meta-analysis, Hunter (1980) found that the three composite scores of the GATB were valid predictors of success in all jobs. He also found that the relationship between the aptitudes and job performance was linear, indicating that as test scores increased so did ratings of job performance. Hence, the best workers had the highest test scores. Thus, the term *validity generalization* refers to the findings that the same test score data may be predictive for all jobs. The implication of this research is that if a test is valid for a few occupations, the test is valid for all jobs in that cluster. Therefore, these researchers found evidence that validity coefficients could be generalized to other occupations.

Hunter (1982) further demonstrated that the GATB composites could be weighted to predict to five job families that included all occupations listed by the Department of Labor. For example, Job Family 1 was 59% Cognitive, 30% Perceptual, and 11% Psychomotor; the other four job families had different weightings on these same three factors. Hunter went on to suggest that these weighted scores should be used for top-down hiring, meaning an employer should hire the applicant with the highest-weighted score because he or she would be the most proficient worker out of the applicant pool. Many local employment service offices began using the Job Family method and provided employers with a rank ordering of applicants based on the weighted scores for the five Job Families. Previous research, however, had shown that African Americans, Hispanics, and Native Americans tend to get lower scores than others on the GATB. Therefore, some argued that using validity generalization and the GATB adversely affected these groups (Hartigan & Wigdor, 1989). Research on validity generalization and whether tests of general ability predict occupational success is ongoing, so it is anticipated that debate regarding intelligence testing and personnel selection will continue.

Is Intelligence Hereditary?

This is one of the most controversial issues in intelligence testing, for the question is essentially asking how much of measured intellectual ability is innate and how much is due to environmental factors. There are many traits that vary among people (e.g., weight, propensity for some diseases, or aspects of personality), and scientists have attempted to discern the amount of variation that is attributable to genetics and the amount that is due to environmental factors. A *heritability index* (h^2) is intended to provide an estimate of the proportion of variance associated with genetic differences. The reverse then applies, with $1\text{-}h^2$ being an indicator of the amount of variance due to environmental factors. Determining estimates of the genetic contribution to intelligence is, at this point, difficult. Some of the studies have examined the differences between monozygotic (MZ) twins and dizygotic (DZ) twins who have been raised together and those who were adopted and raised apart. MZ twins have the same genetic makeup, and DZ twins have half of their genes in common. Other studies involved several kinds of kinship and the influences of genetics on intelligence.

In general, the heritability indexes for intelligence tend to be approximately .50 (Chipuser, Rovine, & Plomin, 1990; Loehlin, 1989). McGue, Bouchard, Iacono, and Lykken (1993) argued that this h^2 figure would probably be larger (i.e., approximately .80) if researchers only included studies with adult samples. Although genes appear to have a substantial influence on performance on intelligence tests, this effect is not sufficiently large enough to indicate that intelligence is inexorably set at conception. Environmental factors also have a significant effect on intellectual development. Neisser et al. (1996), in their extensive review of research in this area, concluded that variation in the unique environments of individuals and between-family factors significantly influence IQ scores of children. IQ scores seemed to be most related to the interaction between an individual's genetic makeup and environmental influences. A child is born with certain capabilities, but the degree to which those capabilities is realized is significantly influenced by the environment surrounding that child.

What Environmental Factors Influence Intelligence?

Many environmental factors influence the intellectual development of an individual, but it is clear that the *cultural* environment in which a person matures has a significant influence on a person's intellectual development. Postmodern philosophy has stressed the influences of culture and language in the overall development of an individual (Gergen, 1985). A child of Indian descent growing up in rural Malaysia has different experiences than an upper-middle class Caucasian child growing up in San Francisco. Cultures differ in a multitude of ways that are both overt and subtle; therefore, we are unable to directly identify all the cultural factors that influence performance on intelligence tests. Even within a population, there are subgroups with cultural variations, such as the many different Native Americans tribes in the United States. For example, the culture of the Arapahos is different from the culture of the Shoshones, even though the two tribes share a reservation in Wyoming.

Although intelligence tests try to eliminate the effects of schooling, attendance at school does influence performance on intelligence tests (Ceci, 1991). Children who attend school regularly have higher test scores than children who attend intermittently. If we examine differences between children who are the same age but, because of birthday deadlines, vary in the number of years attending school, those who have attended longer will have higher IQ scores. Precisely how schooling influences intelligence test performance is difficult to determine. Certainly, many intelligence tests incorporate information items, such as "Who is Madame Curie?" The probability of being exposed to this information increases with attendance at school. Children in school are also more likely to be exposed to manipulation of objects and puzzles. Furthermore, schools promote problem-solving skills and abstract thinking. It must be noted that not all schooling is alike and that the quality of the school experience also influences IQ scores. Those who attend poor-quality schools will not receive the same instruction, and their intelligence scores will reflect this deficiency (Neisser et al., 1996).

Family environments have an influence on many aspects of development, including cognitive development. Early research indicated that intelligence scores were directly influenced by parents' interest in achievement (Honzik, 1967) and methods of disciplining (Baldwin, Kalhorn, & Breese, 1945; Kent & Davis, 1957). Research has since questioned these early findings (Scarr, 1992, 1993). Severely neglectful or abusive environments, however, can negatively affect children's cognitive development. For example, prolonged malnutrition in childhood impedes cognitive development. After a child is provided a minimally nurturing environment, it is difficult to determine what other factors may contribute to performance on intelligence tests.

Environmental factors that can affect intelligence also include exposure to certain toxins. The negative consequences of exposure to lead have been well documented (Baghurst et al., 1992; McMichael et al., 1988). Prenatal exposure to large amounts of alcohol can produce deleterious effects on the child, termed *fetal alcohol syndrome* (Stratton, Howey, & Battaglia, 1996). Mental retardation is often associated with fetal alcohol syndrome. There is conflicting research about the effects on cognitive development related to prenatal exposure to small amounts of alcohol, caffeine, over-the-counter pain medication, and antibiotics.

Are There Group Differences in Intelligence?

Probably the most controversial issue related to the testing of intelligence concerns ethnic and gender group differences. Before we begin a discussion of these group differences in intelligence, it is important to remember that research has continually shown that within-group variance is greater than between-group variance. This means that within any ethnic group, the variation in scores is quite large; in fact, the variation *within* the group is greater than *between* groups. Hence, there is overlap among the groups that challenges the conclusions about the superiority or inferiority of one group compared with another. Furthermore, because of the large variation in intelligence scores, it is inappropriate to stereotype any individual based on group performance scores.

Are There Gender Differences in Intelligence?

Although there do not appear to be general intellectual differences between males and females, there are some differences on specific tasks or abilities. Men appear to be better in visual-spatial ability, which involves tasks that require the individual to visualize and mentally rotate objects. In a meta-analytic study, Masters and Sanders (1993) found an effect size of .90, indicating that men in general score almost a standard deviation higher than females on visual-spatial tests. On the other hand, females appear to have the advantage over males in terms of some verbal tasks. On synonym generation and verbal fluency, females score higher than males, with the effect sizes ranging from .50 to 1.20 (Gordon & Lee, 1986; Hines, 1990). Thus, females' scores on tests of verbal tasks tend to be between a half a standard deviation to more than a full standard deviation higher than those of males.

Are There Ethnic Group Differences in Intelligence?

In general, African Americans, Hispanics, and Native Americans tend to score lower on intelligence tests than European Americans or Asian Americans. African Americans tend to score about one standard deviation (15 points) below Caucasians (Jensen, 1980; Reynolds, Chastain, Kaufman, & McLean, 1987). African Americans tend to do poorly on both the verbal and nonverbal subtests that have a high correlation with general intelligence (Jensen, 1985). Socioeconomic factors seem to have some influence on test scores; however, Black/White differences are reduced, though not eliminated, when socioeconomic factors are controlled for (Loehlin, Lindzey, & Spuhler, 1975). Chapter 15 addresses questions of test bias, which some researchers have argued contributes to the disparity in IQ means between African Americans and Caucasians. Some research does indicate that the difference between African Americans and Caucasians on IQ scores is decreasing, but more definitive studies are needed before this can be considered an established finding (Neisser et al., 1996).

Hispanic Americans' average intelligence test scores are typically between those of African Americans and Caucasians (Neisser et al., 1996). Counselors need to be aware that linguistic factors may influence Hispanic individuals' performance on intelligence tests. Hispanic children often score higher on the performance subtests than on the verbal subtests (Kaufman, 1994). For many Hispanic children, English is not their first language, which may partially explain the discrepancy between performance and verbal scores. Dana (1993) contended that translation of standard intelligence tests into Spanish does not resolve these problems.

Concerning Native Americans' performance on intelligence tests, counselors need to be careful not to generalize due to the multitude of distinct tribes within this population. The traditions and cultures of the Native American tribes vary; thus, performance on aspects of intelligence tests also tends to vary. A general finding is that Native American children, like Hispanic children, seem to score lower on the verbal scales as compared with the performance scales (Neisser et al., 1996). In addition to cultural differences, McShane and Plas (1984) suggested that Native American children are also plagued by chronic middle-ear infections that can negatively affect their development in the verbal area. The behavior of Native Americans during testing may also be misinterpreted by examiners. Native Americans tend to be deferential to a Caucasian examiner, which examiners may perceive as a lack of motivation.

There is some debate concerning the average intelligence scores for Asian American children, with studies reporting averages from around 100 to 110. A general finding is that Asian Americans achieve substantially more, both academically and occupationally, than their intelligence scores would predict (Flynn, 1991). Asian Americans tend to do well in school, and a higher proportion of them are employed in managerial, professional, and technical occupations than would be expected based on their intelligence scores. This "overachievement" demonstrates some of the problems with IQ-based predictions (Neisser et al., 1996). It should be noted that there is also great diversity among Asian Americans (e.g., Chinese, Korean, and Vietnamese).

The ethnic group difference in intelligence test performance does not appear to be related to any one factor, such as heredity or language differences. Neisser et al. (1996) concluded that researchers have not yet been able to explain these differences.

Therefore, simple conclusions about the differences in intelligence among ethnic groups are probably based more on political or social views than on scientific evidence. In counseling individuals, counselors need to remember that there is great variation in intelligence within all ethnic groups and that a counselor cannot predict a client's level of cognitive abilities based on ethnicity. Stereotypes concerning any individual, based on his or her ethnic, gender, or any type of group is detrimental.

What Is the Flynn Effect?

As this section of the chapter is devoted to issues in intelligence testing, it is important to note the steady rise of intelligence scores in recent years. This rise in intelligence score is often called the "Flynn effect" after James Flynn (1984, 1987), who was one of the first researchers to identify this trend. In the past 50 years, the average IQ score has increased more than a full standard deviation. The average gain is about three IQ points each decade. Interestingly, these gains in IQ scores are not reflected in gains in achievement; for example, scores on the SAT declined between the mid-1960s and the early 1980s (Neisser et al., 1996). There are numerous possible explanations for the Flynn effect, such as improvement in nutrition, more test sophistication, changes in education and educational opportunities, and changes in parenting practices.

Although the increases in intelligence scores are well documented, the reasons for this rise are debated within the field. There are also differing opinions about whether this trend will continue or if there will be a leveling-off of average IQ scores.

Summary

Intelligence is a word used in everyday conversation (e.g., "John is intelligent" or "Someone is not very intelligent"). In addition, intelligence testing has a rich and substantial history, with certain instruments having been used extensively in a variety of settings. Given these factors, one might expect more agreement on the definition and theoretical basis for intelligence. Numerous theorists contend that a psychometric or factorial approach best explains the construct of intelligence. These individuals suggest that intelligence is composed of one or more factors. There is some debate about whether intelligence can best be described as one general factor (*g*) that affects all cognitive performance. Many intelligence tests have a composite score or a full-scale IQ score that represents a measure of *g*. Other factor theorists contend that intelligence can be better explained by focusing on lower-order factors, such as the differences between fluid and crystallized intelligence. Developmental theorists suggest that intelligence can be better understood by examining how the structure of intelligence develops. Certainly, the most influential theorist in this developmental area is Piaget. Rather than studying the structures or development of intelligence, Luria's information-processing model concerns how individuals perceive information and make sense of that information. A number of researchers currently hope that by analyzing how the brain works, they will understand the phenomenon of intelligence. Finally, there are new models of intelligence that propose expanding the methods of testing intelligence. The models of Sternberg and Gardner, for example, are influencing how the field considers and conceptualizes intelligence.

Theories of intelligence have influenced the development of some of the most commonly used intelligence tests. To assess a person's cognitive capabilities, an individually administered intelligence assessment may be conducted. The most frequently used instruments are those developed by Wechsler. The various Wechsler intelligence tests are similar in content, but each has been specifically designed for and standardized for a specific age range. The Wechsler Adult Intelligence Scale—III (WAIS-III) is for adults, the Wechsler Intelligence Scale for Children—IV (WISC-IV) is for children ages 6 years, 0 months through 16 years, 11 months old, and the Wechsler Preschool and Primary Scale of Intelligence—III (WPPSI-III) is for children ages 2 years, 6 months through 7 years, 3 months old. Another historically significant scale, the Stanford-Binet, is currently in its fifth edition. The authors of the Kaufman Assessment Battery for Children, Second Edition (KABC-II) designed their test to be appropriate for children from diverse ethnic groups. Although group intelligence tests are easier to administer, they cannot provide the degree of information that individually administered intelligence tests provide. Furthermore, performance on group intelligence tests is highly dependent on the examinees' reading abilities. It also should be noted that cognitive, or general ability, tests are less reliable with younger children than they are with adolescents and adults.

Numerous issues relate to the use of intelligence tests. Information from intelligence tests can be helpful in counseling clients, particularly in terms of educational and career decisions. A skilled clinician, however, must be aware of the strengths and limitations of these measures. Multicultural factors are particularly important to consider when results from intelligence tests are used in decision making. Intelligence test results can provide information about a client's cognitive abilities, but that information needs to be integrated with other contextual factors to give a more thorough understanding of the client.

CHAPTER 8

Assessing Achievement and Aptitude: Applications for Counseling

Anna is a 17-year-old high school senior who is unsure about her college plans. Her parents both graduated from Ivy League schools and want Anna to attend one of those institutions. Anna had planned on going to an Ivy League school but is now wondering if she is smart enough. Anna indicated that she was involved in many high school activities in her freshman, sophomore, and junior years; however, she has dropped out of these activities during her senior year. In addition, Anna and her mother have been arguing about Anna's "lack of motivation." Anna's grades continue to be mostly As with some Bs. Her parents have insisted she go to counseling to improve her attitude and get back to preparing for a "good" college. Anna has provided you, her counselor, with her scores on both the SAT and the ACT. Her SAT Reasoning Test scores were 570 for the Critical Reading section, 590 for the Mathematical score, and 500 for the Writing section. On the ACT, Anna received 22 in English, 24 in Mathematics, 21 in Reading, 23 in Science, and a Composite score of 23. Anna and her parents want your advice on whether she is "bright enough" to go to a selective college. Based on these scores, what might you tell them? In addition, what other information might you collect that would be helpful in providing feedback to Anna about her academic potential? Anna also states that she has a severe case of test anxiety and wants help in improving her scores. Hence, you are considering interventions that might help her test anxiety and wondering if these interventions could significantly improve her performance.

As you will remember from Chapter 1, achievement tests provide information about what individuals have learned or knowledge they have acquired. Anna's case is but one example of an instance when it would be helpful for a counselor to have an understanding of achievement and aptitude assessment. Another example is a situation in which the parents of a girl in second grade were very disappointed in her academic performance. The parents perceived the child to be an "academic failure" and provided evidence of poor spelling in stories and letters the daughter had written to relatives. These parents, however, were not particularly knowledgeable about child development and had unrealistic expectations concerning what a second grader should be able to spell. The results of an achievement test the daughter had taken in school helped the parents understand that their child was not an academic failure. The daughter's lowest achievement score was indeed in spelling, but it was at the 62nd percentile. In this case, interpreting the girl's achievement scores to her parents helped them understand their daughter better and provided a more realistic understanding of their child's academic strengths and limitations.

Knowledge of aptitude assessment can also be useful to counselors. Aptitude tests *predict* future performance or ability to learn. Clients often come to counseling because they are trying to make a decision about their futures (e.g., seek a new job, go back to school, decide on a career), and aptitude tests can provide some useful information in these decisions. In fact, many of us have probably wondered at some point in our lives if we had the aptitude for a particular task. Many aptitude tests are used for selection purposes, such as employers selecting employees and college admissions personnel deciding which students should be admitted to certain colleges. Some of these same aptitude assessments, however, can be used in counseling situations to assist clients in making better-informed decisions about their futures. In general, achievement tests measure acquired learning, whereas aptitude tests measure potential or ability to learn new tasks. Although there are a number of different types of both achievement and aptitude tests, sometimes the differences between them are somewhat ambiguous. The contrast between achievement and aptitude tests is one of purpose more than of content. For example, the same math problems might be used to determine if someone has learned a mathematical concept (achievement) or to predict future performance in jobs requiring some mathematical knowledge (aptitude). This chapter briefly discusses some of the achievement and aptitude tests commonly used by counselors.

Assessment of Achievement

There are many types of achievement tests. Thus, it is important that counselors understand the distinction among the tests and the objectives of each category of achievement tests.

1. *Survey achievement batteries*. These instruments assess individuals over a wide range of subjects. The batteries often measure knowledge in the areas of reading, mathematics, language arts, science, and social studies. Survey achievement batteries can be norm-referenced or a combination of norm-referenced and criterion-referenced instruments. Recent years have seen an increase in the use of these survey achievement batteries to measure student progress as well as the quality of schools.

2. *Individual achievement tests and diagnostic achievement tests.* These achievement instruments, which are administered individually, are often used for diagnostic purposes (e.g., diagnosis of a learning disability) or to measure whether an individual has made academic progress. Many individual achievement tests cover the areas of reading, mathematics, and spelling.
3. *Criterion-referenced tests and minimum-level skills assessments.* These instruments measure knowledge or comprehension and determine if a certain criterion or standard has been met. In minimum-level skills assessment, a criterion is set that establishes the base level at which a person must perform to; for example, advance to another grade, enter an occupation, or graduate from high school.
4. *Subject area tests.* Many achievement tests measure knowledge in specific subject matter. An example of a subject area assessment is a test that covers knowledge of assessment strategies in counseling.

Survey Achievement Tests

Survey achievement tests are administered to thousands of students in multiple school districts throughout the nation and are frequently designed for kindergarten through grade 12. These batteries of achievement tests typically have a number of subtests that measure achievement in certain academic areas (e.g., reading, mathematics, and language arts). These survey achievement tests can help a counselor understand where a child's or an adolescent's strengths and limitations are within the different achievement areas. Furthermore, the results from these tests can provide information about a student's progress from year to year. For instance, school counselors may want to intervene with students whose scores are generally consistent for a couple of years and then begin to decrease. The same applies to mental health counselors who may want to request achievement testing results to better understand the child or adolescent client and examine trends in terms of academic performance.

Numerous achievement batteries are available for academic uses. Table 8.1 provides a sample of some of the commonly used ones and the appropriate grade levels for those instruments. These achievement batteries cover multiple achievement areas so that a counselor can identify both strengths and limitations. Many of these batteries are constructed so that a child's progress can be continually charted from kindergarten through grade 12. Many of these batteries are concurrently normed with tests of academic intelligence or general ability, for example, the *Otis-Lennon School*

TABLE 8.1 *Achievement batteries and grade ranges*

Instrument	Grade Levels
Iowa Test of Basic Skills	K–9
Iowa Test of Educational Development	9–12
Metropolitan (8th edition)	K–12
Stanford Achievement Test Series (10th edition)	K–12
TerraNova, The Second Edition (CAT6)	K–12

Ability Test can be given simultaneously with either the Metropolitan Achievement Tests or the Stanford Achievement Test Series to get estimates of ability/achievement comparisons. The measure of intelligence that corresponds to the *Iowa Tests of Basic Skills* and the *Iowa Tests of Educational Development* is the *Cognitive Abilities Test* (CogAT). Likewise, a new measure, *InView*, can accompany the TerraNova. If major discrepancies are identified between ability and achievement with one of these achievement batteries, then additional testing that is more thorough and individually administered may be warranted.

There are also achievement batteries available for adults because some adults seek information about their current level of achievement in order to upgrade their skills.

For example, a high school dropout may want to know where his academic deficiencies are so that he can learn those skills that were missed. An example of an adult achievement battery is the *Test of Adult Basic Education* (TABE), which includes both a Survey Version and a Complete Battery. The Survey Version can be used for screening and placing, whereas the Complete Battery provides much more thorough information for determining educational interventions. The TABE Complete Battery, which is designed to correspond to the 2002 *General Education Development* (GED) test, assesses the academic areas of vocabulary, reading, language, language mechanics, mathematics, and spelling. The TABE can also be used for other purposes and indicates whether an adult has made progress in literacy education or learning English. The TABE is also used in programs related to workforce development, because it measures work-related basic skills and work-related problem-solving skills. The different levels of the TABE (i.e., Limited Literacy, Easy, Medium, Difficult, and Advanced) enable examiners to assess the basic skills of adults at various levels of literacy.

TerraNova, The Second Edition. The following discussion of the *TerraNova, The Second Edition* (TN2) is intended to provide a detailed example of a current achievement battery. The TerraNova, The Second Edition serves as a good example because it evolved from the *Comprehensive Tests of Basic Skills* (CTBS) and the *California Achievement Tests* (CAT), both of which are achievement tests with long histories. In fact, the TerraNova, The Second Edition is the sixth edition of the CAT, so it is also referred to as the TerraNova (CAT). The TerraNova, The Second Edition is also a good example because it incorporates both norm-referenced interpretation and criterion-referenced interpretation based on item response theory. The TerraNova, The Second Edition is a modular series that offers multiple measures of achievement. School districts can select from the TerraNova CAT Multiple Assessment, which includes both selected-response items and constructed responses, or the TerraNova CAT Complete Battery, which involves only selected-response items. The TerraNova CAT Survey, which takes less time to administer, is also available. All of these options assess reading/language arts, mathematics, science, and social studies, and the results include norm-referenced scores, criterion-referenced objective mastery scores, and performance-level information. However, the amount of information contained in the results varies among the three options. Each of these options (i.e., the Multiple Assessment, Complete Battery, and Survey) can be expanded to measure students' basic skills and to assess word analysis, vocabulary, language mechanics, spelling, and mathematics. In addition, for students who have completed an Algebra I course, there is the TerraNova Algebra test. Finally, a Spanish version of the first edition of the TerraNova, called the SUPERA, compares Spanish-speaking test takers with a national sample of Spanish-speaking students (CTB/McGraw-Hill, 2000). Cizek (2005) suggested that the broad array of options and products related to the TerrraNova can be somewhat confusing.

In the general area of achievement assessment, there are concerns about whether a multiple-choice format (or selected-response items) is always the best approach for measuring students' knowledge. A selected-response format is restricted in terms of the types of questions that can be asked; for example, a student cannot be asked to write a sentence. With selected-response items, guessing or "bubbling" errors can influence scores. Hence, many achievement publishers are incorporating constructed-response items wherein the students must create a short response to answer a question. The problem with constructed-response items is that they often cannot be machine-scored (e.g., computers cannot determine whether a student's written sentence contains grammatical errors). For the TerraNova Multiple Assessment, which contains constructed-response items, these items are scored by a team of evaluation experts. Having different individuals score an assessment can present problems with interrater reliability, because it is difficult for two people to evaluate an answer in the same manner. In the TerraNova Multiple Assessment, evaluators are trained, and their scoring is continually compared with that of other team members and testing professionals (CTB/McGraw-Hill, 2000).

The publishers of the TerraNova, The Second Edition (TN2) claim that items were developed using national standards for curriculum areas, curriculum frameworks, and major basal readers or textbooks (CTB/McGraw-Hill, 2002). Johnson and Mazzie (2005) contended that one of the strengths of the TN2 is the extensive curriculum review conducted by the developers to ensure that the instrument assessed materials that were being taught. Another major goal was to develop materials that students are likely to find to be highly similar to the kinds of materials they regularly encounter in the classroom (Cizek, 2005). Twice as many items as were needed were originally developed, and these items were then "tried out" to empirically evaluate each one. The construction of the TerraNova involved item response theory. Because TerraNova includes both selected-response and constructed-response items, different models of item response theory were employed. Each item was evaluated in terms of its content and its psychometric specifications. Readers interested in the implementation of item response theory should see the *TerraNova, The Second Edition: CAT technical bulletin 1* (CTB/McGraw-Hill, 2002). As discussed in Chapter 4, the intent of item response theory is to calibrate the item to the appropriate grade level. Thus, the TerraNova items were given to several grade levels (e.g., grades 4, 5, and 6) in the process of selecting items for the final version of the instrument. Furthermore, the developers of TerraNova used a sophisticated method to examine each item's differential item functioning (DIF) to detect if there were ethnic group differences on the performance of each item.

The developers of TerraNova used two different stratified random sampling procedures to obtain a sample representative of the U.S. school population. Both public and parochial/private schools were stratified by region, community type, and socioeconomic status (CTB/McGraw-Hill, 2002). At least 264,000 K–12 students participated in the norming process for the TerraNova, The Second Edition. The proportions of students in the stratified cells were determined using national census data. Schools used in the standardization process were also asked to test all students, including those who would need accommodations based on special needs. A total of 1,320 schools from 778 districts participated in the standardization of the TerraNova, The Second Edition.

Figures 8.1 and 8.2 are examples of the TerraNova Individual Profile Report, which typically is kept in the student's educational file and can be seen by school personnel. The Performance on Objectives section (see Figure 8.1) provides the criterion-referenced information as well as information on the student's degree of mastery of each objective measured by the test. The Objective Performance Index (OPI) scores indicate the projected number of items a student would get correct if there were 100 items in this specific area (CTB/McGraw-Hill, 2001). For each objective, the Individual Profile Report provides the student's OPI, the National Average OPI, and the difference (DIFF) between the student's OPI and the National Average OPI. The circles that are fully darkened, half-darkened, or blank indicate the level of mastery—low degree of mastery is indicated by a blank circle; moderate degree of mastery is in-

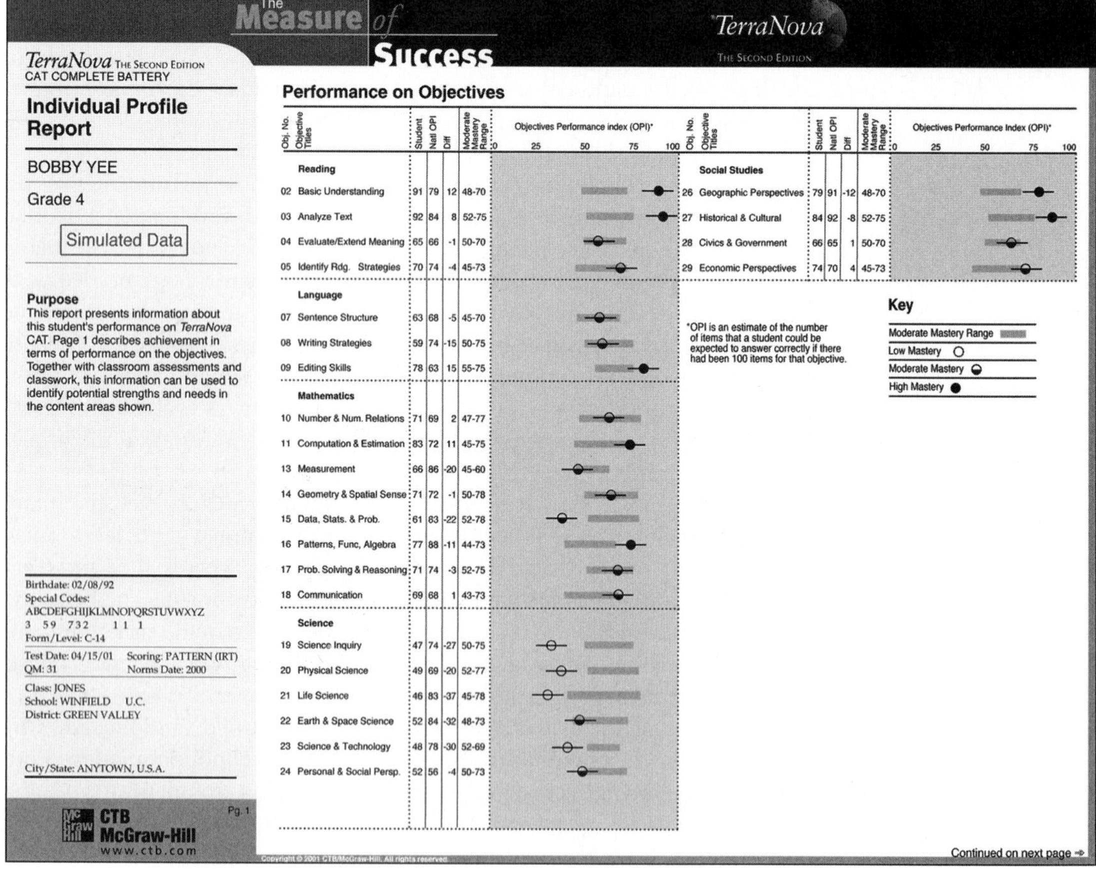

The Measure of Success

TerraNova THE SECOND EDITION

TerraNova THE SECOND EDITION
CAT COMPLETE BATTERY

Individual Profile Report

BOBBY YEE

Grade 4

Simulated Data

Purpose
This report presents information about this student's performance on *TerraNova* CAT. Page 1 describes achievement in terms of performance on the objectives. Together with classroom assessments and classwork, this information can be used to identify potential strengths and needs in the content areas shown.

Birthdate: 02/08/92
Special Codes:
ABCDEFGHIJKLMNOPQRSTUVWXYZ
3 59 732 11 1
Form/Level: C-14

Test Date: 04/15/01 Scoring: PATTERN (IRT)
QM: 31 Norms Date: 2000

Class: JONES
School: WINFIELD U.C.
District: GREEN VALLEY

City/State: ANYTOWN, U.S.A.

CTB McGraw-Hill
www.ctb.com

Pg. 1

Performance on Objectives

Obj. No.	Objective Titles	Student	Natl OPI	Diff	Moderate Mastery Range
	Reading				
02	Basic Understanding	91	79	12	48-70
03	Analyze Text	92	84	8	52-75
04	Evaluate/Extend Meaning	65	66	-1	50-70
05	Identify Rdg. Strategies	70	74	-4	45-73
	Language				
07	Sentence Structure	63	68	-5	45-70
08	Writing Strategies	59	74	-15	50-75
09	Editing Skills	78	63	15	55-75
	Mathematics				
10	Number & Num. Relations	71	69	2	47-77
11	Computation & Estimation	83	72	11	45-75
13	Measurement	66	86	-20	45-60
14	Geometry & Spatial Sense	71	72	-1	50-78
15	Data, Stats. & Prob.	61	83	-22	52-78
16	Patterns, Func, Algebra	77	88	-11	44-73
17	Prob. Solving & Reasoning	71	74	-3	52-75
18	Communication	69	68	1	43-73
	Science				
19	Science Inquiry	47	74	-27	50-75
20	Physical Science	49	69	-20	52-77
21	Life Science	46	83	-37	45-78
22	Earth & Space Science	52	84	-32	48-73
23	Science & Technology	48	78	-30	52-69
24	Personal & Social Persp.	52	56	-4	50-73
	Social Studies				
26	Geographic Perspectives	79	91	-12	48-70
27	Historical & Cultural	84	92	-8	52-75
28	Civics & Government	66	65	1	50-70
29	Economic Perspectives	74	70	4	45-73

Objectives Performance Index (OPI)* 0 25 50 75 100

*OPI is an estimate of the number of items that a student could be expected to answer correctly if there had been 100 items for that objective.

Key
Moderate Mastery Range
Low Mastery
Moderate Mastery
High Mastery

Continued on next page

FIGURE 8.1 *Example of TerraNova Individual Report (page 1)*
From TerraNova, CTB/McGraw-Hill. Reprinted by permission of The McGraw-Hill Companies.

dicated by a half-darkened circle, and high degree of mastery is indicated by a fully darkened circle. The classifications of low, moderate, or high degree of mastery are based on teachers' judgments about what students should know and be able to do in each content area. The information in this section of the profile is designed to help teachers and parents identify specific content areas that need remediation. The lines to each side of the circles indicate standard error of measurement and the confidence bands. It should be noted that some OPI scores are based on only four questions; thus, there are questions about these scores adequately representing the specific academic area (CTB/McGraw-Hill, 2001).

The second page of the Individual Profile Report (see Figure 8.2) contains norm-referenced information. The section labeled "Norm-Referenced Scores" compares the individual test taker with individuals at the same grade level and with national percentile scores (NP). NP ranges are always provided. The NP ranges are based on standard error of measurement and provide an indication of the range of average scores. Other scores, such as national stanines, grade equivalents, or local percentiles, can also be presented. The text under the graph is designed to summarize the student's performance in the specific content area. Counselors can use this text to provide parents with detailed information on a student's academic strengths and limitations (CTB/McGraw-Hill, 2001).

FIGURE 8.2
Example of TerraNova Individual Report (page 2)
From TerraNova, CTB/McGraw-Hill. Reprinted by permission of The McGraw-Hill Companies.

TerraNova THE SECOND EDITION

CAT COMPLETE BATTERY

Individual Profile Report

KEN JONES

Grade: 4

Simulated Data

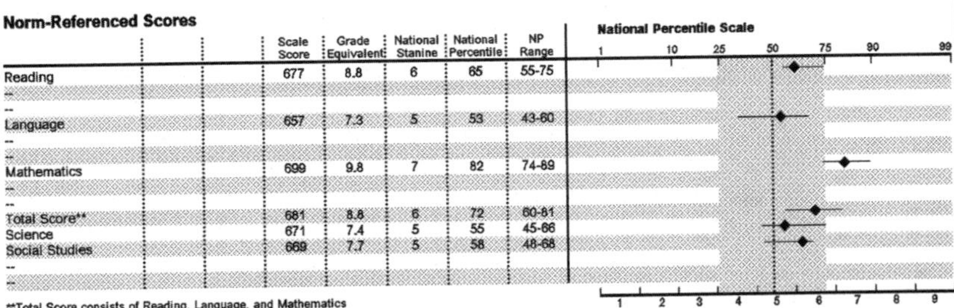

Norm-Referenced Scores

			Scale Score	Grade Equivalent	National Stanine	National Percentile	NP Range
Reading			677	8.8	6	65	55-75
--							
--							
Language			657	7.3	5	53	43-60
--							
--							
Mathematics			699	9.8	7	82	74-89
--							
--							
Total Score**			681	8.8	6	72	60-81
Science			671	7.4	5	55	45-66
Social Studies			669	7.7	5	58	48-68
--							
--							

**Total Score consists of Reading, Language, and Mathematics

Purpose
Page 2 of this report presents norm-referenced information as well as descriptions of the kinds of knowledge, skills, and abilities assessed on the *TerraNova* CAT achievement test. In the descriptions, statements describing written responses refer only to the Multiple Assessments edition of the test.

The following are content area descriptions of the kinds of knowledge, skills, and abilities assessed on the *TerraNova* CAT achievement test.

In Reading...
The student demonstrated most of the following knowledge, skills, and abilities assessed in this content area.
Students read thematically linked passages of varying degrees of difficulty, including short selections from classic and contemporary children's fiction, informative articles from children's books or periodicals, and several poems. Students show knowledge of grade-level vocabulary and comprehension of literal meaning and sequence. They restate main ideas and themes, analyze texts, compare elements within a text, demonstrate some understanding of literary techniques, and read critically to evaluate fictional and factual materials. They also apply reading strategies, using context clues to understand unfamiliar vocabulary and interpreting time lines, charts, or idea webs. In the writing section, students explain imagery and character motivation, recall similar elements in different stories, and draw a simple diagram of what happens in a reading passage.

In Language Arts...
The student demonstrated most of the following knowledge, skills, and abilities assessed in this content area.
Students show an understanding of language skills in single items as well as items in contexts. Contexts are usually paragraph-long book reports, first-person narratives, or informational passages; vocabulary is on or below grade level. Students recognize complete and concise sentences and determine the best way to combine simple sentences. They demonstrate knowledge of paragraph development--for example, choosing appropriate topic and supporting sentences. Students recognize the correct use of verbs, pronouns, adjectives, and letter conventions, such as salutation and closing. In the writing section, students respond to a given topic and proofread a given paragraph and their own writing for sentence structure, usage, spelling, capitalization, and punctuation.

In Mathematics...
The student demonstrated most of the following knowledge, skills, and abilities assessed in this content area.
Students recognize numbers to 1000; identify odd, even, and ordinal numbers; identify common fractions; recognize equivalent forms of numbers; use a number line; add and subtract whole or decimal numbers with or without regrouping; multiply and divide by one-digit numbers; estimate with numbers and money; solve one-step addition and subtraction word problems; use appropriate measurement units and tools; measure lengths to the nearest inch; tell time to the nearest fifteen minutes; find perimeter; recognize/subdivide common shapes; recognize congruency and symmetry; identify coordinates on a grid; identify geometric transformations; read and complete tables and graphs and draw conclusions; find probabilities; find missing elements and extend numerical or geometric patterns; apply logical reasoning; explain mathematical ideas or processes using words or symbols.

In Science...
The student demonstrated most of the following knowledge, skills, and abilities assessed in this content area.
Students demonstrate introductory knowledge of basic science concepts, such as classification and characteristics of organisms, habitats and adaptations, food webs and other aspects of ecology, force and motion, energy, the solar system, rock types, the water cycle, and weather; knowledge of science inquiry, including the ability to design very simple experiments, to read and interpret data presented in tables, charts, and graphs, and to infer the purpose of an experiment from the data collected for the experiment; introductory knowledge of technological design issues and the uses of new kinds of technology; and knowledge of personal and social aspects of science such as health and nutrition, recycling and resource management, and environmental issues.

In Social Studies...
The student demonstrated most of the following knowledge, skills, and abilities assessed in this content area.
Students use a variety of maps; identify regions of the U.S. and major geographic features and states within those regions; associate countries with continents; know how the environment affects peoples' lives; use time lines and different historical sources to compare past and present, recognize examples of change; know some historic events and documents; identify reference sources; use flow charts and diagrams to show knowledge of the election process, the responsibility of voters and elected officials, the basic differences between local, state, and national governments; understand how goods are produced and distributed, the concept of supply and demand, the role of budgeting in everyday life. In their written responses, students are asked to complete bar graphs and time lines, make comparisons, combine information from different sources, give explanations.

For more information, refer to the *Guide to the Individual Profile Report*, or visit CTB's website, www.ctb.com.

Birthdate: 02/08/86
Special Codes:
ABCDEFGHIJKLMNOPQRSTUVWXYZ
3 5 9 7 3 2 1 1 1
Form/Level: C-14

Test Date: 04/15/01 Scoring: PATTERN (IRT)
QM: 31 Norms Date: 2000

Class: JONES
School: WINFIELD
District: GREEN VALLEY

City/State: WINFIELD, CA

CTBID: 01075M016155002-02-00001

CTB McGraw-Hill

Page 2

The estimates of reliability for the TerraNova vary by the length of the test, the content domain, and the grade level of the assessment. In general, the reliability coefficients range from the low .70s to the middle .90s. In terms of validation evidence, the instrument's authors documented that the assessments were developed to correspond to national trends in terms of curriculum at each grade level. Furthermore, there is substantial information on convergent and discriminant validity, which primarily involved correlating the TerraNova scores with other measures of achievement and cognitive ability (CTB/McGraw-Hill, 2002).

Individual Achievement Tests and Diagnostic Achievement Tests

The second type of achievement tests concerns those instruments that are administered individually. These achievement tests are often used in psychoeducational evaluations in which children are screened for learning disabilities, mental handicaps, or behavioral disorders or for other academic referrals (Sattler, 2002). For example, frequently an individual achievement test is given in conjunction with a general abilities measure to diagnose learning disabilities. Some of these achievement instruments are appropriate for adults and can be used to provide retraining for adults (e.g., vocational rehabilitation) to assess the academic skills a person has retained.

An individually administered achievement test is the *Kaufman Test of Educational Achievement—Second Edition* (KTEA-II; Kaufman & Kaufman, 2004). This test comes in two forms: the Brief Form and the Comprehensive Form. The Brief Form covers reading, spelling, and mathematics. The Comprehensive Form is more extensive and was expanded, particularly related to reading, from the earlier version (i.e., the KTEA). The Reading Composite is comprised of two subscales, which are the Letter and Word Recognition and Reading Comprehension. There are six additional Reading-Related Subtests: Phonological Awareness, Nonsense Word Decoding, Word Recognition Fluency, Decoding Fluency, Associational Fluency, and Naming Facility. Bonner (2005) evaluated this grouping of reading scores to be appropriate because the Reading Composite is a measure of reading outcome and the reading-related subscales can help identify reading-related tasks that may need remediation. The KTEA-II also includes a Math Composite score that consists of two subscales: Math Concepts and Applications, and Math Computation. The fourth composite is Written Language and includes Written Expression and Spelling. There is also a fifth composite called Oral Language, which assesses Listening Comprehension and Oral Expression. The final score is a Comprehensive Achievement Composite. The comprehensive form of the KTEA-II, which is appropriate for individuals ages 4–6 through 25, was co-normed with KABC-II (see Chapter 7). There are two alternate forms of KTEA-II so that progress can be monitored, which is an asset particularly as it relates to the Individuals with Disabilities Education Act (IDEA, see Chapter 14).

There is also a major individual achievement test that is associated with a family of well-respected instruments—the *Wechsler Individual Achievement Test-Second Edition* (WIAT-II; Wechsler, 2001). The WIAT-II is standardized with the widely used Wechsler intelligence instruments (i.e., WISC-IV, WPPSI-III, WAIS-III). The WIAT-II can be used with individuals from 4 years old through adulthood. The WIAT-II contains 10 subtests: Oral Language, Listening, Comprehension, Written Expression, Spelling, Pseudoword Decoding, Word Reading, Reading Comprehension, Numerical Operations, and Mathematics Reasoning. Every examinee does not need to take all of the subtests. There is also a shortened version (*Wechsler Individual Achievement Test II—Abbreviated*, WIAT-II-A), which takes about 10 to 20 minutes to administer. The WIAT-II-A measures the subtests of Spelling, Word Reading, and Numerical Operations. The nonabbreviated form of the WIAT-II is designed to be used with individuals ranging in age from 4 to 85. Doll (2003) contended that the authors of the WIAT-II should be commended for their decision to align this achievement test with timely research in learning and assessment of academic knowledge. Doll argued, however, that many users of the WIAT-II will be challenged by this level of conceptual sophistication and more materials are needed to educate users about the research and implications of using the WIAT-II.

Earlier versions of the Wide Range Achievement Test have often been used and a new version, the *Wide Range Achievement Test 4* (WRAT4; Wilkinson & Robertson, 2007), has recently been released. The WRAT4 assesses achievement in the areas of reading, spelling, and arithmetic. The WRAT4 was developed to assess the basic academic skills of individuals ages 5 through 94. Consistent with other individually administered achievement tests, Robertson (2002) developed an expanded version of the WRAT and it is anticipated that an expanded version of the WRAT4 will also be developed. The current WRAT-Expanded has two forms: Form G for group administered assessment and Form I for individually administered assessment.

As has been alluded to, individual achievement tests are often used concurrently with individual intelligent tests to diagnose learning disabilities. As will be discussed shortly, this is often called the discrepancy model and the Woodcock-Johnson was developed to examine these discrepancies. The *Woodcock-Johnson III Complete Battery*, an updated version of the widely used *Woodcock-Johnson Psycho-Educational Battery—Revised*, assesses general intellectual ability, specific cognitive abilities, scholastic aptitude, oral language, and academic achievement for individuals ages 2 through 90 (McGrew & Woodcock, 2001). The Woodcock-Johnson III (WJ-III) is actually comprised of two co-normed batteries (the Woodcock-Johnson Tests of Cognitive Abilities and the Woodcock-Johnson Tests of Achievement). The WJ-III Tests of Cognitive Abilities (WJ-III-COG) measures general and specific cognitive functions; whereas, the purpose of the WJ-III Tests of Achievement (WJ-III-ACH) is to determine the individual's present academic strengths and limitations. When administered in tandem, the comprehensive battery provides information on over/underachievement and patterns of discrepancies among cognitive or achievement areas (Cizek, 2003). Standard and extended versions exist for both the WJ-III-COG and the WJ-III-ACH. The standard version of the WJ-III-COG involves 10 subtests, which can be supplemented in the extended version by another 10 subtests. The WJ-III-ACH has two parallel forms; if an examiner wants the extended version, then both versions can be administered.

The WJ-III used the Cattell, Horn, and Carroll model as the foundation for the assessment of cognitive ability. Because of co-norming of the WJ-III-ACH and the WJ-III-COG, the WJ-III instrument is often used to examine intra-individual discrepancies in achievement, variations in ability areas (e.g., verbal vs. thinking), and differences between ability and achievement (McGrew & Woodcock, 2001). Using the standard version of the WJ-III-ACH and WJ-III-COG, intra-individual comparisons are examined among the clusters of Verbal Ability, Thinking Ability, Cognitive Efficiency, Broad Reading, Broad Math, Broad Written Language, and Oral Language. Additional discrepancies can be examined with the use of the extended version of either assessment. Because examiners can choose from many different derived scores, counselors could read a report that includes one or more of the following: age equivalents, grade equivalents, relative master indices, percentile ranks, extended percentile ranks, standard scores, and extended standard scores. Counselors working in post–secondary school settings can use the WJ-III-ACH and WJ-III-COG to provide information on the abilities of nonnative speakers of English to function in informal and academic settings. There is also an instrument for bilingual assessment, the Bilingual Verbal Ability Tests (Munoz-Sandoval, Cummins, Alvarado, & Ruef, 1998) that uses subtests from the WJ-R.

Both Cizek (2003) and Sandoval (2003) positively evaluated the WJ-III. Cizek indicated that the internal consistency reliability estimates appear to be uniformly high, with major ability and achievement clusters falling in the .90s and with most of the subtests having reliability coefficients higher than .80. The normative sample included 8,818 individuals who were selected to be representative of the U.S. population.

The WJ-III is often used to assess college students with possible learning disabilities because the norming group is appropriate for that age group. The validity information is quite extensive (McGrew & Woodcock, 2001), which contributes to the use of this diagnostic instrument.

Counselors in many settings, particularly school counselors, need some understanding of the process related to assessing and identifying individuals with learning disabilities. The U.S. Department of Education (1999) reported that approximately one-half of students receiving special education services were diagnosed with a learning disability. Although most counselors will not be the clinicians performing the testing and diagnosing the disability, they should still have an understanding of some of the issues related to identifying learning disabilities. Fletcher, Lyon, Fuchs, and Barnes (2007) asserted that a significant difficulty in assessing learning disabilities concerns the findings that learning disabilities are not a homogeneous group of disorders and, therefore, it is difficult to use a one-size-fits-all model of assessment. Historically, the discrepancy model has been prevalent and continues to be used (Hallahan & Kauffman, 2002). Using the discrepancy model, the focus is on examining the differences between IQ and achievement. In the diagnosis of a learning disability, an individual is often given an individual intelligence test and an achievement test, with the intent of examining discrepancy. With the discrepancy model, a learning disability is indicated when a person is not achieving at a level consistent with his or her abilities or intelligence. Previously, if there was a difference of two standard deviations between the achievement level and intellectual level, then a learning disability was diagnosed. There has been significant debate about whether the discrepancy models accurately assesses individuals with specific learning disabilities, and Fletcher, Francis, Morris, and Lyon (2005) documented both reliability and validity problems that exist with some of the instruments often used with a discrepancy approach to diagnosing a learning disability. The 2004 reauthorization of the Individuals with Disabilities Education Act (IDEA) explicitly states that schools are *not* required to use a severe discrepancy between achievement and intellectual abilities to find that a child has a specific learning disability (see Chapter 14).

Low achievement models are another common approach to diagnosing learning disabilities (Fletcher et al., 2007). Psychologists who use this approach would assess individuals related to specific areas and, thus, counselors may also read psychological reports that involve content-specific assessments. Examples of diagnostic reading instruments are the *Stanford Diagnostic Reading Test, Fourth Edition*; the *Nelson-Denny Reading Test*; and the *Classroom Reading Inventory*. In the mathematics areas, counselors may see a report that used the *KeyMath—Revised*, the *Sequential Assessment of Mathematics Inventories*, or the *MAT6 Mathematics Diagnostic Tests*.

Flecher et al. (2007) contended that historically the underpinning of learning disabilities is unexpected underachievement. Thus, professionals cannot know if there is unexpected underachievement until the individual has had a chance to learn and then is assessed to determine if the achievement is less than would be expected. Hence, they argue that a diagnosis of learning disability cannot occur outside the realm of instruction. They contended that "No person can be defined as learning disabled in the absence of evidence of a lack of adequate response to instruction that is effective with most students" (p. 5). Bradley, Danielson, and Hallahan (2002) supported a model of identification that includes three components: (1) inadequate response to appropriate instruction; (2) poor achievement in reading, mathematics, and/or written expression; and (3) evidence that other factors, such as sensory disorders, inadequate instruction, mental retardation, and limited proficiency in the language used for instruction, are not the cause of the low achievement.

Fletcher et al. (2007) argued that the diagnosis of learning disabilities should not be a one-step process, where an individual is tested once and diagnosed. They contended that models involving Response to Interventions (RTI) better assess the complexities of learning disabilities. There are many models of RTI, which were adapted from public health models related to disease prevention and early intervention. In these models, assessments are used for screening and for monitoring progress related to interventions. With RTI models there are multiple assessments over time so that monitoring of unexpected underachievement can be examined more closely. In addition, the impact of different types of interventions can also be monitored to determine what is helping the student learn. In many school settings, counselors should be aware of the Response to Interventions approach because these interventions could become part of the interventions provided to the student with a learning disability. The RTI model is based on an understanding that there are many influences on students, and the goal is to identify interventions that will be most effective in helping students succeed. Hence, school counselors are likely to be involved in these RTI teams because school counselors are responsible for students' academic, career, and personal social development.

Criterion-Referenced Tests and Minimum-Level Skills Assessments

Criterion-referenced achievement tests are instruments designed to determine if a certain academic standard is met. Many tests you have taken for academic courses are criterion-referenced where a score at or above a certain mark merits an *A*, a lower range of scores earns a *B*, and so on. These tests are only criterion-referenced if the criterion or standard is set before the test is taken. Many times criterion-referenced tests are equated with mastery tests. In mastery tests, the person must reach a certain level of mastery before proceeding. For example, a child must be able to add one-digit numbers before advancing to a test that measures the ability to add two-digit numbers. The distinction between a criterion-referenced achievement test and a diagnostic or subject area test is sometimes quite gray, and they should not be viewed as being mutually exclusive. School districts and state departments of education have developed a number of criterion-referenced tests. In addition, some publishers have developed criterion-referenced achievement tests, such as the *TerraNova, The Second Edition*, which provides both criterion-referenced and norm-referenced information. The increasing focus within education on standards and accountability has brought about increases in the number of criterion-referenced achievement tests (Linn, Baker, & Betebenner, 2002). As will be discussed later in this chapter, federal regulations mandate that all students in third grade through eighth grade will need to be assessed each year in at least math and reading so that their progress can be measured against state standards. Another example of a criterion-referenced achievement test is the *Texas Assessment of Knowledge and Skills* (TAKS), which is designed to assess the statewide curriculum. Student knowledge of the reading curriculum in reading is assessed annually in grades 3–9. TAKS also involves testing student writing at grades 4 and 7; English/language arts at grades 10 and Exit Level; mathematics at grades 3–10 and Exit Level; science at grades 5, 10, and Exit Level; and social studies at grades 8, 10, and Exit Level. Spanish versions of the TAKS can be administered in reading and mathematics for grades 3–6, in writing at grade 4, and in science at grade 5. Currently, third graders attending public schools in Texas must pass the Grade 3 TAKS in reading before they are allowed to be promoted to the fourth grade. Fifth graders in public schools must also pass the Grade 5 TAKS in reading and mathematics before they can be promoted to sixth grade. Also, students cannot receive a high school diploma until they have passed the Exit Level TAKS test in English language arts, mathematics, science, and social studies. There are also alternative assessments such as the *Texas Assessment of Knowledge and Skills-Inclusive*, which is designed for some students who receive special education services and for whom the TAKS, even with allowable accommodations, is not appropriate. Students receiving special education services who have a curriculum that does not correspond to the state's standard would take the *State-Developed Alternative Assessment II*. There are also the *Texas English Proficiency Assessment System* and *Texas Assessment of Academic Skills* (TAAS). The TAAS is for students who have completed their graduation requirements but who are not currently enrolled in high school (e.g., adult learners).

Some authorities in the area of assessment make a distinction between criterion-referenced tests and minimum-level skills tests, although it could be argued that all minimum-level tests are criterion-referenced tests with the minimum level being the criterion for passing. The minimum-level achievement tests that have received the most attention and discussion are those that many states require for high school graduation. For example, satisfactory performance on the TAKS at grade 11 (Exit Level) is a prerequisite to a high school diploma in Texas. Over the years, there has been concern about students graduating from high school without minimum competencies. These concerns led many states to require students to pass a minimum competency examination before a high school diploma could be awarded. However, states vary widely in what they require and at what grade level students are tested. Another issue concerns the relationship between the instrument and the curriculum. Because these are achievement tests, minimum competency examinations need to be related to the curriculum. This is not always easy, because even students within the same high school can take very different academic courses. There is also some controversy concerning the minimum competencies expected of high school graduates. For example, there are diverse views on the minimum reading level for a high school graduate. In addition, some students have learning disabilities that might affect their performances on a portion of the tests even though they can do very well in other academic areas. Consequently, numerous difficulties exist in developing and implementing minimum competency examinations.

Subject Area Tests

Single subject tests, developed by teachers, constitute the largest area of achievement tests. These instruments vary in quality, with some teachers developing quite refined assessments and other teachers designing instruments with major flaws. In addition, many textbooks now provide test item banks for which the publishers develop numerous test questions that assess material covered in the text. Whether teachers develop their own items or incorporate items from a test bank, content validity must be considered. Teachers need to ensure that the tests they use adequately reflect the behavior domains being measured. The steps toward ensuring content validity, discussed in Chapter 4, need to be incorporated in developing a subject area test. For example, teachers who develop a test specifications table before the items are written are more likely to develop a sound examination because the test will follow this framework rather than being randomly assembled.

As mentioned earlier, advocates of authentic assessment and performance assessment have had a major influence on teacher-developed subject area tests (Oosterhof, 1994). Authentic and performance assessments strive for greater realism and complexity of tasks. The belief is that simplistic assessments with one correct answer are not adequate measures because real-life problems can often be solved in multiple ways. Hence, in performance assessment there are often multiple solutions. In addition, those who support changing achievement testing argue that one short test cannot adequately measure an individual's abilities. They suggest that multiple measures gathered over a period time provide a more authentic assessment of the individual's achievement level or ability to perform. Starting in the early 1990s there was a movement toward *portfolio assessment*, in which teachers systematically collect multiple indicators of performance.

The assessment then focuses on the total evaluation of the products in the portfolio. The rationale is that with evidence of performance on multiple tasks, better evaluation of the student's strengths and limitations can occur (Gronlund, 1998). Authentic or performance assessment, however, is not simple to implement, and implementing it appropriately requires a substantial commitment of time.

Issues in Achievement Testing

One of the major issues in achievement testing is the increases of standardized achievement testing in all 50 states (Tindal, 2002). This testing has sometimes been labeled high stakes testing because of how the assessment information may be used. Although some states began instituting "high stakes," in the early 1990s, with the passage of the No Child Left Behind Act (NCLB) of 2001, all states needed to institute an assessment program. This law focuses on educational accountability by examining the progress of individual students (Dollarhide & Lemberger, 2006). In terms of accountability, the law stipulates that all students in grades 3 through 8 (not just Title I students) must be assessed annually in at least math and reading so that their progress can be measured against state standards (Linn, Baker, & Betebenner, 2002). Each state must develop measurable adequate yearly progress (AYP) objectives to ensure that students have reached the determined objectives. Furthermore, there must be objectives for specific groups, such as economically disadvantaged students, students from major racial and ethnic groups, students with disabilities, and students with limited English proficiency. The adequate yearly progress objectives are measured at the school level, and schools that do not meet the state objectives for two years are identified as needing improvement. The states were given 12 years (i.e., the end of the 2013–2014 school year) to show that 100% of their students are performing at the proficient level or above. However, they had to have the annual reading and math testing for grades 3 through 8 in place by the 2005–2006 school year. According to Linn et al. (2002), one of the issues with this act is the variation among states in terms of performance standards and the lack of uniformity in measures to determine if students are making adequate progress. Consequently, states will most likely vary significantly in terms of the percentage of students who are proficient in, for example, reading at the eighth-grade level. To address this issue and verify state assessments, a sample of students in grades 4 and 8 will be required to take the National Assessment of Educational Progress (NAEP) in reading and mathematics.

The NAEP, also known as "the Nation's Report Card," is the only national assessment of students' knowledge and performance in various subject areas. Since its inception in 1969, it has been used periodically to assess student achievement nationally in reading, mathematics, science, writing, U.S. history, civics, geography, and the arts. The NAEP does not provide evaluation of individual students or even schools because the original intent of the NAEP was to report on the achievement of the nation, to examine performance of demographic subgroups, and to track trends in educational progress over time (National Center for Education Statistics, 2003). Only since 1990 has the NAEP been used to provide feedback to participating states. Before the No Child Left Behind (NCLB) legislation, the purpose of NAEP was to survey what students knew and were able to do. State and school participation was voluntary.

After NCLB, the NAEP assessments have taken on a new role, and states and school districts, if selected, must participate in reading and math assessment every two years. It should be noted that when states are assessed, only a sample of students will be required to participate. The student sample for a state is drawn to be representative of that state, and minority students and students attending private schools are oversampled to provide a sufficient sample size for mandated subgroup analyses (Hombo, 2003). The NAEP uses both objective and constructed response items. Sample questions are available to school districts. After each administration of the assessment, about 30% of the items are replaced. Although item pools are not identical from year to year, item response theory is used to ensure comparable items and to ensure that subject area and content subdomains are assessed consistently over time.

The intent of the NCLB law is to hold schools accountable for student learning and to ensure that all students are proficient in the areas of reading and math. As mentioned earlier, there are some concerns with high-stakes testing and the effects it could have on individuals. One concern relates to schools labeled as "needing improvement" and the stigma attached with that designation. Many parents, particularly those with financial means, may transfer their children out of those schools into private schools; thus, leaving those schools with students primarily from lower socioeconomic backgrounds. In general, students from lower socioeconomic backgrounds do not perform as well on achievement tests because they often do not have the access to the same activities that families from higher-income levels have (e.g., computers at home, private tutors, summer enrichment programs). Hence, schools labeled as needing improvement may have a higher percentage of lower-achieving students, which increases the possibility that the students' scores will continue to be lower. It is difficult to ascertain the impact on students who are attending a school that "needs improvement" because it may influence their motivation and attitude toward their school. It may also have an influence on parents and their feelings about sending their children to a school that is considered substandard.

Another issue concerns students who do not pass or meet the criterion established by the state. As indicated earlier, in Texas, third grade students who do not pass the reading portion of the state test (i.e., the TAKS) cannot be promoted to the fourth grade. The American Psychological Association (2001) has taken a stand on this type of testing:

> Measuring what and how well students learn is an important building block in the process of strengthening and improving our nation's schools. Tests, along with student grades and teacher evaluations, can provide critical measures of students' skills, knowledge, and abilities. Therefore, tests should be part of a system in which broad and equitable access to educational opportunity and advancement is provided to all students. Tests, when used properly, are among the most sound and objective ways to measure student performance. But, when test results are used inappropriately or as a single measure of performance, they can have unintended adverse consequences. (p.1)

Some states (e.g., Illinois, Indiana, Florida) are moving beyond testing only in mathematics and reading and now test students in other curriculum areas, such as science, social studies, and writing. In most of these states, not every academic area is tested every year; however, the legislatures of these states have voted to gather more testing information than that required by NCLB. I believe this trend reflects a general interest in what children have learned and the belief that schools and teachers must be monitored closely to ensure they are doing a good job. The pertinent question is whether these increases in achievement tests actually benefit children's learning.

One of the concerns voiced by the National Research Council's Committee on the Foundations of Assessment (2001) is that there is a disconnect between large-scale assessment of academic achievement and current knowledge about human cognition and learning. Their vision is that assessment at all levels (i.e., from classroom to state) will work together in a system that is comprehensive, coherent, and continuous. Furthermore, these assessments will be linked back to the same underlying model of student learning.

There are also questions related to high-stakes testing about students who are not performing well and whether one test will be used for decisions such as promotion and graduation (Horn, 2003). As indicted earlier, many states already have minimum competencies examinations that students must pass to graduate from high school. The American Educational Research Association (2000) issued a position statement concerning high-stakes testing in pre-K–12 education. This statement is based on the *Standards for Educational and Psychological Testing* (AERA, APA, & NCME, 1999), which represents a professional consensus concerning sound and appropriate test use in education and psychology and which is discussed more thoroughly in Chapter 14. Central to AERA's (2000) argument is the premise that decisions that affect an individual student's life chances or educational opportunities should not be based on one test score, which is consistent with APA's position that was mentioned earlier. Furthermore, AERA contended that all high-stakes achievement testing programs in education should meet the conditions of (1) adequate resources and opportunities to learn; (2) validation for each separate intended use; (3) full disclosure of likely negative consequences of high-stakes testing programs; (4) alignment between the test and the curriculum; (5) validity of passing scores and achievement levels; (6) opportunities for meaningful remediation for examinees who fail high-stakes tests; (7) appropriate attention to language differences among examinees; (8) appropriate attention to students with disabilities; (9) careful adherence to explicit rules for determining which students are to be tested; (10) sufficient reliability for each intended use; and (11) ongoing evaluation of intended and unintended effects of high-stakes testing. In conclusion, it is clear that achievement testing will continue to have a major role in educational decisions and policies and that the debates about high-stakes testing will continue. The reauthorization process of the No Child Left Behind Act is in the beginning stages at the writing of this book and counselors in diverse settings need to be aware of changes in this type of legislation.

Aptitude Assessment

Because this chapter addresses both achievement and aptitude assessment, it is important to begin a discussion on aptitude assessment that emphasizes that the purposes of aptitude assessments are quite different from achievement testing.

Achievement testing provides information on what the individual has learned to-date, whereas aptitude testing provides an indication of how the individual will perform in the future. Clients often seek counseling to make decisions about the future; thus, knowledge of aptitude testing is often useful. Some aptitude instruments predict the ability to acquire a specific type of skill or knowledge, and others predict performance in a certain job or career. Aptitude instruments are frequently used to predict future academic performance (e.g., success in college). The pertinent issue with any aptitude instrument is the degree to which it predicts relative to the criterion of interest.

Scholastic Aptitude Tests

Hood and Johnson (2007) argued that counselors in a variety of settings (e.g., mental health agencies, elementary schools) need to be knowledgeable about the predominant scholastic aptitude tests. They contended that counselors in most settings are consulted by friends, relatives, and colleagues whose children are applying to colleges and universities. Traditionally, the public has expected counselors to be knowledgeable of these prevalent instruments. Hence, counselors who do not have at least a working knowledge of these instruments may not be viewed as credible by some individuals.

Scholastic Assessment Test. The Scholastic Assessment Test (SAT) is a well-established and widely used predictor of college performance. In 1994, the Scholastic Aptitude Test, which had been around since 1926, was revised and renamed the Scholastic Assessment Test. Part of the reason for changing the name of the SAT was to move away from any reference that might imply that the instrument measures innate aptitudes. The College Board SAT program of assessments includes the SAT Reasoning Test and the SAT Subject Test.

The SAT Reasoning Test is designed to measure critical thinking skills that are needed for academic success in college. The SAT is the most widely used assessment for college admissions (College Board SAT, 2007). It is typically taken during students' junior and senior years in high school. The instrument originated to provide a common standard to which students could be compared because subject matter of high school courses and grading procedures varied so widely.

The SAT Reasoning Test consists of nine sections, including a 25-minute essay. The academic areas assessed and the numbers of items pertaining to the content areas are listed in Table 8.2 on the next page. Students' scores range from 200 to 800. The scores on the critical reading, math, and writing sections have a mean of 500 and a standard deviation of 100. The scores on the Critical Reasoning and Mathematics section are comparable to the Verbal and Mathematics sections of the earlier version of the SAT. The current version, SAT Reasoning, includes a Writing section where, in addition to other subtests, the students write an essay. If a student takes the SAT more than once, their scoring report will include up to six previous scores. These cumulative scoring reports will be sent to a student's high school and colleges to which a student has applied (College Board SAT, 2007).

TABLE 8.2
Content of SAT Reasoning Test

Section	Content	Number of Questions	Time
Critical Reading	Extended Reasoning	36–40	70 minutes (two 25-minute sections and one 20-minute section)
	Literal Comprehension	4–6	
	Vocabulary in Context	4–6	
	Sentence Completions	19	
	Total	**67**	
Mathematics	Number and Operations	11–14	70 minutes (two 25-minute sections and one 20-minute section)
	Algebra and Functions	19–22	
	Geometry and Measurement	14–16	
	Data Analysis, Statistics, and Probability	5–8	
	Total	**54**	
Writing	Essay	1	60 minutes (one 25-minute essay, one 25-minute multiple-choice section, and one 10-minute multiple-choice section)
	Improving Sentences	25	
	Identifying Sentence Errors	18	
	Improving Paragraphs	6	
	Total	**50**	

Educational Testing Service (ETS) uses a complex equating process that adjusts for variation in difficulty from one edition to the next. In addition, counselors can find significant free resources on the CollegeBoard website (http://www.collegeboard.org) to assist students in preparing for the SAT Reasoning Test. The SAT report includes an overall Writing score and subscores on the Multiple Choice and Essay sections. These scores indicate possible strengths and limitations because a student could score well on the multiple-choice items but get a low score on his or her essay. The scores on Multiple Choice range from 20 to 80 and the essay subscores range from 2 to 12.

This report provides information about the institutions to which the student requested his or her SAT scores be sent and matches it with information the student reported (e.g., grade point average, desired size of school). Counselors can also use the Personal and College Profiles, which are sent to students and their high schools. The Personal and College Profiles are also sent to colleges. These profiles provide personal information (e.g., courses taken while in high school) and information about the colleges the student has selected so that school counselors have information readily available.

The SAT Subject Tests are designed to measure students' knowledge in a specific area. These assess not just content knowledge; they also measure whether students can apply the concepts pertinent to the particular areas. Students can take assessments in the areas of English, mathematics, science, and foreign languages. In the foreign languages tests, the students both listen and read in the tested language. Students are required to bring an acceptable CD player with earphones.

An instrument related to the SAT is the Preliminary SAT/National Merit Scholarship Qualifying Test (PSAT/NMSQT). The PSAT/NMSQT provides students with an estimate of how they will perform on the SAT and is used for national scholarship and recognition programs. Students typically take the PSAT/NMSQT during their junior year in high school. Scores range from 20 to 80 and are designed to be comparable to the SAT by adding a zero (e.g., a score of 55 on the Verbal section of the PSAT/NMSQT would be predictive of a score of 550). The PSAT/NMSQT can be an effective tool in counseling students who are facing decisions about college. For instance, a counselor may want to talk with a student who is planning to attend a very selective college but who has low scores on the PSAT/NMSQT. A publication entitled *Guidelines on the Uses of College Board Test Scores and Related Data* (College Entrance Examination Board, 2002) is designed for school counselors who need to be knowledgeable about the SAT, the PSAT/NMSQT, and other College Board assessments, such as the Advanced Placement Program and the College-Level Examination Program. This helpful resource, which can be retrieved from the College Board website (http://www.collegeboard.com), addresses counselors' responsibilities in using these assessments.

ACT Inc. The other major nationally administered college admissions testing program is the ACT. The ACT is the test students often take in either eleventh or twelfth grade, and many colleges use these scores in making decisions about admission. The ACT is part of ACT's Educational Planning and Assessment System (EPAS), which provides a series of assessment programs for students. EXPLORE, which includes achievement tests in English, mathematics, reading, and science, is for eighth-grade students. In addition to these tests, EXPLORE also includes an interest inventory, a study skills checklist, and a coursework planner. PLAN, a similar instrument designed for tenth-grade students, tests academic achievement and facilitates postsecondary planning. The tool for eleventh and twelfth-graders is the ACT. Although it is not part of the EPAS, ACT also publishes Work Keys, an instrument designed to assess workplace skills rather than more traditional academic skills. Work Keys can be used by schools or businesses and can be helpful in tech-prep, school-to-careers, and workforce development initiatives.

The developers of the ACT have attempted to measure as directly as possible the knowledge and skills students will need to perform college-level work (ACT, 2005). The content of the ACT is curriculum-based and tests students' knowledge in English, mathematics, reading, and science. There is an optional writing subtest. In 2002–2003 ACT (ACT, 2003) sought to improve the content of the test and conducted a review of 49 states' standards, surveyed 16,363 school teachers and 10,565 postsecondary faculty who teach entry-level courses, and convened a panel of experts.

An example of the *ACT Plus Writing Student Report* is included in Figure 8.3 on pages 192–193. As can be seen from scores in the upper left portion of the front of the report, students' performance is reflected in a Composite Score and the four major areas of English, mathematics, reading, and science. On these scales the scores range from

FIGURE 8.3

A sample of ACT results

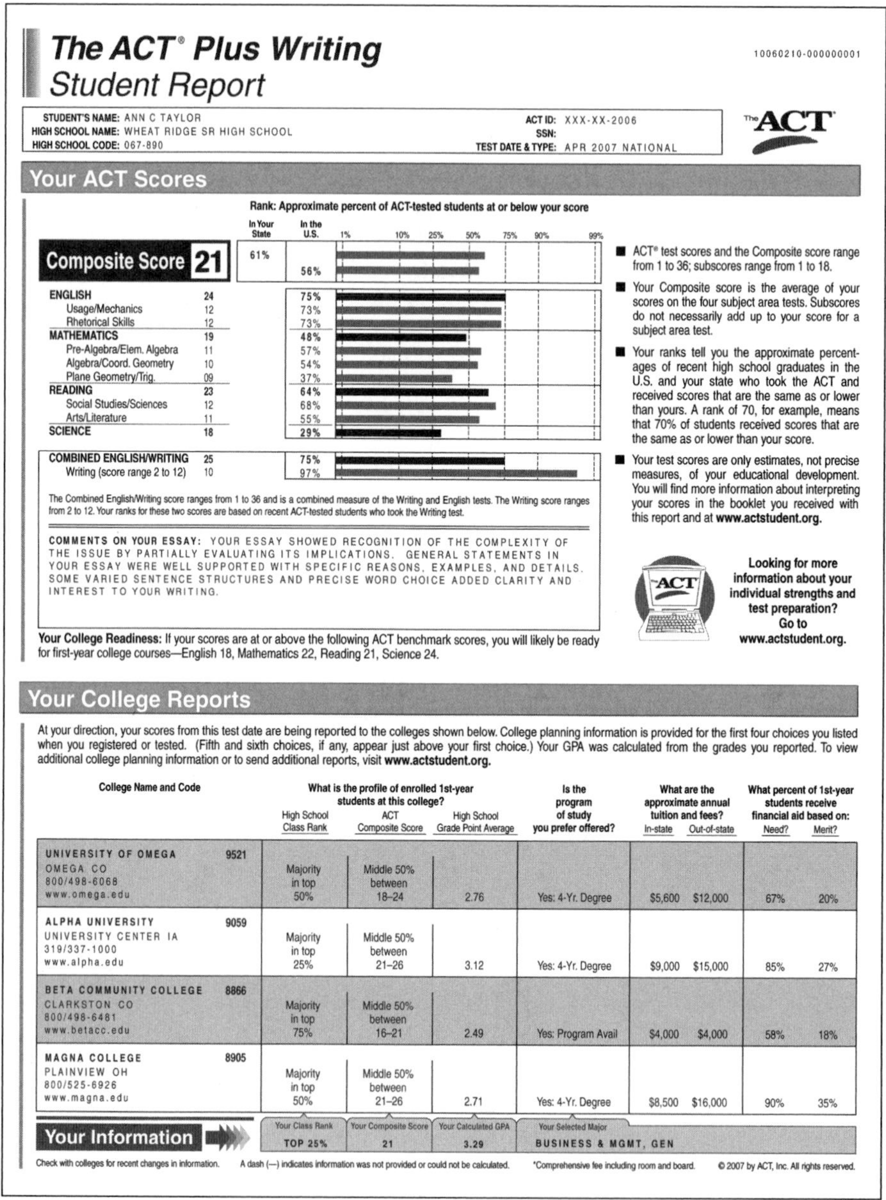

The ACT® Plus Writing
Student Report

10060210-000000001

STUDENT'S NAME: ANN C TAYLOR
HIGH SCHOOL NAME: WHEAT RIDGE SR HIGH SCHOOL
HIGH SCHOOL CODE: 067-890
ACT ID: XXX-XX-2006
SSN:
TEST DATE & TYPE: APR 2007 NATIONAL

The ACT

Your ACT Scores

Rank: Approximate percent of ACT-tested students at or below your score

	Score	In Your State	In the U.S.
Composite Score	21	61%	56%
ENGLISH	24		75%
Usage/Mechanics	12		73%
Rhetorical Skills	12		73%
MATHEMATICS	19		48%
Pre-Algebra/Elem. Algebra	11		57%
Algebra/Coord. Geometry	10		54%
Plane Geometry/Trig.	09		37%
READING	23		64%
Social Studies/Sciences	12		68%
Arts/Literature	11		55%
SCIENCE	18		29%
COMBINED ENGLISH/WRITING	25		75%
Writing (score range 2 to 12)	10		97%

The Combined English/Writing score ranges from 1 to 36 and is a combined measure of the Writing and English tests. The Writing score ranges from 2 to 12. Your ranks for these two scores are based on recent ACT-tested students who took the Writing test.

COMMENTS ON YOUR ESSAY: YOUR ESSAY SHOWED RECOGNITION OF THE COMPLEXITY OF THE ISSUE BY PARTIALLY EVALUATING ITS IMPLICATIONS. GENERAL STATEMENTS IN YOUR ESSAY WERE WELL SUPPORTED WITH SPECIFIC REASONS, EXAMPLES, AND DETAILS. SOME VARIED SENTENCE STRUCTURES AND PRECISE WORD CHOICE ADDED CLARITY AND INTEREST TO YOUR WRITING.

Your College Readiness: If your scores are at or above the following ACT benchmark scores, you will likely be ready for first-year college courses—English 18, Mathematics 22, Reading 21, Science 24.

- ACT® test scores and the Composite score range from 1 to 36; subscores range from 1 to 18.
- Your Composite score is the average of your scores on the four subject area tests. Subscores do not necessarily add up to your score for a subject area test.
- Your ranks tell you the approximate percentages of recent high school graduates in the U.S. and your state who took the ACT and received scores that are the same as or lower than yours. A rank of 70, for example, means that 70% of students received scores that are the same as or lower than your score.
- Your test scores are only estimates, not precise measures, of your educational development. You will find more information about interpreting your scores in the booklet you received with this report and at **www.actstudent.org.**

Looking for more information about your individual strengths and test preparation? Go to www.actstudent.org.

Your College Reports

At your direction, your scores from this test date are being reported to the colleges shown below. College planning information is provided for the first four choices you listed when you registered or tested. (Fifth and sixth choices, if any, appear just above your first choice.) Your GPA was calculated from the grades you reported. To view additional college planning information or to send additional reports, visit **www.actstudent.org.**

College Name and Code		What is the profile of enrolled 1st-year students at this college? High School Class Rank	ACT Composite Score	High School Grade Point Average	Is the program of study you prefer offered?	What are the approximate annual tuition and fees? In-state	Out-of-state	What percent of 1st-year students receive financial aid based on: Need?	Merit?
UNIVERSITY OF OMEGA, OMEGA CO, 800/498-6068, www.omega.edu	9521	Majority in top 50%	Middle 50% between 18–24	2.76	Yes: 4-Yr. Degree	$5,600	$12,000	67%	20%
ALPHA UNIVERSITY, UNIVERSITY CENTER IA, 319/337-1000, www.alpha.edu	9059	Majority in top 25%	Middle 50% between 21–26	3.12	Yes: 4-Yr. Degree	$9,000	$15,000	85%	27%
BETA COMMUNITY COLLEGE, CLARKSTON CO, 800/498-6481, www.betacc.edu	8866	Majority in top 75%	Middle 50% between 16–21	2.49	Yes: Program Avail	$4,000	$4,000	58%	18%
MAGNA COLLEGE, PLAINVIEW OH, 800/525-6926, www.magna.edu	8905	Majority in top 50%	Middle 50% between 21–26	2.71	Yes: 4-Yr. Degree	$8,500	$16,000	90%	35%
Your Information		Your Class Rank: TOP 25%	Your Composite Score: 21	Your Calculated GPA: 3.29	Your Selected Major: BUSINESS & MGMT, GEN				

Check with colleges for recent changes in information. A dash (—) indicates information was not provided or could not be calculated. *Comprehensive fee including room and board. © 2007 by ACT, Inc. All rights reserved.

1 to 36 and percentile scores are included in the report. For the Composite Score, both state and national percentile scores are provided. There are also subscale scores in English, Mathematics, and Reading, which are designed to provide more detailed information about strengths and limitations in those areas. The subscale scores range from 1 to 18 and percentiles are reported for each of the subscales. If students take the optional Writing Test, which is often required for college entrance and/or course

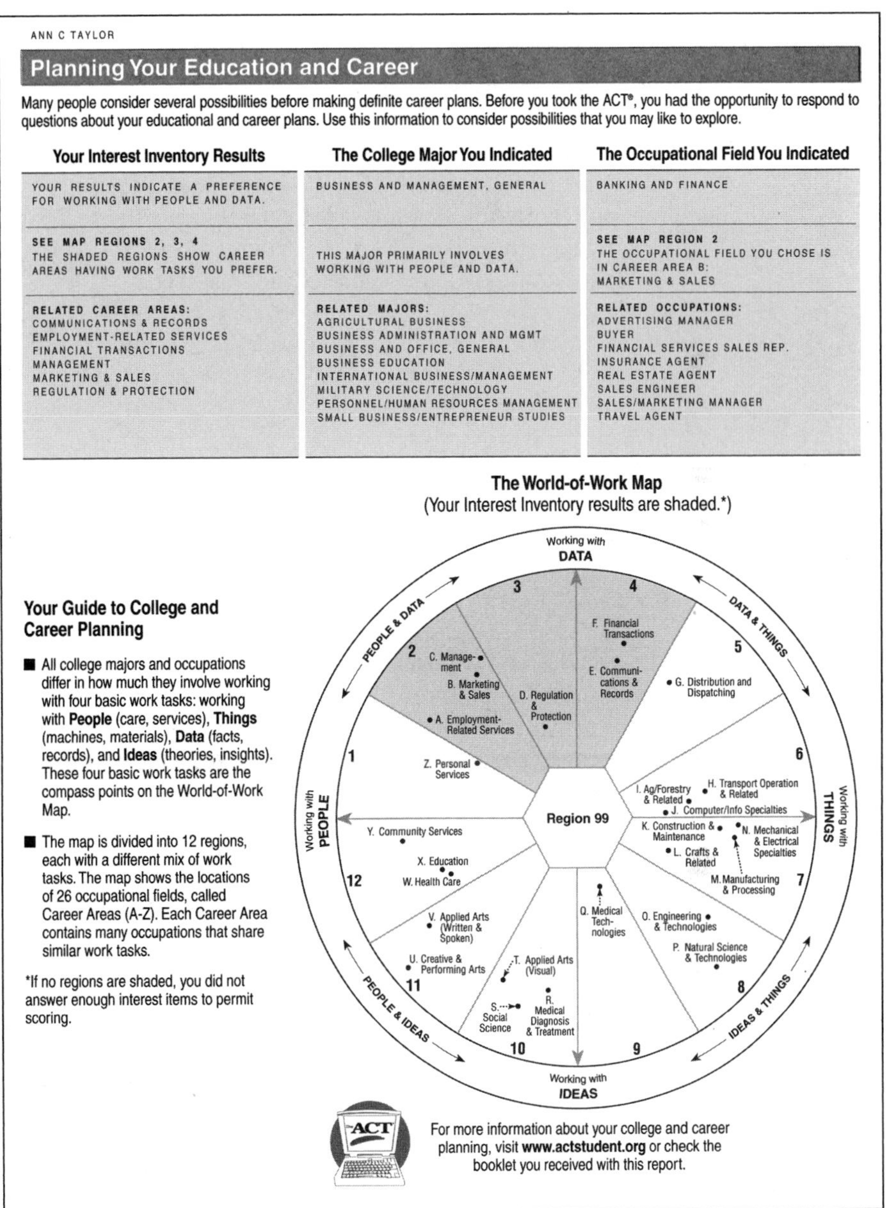

ANN C TAYLOR

Planning Your Education and Career

Many people consider several possibilities before making definite career plans. Before you took the ACT®, you had the opportunity to respond to questions about your educational and career plans. Use this information to consider possibilities that you may like to explore.

Your Interest Inventory Results	The College Major You Indicated	The Occupational Field You Indicated
YOUR RESULTS INDICATE A PREFERENCE FOR WORKING WITH PEOPLE AND DATA.	BUSINESS AND MANAGEMENT, GENERAL	BANKING AND FINANCE
SEE MAP REGIONS 2, 3, 4 THE SHADED REGIONS SHOW CAREER AREAS HAVING WORK TASKS YOU PREFER.	THIS MAJOR PRIMARILY INVOLVES WORKING WITH PEOPLE AND DATA.	SEE MAP REGION 2 THE OCCUPATIONAL FIELD YOU CHOSE IS IN CAREER AREA B: MARKETING & SALES
RELATED CAREER AREAS: COMMUNICATIONS & RECORDS EMPLOYMENT-RELATED SERVICES FINANCIAL TRANSACTIONS MANAGEMENT MARKETING & SALES REGULATION & PROTECTION	RELATED MAJORS: AGRICULTURAL BUSINESS BUSINESS ADMINISTRATION AND MGMT BUSINESS AND OFFICE, GENERAL BUSINESS EDUCATION INTERNATIONAL BUSINESS/MANAGEMENT MILITARY SCIENCE/TECHNOLOGY PERSONNEL/HUMAN RESOURCES MANAGEMENT SMALL BUSINESS/ENTREPRENEUR STUDIES	RELATED OCCUPATIONS: ADVERTISING MANAGER BUYER FINANCIAL SERVICES SALES REP. INSURANCE AGENT REAL ESTATE AGENT SALES ENGINEER SALES/MARKETING MANAGER TRAVEL AGENT

Your Guide to College and Career Planning

- All college majors and occupations differ in how much they involve working with four basic work tasks: working with **People** (care, services), **Things** (machines, materials), **Data** (facts, records), and **Ideas** (theories, insights). These four basic work tasks are the compass points on the World-of-Work Map.
- The map is divided into 12 regions, each with a different mix of work tasks. The map shows the locations of 26 occupational fields, called Career Areas (A-Z). Each Career Area contains many occupations that share similar work tasks.

*If no regions are shaded, you did not answer enough interest items to permit scoring.

The World-of-Work Map
(Your Interest Inventory results are shaded.*)

For more information about your college and career planning, visit **www.actstudent.org** or check the booklet you received with this report.

FIGURE 8.3
(continued)

placement, then their report will include an English/Writing composite score using the same range of 1–36. In addition, there is a Writing subscale score and some comments related to the student's essay. In providing information on methods for using results, ACT (2007) recommended interpreting scores for the four major academic areas by using a range based on a standard error of measure of 2. For the Composite Score, they indicated the standard error of measure was 1 point. There are some minor fluctuations in terms of the mean Composite Score. In addition, ACT (2007) provided benchmark scores for each of the four major academic areas in regards to the chances of getting a B or C in related coursework at the college level.

Some counselors will primarily focus on the ACT academic test scores. The ACT report, however, includes other pertinent information that can provide admissions-related information regarding institutions the student ranked as his or her top four choices. This information enables students and parents to easily see how a particular student's performance compares to those who have been accepted at that institution. The reverse side of the ACT report addresses planning the student's education and career. While students are taking the ACT, they also take an interest inventory and those results are summarized in the "Planning Your Education and Career" section of the report. This section also includes a list of college major and occupational fields that correspond to the student's interests. The World of Work Map also provides a visual representation of the student's interests and can be used by counselors to assist students in exploring careers that are related to their particular interests. The World of Work schemata has been extensively researched and represents students' preferences regarding working with data, ideas, people, and things. Within the map are occupations so that students can easily identify occupations to explore.

Graduate Record Examination. Another scholastic aptitude test is the Graduate Record Examination (GRE). Unlike the other assessments, the GRE is designed to predict performance in graduate school as compared with undergraduate college performance. The GRE General Test is a generic test for prospective graduate students. Many academic programs want to recruit students who already have knowledge about the discipline, and to do so they use one of the GRE subject tests to assess this knowledge. Other tests that have been developed in specific disciplines for the selection of students into professional schools include the Medical College Admissions Test (MCAT), the Dental Admission Test (DAT), the Law School Admission Test (LSAT), and the Graduate Management Admission Test (GMAT).

This discussion covers only the Graduate Record Examination General Test, which will be referred to as the GRE. The GRE consists of three sections: Verbal, Quantitative, and Analytical Writing (Graduate Record Examination Board, 2007). The Verbal test assesses an individual's ability to analyze and evaluate written material, synthesize information from written material, analyze sentences, and recognize relationships between words and concepts. The Quantitative section tests understanding of arithmetic, algebra, geometry, and data analysis, as well as qualitative reasoning and problem solving. Both the Verbal and Quantitative tests have a mean of 500 and a standard deviation of 100 (Graduate Record Examination Board, 2007). In October 2002, the Analytical test was altered to focus more on writing, and it was renamed Analytical Writing. The Analytical Writing section is designed to measure how effectively an individual can articulate complex ideas, evaluate accompanying evidence, support ideas appropriately, provide a coherent discussion, and control the elements of standard written English. An individual's essay is evaluated by two trained readers using a 6-point rating scale.

The GRE is offered as a computer-based assessment in the United States, Canada, and many other countries. The paper-based version is available in countries where computer-based testing is not available. There are numerous testing sites throughout the United States. Individuals can schedule to take the GRE at a time convenient to them and, therefore, do not need to wait until a scheduled testing date. The GRE was one of the first assessments to take advantage of computer-adaptive assessment; in other words, the computer adapts the test to the individual taking the GRE. At the beginning of the test, the test taker is presented with questions requiring average ability. As the individual answers questions, the computer analyzes the answers to determine the difficulty of the next question. The scoring of the test takes into consideration the number of correct responses and the difficulty of the items. The advantages and disadvantages of computer assessment are discussed in Chapter 16.

Validity of scholastic aptitude tests. The most pertinent questions about scholastic aptitude tests relate to how well they predict collegiate performance. These tests are used to make decisions that often have a significant influence on people's lives; therefore, the validity of these instruments deserves analysis. In general, research indicates that the validity of the SAT and the ACT are about the same. Many of the studies indicate that the correlation between scores on these tests and freshman grade point average (GPA) is in the .30 to .50 range. According to the College Entrance Examination Board (2007), the average correlation between high school grades and freshman year grades is .58; whereas, the correlation between SAT scores and freshman grades is .55. The best predictor, however, is a combination of high school grades and scholastic aptitude test scores, which has an average correlation of .65. These two measures seem to balance each other—grades take into consideration persistence and hard work, whereas the scholastic aptitudes tests are not influenced by partiality or teacher bias.

The same trend applies to predicting graduate school performance—multiple predictors are better than any one single predictor. In a meta-analysis of 1,753 independent correlations, Kuncel, Hezlett, and Ones (2001) found that the relationship between GRE scores and first year graduate GPA, comprehensive exam scores and faculty ratings were significant and the average correlational coefficients ranged from .26 to .47. They also found across most disciplines that the combination of GRE scores and undergraduate GPA tended to predict better than GRE scores alone. Although many of the studies on the GRE have assessed students' GPAs during their first year in graduate school, Burton and Wang (2005) found that GRE scores were significantly related to cumulative GPA. Consistent with other researchers, Burton and Wang found that combining GRE scores with undergraduate grade point average was better at predicting cumulative GPA. The Graduate Record Examination Board (2007) also recommended combining the GRE-Verbal, GRE-Quantitative, and GRE-Analytical Writing scores rather than using just one score to assess a student's ability.

Institutions vary in the degree to which scholastic aptitude test scores influence admissions decisions. To counsel college-bound individuals effectively, counselors need to have knowledge about admissions requirements and typical test score performance.

For counselors working with scholastic aptitude tests, it is important to remember these instruments do provide some information but that information should be evaluated in a broader context. Publishers of scholastic aptitude assessments suggest that scores from these instruments be combined with other information (College Entrance Examination Board, 2002; Graduate Record Examination Board, 2007). Counselors need to help clients sort out the meaning of their scores, a task that can be facilitated by incorporating other germane information into the interpretation of scholastic aptitude assessments.

Vocational/Career Aptitude Tests

As mentioned earlier, aptitude tests are often used to predict academic or vocational/career performance. In addition to the scholastic aptitude tests we have discussed, numerous vocational aptitude tests are used in career counseling to predict job or occupational performance. Although these vocational or career aptitude instruments are discussed here rather than in the chapter on career assessment, they should also be considered when selecting assessment tools in career counseling.

There are also vocational aptitude assessments in which the primary purpose is not for use in counseling but rather for employment selection purposes. Effective selection requires that an instrument accurately predict successful performance of job duties. This is a difficult task because job duties within an occupation vary depending on the organization and the setting. In addition, if the instrument is used to predict performance in an occupation, then the test needs to be validated with information from people who are performing successfully in that occupation. This necessitates a precise definition of what constitutes performing "successfully" in that occupation—simply being employed in a job does not guarantee success or competence. This matter is further complicated by the fact that job performance can rarely be measured in a unidimensional manner. Most occupations are complex, and some authorities in the field contend that multifaceted methods of evaluating job performance must be utilized (Campbell, 1994). Therefore, all of these factors make validating an instrument designed to predict job performance a difficult and time consuming task. The difficulty in gathering information on job performance increases the difficulty in getting large norming groups. This problem is magnified when test developers want to create an instrument that predicts performance for a number of occupations. A test developer needs a sufficient number of individuals successfully performing in each occupation to have an adequate norming group.

Some vocational aptitude tests are designed to measure one aptitude or to predict performance in a single occupational area. For example, psychomotor tests are single-purpose aptitude tests that were originally thought to be predictive of many occupations. These instruments are predictive of lower-level manual skills, but they are not good predictors of higher-order abilities (Anastasi, 1988). Clerical aptitude and mechanical aptitude tests are examples of single-purpose vocational aptitude tests that can predict success in certain occupations. However, clients frequently want to know their strengths and limitations and how they might perform in various occupations. Because most clients do not want to spend time taking numerous single-purpose aptitude tests, aptitude *batteries* can be helpful. Aptitude batteries assess multiple aptitudes and predict performance in various occupations. These aptitude batteries can assist clients in examining their strengths and limitations, and also assess potential in a variety of career areas.

Armed Services Vocational Aptitude Test Battery. The *Armed Services Vocational Aptitude Test Battery* (ASVAB), a part of the ASVAB Career Exploration Program, is the most widely used aptitude test in the United States. The Department of Defense offers the ASVAB Career Exploration Program, free of charge, to students in secondary and postsecondary schools. The ASVAB Career Exploration Program consulted with a number of noted researchers in the field of vocational psychology and produced a comprehensive career program that is competency-based. The redesigning of the ASVAB Career Exploration Program began in 2001 and this new program provides students with a more comprehensive career exploration and planning program (U.S. Department of Defense, 2007). The program is targeted for all students in the tenth, eleventh, and twelfth grades along with individuals in postsecondary schools. Web-based and printed materials are designed to assist students in exploring their results and possible career options. There are also structured activities that counselors can use to facilitate the career exploration program.

The Career Exploration Program begins with students taking the ASVAB. Typically a school counselor will arrange for a post-session that focuses on the students' ASVAB scores. This session, typically conducted by a Department of Defense (DoD)

FIGURE 8.4
ASVAB Summary Results Sheet

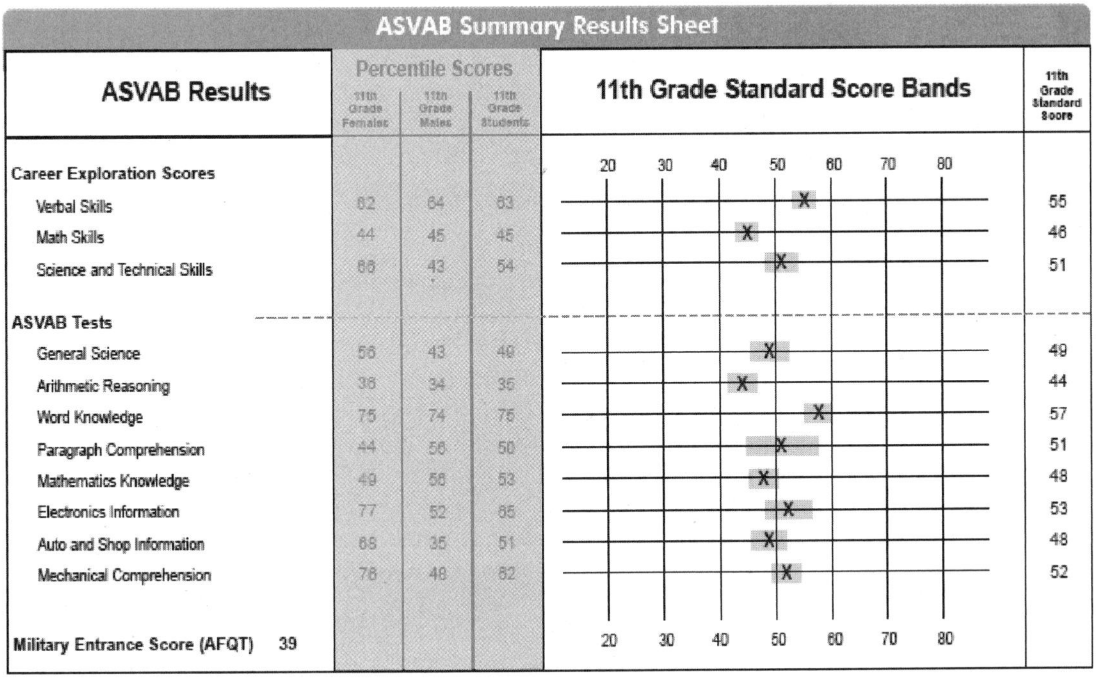

ASVAB Summary Results Sheet

ASVAB Results	Percentile Scores: 11th Grade Females	11th Grade Males	11th Grade Students	11th Grade Standard Score Bands (20 30 40 50 60 70 80)	11th Grade Standard Score
Career Exploration Scores					
Verbal Skills	62	64	63		55
Math Skills	44	45	45		46
Science and Technical Skills	66	43	54		51
ASVAB Tests					
General Science	56	43	49		49
Arithmetic Reasoning	36	34	35		44
Word Knowledge	75	74	75		57
Paragraph Comprehension	44	56	50		51
Mathematics Knowledge	49	56	53		48
Electronics Information	77	52	65		53
Auto and Shop Information	68	35	51		48
Mechanical Comprehension	76	48	62		52
Military Entrance Score (AFQT) 39					

education service specialist, also includes administering, scoring, and interpreting the Find Your Interest (FYI) inventory. The FYI is based on Holland's model of career interests. The students also learn how to use *Exploring Careers: The ASVAB Career Exploration Guide*. In addition, the students are shown how to use their results with OCCU-Find, which assists students in identifying occupations that correspond to their interest. Counselors can also facilitate a comprehensive career exploration program—additional materials supplement these activities. Additional details can be obtained from the ASVAB website at www.asvabprogram.com. With most schools, the military recruiters cannot contact students until seven business days after the school receives the results. These seven days enable school counselors the opportunity to interpret the results and provide counseling to the students.

Ryan Krane and Tirre (2005) contended that the ASVAB is distinguished by its superior norms, thorough investigation of fairness, and substantial evidence of criterion-related validity. The national sample for the ASVAB was obtained from aptitude test data collected as a portion of the Profile of American Youth (PAY97) project. Two samples were drawn for the: (a) Enlisted Training Program and (b) Career Exploration Program. The Enlisted Training Program sample was 6,000 individuals and is used to screen youth for services in the military. The Career Exploration Programs involved 4,700 students in high school and provides the norms for students taking the ASVAB in grades 10, 11, and 12. The reliability estimates were derived based on Item Response Theory, and the coefficients for the composite scores on Verbal Skills, Math Skills, and Science and Technical Skills ranged from .88 to .91 (U.S. Department of Defense, 2007). A copy of a technical manual related to the ASVAB is available at www.asvab.com. Rogers (2002) rated the ASVAB Career Exploration Program as excellent, with attractive and durable test booklets that have attention to detail, are easily readable, and contain colorful graphics. Rogers did, however, express some concerns about the average score differences between minority and nonminority examinees. The ASVAB is evolving, and numerous studies of job performance are continuing to be performed on this widely used instrument. In addition, the Department of Defense is in the process of developing a computer-adapted version that will shorten the time required for taking the ASVAB.

O*NET Ability Profiler. The *O*NET Ability Profiler* is an assessment that replaces the *General Aptitude Test Battery (GATB)*, which was a commonly used vocational aptitude assessment. The O*NET Ability Profiler is one of three assessments linked to O*NET, the Occupational Information Network, which is a comprehensive database of workers' attributes and job characteristics. The network is designed to be the nation's primary source of occupational information and replaces the *Dictionary of Occupational Titles* (DOT). The O*NET Ability Profiler is designed primarily for adults (individuals 16 years and older) who can read at least at a sixth-grade level. The O*NET Ability Profiler contains 11 parts or exercises, with 5 of the exercises involving psychomotor assessment (U.S. Department of Labor, 2002). Although the paper-and-pencil and psychomotor sections can be administered separately, the Department of Labor recommends all 11 subtests, which take approximately 2.5 hours to administer. Typically, the O*NET Ability Profiler is administered to a group of examinees, with the psychomotor sections being administered to group of five or fewer. The O*NET Ability Profiler is scored on the following nine factors: verbal abilities, arithmetic reasoning, computation, spatial ability, form perception, clerical perception, motor coordination, finger dexterity, and manual dexterity. The score report provides both percentile scores and number of correct responses. Included in the profile are occupations linked to the individual's results, with an explanation of the five job zones.

In addition to measuring abilities, the O*NET Career Exploration Tools include assessments that measure interests and work values. The Interest Profiler measures interests using Holland's (1997) six areas of interests (i.e., Realistic, Investigative, Artistic, Social, Enterprising, and Conventional). The Work Importance Profiler assesses the work values of achievement, independence, recognition, relationships, support, and working conditions. There are print versions of the Ability Profiler, Interest Profiler, and Work Importance Profiler, although the print version is called the Work Importance Locator. Tests and their supporting documents (e.g., score reports, master lists of occupations, combined lists, and user's guides) are available for purchase from the U.S. Government Printing Office. The O*NET website (http://www.onetcenter.org) contains substantial information about the Ability Profiler, Interest Profiler, Computerized Interest Profiler, Work Importance Locator, and Work Importance Profiler tools. The O*NET instruments have evolved from other established instruments (e.g., the GATB). Currently, however, there is not much information available about the psychometric qualities of the O*NET instruments, but this information will be forthcoming.

Differential Aptitude Test. The last test to be discussed as an example of aptitude assessments is the *Differential Aptitude Test* (DAT; Bennett, Seashore, & Wesman, 1990). In my opinion, although the DAT was frequently used in the past, its use has recently decreased somewhat in popularity. The DAT is designed for students in grades 7 through 12 but can also be used with adults. This instrument can be used alone or in conjunction with the Career Interest Inventory. A computer-adaptive version of the DAT takes about 90 minutes, whereas the paper-and-pencil version takes about 3 hours. The aptitudes measured, which are similar to those measured by many other instruments, include verbal reasoning, numerical reasoning, abstract reasoning, mechanical reasoning, space relations, spelling language usage, and clerical speed and accuracy. The Verbal Reasoning and Numerical Reasoning scores are combined to produce the Scholastic Aptitude score. The DAT uses separate norms for males and females. The use of separate gender norms is related to findings that males and females tend to score differently on a few of the DAT scales. The norming groups for the DAT are large and were stratified to match the 1980 census information. The reliability coefficients are in the .80 to .90 range (Psychological Corporation, 1991). If results are computer-scored, rather than hand-scored, the scores appear with confidence bands.

Critics of the Differential Aptitude Tests focus on the instrument's validity. Willson and Stone (1994) pointed out that predictive validity information is conspicuously absent. In addition, there is very little differential validity evidence. The term used in the composite score, *scholastic aptitude*, is important because the DAT has been found to be highly correlated with achievement tests and high school and college grade point average (Psychological Corporation, 1991). A counselor can use the DAT to predict academic performance but should be very cautious in using the instrument to predict vocational or occupational performance. In addition, Wang (2002) noted the need for norms for ethnic minorities and methods for using the DAT norming samples with clients of color.

Test Preparation and Performance

Before concluding our discussion of achievement and aptitude testing, it is important to examine briefly the research related to the effects of test preparation. You have probably seen advertisements selling a set of workbooks or a CD-ROM or a special workshop guaranteed to give individuals higher scores on certain tests (e.g., the SAT or the MCAT). You may have questioned whether these programs or products actually improve scores significantly. The answer to that question is that it depends on the program. Before exploring which types of training programs have an impact on scores, some terms need to be defined. *Test sophistication* is a term applied to an individual's level of knowledge in test-taking skills. Test sophistication is not related to knowledge of the content but rather to the format of the tests and the skills required for maneuvering through that format. A distinction also needs to be made between the terms *coaching* and *education*, which are both related to instruction in the content of the examination. *Coaching* involves training or practice on questions that are the same as or similar to the items on the test. The intent is to help the test taker do well on the test, not necessarily to learn the content. *Education* occurs when the domain or area is covered more broadly, with the intent of helping the test taker learn the content or information.

Test Sophistication and Training

The question here is "Do programs that provide practice on the testing format make a significant difference?" Some research indicates that test scores do improve when individuals retake an alternate form of the test (Donlon, 1984). Furthermore, individuals with extensive experience in taking standardized tests have an advantage. However, short orientation and practice sessions tend to bring individuals without extensive experience equal to those who have had more exposure to tests (Anastasi, 1981). These findings indicate that those who can afford test sophistication training have an advantage over those who cannot afford it. In the past few years, the registration materials for a number of tests (e.g., SAT, GRE) have included booklets that address test-taking strategies, explain item formats, and include sample test questions. These booklets are designed to provide those who cannot afford test sophistication training the same sort of experiences as those who can, thus producing "a more level playing field." In addition, many schools provide instruction related to test-taking skills so that all students can use that information.

Coaching

If a program involves coaching, then it involves more than just test sophistication skills. The effects of coaching have been investigated for many years. Some research findings have found that coaching programs can make a significant difference in scores. Some of this research, however, has methodological flaws, particularly related to the equivalence of the treatment and control groups (Bond, 1989). There can be significant differences in scores if a researcher simply compares those who participated in these expensive coaching programs with those who did not. There are other significant differences between these two groups. For example, the members of the group that can afford the coaching program are probably more affluent and have access to other resources that may increase their scores (e.g., tutoring, travel experiences, trips to museums). In general, the studies on coaching have found mixed and inconsistent results concerning the effectiveness of these programs.

One consistent finding is that the closer the resemblance of the coaching material is to the actual test content, the greater the improvement in test scores. A "teaching to the test" approach is one in which the focus is on learning the correct answer to individual questions rather than teaching the broader domain that the test is attempting to measure. Teaching to the test becomes more difficult with instruments such as the SAT because the Truth in Testing legislation has resulted in the need for many new questions for each administration. According to the College Entrance Examination Board (2002), studies that have examined coaching on the SAT indicate that coaching has a modest effect on scores. A recent study indicated that the effect of coaching on the SAT, above the expected gain, was only about 26 points, with the average gain being greater on the Mathematics section (18 points) as compared with the Verbal section (8 points). Powers (1993) found that programs claiming to increase SAT scores by 100 points are questionable and that their claims are probably not accurate. There are also some indications that longer coaching programs result in higher gains as compared with shorter programs. Once again, this make sense in that the more time individuals spend reviewing the material, the more likely it is that they will cover material that will be on the test. The general conclusions are that coaching programs may increase scores slightly, but significant changes occur only if the programs are longer and the content is closely aligned with the material on the test. For many clients, reviewing material on their own can be as effective as these programs and significantly less expensive.

Summary

At some point in their professional lives, counselors can expect to be called upon to have knowledge of both achievement and aptitude assessment. The distinction between an achievement test and an aptitude test is that the former measures past learning, and the latter predicts potential ability to learn or perform. To interpret the results of any achievement test, a counselor first needs to understand whether the instrument is criterion-referenced or norm-referenced. Achievement tests can be developed in many forms, including survey achievement batteries, individual achievement tests, diagnostic tests, criterion-referenced tests, minimum-level skills tests, and subject area tests. Any achievement assessment measures whether an individual has learned some content; therefore, evaluation of the instrument's content validation evidence is paramount. Because achievement tests measure learning, it is not appropriate to assess achievement unless the individual has been exposed to the relevant content.

Aptitude assessment is performed to make predictions about the future. Often aptitude assessments predict educational or vocational/career performance. In the educational area, scholastic aptitude assessment frequently involves predicting performance in college, such as the Scholastic Assessment Test and the American College Testing program. Scholastic aptitude assessment instruments are often used for student selection and placement decisions. They can also serve as an effective counseling tool and assist clients in making decisions. There are also a number of vocational/career aptitude assessments. Professional counselors need to understand the strengths and limitations of any aptitude tool they use. It is particularly important to know how good a predictor the instrument is and what precisely is being predicted (e.g., freshman grade point average, success in a training program, job performance). If counselors do not understand the norming group and the validation information for an aptitude test, they may provide the client with misinformation that could be a disservice to that client.

CHAPTER 9

Assessment in Career Counseling

Enrico is a 24-year-old, Latino male whose parents emigrated from Argentina to the United States when he was 3 years old. Enrico received mostly As and Bs in high school, and his parents strongly encouraged him to go to college and major in medicine. He followed their advice and was admitted to a large Midwestern university. Enrico, however, struggled with both biology and chemistry at the college level and changed his major to business after the first semester. In his second semester, Enrico took an accounting course, which he found boring, so he stopped attending class after a few weeks. He once again decided to change his major and selected Spanish, which was the language often spoken at his parents' home. Enrico's parents, however, were disappointed in his selection of Spanish as a major and encouraged him to return to either medicine or business. An advisor in the on-campus academic advising center suggested that Enrico seek career counseling to help him select a major and determine a career direction. Enrico, frustrated by his indecision about a major, sought career counseling with the hopes of finding a stable career direction.

If you were Enrico's counselor, you might consider incorporating career assessment into the counseling process. Although some individuals believe that career counseling always involves formal assessments, that is not always the case. The question is whether an assessment or assessments would assist Enrico and, further, how these assessments could be used in the counseling process to provide Enrico with pertinent information. Sometimes, potential clients like Enrico believe there exists a standard battery of career tests that are given to clients to provide definitive information on the "best" career for an individual. There is not, however, a standard battery of career assessments that is appropriate for all clients. Therefore, as Enrico's counselor, you must be informed on the array of assessments available so that you can make sound

decisions about which assessments are most appropriate. Furthermore, using career assessments requires interpretative skills and clinical competence. The choice of appropriate career assessments is important because the selection of an occupational direction can affect whether individuals are employed or unemployed, whether they are successful in their occupational pursuits, and how satisfied they are with activities that typically involve at least eight hours a day.

Historically, assessment has been considered an integral part of career counseling. Career assessment has a long history, and many career counselors trace its origins back to Frank Parsons. Parsons (1909) encouraged career assessment in his three-step model of career counseling. In fact, the first step was to study or measure the individual, which often involved testing the client. Some people still view career counseling as solely consisting of testing and then providing occupational information. This "test and tell" approach is not reflective of the current status of this counseling area, because research has shown that career counseling is not separate from personal counseling (Whiston & Raharja, in press). Assessment, however, is often involved in career counseling, and numerous instruments are routinely used to help individuals explore career directions and to make effective career decisions. Spokane (1991) proposed that the purposes of career assessments are to unearth career possibilities congruent with the client's attributes, to assess conflicts and problems, to motivate constructive behavior, to acquire a cognitive structure for evaluating career alternatives, to clarify expectations and plan interventions, and to establish the range of abilities. As reflected in Spokane's description, career assessment has diverse goals and covers a wide variety of areas. Although this chapter focuses on some commonly used career instruments, career assessment should not be viewed as a discrete set of instruments. The American Psychological Association (APA) Task Force on Test Users Qualification argued that test users in a career/vocational area must also be able to assess personality and mental health problems that may impede successful career development (Turner, DeMers, Fox, & Reed, 2001).

Following the lead of Betz (1992), this chapter divides career assessment into two major categories: tools used to assess individual differences and tools used to assess the career-development process. The first category of career assessments is designed to measure different aspects of an individual, such as interests, abilities, values, and needs. These measures of individual differences are useful in career counseling because of their relationship to effective career choices or decisions. The second category of instruments relates to the process of career choice. The focus of these instruments is not on the individual attributes of a client but rather on where the client is in the process of selecting a career. In terms of the career-choice process, most instruments assess either the client's level of indecision or the client's stage of career maturity.

Computers have had a significant influence on career assessment and the dissemination of career information. As technology has increased in sophistication, it has become possible for clients to complete career assessments on a computer and then immediately have access to information about occupations and career preparation based on their results. Some of these computerized programs are interactive and incorporate assessment of clients' interests, values, and skills or abilities.

This chapter includes an overview of two of the major computer-assisted career-assessment programs.

This chapter also addresses issues in career assessment. One of these issues is related to structuring inventories in a way that minimizes gender stereotypes. Research indicates that counselors need to interpret career measures with a sensitivity to sex-role socialization and to encourage clients to explore nontraditional occupations that may correspond to their attributes. There are also ethnic and racial issues related to career assessments. Racial differences on general ability and aptitude assessments must also be reexamined because many of the instruments discussed in previous chapters are used in career counseling. Furthermore, racial and ethnic issues are also pertinent to other types of career assessments used by counselors.

Assessing Individual Differences

Interests

Interest inventories are often used in career counseling because they can be helpful in describing an individual's general occupational interests. Yet, Crites (1999) indicated that using interest inventories is not the only method for assessing interests. Counselors can also assess interests by using measures of expressed or manifest interests. Exploring *expressed interest* involves simply asking clients about their interests and can be a very useful indicator of vocational interests, particularly with adults. *Manifest interests*, on the other hand, are those interests identified by examining how clients choose to spend their time and the activities they select. Assessing both expressed and manifest interests can be a good method for identifying vocational interests. In particular, research has found that expressed and measured interests are equally good at predicting occupational choice (Betsworth & Fouad, 1997). The relationship between expressed and measured interests is significant, with the average correlation being around .46 (Athanasou & Cooksey, 1993). Although these methods of assessing interests can provide sound information, there are some advantages to using more formal interest inventories. Interest inventories have been found to promote career exploration (Herr, Cramer, & Niles, 2004), and many interest inventories connect the client's interests to specific occupations. Some clients have a general idea about their interests but may not know which occupations are related to those interest areas.

In assessing interests, it is important for the counselor to understand the relationship between interests and certain career variables. For example, some clinicians believe that if clients are highly interested in a specific field, then those clients will be successful in that career area. Strong interests do not guarantee occupational success (Betsworth & Fouad, 1997). When explaining the results of an interest inventory, the counselor should stress that these instruments are measuring only interests and do not provide an indication of ability. In summarizing existing research on the relationship between interests and abilities, Lent, Brown, and Hackett (1994) reported a small but significant relationship between them. The relationships between interests and occupational satisfaction have also been found to be small (Transberg, Slane, & Ekeberg, 1993). These small relationships probably result from the fact that work satisfaction involves multiple variables (e.g., monetary rewards, colleagues). Interests are, however, good predictors of career direction (Pryor & Taylor, 1986). Although interest inventories have been found to be good predictors of future academic and career choices, interest alone does not guarantee that once people are in an occupation, they will find it satisfying.

Strong Interest Inventory. One of the most widely used interest inventories is the *Strong Interest Inventory*® (SII®; Donnay, Morris, Schaubhut, & Thompson, 2005), which can trace its roots to the 1927 publication of the Strong Vocational Interest Blank®. The Strong Interest Inventory® assessment, today often simply called the Strong, was called the Strong-Campbell Interest Inventory before 1985. The evolution of this instrument over the past 50 years has resulted in a widely used and respected instrument. Not only is the Strong Interest Inventory® commonly used in career counseling (Watkins, Campbell, & Nieberding, 1994), but it is also often cited as one of the most widely used instruments in counseling in general (Bubenzer, Zimpfer, & Mahrle, 1990; Elmore et al., 1993). In addition, the Strong inventory is one of the more researched instruments in counseling, with hundreds of studies having been performed.

The Strong Interest Inventory® compares individuals' responses to items with the response patterns of people in different occupations. This tool is appropriate for high school students, college students, and adults. The 2004 version of the Strong Interest Inventory® contains 291 items, which are at the eighth- to ninth-grade reading level. Individuals respond to items using a five-point scale (i.e., Strongly Like, Like, Indifferent, Dislike, Strongly Dislike). The items on the 2004 edition are in six sections that address preferences in occupations, subject areas, activities, leisure activities, people, and about their characteristics.

Users can choose from a number of different Strong Interest Inventory® reports such as ones geared toward college or high school students. Figure 9.1 provides a sample of the Standard Report, which is nine pages. Before interpreting a Strong report, a counselor should consider the validity of the profile. This can be accomplished, to a degree, by checking the Item Response Percentages at the bottom of page 9 of the sample profile (see Figure 9.1, page 215). The first step is for the clinician to check the client's total number of responses. This is listed after "Your Response Total." If the client answers less than 276, a report will not be generated for that client (Donnay et al., 2005). The second check of a profile's validity would be to examine the typicality index, which measures the number of unusual responses given by the client. There are 24 paired items that one would expect individuals to respond to similarly (e.g., liking the occupation of actor/actress and also liking the activity of acting). If the typicality index is less than 17, then the counselor should explore why there are so many unusual responses. If an explanation cannot be identified, then the counselor should be cautious in interpreting the results. The third check on the profile's validity involves analyzing the Item Response Percentages. The Item Response Percentages are examined to determine if there are trends such as high percentages of Dislike and Strongly Dislike responses or high percentages of items that were marked Indifferent. Extreme response percentages can be useful in interpreting the results and in providing clinical information.

Strong Interest Inventory® Profile

JOHN SAMPLE	Date taken 1.1.2007 M

HOW THE STRONG CAN HELP YOU

The *Strong Interest Inventory*® instrument is a powerful tool that can help you make satisfying decisions about your career and education. Whether you are just starting out in your career, thinking about a change, or considering education options for career preparation, you can benefit from the wealth of information reflected in your *Strong* results. Understanding your *Strong* Profile can help you identify a career focus and begin your career planning and exploration process.

Keep in mind that the *Strong* measures interests, not skills or abilities, and that the results can help guide you toward rewarding careers, work activities, education programs, and leisure activities—all based on your interests. As you review your Profile, remember that managing your career is not a one-time decision but a series of decisions made over your lifetime.

HOW YOU WILL BENEFIT

The *Strong* can be a valuable tool in helping you identify your interests, enabling you to

- Achieve satisfaction in your work
- Identify career options consistent with your interests
- Choose appropriate education and training relevant to your interests
- Maintain balance between your work and leisure activities
- Understand aspects of your personality most closely associated with your interests
- Determine your preferred learning environments
- Learn about your preferences for leadership, risk taking, and teamwork
- Use interests in shaping your career direction
- Decide on a focus for the future
- Direct your own career exploration at various stages in your life

HOW YOUR RESULTS ARE ORGANIZED

Section 1. General Occupational Themes
Describes your interests, work activities, potential skills, and personal values in six broad areas: Realistic (R), Investigative (I), Artistic (A), Social (S), Enterprising (E), and Conventional (C).

Section 2. Basic Interest Scales
Identifies specific interest areas within the six General Occupational Themes, indicating areas likely to be most motivating and rewarding for you.

Section 3. Occupational Scales
Compares your likes and dislikes with those of people who are satisfied working in various occupations, indicating your likely compatibility of interests.

Section 4. Personal Style Scales
Describes preferences related to work style, learning, leadership, risk taking, and teamwork, providing insight into work and education environments most likely to fit you best.

Section 5. Profile Summary
Provides a graphic snapshot of Profile results for immediate, easy reference.

Section 6. Response Summary
Summarizes your responses within each category of *Strong* items, providing interpretive data useful to your career professional.

Note to professional: Check the Response Summary on page 9 of the Profile before beginning your interpretation.

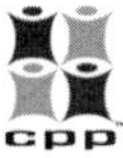

CPP, Inc. | 800-624-1765 | www.cpp.com

Page 1

FIGURE 9.1

Strong Interest Inventory® Standard Profile

Reproduced by special permission of the Publisher, CPP, Inc., Palo Alto, CA 94303 from Strong Interest Inventory of the Strong Vocational Interest Blanks, Form T317. Copyright (c) 1933, 1938, 1945, 1946, 1966, 1968, 1974, 1981, 1985, 1994 by the Board of Trustees of the Leland Stanford Junior University. All rights reserved.

Strong Interest Inventory® Profile JOHN SAMPLE | Page 2

GENERAL OCCUPATIONAL THEMES — SECTION 1

The General Occupational Themes (GOTs) measure six broad interest patterns that can be used to describe your work personality. Most people's interests are reflected by two or three Themes, combined to form a cluster of interests. Work activities, potential skills, and values can also be classified into these six Themes. This provides a direct link between your interests and the career and education possibilities likely to be most meaningful to you.

Your *standard scores* are based on the average scores of a combined group of working adults. However, because research shows that men and women tend to respond differently in these areas, your *interest levels* (Very Little, Little, Moderate, High, Very High) were determined by comparing your scores against the average scores for your gender.

THEME DESCRIPTIONS

THEME	CODE	INTERESTS	WORK ACTIVITIES	POTENTIAL SKILLS	VALUES
Realistic	R	Machines, computer networks, athletics, working outdoors	Operating equipment, using tools, building, repairing, providing security	Mechanical ingenuity and dexterity, physical coordination	Tradition, practicality, common sense
Conventional	C	Organization, data management, accounting, investing, information systems	Setting up procedures and systems, organizing, keeping records, developing computer applications	Ability to work with numbers, data analysis, finances, attention to detail	Accuracy, stability, efficiency
Investigative	I	Science, medicine, mathematics, research	Performing lab work, solving abstract problems, conducting research	Mathematical ability, researching, writing, analyzing	Independence, curiosity, learning
Enterprising	E	Business, politics, leadership, entrepreneurship	Selling, managing, persuading, marketing	Verbal ability, ability to motivate and direct others	Risk taking, status, competition, influence
Artistic	A	Self-expression, art appreciation, communication, culture	Composing music, performing, writing, creating visual art	Creativity, musical ability, artistic expression	Beauty, originality, independence, imagination
Social	S	People, teamwork, helping, community service	Teaching, caring for people, counseling, training employees	People skills, verbal ability, listening, showing understanding	Cooperation, generosity, service to others

YOUR HIGHEST THEMES
Realistic, Conventional, Investigative

YOUR THEME CODE
RCI

THEME	CODE	STANDARD SCORE & INTEREST LEVEL (< 30, 40, 50, 60, 70 >)	STD SCORE
Realistic	R	HIGH	63
Conventional	C	HIGH	59
Investigative	I	HIGH	59
Enterprising	E	MODERATE	47
Artistic	A	LITTLE	39
Social	S	VERY LITTLE	35

The charts above display your GOT results in descending order, from your highest to least level of interest. Referring to the Theme Descriptions provided, determine how well your results fit for you. Do your highest Themes ring true? Look at your next highest level of interest and ask yourself the same question. You may wish to highlight the Theme descriptions on this page that seem to fit you best.

FIGURE 9.1
(continued)

The information on the Strong profile is designed so that interpretation can progress from general to more specific information. Donnay et al. (2005) suggested explaining the Strong's purpose to the client before interpreting the results so that the client understands that the instrument explores interest not abilities. In discussing interpretation of the 1994 version of the SII, Prince and Heiser (2000) encouraged

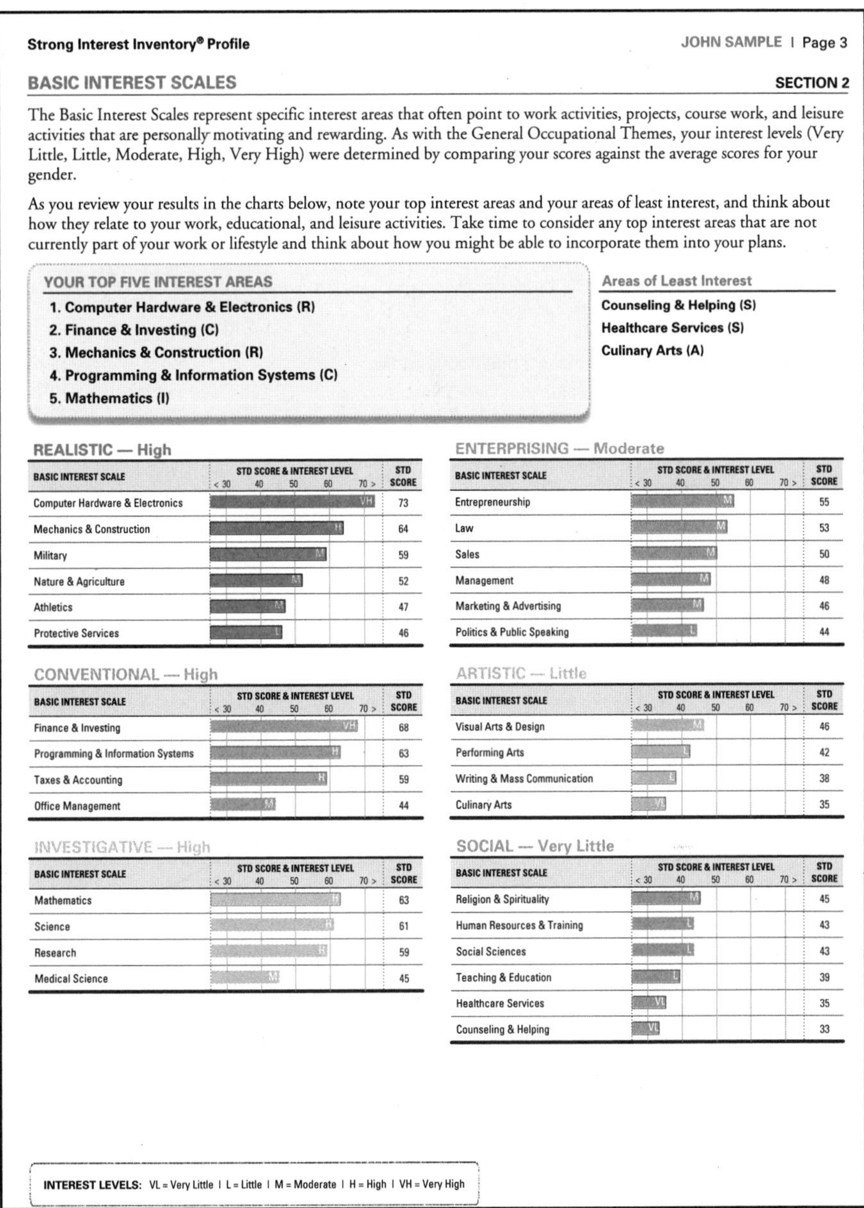

Strong Interest Inventory® Profile JOHN SAMPLE | Page 3

BASIC INTEREST SCALES **SECTION 2**

The Basic Interest Scales represent specific interest areas that often point to work activities, projects, course work, and leisure activities that are personally motivating and rewarding. As with the General Occupational Themes, your interest levels (Very Little, Little, Moderate, High, Very High) were determined by comparing your scores against the average scores for your gender.

As you review your results in the charts below, note your top interest areas and your areas of least interest, and think about how they relate to your work, educational, and leisure activities. Take time to consider any top interest areas that are not currently part of your work or lifestyle and think about how you might be able to incorporate them into your plans.

YOUR TOP FIVE INTEREST AREAS

1. **Computer Hardware & Electronics (R)**
2. **Finance & Investing (C)**
3. **Mechanics & Construction (R)**
4. **Programming & Information Systems (C)**
5. **Mathematics (I)**

Areas of Least Interest

Counseling & Helping (S)
Healthcare Services (S)
Culinary Arts (A)

REALISTIC — High

BASIC INTEREST SCALE	STD SCORE & INTEREST LEVEL (< 30 40 50 60 70 >)	STD SCORE
Computer Hardware & Electronics	VH	73
Mechanics & Construction	H	64
Military	M	59
Nature & Agriculture	M	52
Athletics	M	47
Protective Services	L	46

ENTERPRISING — Moderate

BASIC INTEREST SCALE	STD SCORE & INTEREST LEVEL (< 30 40 50 60 70 >)	STD SCORE
Entrepreneurship	M	55
Law	M	53
Sales	M	50
Management	M	48
Marketing & Advertising	M	46
Politics & Public Speaking	L	44

CONVENTIONAL — High

BASIC INTEREST SCALE	STD SCORE & INTEREST LEVEL (< 30 40 50 60 70 >)	STD SCORE
Finance & Investing	VH	68
Programming & Information Systems	H	63
Taxes & Accounting	H	59
Office Management	M	44

ARTISTIC — Little

BASIC INTEREST SCALE	STD SCORE & INTEREST LEVEL (< 30 40 50 60 70 >)	STD SCORE
Visual Arts & Design	M	46
Performing Arts	L	42
Writing & Mass Communication	L	38
Culinary Arts	VL	35

INVESTIGATIVE — High

BASIC INTEREST SCALE	STD SCORE & INTEREST LEVEL (< 30 40 50 60 70 >)	STD SCORE
Mathematics	H	63
Science	H	61
Research	H	59
Medical Science	M	45

SOCIAL — Very Little

BASIC INTEREST SCALE	STD SCORE & INTEREST LEVEL (< 30 40 50 60 70 >)	STD SCORE
Religion & Spirituality	M	45
Human Resources & Training	L	43
Social Sciences	L	43
Teaching & Education	L	39
Healthcare Services	VL	35
Counseling & Helping	VL	33

INTEREST LEVELS: VL = Very Little | L = Little | M = Moderate | H = High | VH = Very High

FIGURE 9.1
(continued)

counselors to provide an overview of Holland's (1997) theory early in the interpretation process. The interpretation should focus on three areas: the General Occupational Scales (GOTs), the Basic Interest Strong, and the Occupational Scales. Donnay et al. (2005) stated that after discussing Holland's theory, the counselor should interpret the client's results on General Occupational Scales (GOTs) and their results in the six

Strong Interest Inventory® Profile JOHN SAMPLE | Page 4

OCCUPATIONAL SCALES **SECTION 3**

This section highlights your Profile results on the Occupational Scales of the *Strong*. On the next three pages you will find your scores for 122 occupations. The 10 occupations most closely aligned with your interests are listed in the summary chart below. Keep in mind that the occupations listed in your Profile results are just *some* of the many occupations linked to your interests that you might want to consider. They do not indicate those you "should" pursue. It is helpful to think of each occupation as a single example of a much larger group of occupational titles to consider.

Your score on an Occupational Scale shows how similar your interests are to those of people of your gender who have been working in, and are satisfied with, that occupation. The higher your score, the more likes and dislikes you share with those individuals. The Theme Codes associated with each occupation indicate the GOTs most commonly found among people employed in that occupation.

YOUR TOP TEN STRONG OCCUPATIONS

1. Chemist (IR)
2. Engineer (RI)
3. Technical Support Specialist (IRC)
4. Computer Scientist (ICR)
5. Geologist (IRA)
6. Computer & IS Manager (RIC)
7. Computer Systems Analyst (CRI)
8. R&D Manager (IRC)
9. Forester (RI)
10. Actuary (CI)

Occupations of Dissimilar Interest

- Art Teacher (AS)
- Public Relations Director (AE)
- Physical Therapist (SIR)
- English Teacher (ASE)
- Medical Illustrator (AIR)

As you read through your Occupational Scales results on this and the following pages, note the names of those occupations for which you scored "Similar." Those are the occupations you might want to explore first. If you have no scores in this range, take a look at those in the midrange and begin there. You might also consider occupations of least interest or for which you scored "Dissimilar"; however, keep in mind that you are likely to have little in common with people in those types of work and probably would contribute to such occupations in a unique way. Your career professional can guide you further in this process.

You can learn about occupations from information found in a public library, in the career library of a college or university near you, in a professional career center, or on the Internet. A recommended online source for occupational information is the O*NET™ database at http://online.onetcenter.org. You can also learn a lot about an occupation by talking to people who are working in that particular occupation. These people can describe their day-to-day work and tell you what they like and dislike about it.

FIGURE 9.1
(continued)

interest areas of Realistic, Investigative, Artistic, Social, Enterprising, and Conventional. After discussing the GOT themes, the counselor should then relate the scores and meanings of the Basic Interest Scales (BISs) under each theme. The 30 BISs can be viewed as subdivisions of the GOTs. For example, under the Social theme—which is related to helping, instructing, and caregiving—the BISs are Religion and Spirituality, Human Resources and Training, Social Sciences, Teaching and Education, Healthcare Services, and Counseling and Helping. The BISs can help clients understand their underlying interests as related to the six GOTs. For both the GOTs and BISs, the *standard scores* are determined using a norming sample combined of both men and women. However, the distinctions Very Little, Little, Moderate, High, and Very High are determined using either male or female samples. As will be discussed later, there

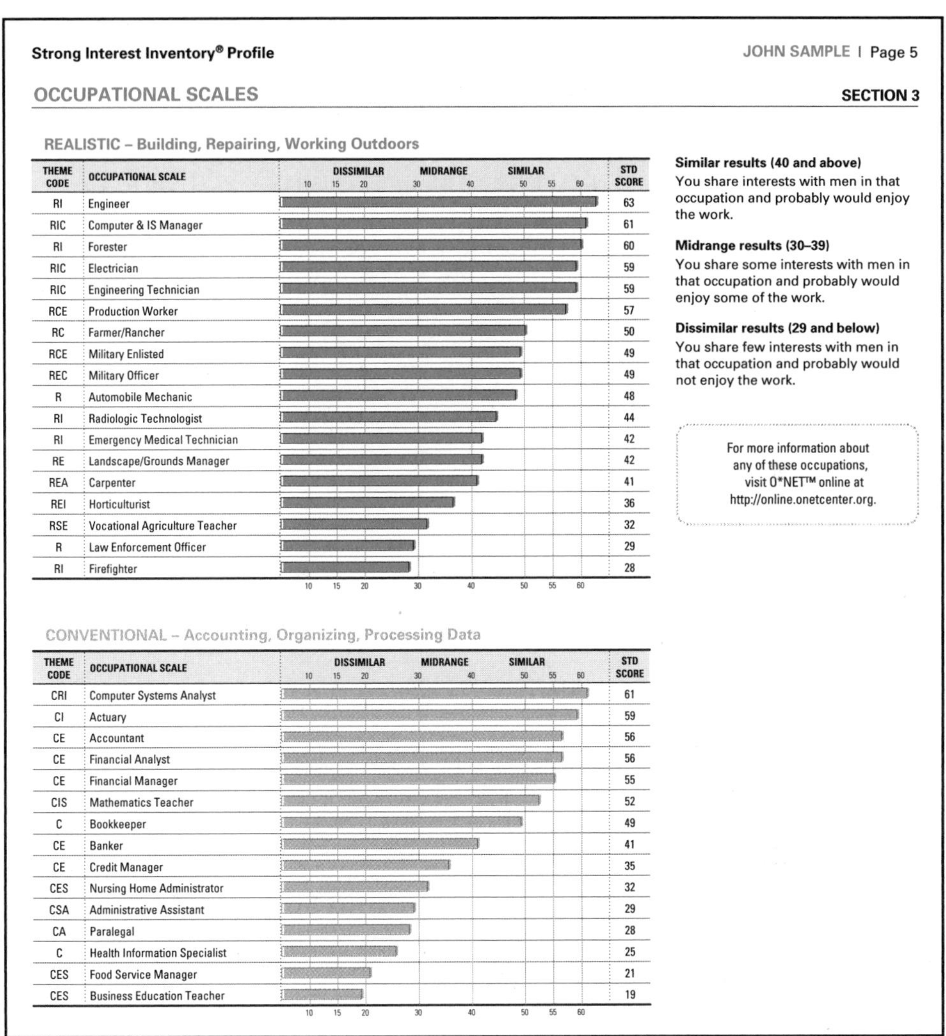

Strong Interest Inventory® Profile

JOHN SAMPLE | Page 5

OCCUPATIONAL SCALES

SECTION 3

REALISTIC – Building, Repairing, Working Outdoors

THEME CODE	OCCUPATIONAL SCALE	DISSIMILAR · MIDRANGE · SIMILAR (10 15 20 30 40 50 55 60)	STD SCORE
RI	Engineer		63
RIC	Computer & IS Manager		61
RI	Forester		60
RIC	Electrician		59
RIC	Engineering Technician		59
RCE	Production Worker		57
RC	Farmer/Rancher		50
RCE	Military Enlisted		49
REC	Military Officer		49
R	Automobile Mechanic		48
RI	Radiologic Technologist		44
RI	Emergency Medical Technician		42
RE	Landscape/Grounds Manager		42
REA	Carpenter		41
REI	Horticulturist		36
RSE	Vocational Agriculture Teacher		32
R	Law Enforcement Officer		29
RI	Firefighter		28

Similar results (40 and above)
You share interests with men in that occupation and probably would enjoy the work.

Midrange results (30–39)
You share some interests with men in that occupation and probably would enjoy some of the work.

Dissimilar results (29 and below)
You share few interests with men in that occupation and probably would not enjoy the work.

For more information about any of these occupations, visit O*NET™ online at http://online.onetcenter.org.

CONVENTIONAL – Accounting, Organizing, Processing Data

THEME CODE	OCCUPATIONAL SCALE	DISSIMILAR · MIDRANGE · SIMILAR (10 15 20 30 40 50 55 60)	STD SCORE
CRI	Computer Systems Analyst		61
CI	Actuary		59
CE	Accountant		56
CE	Financial Analyst		56
CE	Financial Manager		55
CIS	Mathematics Teacher		52
C	Bookkeeper		49
CE	Banker		41
CE	Credit Manager		35
CES	Nursing Home Administrator		32
CSA	Administrative Assistant		29
CA	Paralegal		28
C	Health Information Specialist		25
CES	Food Service Manager		21
CES	Business Education Teacher		19

FIGURE 9.1
(continued)

are differing opinions on addressing nontraditional interests for men and women and whether to use combined or separate norms.

In the spirit of going from general to specific, after interpreting the more general interest measures, the counselor can begin to explore the specific Occupational Scales (OSs). These scales reflect the similarity of the client's interest to the interests of individuals actually working in different occupations. Using people who actually work in the occupations is one of the strengths of the Strong (Busch, 1995). The current Occupational Scales in the SII compare interests of the client to either men or women

Strong Interest Inventory® Profile JOHN SAMPLE | Page 6

OCCUPATIONAL SCALES

SECTION 3

INVESTIGATIVE – Researching, Analyzing, Inquiring

THEME CODE	OCCUPATIONAL SCALE	STD SCORE
IR	Chemist	63
IRC	Technical Support Specialist	63
ICR	Computer Scientist	62
IRA	Geologist	62
IRC	R&D Manager	61
IRC	Network Administrator	59
IAR	Software Developer	59
IRA	Physicist	58
IAS	University Professor	53
IRC	Medical Technologist	46
ICA	Mathematician	44
IRE	Medical Technician	42
IA	Biologist	41
IR	Optometrist	39
IAR	Physician	39
IA	Psychologist	35
IRS	Science Teacher	33
ICE	Pharmacist	29
IA	Geographer	26
IRS	Respiratory Therapist	26
IR	Veterinarian	25
IR	Dentist	20
ISA	Chiropractor	11

Scale: DISSIMILAR 10 15 20 | MIDRANGE 30 40 | SIMILAR 50 55 60

Similar results (40 and above)
You share interests with men in that occupation and probably would enjoy the work.

Midrange results (30–39)
You share some interests with men in that occupation and probably would enjoy some of the work.

Dissimilar results (29 and below)
You share few interests with men in that occupation and probably would not enjoy the work.

For more information about any of these occupations, visit O*NET™ online at http://online.onetcenter.org.

ENTERPRISING – Selling, Managing, Persuading

THEME CODE	OCCUPATIONAL SCALE	STD SCORE
ECI	Investments Manager	58
ER	Optician	48
E	Operations Manager	37
ECS	Housekeeping/Maintenance Manager	33
ECA	Travel Consultant	32
E	Top Executive	31
ECR	Purchasing Agent	30
E	Realtor	29
ECR	Restaurant Manager	27
E	Life Insurance Agent	26
EA	Marketing Manager	25
EAC	Florist	23
ES	Human Resources Manager	23
ES	Sales Manager	23
ECS	Retail Sales Manager	22
ESI	Technical Sales Representative	20
E	Retail Sales Representative	19
ER	Chef	12
EAS	Flight Attendant	12
EA	Cosmetologist	11
EC	Buyer	10
ESA	Elected Public Official	3

Scale: DISSIMILAR 10 15 20 | MIDRANGE 30 40 | SIMILAR 50 55 60

FIGURE 9.1
(continued)

Strong Interest Inventory® Profile JOHN SAMPLE | Page 7

OCCUPATIONAL SCALES

SECTION 3

ARTISTIC – Creating or Enjoying Art, Drama, Music, Writing

THEME CODE	OCCUPATIONAL SCALE	STD SCORE
ARI	Architect	34
A	Librarian	32
AI	Translator	30
ARE	Photographer	29
AI	Urban & Regional Planner	29
A	Musician	26
AES	Corporate Trainer	21
A	Artist	18
A	Attorney	17
AI	Technical Writer	16
A	Graphic Designer	15
AE	Interior Designer	12
ASE	Public Administrator	12
AI	Sociologist	9
AI	Editor	6
ASI	ESL Instructor	6
AE	Broadcast Journalist	4
A	Reporter	-1
AE	Advertising Account Manager	-3
AIR	Medical Illustrator	-11
ASE	English Teacher	-12
AE	Public Relations Director	-21
AS	Art Teacher	-23

DISSIMILAR 10 15 20 — MIDRANGE 30 40 — SIMILAR 50 55 60

SOCIAL – Helping, Instructing, Caregiving

THEME CODE	OCCUPATIONAL SCALE	STD SCORE
SE	Parks & Recreation Manager	20
S	College Instructor	19
SIR	Athletic Trainer	18
SCE	Licensed Practical Nurse	17
SEC	School Administrator	16
SA	Foreign Language Teacher	14
SEC	Dietitian	12
SAI	Rehabilitation Counselor	10
SEA	Social Science Teacher	10
SE	Community Service Director	8
SE	School Counselor	8
SA	Social Worker	4
SA	Minister	1
SA	Speech Pathologist	1
SR	Physical Education Teacher	-1
SAR	Recreation Therapist	-1
SEA	Special Education Teacher	-1
SAI	Registered Nurse	-6
S	Elementary School Teacher	-7
SA	Occupational Therapist	-8
SIR	Physical Therapist	-13

DISSIMILAR 10 15 20 — MIDRANGE 30 40 — SIMILAR 50 55 60

Similar results (40 and above)
You share interests with men in that occupation and probably would enjoy the work.

Midrange results (30–39)
You share some interests with men in that occupation and probably would enjoy some of the work.

Dissimilar results (29 and below)
You share few interests with men in that occupation and probably would not enjoy the work.

For more information about any of these occupations, visit O*NET™ online at http://online.onetcenter.org.

FIGURE 9.1
(continued)

Strong Interest Inventory® Profile JOHN SAMPLE | Page 8

PERSONAL STYLE SCALES

SECTION 4

The Personal Style Scales describe different ways of approaching people, learning, leading, making decisions, and participating in teams. Personal Style Scales help you think about your preferences for factors that can be important in your career, enabling you to more effectively narrow your choices and examine your opportunities. Each scale includes descriptions at both ends of the continuum, with scores indicating your preference for one style versus the other.

Your scores on the Personal Style Scales were determined by comparing your responses to those of a combined group of working men and women.

YOUR PERSONAL STYLE SCALES PREFERENCES

1. **You are likely to prefer working alone**
2. **You seem to prefer to learn by doing and through lectures and books**
3. **You probably prefer to lead by example**
4. **You may be comfortable taking some risks**
5. **You probably enjoy both team roles and independent roles**

Clear Scores
(Below 46 and above 54)
You indicated a clear preference for one style versus the other.

Midrange Scores (46–54)
You indicated that some of the descriptors on both sides apply to you.

PERSONAL STYLE SCALE		CLEAR < 25 35 / MIDRANGE 45 55 / CLEAR 65 75 >		STD SCORE
Work Style	Prefers working alone; enjoys data, ideas, or things; reserved	◆	Prefers working with people; enjoys helping others; outgoing	28
Learning Environment	Prefers practical learning environments; learns by doing; prefers short-term training to achieve a specific goal or skill	◆	Prefers academic environments; learns through lectures and books; willing to spend many years in school; seeks knowledge for its own sake	49
Leadership Style	Is not comfortable taking charge of others; prefers to do the job rather than direct others; may lead by example rather than by giving directions	◆	Is comfortable taking charge of and motivating others; prefers directing others to doing the job alone; enjoys initiating action; expresses opinions easily	42
Risk Taking	Dislikes risk taking; likes quiet activities; prefers to play it safe; makes careful decisions	◆	Likes risk taking; appreciates original ideas; enjoys thrilling activities and taking chances; makes quick decisions	54
Team Orientation	Prefers accomplishing tasks independently; enjoys role as independent contributor; likes to solve problems on one's own	◆	Prefers working on teams; enjoys collaborating on team goals; likes problem solving with others	46
		< 25 35 CLEAR / 45 55 MIDRANGE / 65 75 > CLEAR		

FIGURE 9.1
(continued)

Strong Interest Inventory® Profile

JOHN SAMPLE | Page 9

PROFILE SUMMARY

SECTION 5

YOUR HIGHEST THEMES

Realistic, Conventional, Investigative

YOUR THEME CODE

RCI

YOUR TOP FIVE INTEREST AREAS

1. **Computer Hardware & Electronics (R)**
2. **Finance & Investing (C)**
3. **Mechanics & Construction (R)**
4. **Programming & Information Systems (C)**
5. **Mathematics (I)**

Areas of Least Interest

Counseling & Helping (S)
Healthcare Services (S)
Culinary Arts (A)

YOUR TOP TEN STRONG OCCUPATIONS

1. **Chemist (IR)**
2. **Engineer (RI)**
3. **Technical Support Specialist (IRC)**
4. **Computer Scientist (ICR)**
5. **Geologist (IRA)**
6. **Computer & IS Manager (RIC)**
7. **Computer Systems Analyst (CRI)**
8. **R&D Manager (IRC)**
9. **Forester (RI)**
10. **Actuary (CI)**

Occupations of Dissimilar Interest

Art Teacher (AS)
Public Relations Director (AE)
Physical Therapist (SIR)
English Teacher (ASE)
Medical Illustrator (AIR)

YOUR PERSONAL STYLE SCALES PREFERENCES

1. **You are likely to prefer working alone**
2. **You seem to prefer to learn by doing and through lectures and books**
3. **You probably prefer to lead by example**
4. **You may be comfortable taking some risks**
5. **You probably enjoy both team roles and independent roles**

RESPONSE SUMMARY

SECTION 6

This section provides a summary of your responses to the different sections of the inventory for use in interpretation by your career professional.

ITEM RESPONSE PERCENTAGES

Section Title	Strongly Like	Like	Indifferent	Dislike	Strongly Dislike
Occupations	8	10	14	34	34
Subject Areas	4	37	20	28	11
Activities	7	34	24	29	6
Leisure Activities	0	32	18	50	0
People	13	63	0	25	0
Characteristics	11	67	11	11	0
TOTAL PERCENTAGE	**7**	**28**	**17**	**32**	**16**

Total possible responses: 291 Your response total: 291 Items omitted: 0 Typicality index: 23—Combination of item responses appears consistent

Note: Due to rounding, total percentage may not add up to 100%.

FIGURE 9.1
(continued)

working in 122 occupations. One of the goals of revising the Strong Interest Inventory was to encourage individuals to explore a wide range of occupations, including ones that may have been dominated by one gender; therefore, each occupation has norms for both males and females. In the past, the Strong had been criticized for focusing on professional occupations, and many nonprofessional occupations have been added to the recent version. Occupations where the client's interests are similar have standard scores of 40 or more and these are the occupations that are often explored in counseling. It is, however, often beneficial for counselor to also identify occupations for which there is very low interest. If there are no occupations of 40 and above, then the counselor should focus on the occupations where there is the highest interest. The SII is designed to assist counselors in facilitating the identification of interest patterns and examining where the client has interests similar to those working in various occupations. The identification of various occupations is consistent with the current labor and economic market where individuals often change occupations many times in their lives. Donnay et al. (2005) advised counselors, after exploring the Occupational Scales with the client, to return to the third codes from Holland's model that were identified in GOT and begin to generate other possible occupations that fit the client's pattern of interest.

As can be seen in Figure 9.1, on page 8 of the profile, there are the Personal Style Scales of the Strong Interest Inventory®. These scales are designed to help individuals explore how they approach working, learning, leading, making decisions, and participating on teams. The names of the Personal Styles Scales are Work Style, Learning Environment, Leadership Style, Risk Taking, and Team Orientation. The Work Style scale indicates preferences related to working with people as compared with working with ideas, data, or things. The Learning Environment scale indicates an individual's preferred learning environment on the continuum from a preference for academic learning to a preference for a more practically oriented, hands-on environment. The third scale, the Leadership Style, reflects whether people like to lead by example or by directing and persuading others. The Risk Taking scale indicates whether the client prefers to "play it safe" and make careful decisions or takes risks and makes quick decisions. The last scale is Team Orientation, which reflects an individual's preferences related to accomplishing tasks independently or working on a team using a collaborative style. These scales should probably be interpreted more cautiously than other sections of the SII because they are comparatively new and have not been researched as thoroughly as the General Occupational Themes, the Basic Interest Scales, and the Occupational Scales.

Scoring, norms, and psychometric information. The scoring of the Strong Interest Inventory® is somewhat complex and in scoring the profile, the client's responses are compared to various groups. For both the GOTs and the BISs, an individual's responses are compared with a combined General Representative Sample of 2,250 employed adults. The items that measure the 6 GOTs and the 30 BISs were determined by their content and factor analysis. The sample for the 2004 version consists of an equal number of males and females. Furthermore, 30% of the sample is nonwhite and the sample reflects the distribution of racial and ethnic groups in the United States. In terms of reliability, the test-retest coefficients ranged from .80 to .91. Donnay et al. (2005) provided substantial validation information regarding the 6 themes of the GOT. The coefficient alphas for the BIS ranged from .80 to .91 and the test-retest coefficients were .78 to .89. The manual (Donnay et al., 2005) presented some validation evidence regarding the BIS scores such as relationship with college major and previous scores on earlier versions of the SII.

The Occupational Scales were developed using a different norming procedure and a different method of item selection. Items were selected not because of their similarity in content to other items but rather because of their ability to differentiate the interests of those in an occupation from the general sample (i.e., the General Representative Sample). Thus, the scoring of the OSs is built on comparing the interests of people in certain occupations to a broadly based group of the same gender. Items that differentiate between the occupation and the General Representative Sample were identified, and then weights were assigned based on further analyses. The 2004 version has an adequate sample so that interests can be differentiated for men and women separately for all 122 occupations. Sometimes this required oversampling to ensure an equal number of women and men in each occupation and to include as many individuals from various backgrounds as possible.

To be included in the norming sample for *each* occupation, an individual had to (1) be satisfied with his or her work, (2) have at least three years of work experience in the occupation, and (3) perform the job duties that are typical and that clearly represent the occupation. The reliability coefficients for the Occupational Scales varied with the range of times between testings being from 2 to 23 months and the reliability coefficients ranged from .71 to .91. In terms of concurrent validity, Donnay et al. (2005) found that the male and female scores for many of the occupations were highly correlated and they examined overlapping scores from different occupations. In terms of predicting occupational direction, the 2004 version of the Strong Interest Inventory is different from previous editions and readers are encouraged to continue to monitor the accumulation of validation evidence on the Occupational Scales.

The Personal Style Scales have many features similar to the General Occupational Themes and the Basic Interests Scales; however, these scales were first published in the 1994 version of the SII. The Team Orientation scale seems to have the lowest reliability coefficients (e.g., .70 and .74). The Work Style scale has coefficients that range from .90 to .91.

The Strong can be taken on-line or clients' responses can be mailed in. The Strong Interest Inventory® is often considered a model for other interest inventories in terms of its psychometric characteristics. Certainly, it is the most researched of the interest inventories, and its long history has resulted in a well-developed inventory. There are, however, certain limitations to the Strong, and counselors need to consider whether it is appropriate on a case-by-case basis.

Career Assessment Inventory. In the past, the *Career Assessment Inventory* (CAI) was often considered the "working person's Strong." Whereas previous editions of the Strong Interest Inventory® focused primarily on professional occupations, CAI—Vocational Version (CAI-VV), which was the original version of the inventory, focused on careers that require two or fewer years of postsecondary training. The newer version, the CAI—Enhanced Version (CAI-EV), focuses on careers requiring various levels of postsecondary education. Both versions of the CAI (Johansson 1984, 1986) continue to be published. The profiles of both the CAI-EV and the CAI-VV are patterned after the Strong. Clients receive scores on General Themes (Holland's six personality types), Basic Interests, and Occupational Scales. There are also Administrative indexes and Nonoccupational scales (similar to the Strong's Personal Style Scales).

Although in many ways similar to the Strong Interest Inventory®, the CAI has considerably smaller norming samples (e.g., Machinists has 70 males and no females). Miner and Sellers (2002) criticized the use of combined gender norms in the occupational scales of the CAI. The difficulties associated with combined gender norms are discussed in a later section of this chapter. Furthermore, Miner and Sellers suggested that both versions of the CAI need to be updated, in terms of the items and the occupations covered. They also noted a significant shortage of predictive validity studies.

Self-Directed Search. The *Self-Directed Search* (SDS, Holland, Fritzsche, & Powell, 1994) is another inventory that is usually designated as an interest inventory, although its focus is not exclusively interest. The SDS also includes items related to individuals' abilities and competencies. The conceptual base of the SDS is Holland's theory in that the instrument measures the six basic personality types he proposed. There are four versions of the SDS, with each designed for different groups of individuals. Form R is for high school students, college students, and adults; Form E is for adults and older adolescents with limited reading skills; Form CP (Career Planning) is for employees who aspire to greater levels of professional responsibility; and the Career Explorer version is for middle and junior high school students. All of these versions are self-administered and self-scored. The assessment book is accompanied by an *Occupational Finder* that facilitates the exploration of occupations related to the three-letter summary code produced by taking the SDS. There is also a computer version and computerized interpretative reports for Forms R and CP. Ciechalski (2002) suggested that the SDS can be used in numerous ways in counseling and that the different versions are applicable for a wide range of clients.

Unlike most instruments, the SDS uses raw scores in determining results (i.e., the individual counts the responses related to the six personality types, and the three areas with the most responses produce the three-letter summary code). Daniels (1994) criticized the use of raw data because the four sections of the instruments (i.e., Activities, Competencies, Occupations, and Self-Estimates) vary in the number of items that contribute to the raw scores. In addition, there does not seem to be a theoretical or psychometric reason for the disproportionate contributions to the three-letter summary codes. Although percentiles can be calculated for the SDS, this is not a part of the self-scoring instructions.

In conclusion, the SDS can be an inexpensive and relatively easy assessment device to use. Manuele-Adkins (1989) recommended that when using the instrument, counselors be more involved than the manual recommends. As the *SDS Professional User's Guide* (Holland, Powell, & Fritzsche, 1997) indicates, there are problems with the self-scoring; therefore, scoring should be monitored. There are also differences between how occupations are coded between the Occupational Finder of the SDS and those on the Strong Interest Inventory®, which can be confusing for clients who may receive results from both instruments. The SDS scoring is also criticized because it does not provide any consideration of gender differences, so nontraditional interests may be underrepresented. The norming group for Form R is substantial; however, the norming groups for the other forms are smaller (Brown, 2001). Finally, in my opinion, the validation information on the SDS is supportive of using the instrument for career exploration activities, but other assessment tools and information should be incorporated into the counseling process if the goal is career selection or decision making.

Kuder assessments. Fredrick Kuder, similar to E. K. Strong, has had a long and substantial influence on interest assessment. Most recently, his name has been attached to the *Kuder® Career Planning System* (KCPS), an online assessment that combines the use of three instruments (see the overview of integrative career assessments later in this chapter). Two interest assessments with a long history of clinical use and substantial research are the Kuder Occupational Interest Survey, Form DD (KOIS-DD; Kuder & Zytowski, 1991) and the Kuder General Interest Survey (KGIS; Kuder, 1988). The Kuder Occupational Interest Survey, Form DD assesses the interests of high school students, college students, and adults. The reports provide information on 10 general interest areas and 109 occupations. Of the 109 occupations, 33 are normed with both females and males, 32 are normed with males only, and 11 are normed with females only. Hackett and Lonborg (1993) criticized the inclusion of more male occupations than female occupations and the message this may be sending to female clients. There are also College Major Scales in which, once again, there are gender inequities. Another limitation of this instrument is that most of the criterion groups were sampled more than 30 years ago (Kelly, 2002). Another interest inventory developed by Kuder is the *Kuder General Interest Survey* (KGIS; Kuder, 1988). The KGIS is somewhat unique in that it is geared toward younger adolescents—it can be used with individuals as young as grade 6. The purpose of the KGIS is not for career decision making but rather to stimulate career exploration. Similar to the criticisms of the KOIS-DD, Pope (2002) contended that the normative groups for the KGIS are out of date and that the instrument has limited applicability due to the lack of reported culture-specific data.

Other interest inventories. Counselors use many other interest inventories in addition to the ones mentioned previously. Within the career exploration materials compiled by the U.S. Department of Labor, there is an interest assessment that is related to other O*NET products. The O*NET Interest Profiler can be downloaded from the O*Net website at http://www.onetcenter.org/ or paper and pencil versions can be ordered. The O*NET Interest Profiler measures interests by using Holland typology (i.e., Realistic, Investigative, Artistic, Social, Enterprising, and Conventional). The assessment is designed to be self-administered and interpreted, although current research has found that clients gain more when counseling interventions are utilized with counselor-free vocational assessment (Whiston, Brecheisen, & Stephens, 2003). The website also contains information for counselors on how to effectively use the O*NET Interest Profiler.

Another instrument is the *Jackson Vocational Interest Survey* (JVIS; Jackson, 1996), which is a relatively recent contribution to interest assessments and is intended for use with adolescents and adults. The JVIS is unique in that it measures preferences in both work styles and work roles. Work styles concern preferences for work environments and include scales such as Dominant Leadership, Job Security, and Stamina. Roszkowski (2001) recommended that the instrument be used with highly motivated clients because of the length of the survey. A quite recent addition to the area of interest assessment is the *CAPA Interest Inventory*, which was developed by two eminent vocational psychologists (Nancy Betz and Fred Borgan).

Very few interest assessments are published for elementary students. Examples of inventories geared for these younger students are the *Career Finder*, the *Judgment of Occupational Behavior-Orientation* (JOB-O), and the *What I Like to Do* (WILD).

Another method of identifying and assessing career interests is through the use of card sort techniques. In addition to the many commercially available card sorts, practitioners have also developed their own (Hartung, 1999). Hartung concluded that many of the established card sorts are, to varying degrees, theoretically tied to Holland's theory and to the RIASEC (Realistic, Investigative, Artistic, Social, Enterprising, and Conventional) model. Most often, card sorts have occupations listed on cards. The client sorts the cards into three piles: Would Choose, Would Not Choose, and No Opinion. As Williams (1978) contended, card sorts are a creative way of extracting meaningful information from clients, with the added advantage of providing immediate feedback. Card sorts allow for an interactive process between the client and counselor, enabling the counselor to inquire into the reasons for sorting the cards into specific piles. Slaney and MacKinnon-Slaney (1990) maintained that the research on vocational card sorts suggests that they are as effective as other career assessments. The number of research studies on which this conclusion is based, however, is quite small. It may be better to consider card sorts as a supplement to other career assessments. The research does indicate that card sorts should not be self-administered and that the interaction between the client and counselor contributes to the usefulness of the technique.

Some counselors work with clients who have disabilities and special needs. For these clients, the more traditional interest inventories may not always be appropriate. The *Wide Range Interest-Opinion Test* (WRIOT; Jastak & Jastak, 1979) is a commonly used interest inventory in this area. The WRIOT is a pictorial inventory—out of a series of three pictures, the client selects the one they like most and the one they like least. Because the instrument does not involve reading, it is appropriate for clients for whom reading may be a problem. There are, however, some technical limitations with the WRIOT. Other instruments geared for this population are the *Pictorial Inventory of Careers*, the *Reading-Free Vocational Interest Inventory*, and the *Ashland Interest Assessment*.

Conclusion. According to MacCluskie, Welfel, and Toman (2002), there can be an artistic quality in explaining the results of an interest inventory. For interpreting the Strong Interest Inventory®, Prince and Heiser (2000) suggested beginning with an explanation of Holland's theory. Savickas, Taber, and Spokane (2002) found that interest scales intended to measure Holland's typology shared only about 35% common variance; therefore, counselors should not assume that the definitions of the scales are the same. Hence, although counselors should not rely on Holland's definitions, they do need to understand how the scales are defined within the specific interest assessments they are using. When interpreting any interest inventory, counselors also need to be vigilant about ensuring that the client understands that the results represent what the client is interested in but do not represent what the client may be good at. Sometimes, particularly when clients are viewing an attractive computer-generated profile, they believe the profile reflects what their future career direction should be. Counselors need to reinforce that the results of an interest inventory are just one piece of information to be used in the career decision-making process.

Abilities/Skills

In career counseling, Ryan Krane and Tirre (2005) asserted that the assessment of abilities and skills often are conducted to identify occupational possibilities in which the client could be successful. Many of the instruments discussed in Chapter 8 that relate to the assessment of aptitude and achievement can be used in career counseling. Certainly, the Armed Services Vocational Aptitude Battery (ASVAB) and O*NET Ability Profiler have been used for career exploration and decision making. In addition, these instruments have the option of being used in combination with an interest inventory. Therefore, in considering career assessments, counselors should include those measures mentioned in the previous chapter. Aptitude tests are often used in career counseling because they are good predictors of occupational success (Hunter & Schmidt, 1983). This does not mean, however, that aptitude test results should be examined in isolation as the sole determinant of a client's potential in an occupation. Counselors need to gather information about the whole person when assisting clients in their career planning process.

When interpreting aptitude assessment in career counseling, it is important for counselors to verify the results with other information. Verifying the results entails asking the clients if scores are consistent with other information, such as grades, work performance, self-perceptions of abilities, and other types of evaluations. This verification of the results accomplishes two goals. First, it provides a method of identifying any problems that may have occurred during the testing (e.g., the client's ability to read may have influenced performance, or the client was ill when taking the instrument and the results don't reflect his or her ability). Second, the verification process brings more client information into the interpretative process. Thus, the verification process can assist in providing a more holistic view of the client's abilities as well as giving information on other facets of the client's life. Some aptitude publishers have responded to counselors' need to gather more complete client information by combining an aptitude test with an interest inventory. An example of this is the *Unisex Addition of the ACT Interest Inventory* (UNIACT), which is a key component of many ACT services (e.g., ACT, EXPLORE, PLAN). The combination of aptitudes and interests facilitates exploration and leads to a more comprehensive view of the client.

Campbell Interest and Skills Survey. A different method of combining interests and skills or ability assessment is available through the *Campbell Interest and Skills* (CISS; Campbell, 1992). Campbell, the author of this instrument, has a long, distinguished career in vocational assessment and was instrumental in the development of the Strong Interest Inventory's® predecessor, the Strong-Campbell Interest Inventory. The CISS combines the self-assessment of skills with an exploration of interest. This combination encourages the client to examine the interaction between interests and skills and to examine career areas in which the two intersect. As is discussed later, research supports the use of self-estimates of skill level assessment.

The 320 items of the CISS result in scores on 7 Orientation Scales, 29 Basic Interest and Skills Scales, and 58 Occupational Scales. The Orientation Scales roughly correspond to Holland's six themes, except that the Realistic theme is broken down into two categories, the Producing and the Adventuring orientations. The Basic Scales are subcategories of the Orientation Scales and represent various occupational activities. Unlike the Strong, the norms for these two scales and the Occupation Scales are unisex rather than reporting scores for men and women separately. The CISS also includes three procedural checks (a Response Percentage Check, an Inconsistency Check, and an Omitted Items report).

Based on the scores on interests and self-assessment of skill level, the profile provides four categories: Pursue—high interest and high skills; Develop—high interest and lower skills; Explore—lower interest and high skills; and Avoid—lower interest and lower skills. Pugh (1998) recommended that counselors use caution in interpreting the Develop and Explore designations, because a small difference in interests and skills can result in different categorizations. The reference sample of 5,225 seems adequate; however, the sample has substantially more men than women. The median coefficient alpha is .87 for the Orientation Scales and .86 for the Basic Scales. There is more variability in the Occupational Scales, and the skills assessments on the Occupational Scales tend to be less reliable than the interest scores. Validation evidence is growing; it is anticipated that in 10 years, there will be substantially more. Recently, Hansen and Leuty (2007) found approach convergent evidence related to the skills portion of the CISS and that the scores were predictive of different college majors. The interest assessment has a strong empirical base because it comes from Campbell's work on the Strong-Campbell Interest Inventory.

Skills Confidence Inventory. With the revision of the Strong Interest Inventory®, there has also been a revision of the *Skills Confidence Inventory* (SCI; Betz, Borgen, & Harmon, 2005). The Skills Confidence Inventory measures perceptions of one's capabilities in performing activities that correspond to Holland's six interest themes and it is often used in conjunction with the Strong Interest Inventory®. This 60-item instrument is designed to measure an individual's self-perceived ability or self-efficacy expectation in successfully completing a variety of tasks, activities, and coursework. Scores on the six scales range from 1 to 5. The SCI was designed to be used in conjunction with the Strong Interest Inventory® so that individuals can examine their interests and perceived abilities simultaneously.

Betz and Borgan (2005) developed the *CAPA Confidence Inventory*, which is a 190-item instrument designed to measure confidence by examining more specific activities within Holland's six categories. The Enterprising theme has the most confidence areas, which include Public Speaking, Law, Politics, Management, Marketing & Advertising, Entrepreneurship, and Sales. The Investigative theme has three confidence areas: Math, Science, and Medical Science. The CAPA Confidence Inventory is an interactive program in which clients take the assessment on-line and results are provided immediately. Both Betz and Borgan have been instrumental in many career assessments and this instrument holds great promise.

Self-estimates of abilities. In considering methods for assessing skills and abilities, counselors may want to consider the use of self-estimates. Westbrook, Sanford, Gilleland, Fleenor, and Merwin (1988) found a significant relationship between self-appraisal estimates of abilities and measured abilities. They also found, however, that adolescents generally tended to overestimate their abilities. Their research indicates that counselors can use self-appraisals in career counseling. Prediger (1999) recommended using "informed self-estimates" of abilities, which draw upon clients' experiences.

When using self-estimates of abilities, counselors need to consider the client's self-efficacy beliefs. Self-efficacy concerns clients' beliefs about their ability to perform a specific task or behavior. Substantial research has shown that self-efficacy beliefs mitigate tasks approached, academic pursuits, and career choice. There are, however, significant gender differences in many areas of self-efficacy. For example, women tend to have lower math self-efficacy than do men, and those perceptions of being less efficacious in math influence women's reluctance to pursue scientific and technical careers (Betz, 2000). In considering self-estimates and self-efficacy, Tracey and Hopkins (2001) suggested an important distinction between them. They contended that self-efficacy beliefs concern future performance with the client possibly using a criterion-reference framework. On the other hand, self-estimates tend to involve current levels of abilities and often involve an implicit assumption that one is comparing one's abilities to others. Although there may be some distinctions between self-estimates and self-efficacy, there also probably some overlap. This notion can be translated into practice by asking clients about the information they are using when asked to provide self-estimates of their abilities. The counselor can then assist the client in exploring whether their self-estimates of their abilities are based on multiple sources of documented information or on somewhat vague and isolated experiences.

Values

In the area of career assessment, the exploration of values is sometimes neglected, even though it is often a critical aspect of the career-counseling process. Rounds and Armstrong (2005) contended that values should play a vital role in career decision-making. Osborne, Brown, Niles, and Miner (1997) indicated that "The understanding of an individual's values is, perhaps, the most important element of the decision-making process. Values serve as the basis for which life goals are established and provide a guide for individuals in making personally consistent and meaningful decisions about the future" (p. 82).

Work values are more highly correlated than interest with work satisfaction (Rounds, 1990). Some of the instruments typically associated with the assessment of values in the career area use terms such as *needs* or *preferences*. Although there are some discrepancies in the definitions of these dimensions, Betz (1992) indicated that they seem to measure an overlapping set of variables.

If a counselor is using a values inventory, the practitioner should remember that no inventory is inclusive of all possible values. In other words, a client may value something that is not assessed on the instrument being used. Chartrand and Walsh (2001) argued that those career assessments in which the focus is only on work values are insufficient because many people may want to examine their values across multiple life roles. Counselors need to supplement the use of a values inventory with an exploration of other possible values, which can be accomplished by asking the client questions about personal values not otherwise assessed or by exploring the client's lifestyle.

Minnesota Importance Questionnaire. The *Minnesota Importance Questionnaire* (MIS; Weiss, Dawis, & Lofquist, 1981) relates to the theory of work adjustment but is also used as an assessment of values or needs in career counseling. It measures 20 vocational needs (e.g., Ability Utilization, Compensation, Coworkers, Recognition) and six underlying work values (Achievement, Altruism, Autonomy, Comfort, Safety, and Status). Needs are indicated by the number of times an individual selects a statement as being important relative to other statements and values are defined as a cluster of related needs. Brooke and Ciechalski (1994) rated its psychometric qualities positively and the instrument has been heavily researched.

O*NET Work Importance Profiler. In addition to measuring interests and abilities, the O*NET Career Exploration Tools include assessments that measure work values. The Work Importance Profiler is a new computerized self-assessment that encourages individuals to focus on what is important to them in their work. The O*NET Work Importance Profiler assesses work values in the areas of achievement, independence, recognition, relationships, support, and working conditions. Individuals can download the Work Importance Profiler from the O*NET website (http://www.onetcenter.org). This website also contains information related to how to use and interpret the results of the Work Importance Inventory. The development of the O*NET Work Importance Profiler began with a critical examination of the Minnesota Importance Questionnaire. There is also a paper version entitled the Work Importance Locator. The advantage of these assessments is that they are linked to occupations and occupational information.

Values Scale. The *Values Scale* (Nevill & Super, 1989) is a measure of both work-related values and general values. The 106 items produce scores on 21 values (e.g., Ability Utilization, Achievement, Economic Security, and Personal Development). The authors of this scale have labeled it the Research Edition to indicate that clinicians should be cautious in using it. There is a normative sample, but the authors recommend using an ipsative interpretation. With *ipsative interpretation*, the variables are compared with each other without reference to whether the client's values in that area are high or low as compared with values of other people. Slaney and Suddarth (1994) wondered if this cautious approach is even warranted given the lack of predictive validation studies; however, Schoenrade (2002) considered the content validation evidence to be respectable. Hackett and Watkins (1995) agreed that there were drawbacks with the instrument but suggested it had cross-cultural applications and did not appear to be gender-biased. The Value Scale is one of the instruments administered in Super's Career Development, Assessment, and Counseling (C-DAC) model (Osborne et al., 1997).

Salience Inventory. The *Salience Inventory* (Nevill & Super, 1986) scale focuses on the *roles* valued by individuals. This scale is based on Super's concept that the saliency of different roles varies throughout an individual's life cycle. Super (1980) identified five major roles that the Salience Inventory measures: student, worker, homemaker (including spouse and parent), leisurite, and citizen. On the Salience Inventory, each role is assessed three ways: the Commitment Scale, the Participation Scale, and the Value Expectation Scale. This instrument can assist adolescents in examining their current roles and the ones they are interested in committing to in the future. It can also be helpful for women who have issues of multiple roles and possible role overload. The Salience Inventory is also an integral part of Super's C-DAC model (Osborne et al., 1997).

According to Rounds and Armstrong (2005), although assessment of values will often provide clients with important information to consider in career planning, values measures have not received the same attention as other typical career counseling assessments (e.g., interests inventories and ability assessments). They recommended that values assessment be used in a comprehensive strategy that involves occupational information.

Integrative Career Assessment Programs

As noted earlier, a number of interest and aptitude assessments are now offered in conjunction with each other. This section discusses a few of the programs that combine interests, abilities, and values assessments.

Kuder Career Planning System. Building on the historical work of Fredrick Kuder, the Kuder® Career Planning System (KCPS) is an online, interactive program that is the latest in a series of career assessment tools that dates back to the 1930s. The KCPS includes an interest inventory, a skills assessment, and a work values inventory. The easy access of the three assessments on-line is one of the advantages of this package of instruments. In addition, all instruments are available in English and Spanish. There is a charge for these assessments, but it is adjusted for larger groups of individuals. The interest inventory, the *Kuder Career Search with People Match* (KCS), takes a different approach from other interest inventories (Zytowski, nd). It is based on the premise that people employed in an occupation are not a homogeneous group.

Therefore, instead of matching to a specific occupation, individual's responses are compared with the responses of an appropriate norming groups (e.g., middle school boys and girls, high school boys and girls, adult combined gender). Scores on six clusters are given using percentiles, and the clusters are rank-ordered on the profile. The six areas are similar to Holland and include the clusters of Outdoor/Mechanical, Science/Technical, Arts/Communication, Social/Personal Services, Sales/Management, and Business Operations. Furthermore, unlike other interest inventories, the KCS uses the individual's responses to identify the 14 people from the criterion person's pool whose interests most closely match the client's. Based on the 14 person matches identified, the client is then provided not only the job title information, but also information about the actual duties and responsibilities of that person. The intent of the person match information is not to represent an entire occupation but, rather, to find the specific individuals whose interests are most similar to the inventory taker's interests. The KCS has 180 items that are presented in triads and individuals indicate among the three activities which they prefer most, next most, and least.

The *Kuder Skills Assessment* is the skills assessment portion of the Kuder® Career Planning System and it uses self-reports of abilities. The Kuder Skills Assessment (KSA) has recently been revised (Zytowski, Rottinghaus, & D'Archiardi, 2007). The KSA has two levels with one being designed for middle school and high school and another version developed for college students and adults. The results are presented in either 6 skill areas or 16 clusters that are used in some states to assist students in selecting career pathways. As indicated earlier, many of the measures of abilities designed to be used in career counseling have incorporated a self-estimate format. The reports are designed to encourage exploration and interest and abilities are presented to encourage self-reflection. There is also a values assessment in the Kuder® Career Planning System, the *Super's Work Values Inventory-Revised* (Zytowski, 2006). The reading level of the Super's Work Values Inventory-Revised (SWVI-r) is around sixth grade and most middle school and high school students can complete the assessment in less than 20 minutes. The SWVI-r measures 12 work-related values and individuals' results are rank-ordered so that they can better understand their values. The results are also linked to O*NET occupational information so that there is a seamless connection between information about self and the world of work.

In addition to the online version of the *Kuder Career Planning System*, Kuder offers a practical career planning printed guide called the *Kuder Career Planning System: Take Hold of Your Future*, fifth edition, which was written by a well-respected scholar in career development, JoAnn Harris-Bowlsbey. This guide and its supplementary materials focus on identifying interests, skills, and work values. Furthermore, they assist individuals in articulating their goals, creating vocational plans, and identifying steps in implementing those steps. The guide can be used either with individuals or groups.

COPSystem. The *COPSystem* is published by EdITS/Educational and Industrial Testing Services and combines separate interests, abilities, and values inventories. The instruments in this system can be used alone or in tandem with one another. Using the Comprehensive Career Guide, the results from the interests, abilities, and values assessment can be interpreted, with the results from all three assessments using the same occupational classification system. Depending on the client's needs, the practitioner can select from several versions of the COPSystem Interest Inventory (COPS), such as the general form (COPS-Revised), a professional-focused instrument (COPS-P), an instrument appropriate for elementary through high school (COPS-II), and a pictorial instrument (COPS-PIC). The values instrument, the Career Orientation Placement and Evaluation Survey (COPES), was revised in 1995. The COPES instrument measures eight values using a continuum (e.g., Investigative vs. Accepting, Practical vs. Carefree, Independence vs. Conformity). Thus, counselors can use the results to interpret which area is valued over the other on the continuum and identify from the eight areas the ones that are most valued. The ability measure is the Career Ability Placement Survey (CAPS), which consists of eight subtests. Each of the subtests lasts only five minutes and, therefore, is not a comprehensive test of those eight abilities. Each instrument in the COPSystem can be hand-scored by the client, and there are procedures for integrating the results of the three instruments to facilitate a more comprehensive exploration experience. Although the COPSystem continues to be revised and improved, there is limited validation evidence, particularly longitudinal studies. The COPSystem can provide an integrative program for career exploration, but sometimes clients will benefit from more thorough assessments. Although the COPSystem is designed as a self-directed exercise in which clients can take and interpret their results unaided, Wickwire (2002) strongly encouraged counselors to be actively involved in the process.

Integrated assessment and career information systems. These systems include a number of assessments as well as an integration of occupational information. There are many computerized career assessment and information systems, but two of the most widely used are the DISCOVER Program and SIGI-Plus (Garis & Niles, 1990). These programs are widely used, and studies have indicated that students and counselors generally react positively to both of these systems (Kapes, Borman, & Frazier, 1989). *DISCOVER* is one of the predominant computer-assisted career guidance systems and was developed by the American College Testing Program (ACT). There are three versions of DISCOVER: the Internet, Middle School, and Windows. The Internet and Windows versions involve a sequential process in which individuals take interest, abilities, and values assessments, which then lead to planning their occupational and educational futures. Integrated throughout the program is information on occupations and how to prepare for those occupations. The systems include information on post-secondary programs and institutions, and most individuals are able to successfully navigate throughout the system. The Middle School version is designed for younger students and is not quite as detailed. The DISCOVER website (http://www.act.org/discover/overview/index.html) contains information related to using DISCOVER and the research supporting its effectiveness. There is a licensing fee for using DISCOVER and many high schools, colleges and universities, one-stop career centers, and libraries have contracts.

The System of Interactive Guidance and Information, now called SIGI^3, is another extensive educational and career planning program that involves assessments. The current version is consistent with previous versions and their philosophical foundation of focusing on values identification and clarification. Besides values assessment, SIGI[3] also involves interest and abilities assessments, and provides a framework for exploring differing career options and educational training opportunities.

The advantage of these integrated career assessment programs is that they are packaged so that there is an integration of interest, abilities, and values assessments. The disadvantage of the systems, however, is that one of the assessments could be weak and with some of the systems, the clinician cannot "pick and choose" assessment, but must buy all of the assessments together. Furthermore, some of these integrated career assessment programs are designed to be stand-alone systems. Although many of the integrated vocational assessment systems are used, they should not be considered a replacement for career counseling because research has clearly shown that career counseling is more effective if a counselor is involved in the process (Whiston et al., 2003).

Integrating Assessment Information

Integrative assessment does not have to involve only one system, such as the COPSystem; counselors can integrate a number of separate career assessments. The Career Development Assessment and Counseling Approach (C-DAC; Osborne et al., 1997) involves integrating the results from a number of career assessments: the Adult Career Concerns Inventory, the Career Development Inventory, the Strong Interest Inventory®, the Values Scale, and the Salience Inventory. In addition, career assessment does not always have to involve formal assessment instruments; some informal exercises have been shown to be valid tools (e.g., the Occupational Daydream exercise in the Self-Directed Search). Integrating information on interests, abilities, and values should be a part of the career counseling process. In terms of integrative career assessment, Spokane and Jacob (1996) found that there is a renewed interest in portfolio assessment, an approach that could facilitate the integration of interests, abilities, and values assessment. Portfolio assessment also makes sense in terms of career development because students can keep career counseling exercises and results of assessments in their portfolios. School counselors could then use the portfolios to integrate career information gathered from students throughout their academic careers. Hence, an interest inventory taken in middle school could be compared with an interest inventory taken in high school.

Career Choice Process

The previous discussion addressed assessments of individual differences that are used to assist clients in career planning or addressing various issues related to work. These instruments assess various content (e.g., interests, values) that has been shown to be related to sound career choices. This chapter's focus is now moving toward instruments that measure where clients are in the career development or decision-making process. Typical measures of career process variables are related to level of decidedness or certainty and an individual's level of career maturity (Whiston et al., 2003; Whiston, Sexton, & Lasoff, 1998).

Career Decision Making

It is often helpful in career counseling to have an indication of where the client is in terms of career decision or indecision. The interventions a counselor selects would probably be very different for a client who has not made a career decision as compared with individuals who are decided. A distinction should be made between clients who experience normal developmental undecidedness and those who experience indecisiveness. The term *undecided* means the client has not yet made a career decision, whereas the term *indecisiveness* indicates chronic problems with indecision (Betz, 1992). A number of instruments have been found to be useful in assessing clients' progress in the decision-making process or in identifying difficulties clients may be experiencing in making a career decision.

A widely used instrument in this area is the *Career Decision Scale* (CDS; Osipow, 1987). The CDS includes 19 items. The first two items measure the level of certainty the individual feels in making a career decision. The next 16 items measure the level of career indecision. The last item provides an opportunity for individuals to describe their career indecision if none of the other items seemed appropriate. The CDS is generally regarded as a reliable instrument, with validity evidence related to its use as a measure of overall career indecision (Harmon, 1994). It is important to note that the CDS provides a measure of career indecision, but it does not indicate the source or the type of indecision. Another measure often used in this area is Holland, Daiger, and Power's (1980) *My Vocational Situation* (MVS). The MVS has three subscales: the Vocational Identity scale, the Occupational Information scale, and the Barriers scale. The Vocational Identity scale is often considered a measure of indecision and assesses the clarity and stability of one's career-related attributes. Both the CDS and the MVS are used not only to gather information about clients but also to evaluate the effectiveness of career counseling.

An instrument that is increasingly being used in career counseling and outcome research is the *Career Decision-Making Self-Efficacy Scale* (CDMSE; Betz & Taylor, 1994). Often used with college students, the CDMSE measures the confidence individuals have in their ability to make career decisions. This instrument draws from Bandura's (1977) theory of self-efficacy, which proposed that an individual's belief about his or her ability to perform a specific task or behavior significantly affects the individual's choices, performance, and persistence in that task. There is a short version with 25 items, as compared with the longer version, which has 50 items. There are five scales (i.e., Accurate Self-Appraisal, Gathering Occupational Information, Goal Selection, Making Plans for the Future, and Problem-Solving) in both the original and the shortened versions of the CDMSE.

A new instrument that holds potential in identifying or diagnosing decision-making difficulties is the *Career Decision-Making Difficulties Questionnaire* (CDDQ; Gati, Krausz, & Osipow, 1996). The CDDQ was constructed to measure a theory-based taxonomy of decision-making difficulties. The taxonomy includes three major areas of difficulties that are further subdivided into 10 specific difficulty categories, and, finally, into 44 specific difficulties. For example, the first of the three major dimensions is Lack of Readiness, which is subdivided into the categories of lack of readiness due to Lack of Motivation, Indecisiveness, and Dysfunctional Beliefs. The second major dimension is Lack of Information, with the subcategories being Lack of Information about the Career Decision-Making Process, Lack of Information about Self, Lack of Information about Occupations, or Lack of Information about Ways of Obtaining Information. The last dimension is Inconsistent Information, and the categories are Unreliable Information, Internal Conflicts, and External Conflicts. Studies related to the psychometric qualities of the CDDQ have been mostly favorable (Gati, Osipow, Krausz, & Saka, 2000; Osipow & Gati, 1998).

Career Maturity

Betz (1988) defined *career maturity* as the "extent to which the individual has mastered the vocational tasks, including both knowledge and attitudinal components, appropriate to his or her stage of career development" (p. 80). Career maturity is examined developmentally and compares the individual to others in terms of career development. Essentially, career maturity measures the client's level of readiness for mastering career development tasks. In a discussion of the assessment of career maturity, it is important to note some criticisms of the construct and the assumptions that career development is always temporal, unidirectional, and linear (Savickas, 2001). Career maturity measures, however, are often used to identify limitations or deficiencies in terms of an individual's career maturity and as an evaluation tool to determine if career counseling has increased the client's career maturity. The two instruments that are most frequently used in this area are the Career Development Inventory and the Career Maturity Inventory.

The *Career Development Inventory* (CDI; Super, Thompson, Lindeman, Jordaan, & Myers, 1988b) measures career maturity by using Super's theory. The scales of Career Planning, Career Exploration, Decision Making, and the World of Work correspond to Super's theory, with the exception of not including a measure of Reality Orientation. An overall career maturity measure, called the Career Orientation Total, is also available. The CDI does measure a cogent model of career development but some have questioned whether the model still has applicability given the rapid changes in the workforce and global labor market. A somewhat related instrument is the *Adult Career Concerns Inventory* (ACCI; Super, Thompson, Lindeman, Jordaan, & Myers, 1988a), which evolved from the Career Development Scale (Adult Form). Super suggested that the term *career adaptability* is more appropriate for adults than the term *career maturity*. The ACCI, which does not follow the same format as the CDI, focuses solely on the planning dimension of Super's model. The ACCI primarily assess adults' needs for career planning and adaptation, but it should not be used if a counselor desires a measure of adult career competencies, such as decision-making skills or job search skills.

Another common measure of career maturity is the *Career Maturity Inventory* (CMI), which was recently revised (CMI-R; Crites & Savickas, 1995). The CMI was revised to shorten the administration time and to modify the instrument so that it could be used with postsecondary students and adults. The CMI-R is composed of an Attitude Scale, a Competence Scale, and an overall indicator of Career Maturity. Furthermore, the revised edition includes the Career Developer (CDR), which was constructed to interpret each item. Counselors can use the CDR for hand-scoring or to help facilitate greater maturity by allowing the client to learn the correct response to each item. In the CMI-R, the Attitude Scale and the Competence Test both contain 25 items. Currently, there is limited information on the psychometric qualities of the revised edition; however, this instrument has a strong theoretical and empirical foundation.

As you may have noticed, many of the assessments that have been used to assess clients' progress in career development or to evaluate the effectiveness of career counseling were published in the 1980s. As will be discussed in Chapter 13, counselors increasingly need to demonstrate that the services and treatments they provide are worth the time and expense. There is a substantial need for more refined and current assessments that can be used to evaluate the effectiveness of different career assessments and counseling programs.

Qualitative Career Assessment

Some counselors have questioned whether career assessment attempts to objectively measure clients' traits are consistent with postmodern philosophy and constructivism (McMahon, Patton, & Watson, 2003). One of the first professionals to promote qualitative assessment was Goldman (1990), who contended that qualitative assessment can most easily be defined by what it is not. Goldman contended that qualitative assessment is for the most part not standardized tests that usually yield quantitative scores and norm-based interpretation. In Goldman's view, qualitative assessment tends to foster a more active role for the client rather than a more passive interpretation of the results provided by the clinician. Goldman also suggested that qualitative assessment emphasizes a holistic study of the individual compared with relying on more discrete measures of human constructs such as interest, abilities, or personalities.

Qualitative career assessment is not a set of specific assessment instruments or techniques. In discussing career counseling in the postmodern era, Savickas (1993) recommended assisting clients in inventing a workable personal framework for their lives that includes their work role. The career assessment process focuses on stories, enabling the counselor to rely more on autobiographical techniques than interest inventories or other traditional assessments. As Savickas indicated, "Counselors can help clients to interpret life and career by viewing the person as a text. Like hermeneutical scholars who interpret the meaning of a literary passage from the corpus of the work, career counselors may interpret clients' interest, abilities, and work values as an expression of a career pattern or central theme" (p. 213). This process, however, does not involve the counselor simply listening to the client's stories and making interpretative conclusions; rather, the client and counselor act as coauthors and editors in (1) authoring a coherent, continuous, and credible career story; (2) identifying themes and tensions within the story lines and attributing meaning to those concepts; and (3) developing a narrative or plan to learn the skills needed to perform the next episode in the story.

McMahon et al. (2003) also suggested that qualitative career assessments should consist of small, simple, and sequentially logical steps. These small steps should flow logically and provide a focused, yet flexible process that promotes a sense of hope in clients. Furthermore, the qualitative assessment needs to be structured to encourage client-counselor collaboration and cooperative involvement. Finally, McMahon recommended that the instructions that accompany a qualitative career assessment process also include examples of debriefing questions that facilitate learning and generate examination of meaning.

Cohen, Duberty, and Mallon (2004) addressed the importance of social and cultural influences and themes of power and ideology in research using career narratives. Many of these same issues related to attending to social contextual factors as they apply to the use or development of qualitative career assessments. These authors suggested that the construction of narratives needs to elucidate the socially and culturally embedded nature of career and facilitate a greater understanding of the relationship between the individual and the social context. Hence, when one is developing a qualitative career assessment, an emphasis would be placed on social phenomena and the interrelationship with the cultural and historic context of the individual. Schultheiss (2005) suggested assessing and examining the relational influence in career assessment because work and important relationships (e.g., relationships with family members) are complexly interwoven constructs, and sometimes relational influences are ignored by counselors conducting career assessments.

To use qualitative career assessment, a practitioner must understand the philosophical underpinnings of the approach. The philosophical foundations of a narrative approach are different from most career development theories that often have the goal of *predicting* career choice or career-related behaviors (Bujold, 2004). This philosophical distinction is paramount, because in traditional career assessment, a clinician would focus on the degree to which the instrument provides assistance in determining a career direction (Whiston & Rahardja, 2005).

Issues and Trends in Career Assessment

In the area of career or vocational assessment, it is particularly important for counselors to consider current trends and emerging issues. Often in vocational assessment, counselors are assisting individuals in planning their work lives and with the rapid changes that are occurring in our society. This is becoming increasingly more difficult. Technology continually influences the counseling field and this is particularly true in the area of vocational assessment. Many of the instruments that have been discussed in this chapter can be taken over the Internet and clients can receive results within seconds. This evolution in career assessments has many advantages, but there also are some disadvantages and some issues that counselors should consider related to Internet-based career assessment. One issue in particular concerns employment trends and gender and racial group differences regarding career exploration and planning. In using career assessments, counselors need to be aware of issues related to gender, race, and ethnicity to best serve the needs of their clients. Although this is true in every area of assessment, it is particularly true in the area of career assessment where some clients are likely to see the results of a career assessment as being prescriptive and not understand the limits of these instruments.

Technology and Internet-Based Career Assessments

The number of sites on the Internet expands exponentially each day, and this same expansion has occurred in websites on career assessment. In examining instruments included in *A Counselor's Guide to Career Assessments Instruments* (Kapes & Whitfield, 2002), Sampson, Lumsden, and Carr (2002) found that only about 18% of career assessments were available directly on the Internet, whereas today many of the commonly used assessments have Internet versions that can be purchased by individual clients or counseling organizations. They can do so by either purchasing licenses to use the sites or downloading the software from the Internet site.

In one of the first attempts to examine career counseling Internet sites, Oliver and Zack (1999) evaluated 24 no-cost career sites. These researchers found that the content of the sites varied markedly, with many sites deficient in terms of the quality of their assessments and interpretations. They found only one site that reported psychometric data for its measures, and information concerning the development of the sites was not attainable, even when efforts were made to contact the site developers. Oliver and Zack concluded that although they saw considerable potential in the Internet sites, the sites had many shortcomings. Barak (2003) contended that the area of online career assessments may be divided into two groups. The first group includes assessments provided by professionals intended for use by individuals or groups, such as the Self-Directed Search online version (http://self-directed-search.com). The second group includes amateur tests, quizzes, questionnaires, or illegally adapted copies of existing instruments.

Even for existing instruments that were developed by professionals, many authors emphasize the necessity of validating career-counseling instruments and interpretive materials now found on websites (e.g., Oliver & Chartrand, 2000; Sampson, 2000). Although there may be extensive research related to a paper-and-pencil version of an instrument, there still needs to be additional research related to whether the Internet version is comparable to the paper-and-pencil version. For many users of Internet assessments, it is difficult to ascertain whether the instrument is sound and methodologically strong or if it is some quickly developed test with no basis. Although this same criticism can be made of paper-and-pencil assessments, these instruments are typically given by professionals who have the necessary training to use them. The Internet is not regulated; thus, in many ways, the consumer may be purchasing worthless information. In addition to the monetary costs, there are other costs of using online material. For example, an individual might quit a job, enter an expensive training program, or seek unsuitable work based on the results of an instrument developed by a nonprofessional. Hence, Internet career assessment has the potential to harm individuals.

One issue particularly salient to Internet use concerns privacy and keeping results confidential. Although some sites are protected by advanced security procedures, this is not true of all sites. Furthermore, in face-to-face interpretations of test results, the counselor has the opportunity to explain assessment results that may be confusing or upsetting to the client. This ability is completely lost if the interpretative material is provided only over the Internet. Although somewhat dated, the National Career Development Association (NCDA) has developed *Guidelines for the Use of the Internet for the Provision of Career Information and Planning Services* (National Career Development Association, 1997), and the National Board for Certified Counselors (NBCC) has developed *Standards for the Ethical Practice of Web Counseling* (National Board for Certified Counselors, 1998).

Strengths and limitations of internet or technology-assisted career systems. In the previous 20 years, computers and technology have changed career assessments. It may no longer be appropriate to use the simplistic term *computer-assisted career assessment systems* because individuals are now accessing information not just from computers but also from devices other than their computer (e.g., cell phone). In addition, with the explosion of the Internet, career assessments are not necessarily downloaded onto a computer as assessments, and interpretations can often be more efficiently managed through a website. Hence, the term I will use is *technology-assisted career assessments*. Technology-assisted career assessment systems have many advantages. (1) The systems can store large amounts of information that can be easily updated, (2) clients can retrieve information that corresponds to their individual needs, (3) clients can progress through the assessments and information at their own pace, and (4) many of these systems guide clients through a systematic decision-making process that can serve as a framework for future career decisions (Gati, Saka, & Krausz, 2001).

Another problem concerns the perception that these technology- or computer-assisted programs provide "the answer" rather than encouraging the client to explore and make informed career decisions. Because of the nature of computers, some clients are likely to see these programs as being more "scientific" and providing a definitive career decision. Individuals may access career assessments through the Internet and not seek assistance related to interpreting the results. Counselor-free career interventions have not been found to be effective and clients may make poor choices without the assistance of a trained counselor. Computers and other technologies are well-suited to repetitive tasks and computational activities (e.g., administering items, scoring scales, and constructing profiles), which can give clinicians more time to integrate findings, interpret results, and assist clients with career-related issues (Sampson, Lumsden, & Carr, 2002).

In my view, one of the major problems with career assessments on the Internet is the difficulty many individuals may have in telling the differences between legitimate websites and ones constructed in a haphazard manner with little if any attention to the quality of the assessments. Barak and English (2002), in their thorough discussion of the pros and cons of psychological testing on the Internet, have stressed the need for examining the psychometric properties of tests. Reliability and validity data are needed for all online instruments. Some instruments may appear to be legitimate but professionals may not have critiqued those Internet-based career assessments. Whiston and Oliver (2005) encouraged the involvement of counseling professionals in the construction, maintenance, and operation of Internet sites related to career assessment.

Gender and Career Assessment

In recent years, one of the issues in career assessment has been related to gender differences on some career-assessment instruments. Research related to women's career development abounded in the 1980s and 1990s, and as a result, problems with women's career assessment were identified. According to Harmon (1997), "Women who experienced the career assessment process of the 1960s often report that their nontraditional interests were dismissed by their counselors as inappropriate" (p. 467). Although it is obvious that many changes have taken place in this field since the 1960s, career assessment with women still requires specific knowledge about gender differences and current knowledge of assessment research. Interest inventories typically use questions that are reflective of differential experiences. For example, the answers to questions such as "I like to fix car engines" and "I like to take care of children" may be influenced by whether the individual has had opportunities to participate in these activities. Therefore, it is not surprising that interest inventory results show gender differences. When using results from inventories that use Holland's theory, females are more likely to have higher scores on the Social and Artistic themes, whereas males tend to have higher scores on the Realistic and Investigative themes (Hansen, 2005). Females' lower scores on the Realistic and Investigative themes decrease the likelihood that they will explore occupations in the skilled trades, medicine, science, and engineering. Men, on the other hand, will be less likely to identify occupations such as counselor, nurse, teacher, or graphic artist.

Betz (1992) and Hackett and Lonborg (1993) suggested that interest inventories should use same-sex normative scores rather than combined norms. With same-sex norms, females' interests would be compared with those of other females, which would increase the likelihood of nontraditional interests being identified. For example, a female who is interested in a number of Realistic activities may receive a score of moderately high interest in this area when compared with other females, but her score may appear only as average or even below average if half of the norming group is male. Separate norming groups, however, can have a subtle influence on the manner in which clients view their results, and, thus, counselors need to address sexual stereotyping in their interpretations of interest inventories.

To supplement structured interest inventories, Hackett and Lonborg (1994) proposed the use of less-structured assessment methods, such as value clarification exercises. These less-structured assessments can more easily incorporate discussion of gender and cultural issues. Betz (2000) suggested that any type of interest assessment should be guided by exploratory versus confirmatory objectives and that the interpretation should be in line with the "opportunity dominance" versus "socialization dominance" approach. The opportunity dominance approach emphasizes that low interest scores may be a reflection of an individual's restricted learning experiences and opportunities and that new interests can develop if individuals are exposed to new experiences. Hence, low scores in mechanical and building trades occupations may be a reflection of a lack of exposure rather than solely a lack of interest. Betz (1992) therefore proposed that in addition to using same-sex norms or sex-balanced interest inventory scales, counselors have a responsibility to assist women in broadening their experiences, particularly in areas such as the sciences, engineering, and technology.

In assessing career factors with women, it is important to examine both internal and external barriers (Fassinger & O'Brien, 2000). Examples of external barriers include gender-role stereotypes, obstacles in educational systems, a lack of role models, and the "null environment" (Betz, 1994). Higher education is often referred to as a null environment because women are neither supported nor encouraged. Thus, they are in an environment that is void of assistance. Although this external or environment is not overtly discriminatory, the lack of encouragement often results in failure. Environmental barriers are not the only barriers—the socialization process for many women results in such internal barriers as low self-efficacy, performance anxiety, and lower aspirations and expectancies. In general, when using either formal or informal career assessment strategies, the counselor needs to be sensitive to gender issues and cognizant of how stereotypes may be affecting the assessment process.

Ethnic and Cultural Differences in Career Assessment

Although issues related to multicultural assessment are discussed in Chapter 15, some issues are particularly relevant to career assessment. Leong and Hartung (2000) analyzed the literature related to multicultural career assessment and discussed it related to the dimensions of *cultural validity* and *cultural specificity*. Cultural validity addresses the concept of whether instruments that have been developed primarily from a Eurocentric perspective can be used with clients from other cultural backgrounds. Cultural specificity, on the other hand, concerns the extent to which variables, such as worldview, cultural identity, communication style, and decision-making preferences, are addressed in the assessment process.

Career researchers have also examined the appropriate use of interest inventories with racial and ethnic minorities. Although early research cast some doubt on the use of Holland's hexagonal model with ethnic minority samples in the United States (Rounds & Tracey, 1996), later research supported a common vocational interest structure among racial and ethnic minorities (Day & Rounds, 1998; Fouad, Harmon, & Borgen, 1997). The Day and Rounds results are particularly noteworthy because their sample was more than 49,000 and involved large groups of minority students. Their multidimensional scaling analysis provided support for traditional methods of assessing career interests by indicating that individuals from diverse ethnic groups use the same cognitive map or structure of preference when examining career interests. This does not mean, however, that the percentage of individuals from different ethnic groups will be the same for Holland's six areas, because we do see that certain themes tend to have higher representation. For example, African Americans are more likely to have high Social interests, and Asian Americans tend to have higher Investigative interests.

In response to these concerns about multicultural career assessment, Flores, Spanerman, and Obasi (2003) developed a culturally appropriate model of career assessment. The first phase is *culturally encompassing information gathering*. In this initial phase, it is important that the counselor gather information related to identifying the client's career issues and to understanding the client as a cultural being. Flores et al. stressed that given the limitations of many career instruments, in the data collection process it is critical to understand the client along cultural dimensions. The second stage of this model concerns *culturally appropriate selection of instruments*. Within this stage, the counselor should examine scale development, the degree to which the instrument developers addressed multicultural issues, and the use of the instruments with multiple groups. In addition, the counselor should consider measurement issues and evaluate the normative sample. There is also the issue of validation evidence across different ethnic and racial groups. In the third phase of the model, the focus is on *culturally appropriate administration*. According to Flores et al., the development of a strong therapeutic relationship is key to culturally appropriate administration. Multicultural assessment standards (Association for Assessment in Counseling, 2003b) suggest providing information to individuals both before and after test administration to orient and debrief clients. The final phase is *culturally appropriate interpretation of assessment data*. In this phase, all prior information collected during the information gathering and assessment administration stages is synthesized to formulate hypotheses that will inform future career interventions. The counselor needs to be cautious when interpreting test results from culturally diverse clients, particularly when there is limited normative data available. Flores et al. recommended a multilevel, multimethod approach that incorporates information from various sources and includes culturally relevant information (e.g., racial identity, worldview, and acculturation). Finally, it should be noted that all of the phases within this model are embedded in sound counseling practices that include multicultural competencies, career competencies, and general counseling skills.

Summary

Testing and assessment has often been seen as an integral part of career counseling. This chapter reflects many of the common practices in the area of career assessment. When considering career assessment, one should not just consider using formal assessments in isolation; Flores et al. (2003) contended that career assessments should be supplemented by interviewing so that counselors can gather a wide range of information. Turner, DeMers, Fox, and Reed (2001) suggested that career/vocational counselors should be able to integrate comprehensive results that cross the multiple domains of adolescent and adult development, personality, and psychopathology with detailed knowledge related to the assessment of interests, abilities, personality dimensions, and values. Furthermore, Chartrand and Walsh (2001) asserted that personality and cognitive assessments should be considered part of the career assessment domain. Therefore, career assessment and counseling do not involve solely job-related issues; rather, career assessment and counseling concern viewing the individual holistically and integrating career and personal information.

A number of well-developed measures of clients' individual attributes can be used effectively in career assessment. In career counseling, counselors often assess clients' interests, which are a good indicator of career direction or choice. In terms of interest inventories, John Holland's theory has had a significant influence. One of the instruments influenced by Holland is the Strong Interest Inventory®, which is one of the most widely used instruments in counseling. The purpose of the Strong is to identify interest patterns. The Strong Interest Inventory® provides results related to 6 General Occupational Themes, 30 Basic Interest Scales, and 244 Occupational Scales (122 for women and 122 for men). Counselors can have the most confidence in interpreting the General Occupational Themes and the Basic Interest Scales, and less confidence in the results from the Occupational Scales and the Personal Style Scales. There are other interest inventories or methods for assessing that counselors can consider in the career counseling process.

Ability assessment or aptitude testing is often used in career counseling because they are significant predictors of occupational success. There is also research that supports the use of self-estimates of abilities. The exploration of clients' aptitudes and abilities should include an analysis of their self-efficacy beliefs. Because self-efficacy beliefs directly influence the tasks attempted by clients, they should be considered when clinicians are engaged in any therapeutic relationship. The assessment of values is sometimes neglected despite being an important part of the career assessment process. Work values have been found to be highly correlated with work satisfaction. Any values instrument is not inclusive of all values; hence, these assessments need to be supplemented with other exercises when working with clients. There are number of integrated career assessment programs that involve the assessment of interest, abilities, and work values. Some of the more expensive programs also integrate occupational and education information into the programs so that the assessments and germane information are woven together to assist the client.

Counselors may also want to consider qualitative career assessments, which have evolved from a postmodern or constructivist perspective. Qualitative career assessments focus on understanding the client's view with an understanding that a client's perspectives are influenced by cultural, societal, and relational factors. Qualitative career assessment often involves analyzing clients' discourse or stories to identify themes and perspectives. In conducting qualitative career assessments, it is important that counselors understand the philosophical foundations of these techniques.

Rather than focusing on individual differences, some career assessment tools focus on where clients are in the career decision-making process. Typical measures of career process variables are related to the level of decidedness or certainty and degree or stage of career maturity. These instruments can be helpful in selecting career interventions that are appropriate for the client. In addition, these instruments are used to evaluate career counseling to see if clients became more vocationally mature or decided about their occupational choice as a result of the counseling.

Technology has had a significant influence on the area of career assessment and it is anticipated that this trend will continue. Computers are very adept at storing large amounts of information, and some individuals saw that this capacity made computers an excellent tool for combining career assessment with the delivery of career information. A number of systems have been developed that integrate career assessment and career information. Thus, clients can use a computer to take a career assessment, get the results, and then immediately access career information. The number of online career assessments has substantially increased in the past few years. These assessments include both those assessments developed by professionals and those quizzes and surveys developed by lay individuals. In terms of both Internet assessments and computerized systems, these instruments, like more traditional assessments, should be evaluated in terms of the reliability, validity, norms, and suitability for the client.

In conclusion, counselors involved in career assessment must be particularly cognizant of gender issues and of ethnic and racial differences on career instruments. These issues are being addressed in the field, and, in response, instruments are being developed and revised. Although instrument developers are attending to these issues, however, the practitioner still bears the ultimate responsibility for appropriate use of an instrument. Therefore, clinicians must ensure that career assessments are appropriate for each client they assist.

CHAPTER 10

Appraisal of Personality

As a counselor, there is a good possibility that you will occasionally conduct workshops on topics related to counseling. For example, consider that you have been asked by a utilities company with a large number of employees to conduct a two-day workshop on reducing stress and increasing productivity for the clerical staff. As a part of the workshop, they would like for you to give the participants a personality inventory. The company's vice president for human resources believes a personality assessment will help the staff understand themselves better and could identify ways the staff could cope better with the stresses of their jobs. This organization has approximately 60 employees on the clerical staff, so you will need a personality inventory that can be used with a variety of people and that does not focus exclusively on psychopathology. You will also need to select an instrument that is easy to score, as it is only a two-day workshop.

The term *personality* is used in everyday conversation and has certain connotations in the mental health professions. It is not uncommon to hear someone say, "She has a good personality." When we attempt to define personality, we find that it is a somewhat elusive construct. *Personality* comes from the Greek word *persona,* which was a role-play by an actor. Like other psychological constructs, there are varied theoretical views about the facets of personality. Recent research has contributed to a greater understanding of the structure of personality. Although we know more about personality than we did 20 years ago, there is still debate about the precise definition and how to best measure it.

The assessment of personality has existed for thousands of years. The early hunters and gatherers may have assessed each other's personalities to determine who would be a better hunter or who would be a better gatherer. Nonetheless, the field of formal psychological assessment of personality is less than a century old. During the twentieth century, both public sentiments and professional views toward personality assessment varied. While Butcher (1995) predicted that personality assessment was going to increase, Piotrowski's study (1999) found that with the rise of managed care, personality assessment had decreased in use. In the future, the popularity of personality assessments will probably wax and wane based on professional, political, and economic issues.

Incorporating personality assessment into the counseling process can be beneficial. Personality assessment can, at times, provide a shortcut in identifying client problems (Aiken, 1999). In selecting interventions and making decisions about treatment, counselors can frequently benefit from having information about the client's personality. Personality probably influences coping styles, needs and desires, responses to environmental stressors, interpersonal patterns, and intrapersonal sensitivity. Counselors can use client personality information to assist them in structuring the counseling relationship and in selecting specific interventions for that client.

This chapter provides an overview of personality assessment. The information contained in this chapter is not sufficient for anyone to use these assessments without considerable additional training and supervision. Many of the instruments discussed in this chapter can be administered, scored, and/or interpreted by master's level practitioners; however, some formal instruments (e.g., Rorschach) cannot. Nonetheless, counselors often work in multidisciplinary teams and need to have a basic understanding of these instruments.

There are numerous informal and formal personality assessment tools. Within formal personality assessment, there are two major categories: **structured personality instruments** and **projective techniques.** Structured instruments (e.g., the Minnesota Multiphasic Personality Inventory-2) are formalized assessments in which clients respond to a fixed set of questions or items. Projective techniques vary from standardized instruments in that the client is asked to describe, tell a story, or respond in some way to relatively unstructured stimuli. The intent of the personality assessment is less obvious with projective techniques than with a structured inventory. The unstructured format presumably guards against faking because the examinee is not sure what the examiner is evaluating. With projective techniques, clients are believed to "project" their personality characteristics in their responses. Thus, proponents of projective techniques consider them to be an effective method for uncovering latent, hidden, or unconscious aspects of personality.

This chapter examines both informal and formal personality assessment techniques. Informal assessment techniques are frequently used, and clinicians need to understand the reliability and validity of these measures. Informal techniques, just like formal instruments, need to be analyzed for their soundness. Following the discussion of the informal techniques of observation and interviewing, there is a discussion of formal personality instruments. It includes an overview of the most commonly used structured personality inventories and projective techniques.

Informal Assessment Techniques

Observation

When you think of personality assessment, you may only consider formal assessment instruments such as the Minnesota Multiphasic Personality Inventory-2 (MMPI-2). If you believe personality assessment only includes standardized instruments, then you would be ignoring the most common method counselors use to assess personality: observation. When you meet someone, you may begin to make judgments about that person's personality based on such factors as attire, stance, choice of words, and facial expressions. In the same way, counselors observe clients from the first meeting and begin to make clinical judgments based on those initial observations. Counselor training is typically designed to produce individuals with refined observational skills. Social psychology research, however, has found that mental health practitioners tend to be biased when interpreting their observations. When clinical decisions are based on observation, there are problems with selective recall, selective interpretation, and the power of preexisting assumptions (Dawes, 1994). Clinicians often selectively remember certain aspects of what clients say and how clients behave. Practitioners also have "themes" concerning what they remember, and they have been found to recall similar information about a number of different clients. In addition, clinicians tend to be selective in their interpretations and to focus on certain behaviors and draw conclusions based on those behaviors. Social psychological research has also shown that people tend to see things with which they are familiar. Hence, a counselor who works primarily with clients who have eating disorders is more likely to see a new client as having an eating disorder than is a clinician who does not work with this type of client (Dawes, 1994). Subjectivity is a persistent problem in observation. As an example, you have probably experienced subjectivity in observation when a friend or family member holds a very different view of an event that you both witnessed.

Practitioners cannot afford to be subjective in their observations when assessing personality. Observation is an assessment tool; therefore, it should be evaluated in the same manner that we evaluate other assessment tools (e.g., examining the reliability and validity of our observations). Let us consider reliability in terms of observation. *Unsystematic error* has a way of slithering into counselors' observations of their clients. Counselors, like other humans, tend to get an occasional cold, get stuck in traffic, or have a disagreement with a family member. Any of these situations may lead to unsystematic error in their observations. Furthermore, the client may contribute to the unsystematic error. A counselor may perceive a client with sluggish speech and frequent yawns as being disinterested. However, these actions may be more related to the client staying up late the night before than to disinterest. Counselors should examine the reliability of their observational methods, for there may be a high degree of error in these methods. Counselors can adapt some of the traditional methods of determining reliability to examine the consistency of their own observations. For example, counselors could systematically conduct a test-retest situation by noting observations in one session and then comparing these with recorded observations of a second session. A counselor could split a session into halves or systematically attend to observations at specific time intervals in a session to examine the consistency of these observations. Sattler (2002) found that clear and precise definitions of the observed behaviors and a systematic method for observing them could increase reliability. Trained observers also tend to be more reliable in their observations than nontrained observers. Attending to the concept of reliability in observation has the potential to increase the validity of the counselor's observations.

There also can be problems with the validity of counselor observations (Hoge, 1985). When counselors observe, they need to consider the *representativeness* and the *generalizability* of their observation (Sattler, 2002). In terms of representativeness, because the time the client spends with the counselor is not long, the client may not be completely natural with the counselor. Therefore, the validity of the observations may be restricted because only a small sample of behaviors was observed, which might not represent the client's typical behavior. Inadequate observations limit the counselor's ability to generalize to how the client behaves outside of counseling. For example, a client in the counseling sessions may act reserved; yet, when outside of counseling, the client's behavior may be very domineering and aggressive. One method for enhancing the representativeness of the observations is to increase the amount of time the individual is observed. For school counselors, this might be easily accomplished by observing students in the classroom, during lunch, during physical education, or on the playground. In other settings, counselors may want to have clients keep a log, which is essentially a self-observation technique. Another technique to increase the sample of observation is to have another person (e.g., a family member) record certain behaviors.

In conclusion, counselors often use observation to assess personality, and in doing so, they need to consider certain factors. Clinicians need to consider carefully how they organize the observations as well as the conceptual framework they use in determining their conclusions. Furthermore, clinicians should evaluate their working models of personality that may influence this process. Counselors also need to consider how their observations are filtered through their own biases and beliefs.

Interviewing

Interviewing is another widely used method of personality assessment. In this context, an interview is defined as a face-to-face verbal exchange in which the counselor is requesting information or expression from the client. Vacc and Juhnke (1997) found that structured clinical interviews fall into the categories of either *diagnostic assessments* or *descriptive assessments*. The intent of diagnostic interviews is to identify issues and possible disorders consistent with a diagnostic taxonomy (e.g., the *Diagnostic and Statistical Manual of Mental Disorders—Fourth Edition-Text Revision*). Chapter 12 addresses interviews in terms of diagnosis. Descriptive interviews are used when the purpose is to describe aspects of the client. The focus in this chapter is on descriptive interviews with the specific purpose of describing personality.

The same characteristics of a good intake interview (Chapter 6), such as being warm and encouraging, also apply here. The quality of the questions that counselors use in assessing personality has a substantial influence on the value of the assessment. Poorly developed questions that are not conceptually related to personality assessment will probably add little to the counselor's understanding of the client's personality. Sometimes, counselors will use questions related to the client's problems and situation as the primary mechanisms for personality assessment. Questions only peripherally related to personality may not provide clients with the opportunity to explain aspects of their personality. Therefore, when the major purpose is to understand the client's personality, counselors should ask clients questions that directly assess personality. As we will see later in this chapter, there is substantial research supporting a five-factor model of personality, and a structured interview has been developed to assess those factors of personality. The *Structured Interview for the Five-Factor Model of Personality* (Trull & Widiger, 1997) can involve more than 120 questions as the interview frequently requires follow-up questions to clarify the client's responses. In concluding this section on assessing client's personality based on interviewing, it is important to note that many of the same issues related to the discussion of reliability and validity of observation also applies to interviewing.

Structured Personality Inventories

To understand the most commonly used personality instruments in counseling, it is probably valuable to have some foundational information regarding the standard methods used in constructing personality inventories. Anastasi and Urbina (1997) suggested that there are four basic methods of constructing personality inventories. The first method is the *content-related procedure*, in which the focus is on the content relevance of the items. Developers using this method follow a rational approach to item development, with items directly relating to the personality attributes being measured. The content scales of the MMPI-2 are examples of this type of procedure. There are some difficulties with content-related procedures because the instruments are often easy to fake or to have a response set. A response set exists when an individual answers one question a certain way and then falls into the habit of answering similar questions in the same way.

The second method of constructing personality inventories uses *personality theory* as the base for development. Once the instrument is developed, construct validation procedures are implemented to determine if the instrument actually measures the tenets of the theory. Thus, the validation information is interpreted concomitantly with the theory. An example of a theory-related instrument is the Myers-Briggs Type Indicator, which is based on Jungian theory.

Empirical criterion keying is the third method of constructing personality inventories. Items are selected based on their relationship to some external criterion rather than on their content. The MMPI-2 is an example of the empirical criterion keying method, because items were selected that separated people who were considered normal from those who were diagnosed with some form of psychopathology. The Occupational Scales of the Strong Interest Inventory® were also developed using this same method—only items that differentiate between people working in an occupation from people not working in that occupation are used in scoring of each occupation scale.

The last method involves the statistical technique of *factor analysis*. This strategy entails examining the interrelationships of items and determining the similarities of the items that group together. Researchers who have used factor analysis to investigate personality have found five factors (nicknamed the "Big Five"). The NEO Personality Inventory—Revised (NEO-PI-R) is designed to measure these five factors of personality.

The precise number of self-report personality inventories is difficult to determine, but there are at least several hundred. Rather than discuss all of these instruments (which would mean reading this book for a very long time), this section summarizes the instruments most frequently used by counselors. The most widely used structured personality instrument, the Minnesota Multiphasic Personality Inventory 2, will be discussed first. The second instrument to be discussed is the NEO-PI-R, which has a substantial empirical foundation and is increasingly being used by practitioners. Finally, the Myers-Briggs Type Indicator, another popular instrument used in diverse settings will also be reviewed.

Minnesota Multiphasic Personality Inventory 2

The *Minnesota Multiphasic Personality Inventory 2* (Butcher, Dahlstrom, Graham, Tellegen, & Kraemmer, 1989) replaced the original MMPI in order to improve on this widely researched and used instrument. The MMPI-2 subsequently replaced the MMPI as the most widely used personality instrument. Soon after the publication of the MMPI-2, another form was introduced, the *Minnesota Multiphasic Personality Inventory—Adolescent Version* (MMPI-A, Butcher et al., 1992) for children ages 14 to 18. The MMPI and the MMPI-2 are empirical criterion keyed instruments, which means the items were not selected for their content but rather for their relationship to a criterion. The criterion in the original MMPI was the identification of psychopathology: it was designed to differentiate those individuals with psychopathology as compared with normal individuals. The MMPI-2 manual reflected that it is a "broad-based test to assess a number of the major patterns of personality and emotional disorders" (Butcher et al., 1989, p. 2). Therefore, the MMPI-2 is used to diagnose emotional disorders, but it is also intended for use in nondiagnostic activities. Although the MMPI-2 is often cited as the most widely used structure personality assessment, Maruish (2004) has noted a recent decline in use because of its length (i.e., 567 items). On the other hand, the MMPI-2 continues to be actively researched since Graham (2006) found that, since the publication of the MMPI-2 in 1989, there have been approximately 2,800 published journal articles related to the MMPI-2.

The MMPI-2 booklet contains 567 items, and the MMPI-A has 478 items. The items are statements (e.g., I am sure I get a raw deal from life, I cry easily) to which the client responds by indicating whether the statement is true, false, or cannot say. The MMPI-2 has an eighth-grade reading level, although clinicians can purchase an audiocassette version for clients whose reading level is not sufficient. In addition, the MMPI-2 is available in English, French, Hmong, and Spanish.

One of the major reasons for revising the MMPI was that the original norming group had been tested in the 1930s and consisted primarily of white, middle-class individuals from Minnesota. The MMPI-2 norming group, selected to match the 1980 census data, included 2,600 individuals who matched the proportions of ethnic groups, geographic representation, and age distribution of the U.S. population. The MMPI-2 norming group has been criticized, however, for including a high proportion of individuals with advanced educational backgrounds and higher-status occupations. Although there is greater representation of minority individuals in the MMPI-2 than in the MMPI, there continues to be some debate about racial bias (Newmark & McCord, 1996). Graham (1999) and Timbrook and Graham (1994) found that the differences among ethnic groups on the MMPI-2 were not statistically significant. Anyone using the MMPI-2 or the MMPI-A with diverse clients, however, should be knowledgeable about racial and ethnic differences on both the validity and clinical scales to ensure proper interpretation. Furthermore, others have argued that with clients of color, clinicians need to take into account acculturation (Anderson, 1995), socioeconomic status, and education (Long, Graham, & Timbrook, 1994).

The interpretation of the MMPI-2 is complex, and specific training is needed to use the results appropriately. There are seven validity scales and a variety of clinical scales subdivided into three major categories: Basic Scales (10), Content Scales (15), and Special Scales (varying number) (MacCluskie et al., 2002). In addition, some psychologists are particularly interested in the Restructured Clinical Scales that were published in 2003. A proper interpretation involves examining the entire profile as a whole, not just each clinical scale in isolation. Newmark and McCord (1996) argued the MMPI-2 could be dangerous in the hands of the casual user who has not mastered its intricacies. Even though a *T* score of 65 is usually considered the cutoff, a clinician does not consider just one elevated score to indicate the disorder with which that scale is labeled. This is one reason that the basic clinical scales are usually referred to by number rather than by name. For example, an elevated Scale 4 (Psychopathic Deviance) might result from family discord, friction with peers, hostility toward a supervisor, or alienation from self and society. As Groth-Marnat (2003) indicated, a clinician should not interpret an elevated Scale 4 score as always indicating antisocial acting out, as it may be a reflection of family discord.

The purpose of this discussion of the MMPI-2 and MMPI-A is to provide counselors with an introduction to these well-known personality assessments. This discussion, however, does not provide sufficient information on how to interpret or use the MMPI-2 or the MMPI-A, and clinicians would need additional training and supervision before they would be qualified to use these assessments. In analyzing a client's results, one of the initial steps often involves examining how long the individual took to complete the MMPI and whether the client's time is close to the typical time (90 minutes for the MMPI-2 and 60 minutes for the MMPI-A). The clinician should have some concerns if the individual took an extraordinarily long time or completed it very quickly. A common second step involves scoring and plotting the scores on the profile sheet or examining a computer-scored profile. Figure 10.1 shows the computer scored profile, which includes three of the Validity Scales and the ten Basic Scales. There are additional profile sheets for plotting the Content Scales and the Supplementary Scales. In addition, some MMPI-2 or MMPI-A reports will include a Welsh Code, which is a "short-hand" method for indicating performance on the Basic Scales (see Butcher & Williams, 2000). The clinician would then move on to examining the "validity" of the profile using primarily the Validity Scales (see the following section). The scores on the Validity Scales provide an indication of the degree to which the individual may have attempted to distort or skew his or her responses. After the Validity Scales are examined to determine the amount of distortion, the Basic Scales (which are described later in this chapter) are interpreted. Often when two or three Basic Scales are elevated, the interpretation of the profile includes an examination of the Two-Point Codes and Three-Point Codes. Many times interpretations of the MMPI-2 will also include analysis of the 15 Content Scales, which are listed in Table 10.2.

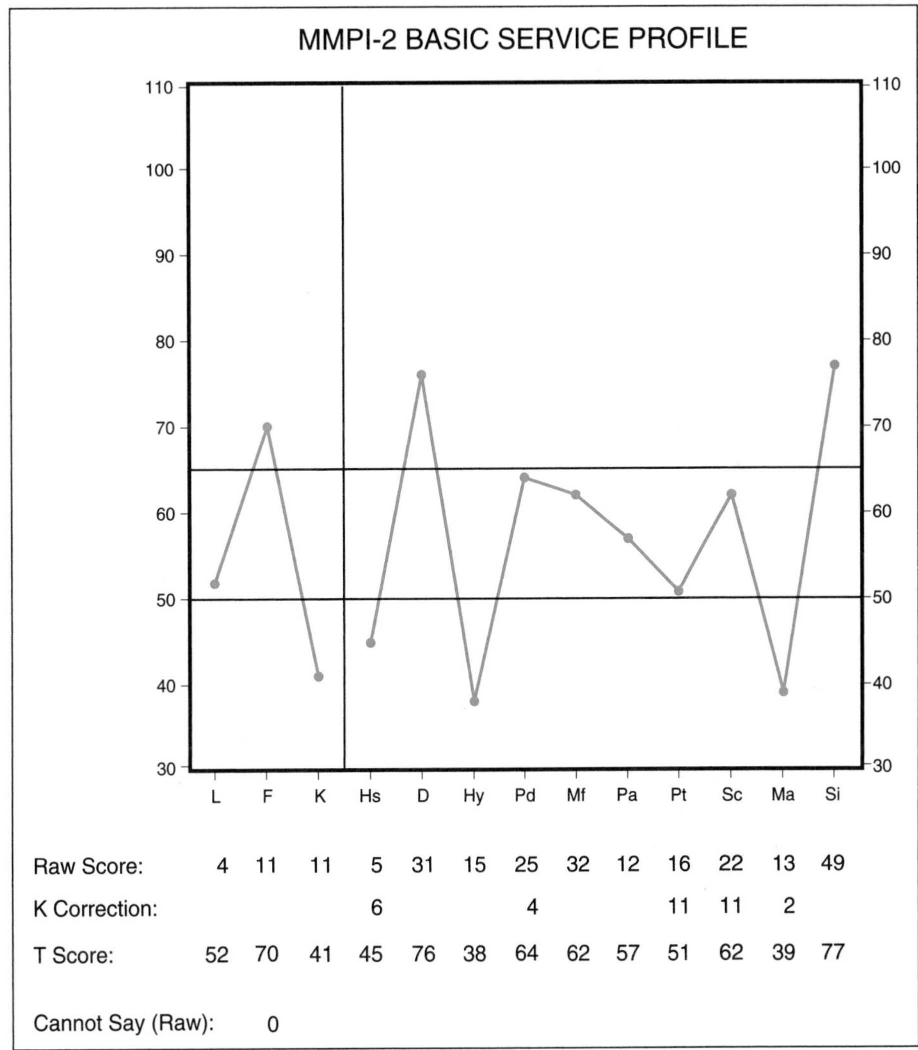

FIGURE 10.1
MMPI-2 Basic Service Profile
MMPI-2 Basic Service Report. Copyright © 1989 Regents of the University of Minnesota. All rights reserved. Portions excerpted from the MMPI-2 Manual for Admimistration, Scoring, and Interpretation. Revised Edition, copyright © 2001 Regents of the University of Minnesota. All rights reserved. "MMPI-2" and "Minnesota Multiphasic Personality Inventory-2" are trademarks of the University of Minnesota.

Validity scales. In interpreting a personality inventory, it is often quite helpful to understand individuals' attitudes while they were taking the inventory. For example, it might be helpful to know if clients are trying to put their "best foot forward," or if someone on trial for murder is attempting to appear psychologically disturbed. The validity scales of the MMPI-2 are designed to provide this type of information; in other words, these scales reflect the validity of the profile. There are several measures of the validity of the MMPI-2 and MMPI-A profile, and it is best to examine many of the measures simultaneously to make clinical judgments about the usefulness of the results. Butcher and Williams (2000) recommended first examining item omissions, inconsistent responding, and fixed responding, which involves the Cannot Say Score (?),

VRIN, and TRIN. They then suggested that a clinician examine measures of random and exaggerated responding, which are the F, Fb, Fp, and FBS scales. Finally, the clinician should examine the scales designed to assess defensiveness and claims of extreme virtue, the L, K, and S scales.

Cannot Say Score (?) The ? scale is simply the total number of items on the MMPI-2 that the individual did not answer. For most clients, the typical number omitted is between zero and six, and Duckworth and Anderson (1997) suggested further investigation if the number of omitted items is seven or more. If a client leaves a large number of items blank on the MMPI-2 or MMPI-A, it is important to explore possible factors that may have contributed to the omissions (e.g., difficulty with reading, confusion, recalcitrance).

VRIN Scale The Variable Response Inconsistency (VRIN) scale examines consistency of response and can be helpful in determining if the person randomly marked answers or had difficulty understanding the items. VRIN consists of paired items in which the content is very similar or opposite. Thus, if responses are not in the expected manner, then the inconsistencies will be reflected in the VRIN score. VRIN can be helpful in interpreting whether a higher F scale relates to responding randomly or attempting to fake.

TRIN Scale The True Response Inconsistency (TRIN) scale is designed to measure "yea-saying" or "nay-saying." These are paired items with consistency indicated by answering true one time and false the other time. This scale identifies those individuals who mark all the items true or all the items false.

F Scale The Infrequency (F) scale concerns whether the individual is faking or attempting to exaggerate symptoms. Endorsing a large number of these items indicates the test taker is presenting an extremely symptomatic picture not found in the general population. In some cases, there may be a tendency to exaggerate symptoms or attempt to "fake bad." However, Duckworth and Anderson (1997) found that in mental health clinics and college counseling centers, a high F scale represents the degree to which an individual's thoughts are different from the general population and only occasionally is it an indication of purposefully faking bad.

FB Scale The Infrequency Back (FB) scale is an extension of the F scale and measures items that are infrequently endorsed by the general population. The majority of validity scales are in the first part of the MMPI-2, in case practitioners use the shortened version; the FB is on the back portion of the MMPI-2 and can verify the score on the F scale. In addition, counselors may also use the score on the FB to determine whether the person may have responded randomly on the second half of the test. The MMPI-2, which has 567 items, is a lengthy instrument, and some test takers may become tired or bored while completing the second half of the assessment.

FP Scale The Psychopathology Infrequency (FP) scale is a comparatively new validity scale that indicates the veracity of the client's negative symptoms. This validity scale is designed to indicate rare or extreme responses in a psychiatric setting as compared with the other F scales, which indicate rare responses in a normal setting.

FBS Scale The Symptom Validity (FBS) Scale has been recently added to the standard validity scales of the MMPI-2, although it was introduced by Lees-Haley, English, and Glenn (1991). It is sometime informally labeled the fake bad scale, but there is substantial research that supports this scale's usefulness in measuring potentially exaggerated claims of disability. This scale should not be interpreted in isolation: it should be interpreted in the context of the setting and in conjunction with the scores of the other validity scales.

L Scale The Lie (L) scale provides an indication of the degree to which the individual is trying to look good. Higher scores indicate that the individual wants to report socially correct behaviors; lower scores suggest the ability to acknowledge general human weaknesses. This scale should not be interpreted to represent overall honesty or the tendency to lie. A high L scale may indicate that the counselor will need to work on being seen as trustworthy to encourage the client to be more self-disclosing. Butcher, Cabiya, Lucio, and Garrido (2007) indicated that is not unusual for Hispanic clients to have slightly elevated L Scales, particularly newer immigrants to the United States, who may feel uncertain about their acceptance in this culture.

K Scale The Correction (K) scale measures defensiveness or guardedness. It is more subtle than the L scale but measures the same dimension of trying to present oneself in an overly positive manner. The context in which the person is taking the MMPI-2 must be considered when interpreting the K scale. For example, one might expect a higher K scale if the MMPI-2 is a part of a hiring process than if it is taken by someone seeking counseling. In counseling situations, an elevated K scale (above 65) may indicate the individual will have difficulty recognizing his or her own contributions to problems (Duckworth & Anderson, 1997).

S Scale The Superlative Self-Presentation (S) scale is another comparatively new validity scale of the MMPI-2 and was designed as an additional measure of defensiveness. In addition to serving as a general measure of defensiveness, it is also possible to obtain subscale scores that provide information on the possible reasons underlying the defensive attitude. These subscales are the Beliefs in Human Goodness, Serenity, Contentment with Life, Patience/Denial of Irritability, and Denial of Moral Flaws.

Basic or clinical scales. After examining the validity scales to determine the validity of the profile, the next typical step is to interpret the Basic or Clinical Scales of the MMPI-2 or MMPI-A. These traditional scales of the MMPI-2 and MMPI-A are drawn from the clinical scales of the MMPI (Butcher & Williams, 2000; Duckworth & Anderson, 1997). Table 10.1 on the following page lists the 10 scales, each with a number, an abbreviation, and a formal name. As with the validity scales, the clinical

TABLE 10.1
The Clinical or Basic Scales of the MMPI-2

Number	Abbreviation	Formal Name
Scale 1	Hs	Hypochondriasis
Scale 2	D	Depression
Scale 3	Hy	Conversion Hysteria
Scale 4	Pd	Psychopathic Deviate
Scale 5	Mf	Masculinity-Femininity
Scale 6	Pa	Paranoia
Scale 7	Pt	Psychasthenia
Scale 8	Sc	Schizophrenia
Scale 9	Ma	Hypomania
Scale 0	Si	Social Introversion

scales are not interpreted in isolation because the entire profile must taken into account when interpreting the MMPI-2. In MMPI-2 interpretation, the term *elevated* is often used to indicate that the *T* score on that scale is above 65. An interpretation may also include the term *moderately elevated*, which generally indicates that the *T* score is between 60 and 65. Sometimes a practitioner focuses only on the scales with elevated scores; however, other scales should also be examined to identify possible strengths and coping skills. The following overview of each clinical scale is designed to provide a basic understanding of the scales and an introduction to how the scales are combined in interpretation.

Scale 1: Hypochondriasis Scale 1 is related to excessive concerns with health, as indicated by reporting the presence of bodily complaints. This scale assumes that there is little or no organic basis for these complaints. If you have a client with a chronic illness or a client who was physically ill while taking the MMPI-2, then you need to be more cautious in your interpretation. It is believed, however, that scale 1 represents a characterological preoccupation with bodily concerns rather than a situational attentiveness to physical complaints. In addition to the physical complaints, elevated scores indicate a tendency to be self-centered, selfish, and pessimistic—although the complaints may center on health issues, they can spread to complaining or whining about other issues. Markedly elevated scores may indicate the tendency to manipulate others with physical complaints and to use these complaints to avoid responsibility and meet dependency needs.

Scale 2: Depression Elevated scores on scale 2 suggest feelings of discouragement, hopelessness, and isolation. Lower scores on the scale indicate the tendency to be optimistic, gregarious, and alert. Duckworth and Anderson (1997) indicated that scale 2 is frequently elevated for people voluntarily seeking counseling. As the scores on scale 2 increase, the client's attitude changes from sadness or gloom to a pervasive pessimism about the world. This pessimism extends to the self, with high scale 2 scores often indicating self-deprecation and overriding feelings of hopelessness.

Scale 3: Conversion Hysteria Scale 3 concerns conversion disorders that are a complex combination of denial and social flamboyancy. Moderate elevation may only reflect a tendency to think positively about people. Elevated scores reflect the tendency to deny issues. Individuals with elevated scores often react to stress and anxiety with physical symptoms. Elevations on scale 3 are also indicative of individuals who are extroverted but somewhat superficial. They have a tendency to lack both insight into their own motivations and actions as well as insight into others' motivations. Rarely is a person with an elevated scale 3 diagnosed as psychotic.

These first three scales of the MMPI and MMPI-2 are often examined in combination. Sometimes they are labeled the "neurotic triad," which is a somewhat misleading title. The configurations among the triad of scales are examined. There is empirical support for certain interpretations based on certain patterns.

Scale 4: Psychopathic Deviate An elevation on scale 4 suggests that the client is "fighting something," but does not identify the specific conflict. Higher scores reflect hostility toward social convention, authority figures, and possibly family members. Descriptors of individuals with elevated scale 4 scores include *moody, irritable, resentful,* and *impulsive.* These individuals tend to blame other people for their troubles. In addition, they often have difficulties with law enforcement and may be incarcerated. It is important for counselors to explore the context of an elevated 4 scale. If the scores are markedly elevated, the prognosis for change in therapy is poor.

Scale 5: Masculinity-Femininity Scale 5 provides a measure of whether the individual's emotions, interests, attitudes, and perspectives on social relationships and work are consistent with men or women in general. This scale is scored separately—men's attitudes are compared with men and women's with women. High scores indicate that a person's general perspective is nontraditional from others of the same gender. Hence, for males, elevated scores are associated with having a wide range of interests, especially aesthetic interests. On the other side, low scores for males indicate more of a "he-man" attitude. Higher scores are also associated with nontraditional attitudes for women, with elevated scores indicating interest in masculine activities, being assertive, competitiveness, and self-confidence. Women with lower scores have endorsed more items indicative of stereotypically feminine interests. Low scores for women on scale 5 may indicate passivity and submissiveness. Any interpretation of scale 5 needs to incorporate the client's ethnicity, socioeconomic status, and educational level.

Scale 6: Paranoia Scale 6 considers whether there is a pattern of suspiciousness, mistrust, delusional beliefs, and marked interpersonal sensitivities. Some of the items also address self-centeredness and insecurity. Moderately elevated scores are characteristic of a sensitive individual. An elevated scale 6 indicates the individual has the tendency to misinterpret the motives and intentions of others. These individuals tend to be suspicious and believe that others' actions are somehow aimed at them. Research on the MMPI-2 indicated that scale 6 was associated with severe pathology. Markedly elevated scores are indicative of disturbed thinking and psychotic behaviors.

Scale 7: Psychasthenia Scale 7 is related to some of the symptoms associated with anxiety and obsessive-compulsive disorders. It is often considered to be a measure of neuroticism and generalized anxiety and distress. Moderate scores may reflect the ability to be methodical, organized, punctual, and have high moral standards. Elevated scores indicate a tendency toward self-blame accompanied by anxiety, rumination, and feelings of insecurity. Extremely high scores are usually associated with some obsession and rigid efforts to control impulses.

Scale 8: Schizophrenia The developers of the original MMPI constructed scale 8 to identify patients manifesting various forms of schizophrenia. Because various forms of schizophrenia are measured with this scale, there are a large number of items that may appear somewhat strange to more typical clients. Scale 8 includes a wide range of strange beliefs, unusual experiences, and emotional problems. Elevated scores reflect an unconventional lifestyle, feelings of alienation, and psychoticism. It may be difficult to follow the individual's train of thought and mental processes. High scores are usually associated with people who are isolated and alienated. These clients are unconventional, eccentric, and nonconforming. Extremely high scores are associated with individuals who show blatantly psychotic symptoms.

Scale 9: Hypomania Scale 9 was constructed to measure manic or hypomanic behaviors, such as being energetic, hyperactive, and euphoric. Moderately elevated scores (not uncommon in graduate school students) suggest highly energetic, involved, and gregarious people. As the scores increase, individuals are expending more energy but are less efficient ("spinning their wheels"). Elevated scores are indicative of overactivity, flight of ideas, and emotional excitement. Clients can be easily frustrated and may fluctuate between euphoria and irritability.

Scale 0: Social Introversion High scores on scale 0 are associated with a preference for being alone; low scores indicate a preference for being with others. With many of the scales of the MMPI-2 and MMPI-A, clinicians have a tendency to assume that low scores are positive and high scores are negative. This conclusion on scale 0 is incorrect because introversion is not necessarily a deficit. Clients with moderately elevated scores on this scale prefer to be alone or with select friends. Increased scores usually indicate more social withdrawal and anxiety associated with being around people. Individuals with high scores have a tendency to worry and be guilt-prone. Examining other scales can provide an indication of the type and level of the social adjustment problems.

Two-point codes and three-point codes. After examining the client's scores on each of the Basic Scales, an interpretation of the MMPI-2 will often include an analysis of the two or three elevated scales that draw from the research on code types (Butcher & Williams, 2000). Butcher and Williams, however, cautioned against using code types when interpreting MMPI-A results. Two-point code types are one of the more researched areas of the MMPI-2 and occur when two Basic Scales scores are in the critical range (*T* scores at or above 65). For example, if an individual's scales 1 and 9 scores were 66 and 70, respectively, this would be a two-point code of 1-9/9-1. Butcher and Williams provided information on 20 different two-point code types and 3 common three-point code types. These descriptions include symptoms and behaviors, personality characteristics, and prediction or dispositions.

Other supplemental scales. Since the original MMPI was published in the 1940s, many other scales have been developed to supplement the original validity scales and clinical scales. The Content Scales have been one of the more widely researched and used scales after the Basic or Clinical Scales of the MMPI-2. As compared with the Clinical Scales, which were empirically developed, the Content Scales were developed by examining item content. Barthlow, Graham, Ben-Porath, and McNulty (1999) provided evidence that the Content Scales significantly add to predicting clients' behavior and personality, even more so than the Clinical Scales. The 15 Content Scales are briefly described in Table 10.2. On the MMPI-A, 11 of the Content Scales are the same as the MMPI-2; however, the scales of Fears, Antisocial Practices, Type A Personality, and Work Interference are replaced by the scales of Alienation, Conduct Problems, Low Aspirations, and School Problems.

The number of supplementary scales that can be derived from the MMPI-2 is substantial. Some of the supplementary scales can be hand-scored; because of the time investment, however, most practitioners use computer-generated supplementary

TABLE 10.2
The Content Scales of the MMPI-2

Content Scale	Descriptors/Symptoms
Anxiety (ANX)	Tension, somatic problems, sleep difficulties, excessive worry, and concentration problems
Fear (FRS)	Specific fears or phobias (excluding general anxiety)
Obsessiveness (OBS)	Rumination and obsessive thinking, difficulties with decisions, and distressed with change
Depression (DEP)	Depression, feeling blue, uninterested in life, brooding, unhappiness, hopelessness, frequent crying, and feeling distant from others
Health Concerns (HEA)	Many physical complaints across body systems, worry about health, and reports of being ill
Bizarre Mentation (BIZ)	Thought disorder that may include hallucinations, paranoid ideation, and delusions
Anger (ANG)	Anger control problems, irritability, being hotheaded, and having been physically abusive
Cynicism (CYN)	Misanthropic beliefs, suspicion of others' motives, and distrustful of others
Antisocial Practices (ASP)	Misanthropic attitudes, problem behaviors in school, antisocial practices, and enjoyment of criminals' antics
Type A Personality (TPA)	Hard-driven and competitive personality, work-oriented, often irritable and annoyed, overbearing in relationships
Low Self-Esteem (LSE)	Negative view of self that does not include depression and anxiety, feeling unimportant and disliked
Social Discomfort (SOD)	Uneasiness in social situations and preference to be alone
Family Problems (FAM)	Family discord, families seen as unloving, quarrelsome, and unpleasant
Work Interference (WRK)	Problems with and negative attitudes toward work or achievement
Negative Treatment Indicators (TRT)	Negative attitude toward physicians and mental health professionals

scales. Clinicians use these additional scales to both augment and confirm their interpretation of the Clinical Scales. Most of the supplemental scales were developed with a specific purpose in mind (e.g., addiction problems, marital distress). The supplemental scales that Butcher and Williams (2000) endorsed as providing the most clinically useful information are the MacAndrew Alcoholism Scale (MAC-R), the Addiction Potential Scale (APS), the Addiction Admission Scale (AAS), the Marital Distress Scale (MDS), and the Hostility (Ho) scale.

MMPI-2 current and future changes. Tellegen et al. (2003) dramatically moved the interpretation of the MMPI-2 away from empirically keyed scales and completely revamped the building of clinical scales based on combining factor-analytic methods with construct-oriented scale development. Tellegen and colleagues called these new scales the Restructured Clinical Scales and these scales have garnered significant clinical attention. These researchers noted that the scales of the MMPI were highly correlated with each other and lacked a theoretical base. They also criticized the empirical keying criterion as some of the criterion groups for the MMPI were often quite small. Tellegen et al. hypothesized that a "general distress" or demoralization factor was underlying a number of the clinical scales that obscured the interpretation of the MMPI-2 clinical scales. The overall goals in developing the Restructured Clinical (RC) Scales were to (a) have nonoverlapping scales, (b) identify scales that were distinct from Demoralization, and (c) identify scales that are relevant to clinical constructs (Rogers, Sewell, Harrison, & Jordan, 2006). The RC scales were developed to provide a roadmap for interpreting the MMPI-2 by measuring more precisely focused and pertinent elements of the Clinical or Basic Scales. The Restructured Clinical Scales are currently included in the MMPI-2 Extended Score Report.

Minnesota Multiphasic Personality Inventory-2 Restructured Form. Evolving from the Restructured Clinical Scales is a new instrument (i.e., the Minnesota Multiphasic Personality Inventory-2 Restructured Form), which will be published in 2008. The MMPI-2-RF is not intended as a replacement of the MMPI-2 but as alternative to it. One of the advantages of the MMPI-2-RF is that it will be composed of only 338 items and will take less time to complete than the MMPI-2. Even experienced users of the MMPI-2 will need training in using the MMPI-2-RF, as interpreting the results is quite different. Furthermore, the results of the MMPI-2-RF will consist of scores on 50 scales (see Table 10.3) and, thus, interpretation is complex. In addition, there will be scoring software, Q Local, which will be able to convert MMPI-2 scored records to the MMPI-2-RF results.

Psychometric qualities. There has been some debate concerning whether the MMPI-2 is equivalent to the MMPI and, as such, whether it was appropriate to build from the vast amount of validation information that existed on the original assessment. In their reviews of the MMPI-2, both Archer (1992) and Nichols (1992) contended that, for better or worse, the instruments are closely related. Certainly, Butcher et al. (1989) provided a compelling case for the comparability of the two instruments. The test-retest reliability coefficients for the clinical scales range between .67 and .92 for men and .58 and .91 for women. Using reliability generalization to analyze MMPI-2 coefficients, Vacha-Haase et al. (2001) found the average reliability coefficients ranged from .64 for Scale 6 to .81 for Scale 0. Already there is substantial validity

Validity Scales

VRIN-r	Variable Response Inconsistency-Revised
TRIN-r	True Response Inconsistency-Revised
F-r	Infrequency-Revised
Fp-r	Infrequency-Psychopathology-Revised
Fs	Infrequency-Somatic
FBS-r	Fake Bad Scale-Revised
L-r	Lie-Revised
K-r	Defensiveness-Revised

Higher-Order Scales

EID	Emotional/Internalizing Dysfunction
THD	Thought Dysfunction
BXD	Behavioral/Externalizing Dysfunction

Restructured Clinical (RC) Scales

RCd	Demoralization
RC1	Somatic Complaints
RC2	Low Positive Emotions
RC3	Cynicism
RC4	Antisocial Behavior
RC6	Ideas of Persecution
RC7	Dysfunctional Negative Emotions
RC8	Aberrant Experiences
RC9	Hypomanic Activation

Somatic Scales

HPC	Head Pain Complaints
NUC	Neurological Complaints
GIC	Gastro-Intestinal Complaints

Interest Scales

AES	Aesthetic-Literary Interests
MEC	Mechanical-Physical Interests

Internalizing Scales

SUI	Suicidal/Death Ideation
HLP	Helplessness/Hopelessness
SFD	Self-Doubt
NFC	Inefficacy
COG	Cognitive Complaints
SNV	Sensitivity/Vulnerability
STW	Stress/Worry
AXY	Anxiety
ANP	Anger Proneness
BRF	Behavior-Restricting Fears
MSF	Multiple Specific Fears

Externalizing Scales

JCP	Juvenile Conduct Problems
SUB	Substance Abuse
AGG	Aggression
ACT	Activation

Interpersonal Scales

FML	Family Problems
IPP	Interpersonal Passivity
SAV	Social Avoidance
SHY	Shyness
DSF	Disaffiliativeness

Personality Psychopathology Five (PSY-5) Scales

AGGR-r	Aggressiveness-Revised
PSYC-r	Psychoticism-Revised
DISC-r	Disconstraint-Revised
NEGE-r	Negative Emotionality/ Neuroticism-Revised
INTR-r	Introversion/Low Profile Emotionality-Revised

TABLE 10.3 *Scales of the MMPI-2 RF*

information concerning the MMPI-2 and, to a lesser extent, the MMPI-A. Archer and Krishnamurthy's (1996) major concern about the MMPI-A is the instrument's ability to detect psychopathology and the possibilities of false negatives (i.e., the instrument indicates clients do not have a psychopathology when they actually do have a disorder). Austin (1994) criticized the MMPI-2 for not responding to recent developments concerning conceptual classification in psychopathology. Chapter 12 addresses diagnosis and some instruments (e.g., Millon Clinical Multiaxial Inventory) that are directly tied to a prominent diagnostic system.

In conclusion, the MMPI-2 and the MMPI-A are widely used instruments that have clinical applications for counselors. A counselor must have in-depth knowledge about this complex instrument to use it appropriately. Computer-generated interpretative reports have almost eliminated hand-scored and interpreted reports. The use of a computer-generated report, however, does not exonerate a clinician from understanding the instrument. Furthermore, knowledge of the MMPI-2 does not mean someone can automatically use the MMPI-A, as there are differences. Ethical guidelines clearly indicate that knowledge of the specific instrument is needed.

Another instrument associated with the MMPI is the *California Psychological Inventory* (CPI). The CPI, which is now in its third edition (Gough & Bradley, 1996), drew almost half of its 434 questions from the MMPI. The CPI scales stress aspects of personality that are more normal as compared with the Clinical Scales of the MMPI. For example, the CPI provides measures of 20 Folk Scales, such as Sociability, Self-Acceptance, Empathy, Well-Being, and Responsibility. It is also possible to obtain scores on five factors of personality: Extroversion, Personal Integrity, Conventionality, Flexibility, and Emotionality. The CPI can be used in many counseling settings with clients 13 years of age and older. The CPI has a rich history and has been researched for more than 40 years. It does not appear, however, to be as currently popular as some other instruments, such as the Myers-Briggs Type Indicator.

Another instrument developed from the MMPI is the *Personality Inventory for Children—Second Edition* (PIC-2, Lachar & Gruber, 2001), which is completed by a child's parent or caregiver. Similar to the MMPI-2, this instrument has validity scales that measure Inconsistency, Dissimulation, and Defensiveness. The adjustment scales are Cognitive Impairment, Impulsivity and Distractibility, Psychological Discomfort, Family Dysfunction, Reality Distortion, Somatic Concern, Delinquency, Social Withdrawal, and Social Skill Deficits. In addition, Lachar and Gruber (1995) published the Personality Inventory for Youth (PIY), which is an extension of the PIC-2. The major difference between the two assessments is that the child or adolescent completes the PIY. The Student Behavior Survey, which is completed by a teacher, complements the other two assessments.

NEO-PI-R

Some exciting advancements in personality research directly pertain to personality assessment and one of the instruments that reflects this research is the revised NEO Personality Inventory (NEO-PI-R; Costa & McCrae, 1992). Substantial research indicates that personality can best be described by five factors (Digman, 1990; Goldberg, 1994; McCrae & John, 1992). Researchers have gathered multiple descriptors of personality, and, using factor analysis, they found that all these different descriptors fall into one of the five factors (e.g., Digman & Takemoto-Chock, 1981; Goldberg, 1992; McCrae & Costa, 1997). The prominence of these five factors has led some researchers to label them the "Big Five." These Big Five factors have traditionally been numbered and labeled as follows: Factor I, *Surgency or Extroversion*; Factor II, *Agreeableness*; Factor III, *Conscientiousness*; Factor IV, *Emotional Stability or Neuroticism*; and Factor V, *Intellect or Openness to Experience*. A mnemonic for remembering the Big Five factors of personality is OCEAN, in which it is: O for Openness, C for Conscientiousness, E for Extraversion, A for Agreeableness, and N for Neuroticism.

Not only is there substantial research that personality can be described by these five factors, but it also appears that the factors may apply across diverse cultures. McCrae and Costa (1997) found, with a particularly large sample, that the American personality factors showed remarkable similarity to the factor structure in German, Portuguese, Chinese, Korean, and Japanese samples. They contended that their findings, in addition to other research, indicate that the structure of personality is universal. These results are encouraging and suggest that instruments based on the Big Five may be appropriate with clients from diverse backgrounds.

Two researchers have been influential in developing instruments that operationalized the five factors. Costa and McCrae (1992) developed the revised NEO Personality Inventory (NEO-PI-R) as well as an abridged version, the NEO Five-Factor Inventory (NEO-FFI). The scales were developed using a combination of rational and factor analytic methods with both normal adults and clinical samples. Although the NEO-PI-R is a comparatively recent addition to the area of personality assessment, it is gaining in prominence. Caprara, Barbaranelli, and Comfrey (1995) found the NEO to be among the personality tests most heavily researched in the 1990s.

There is some debate about the appropriate names for the five factors. In the NEO-PI-R, Costa and McCrae (1992) have labeled their domains Neuroticism, Extroversion, Openness, Agreeableness, and Conscientiousness. The *Neuroticism* (N) scale provides a measure of adjustment or emotional stability. High scores are associated with a general tendency to experience negative feelings, such as fear, sadness, embarrassment, anger, and guilt. Although clinicians make distinctions between types of emotional distress (e.g., anxiety, anger, depression), Costa and McCrae have found that if individuals are prone to one of these emotional states, they are more likely to experience the others. Thus, this domain measures a tendency toward coping poorly with stress, difficulty controlling impulses, and a proclivity toward irrational thoughts.

The *Extroversion* (E) scale concerns the individual's tendency to be sociable, assertive, active, and talkative. High scores are associated with being upbeat, energetic, and optimistic. Costa and McCrae (1992) have found that introverts are not unhappy, hostile, or shy. Their studies indicated that introverts are reserved rather than unfriendly, independent as compared with followers, and even-paced as compared with sluggish.

The third dimension of personality, according to Costa and McCrae (1992), is *Openness* (O). This scale measures the degree of openness to a variety of experiences. Elements associated with openness are an active imagination, aesthetic sensitivity, attentiveness to inner feelings, and intellectual curiosity. This is perhaps the most controversial of the domains on the NEO-PI-R. Other researchers labeled this factor Intellect and contended that the Openness label does not adequately address the factor (Goldberg, 1994; Widiger, 1992). Costa and McCrae argued that this is the most researched scale of the NEO-PI-R and that a preference for the familiar as compared with a preference for novel experiences is one of the five factors.

The *Agreeableness* (A) scale measures a tendency to be sympathetic, a desire to help others, and a belief that others will reciprocate similarly. Low scores on this scale are associated with a tendency to be antagonistic, egocentric, and skeptical of others' intentions. Costa and McCrae (1992) posit that extremes at either end of this scale are problematic. Low scores are associated with narcissistic, antisocial, and paranoid behaviors; high scores are associated with dependency problems.

The last domain is *Conscientiousness* (C), which is related to the individual's ability to control impulses. This domain measures self-control and the ability to plan, organize, and carry out tasks. Low scores are associated with being more lackadaisical in the pursuit of goals. Extremely high scores can indicate fastidious behaviors, compulsive neatness, and workaholic tendencies.

Each of the five domains (N, E, O, A, C) has six facets. As reflected in Figure 10.2, the facets for the Neuroticism domain are Anxiety, Angry Hostility, Depression, Self-Consciousness, Impulsiveness, and Vulnerability. Form S is the self-report version of the NEO-PI-R, which contains 240 items with each facet containing only 8 items. Three statements at the end of the self-report instrument address the validity of the profile. These, however, are simplistic statements (e.g., asking the individual if he or she responded honestly and accurately).

To check the accuracy of an individual's responses, counselors could have someone else (e.g., a family member, friend, or colleague) complete NEO-PI-R Form R, which is the observer-report form. There are two versions of Form R—one for women, and one for men. These observer forms correspond to the self-report version except that the items are in the third person. Form S of the NEO-PI-R has both normal adult norms and college-age norms for men and women, whereas the norms for Form R are only for normal adults.

The NEO-PI-R has some critics. Part of the criticism focuses on the use of the NEO-PI-R in identification of psychopathology, which Costa and McCrae (1992) advocated. Juni (1995) contended that this use is questionable because the instrument was developed with normal adults and the model is based on common characteristics

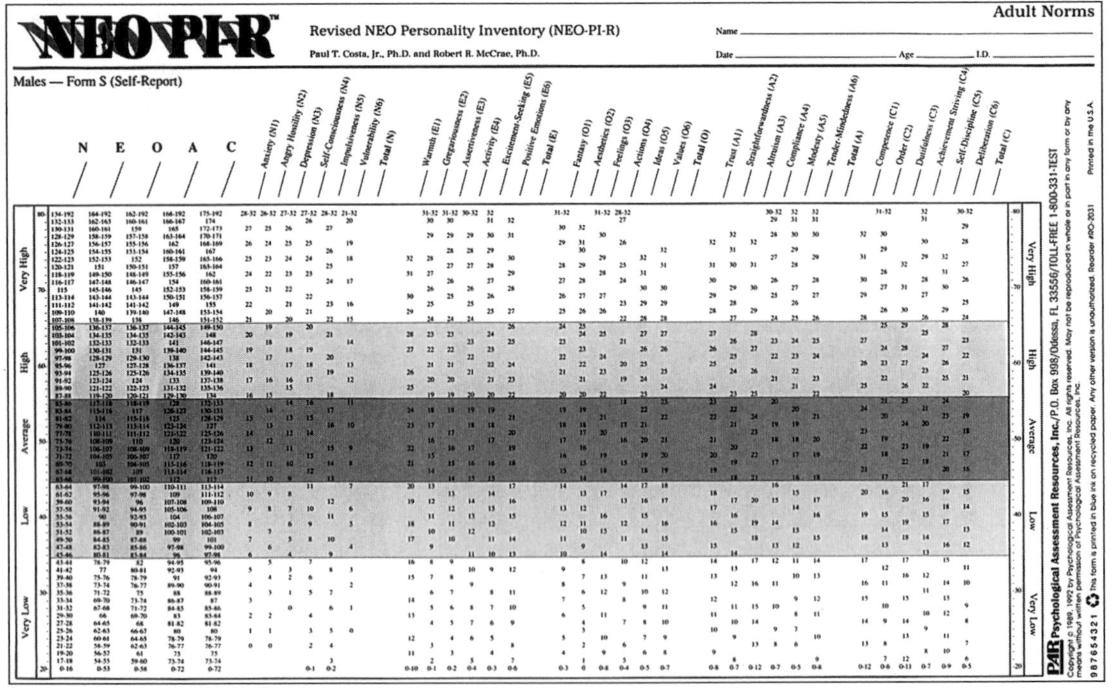
NEO-PI-R™

Revised NEO Personality Inventory (NEO-PI-R)

Paul T. Costa, Jr., Ph.D. and Robert R. McCrae, Ph.D.

Adult Norms

Name

Date Age I.D.

Males — Form S (Self-Report)

N E O A C

Anxiety (N1), Angry Hostility (N2), Depression (N3), Self-Consciousness (N4), Impulsiveness (N5), Vulnerability (N6), Total (N)

Warmth (E1), Gregariousness (E2), Assertiveness (E3), Activity (E4), Excitement-Seeking (E5), Positive Emotions (E6), Total (E)

Fantasy (O1), Aesthetics (O2), Feelings (O3), Actions (O4), Ideas (O5), Values (O6), Total (O)

Trust (A1), Straightforwardness (A2), Altruism (A3), Compliance (A4), Modesty (A5), Tender-Mindedness (A6), Total (A)

Competence (C1), Order (C2), Dutifulness (C3), Achievement Striving (C4), Self-Discipline (C5), Deliberation (C6), Total (C)

Very High — High — Average — Low — Very Low

PAR Psychological Assessment Resources, Inc./P.O. Box 998/Odessa, FL 33556/TOLL-FREE 1-800-331-TEST

This form is printed in blue ink on recycled paper. Any other version is unauthorized. Reorder #RO-2031

987654321 Printed in the U.S.A.

FIGURE 10.2
NEO-PI-R

Reproduced by special permission of the Publisher, Psychological Assessment Resources, Inc., 16204 North Florida Ave, Lutz, Florida 33549, from the NEO Personality Inventory-Revised, by Paul Costa and Robert McCrae, Copyright © 1985, 1989, 1992 by PAR, Inc. Further reproduction is prohibited without permission of PAR, Inc.

of personality, not on pathology. Conversely, in support of the NEO-PI-R, Hogan, Hogan, and Roberts (1996) found that when the five-factor model was measured with a well-developed instrument, such as the NEO-PI-R, it was a valid predictor of performance in virtually all occupations. Furthermore, they found that measuring personality in this way did not result in adverse effects for job applicants from minority groups. Another positive feature of this assessment, according to McCrae and Costa's (1997) research, is that the NEO-PI-R could be used cross-culturally.

Although not related to the NEO-PI-R, there is an instrument for children that measures the five factors of personality. The FFPU-C: Five Factors Personality Inventory-Children (FFPI-C, McGhee, Ehrler, & Buckhalt, 2007) is for children and adolescents (9-0 to 18-11). It assesses the traits of Agreeableness, Extraversion, Openness to Experience, Conscientiousness, and Emotional Regulation.

Myers-Briggs Type Indicator

The Myers-Briggs Type Indicator® inventory, authored by Isabel Briggs Myers and Katharine C. Briggs (MBTI®), is a widely used instrument based on Jungian theory. The theory suggests that variations in behavior are related to basic differences in the ways individuals prefer to perceive and then make judgments about what they have perceived. Furthermore, Jung proposed that individuals have different attitudes (i.e., introversion or extroversion) in which they use their perceptions and judgments. The different forms of the MBTI inventory are designed to assist people in understanding their preferences as measured on four dichotomies (see Figure 10.3 on the following page). The MBTI is a typology instrument in which scores on the four dichotomies result in individuals being categorized into 16 psychological types. The manual indicates the MBTI is appropriate for individuals 14 and older who can read at the eighth-grade level (Myers, McCaulley, Quenk, & Hammer, 1998). The Murphy-Meisgeier Type Indicator for Children (Murphy & Meisgeier, 1987) is an instrument that measures MBTI types for children in grades second through eighth. It contains 70 items and was designed to measure the same four preferences scales as the MBTI.

The first dichotomy, or dimension, on the MBTI indicates preference in attitudes in terms of *extroversion-introversion*. Jung described extroversion and introversion as being complementary attitudes. He suggested that everyone feels a pull between extroversion and introversion; thus, the MBTI is designed to measure an individual's preference along a continuum. The extroverted attitude (E) on the MBTI is not a simple indicator of being socially outgoing. Rather, the extroverted attitude reflects that an individual's attention seems to flow out or be drawn out to people and objects in the environment. An introverted attitude (I) is a preference for drawing energy from the environment and consolidating it within one's own position. Extroverts prefer to focus their energy on the outer world, whereas introverts prefer to focus their energy on the inner world of ideas and concepts.

The preference in terms of perception is indicated on the second dimension, which is labeled the *sensing-intuition* dimension. A higher sensing (S) score indicates a preference for perceiving using the five senses. These individuals use the senses to perceive what exists, and they often develop skills in perceiving detail, observing the situation, and remembering specifics. Those with higher scores on the intuition (N) side of the continuum perceive more by using "hunches" and perceptions of patterns.

FIGURE 10.3
Myers-Briggs Type Indicator Report Form

Reproduced by special permission of the Publisher, CPP, Inc., Palo Alto, CA 94303 from Myers-Briggs Type Indicator Report Form - Form M by Isabel Briggs Myers. Copyright © 1998 by Peter B. Myers and Katharine D. Myers. All rights reserved. Further reproduction is prohibited without the Publisher's written consent.

mbti

STEP I / REPORT FORM **FORM M**

Name ______________________________ Date ______________

The MBTI® instrument reports your preferences on four dichotomies.
There are two opposite preferences on each dichotomy, as shown below.

E–I Dichotomy Where you like to focus your attention	**E Extraversion** You prefer to focus on the outer world of people and things	**I Introversion** You prefer to focus on the inner world of ideas and impressions
S–N Dichotomy The way you like to look at things	**S Sensing** You tend to focus on the present and on concrete information gained from your senses	**N Intuition** You tend to focus on the future, with a view toward patterns and possibilities
T–F Dichotomy The way you like to go about deciding things	**T Thinking** You tend to base your decisions primarily on logic and on objective analysis of cause and effect	**F Feeling** You tend to base your decisions primarily on values and on subjective evaluation of person-centered concerns
J–P Dichotomy How you deal with the outer world	**J Judging** You like a planned and organized approach to life and prefer to have things settled	**P Perceiving** You like a flexible and spontaneous approach to life and prefer to keep your options open

YOUR REPORTED TYPE AND PREFERENCE CLARITY CATEGORY

Your reported type comprises four letters representing the four preferences you chose. Your preference clarity category (pcc) shows how consistently you chose one preference over the other. High points indicate a clear preference; note, however, that the pcc does not measure abilities or development. To determine your pcc, follow these steps:

1. Refer to the "Points" chart on page two of the answer sheet. For each dichotomy, identify the preference with the greater number of points, and record that letter and number in the "Your Reported Type" column.
2. For each dichotomy, circle in the chart below the range that includes the number next to your preference.
3. Identify the preference clarity category ("slight," "moderate," etc.) shown above each circled range and record it below. If you did not answer all of the items, your points may be lower than the lowest range of numbers on the chart. If so, use "slight" as your pcc.

YOUR REPORTED TYPE

PREFERENCE CLARITY CATEGORY
Raw Points Ranges

DICHOTOMY	Slight	Moderate	Clear	Very Clear
E–I	11–13	14–16	17–19	20–21
S–N	13–15	16–20	21–24	25–26
T–F	12–14	15–18	19–22	23–24
J–P	11–13	14–16	17–20	21–22

YOUR PREFERENCE CLARITY CATEGORY

Each type, or combination of preferences, tends to be characterized by its own interests, values, and unique gifts. On the back of this page is a brief description of each of the sixteen types. Find your reported type and see whether the description fits you. If not, the person who administered the MBTI® instrument to you can help you identify a better-fitting type. Whatever your preferences, you may still use some behaviors that are characteristic of contrasting preferences. For a more complete discussion of the sixteen types and applications, see *Introduction to Type®*, 6th ed. (Myers, I. B., 1998, CPP, Inc.) or *Gifts Differing* (Myers, I. B., with Myers, P. B., 1995, Davies-Black® Publishing).

cpp 3803 East Bayshore Road • Palo Alto, California 94303 • 800-624-1765 • www.cpp.com 6134

Those with an intuition preference perceive relationships, meanings, and possibilities. As an example, a sensing person will be able to describe the color of the carpet and the amount of wear on the furniture, whereas the intuitive person will contend that the room had a depressed feel to it.

The third dichotomy on the MBTI concerns how the individual processes or makes judgments about the information brought in through the second dimension. This third dimension measures where individuals prefer to make judgments on the *thinking-feeling* continuum. The thinking (T) function is a preference for processing perceptions using rational, cognitive abilities. A higher T score reflects a preference toward making judgments logically and impersonally. A preference toward feeling (F) indicates that an individual primarily uses personal or social values in making judgments. Individuals with higher F scores are attuned to the values of others, as well as their own, when making decisions.

The last dimension describes the process an individual primarily uses in dealing with the outer world. The MBTI assessment focuses on how individuals perceive information and how they make judgments about that information. Thus, this dimension reflects the *judging-perceiving* preference in dealing with the external world. Those who prefer judging (J) favor arriving at a decision or conclusion (using either thinking or feeling) more quickly than those who prefer perceiving (P). Those who prefer perceiving like to perceive situations and, thus, will favor putting judgments off to spend more time perceiving. The judging-perceiving dimension was not explicitly addressed in Jung's discussions of psychological types, and there are questions about whether it is truly independent from the other dimensions (Hood & Johnson, 2007).

The preferences on the four dimensions of the MBTI assessment result in a four-letter code. The different methods of combining the letters produce 16 personality types. For example, an ESFP reflects an extrovert who uses senses to perceive information and feelings to process the information and whose orientation to the outer world is perception. An INTJ is an introvert who perceives using intuition and makes judgments by thinking and whose orientation to the outer world is judgment. Counselors, however, need to be careful not to pigeonhole clients based on their personality types, because there is wide variation within each of the 16 personality types. There can often be an inherent link between types and stereotypes, and counselors using any kind of typology instrument need also to consider the uniqueness of the individual.

One of the reasons for the popularity of the MBTI inventory rests in its philosophical stance that all types are valuable and that the preferences are not correct or incorrect. The developers of the MBTI stressed that the preferences are simply differences rather than indicators of health or pathology. Myers (with Myers P. B., 1980) explained this concept in detail in *Gifts Differing,* which the MBTI manual suggests as a basic reference for anyone using the instrument. A variety of other resources are also available to aid in the interpretation of MBTI results.

On most personality tests, there are concerns about *social desirability,* or the tendency for individuals to answer questions in a manner that is socially acceptable rather than in a manner that truly reflects their personality. The developers of the MBTI attempted to control for this by weighting items differently depending on measures of the popularity of responses. Item response theory (IRT) has had a significant impact on achievement testing. It also appears to be having a similar impact on personality assessments, as evidenced by the fact that the 1998 revision of the MBTI inventory incorporated item response theory. In this revision, the instrument's developers examined the item characteristic curves (ICC) for each item (refer to Chapter 4). As an example, Figure 10.4 (see following page) contains an example of an ideal MBTI item on the extroversion-introversion dichotomy. In this case, the intent is to examine the response indicating introversion. The vertical axis represents the percentage of people who chose the introversion response, and the horizontal axis represents individuals' scores on the

FIGURE 10.4
Ideal item characteristic curve for the Myers-Briggs Type Indicator

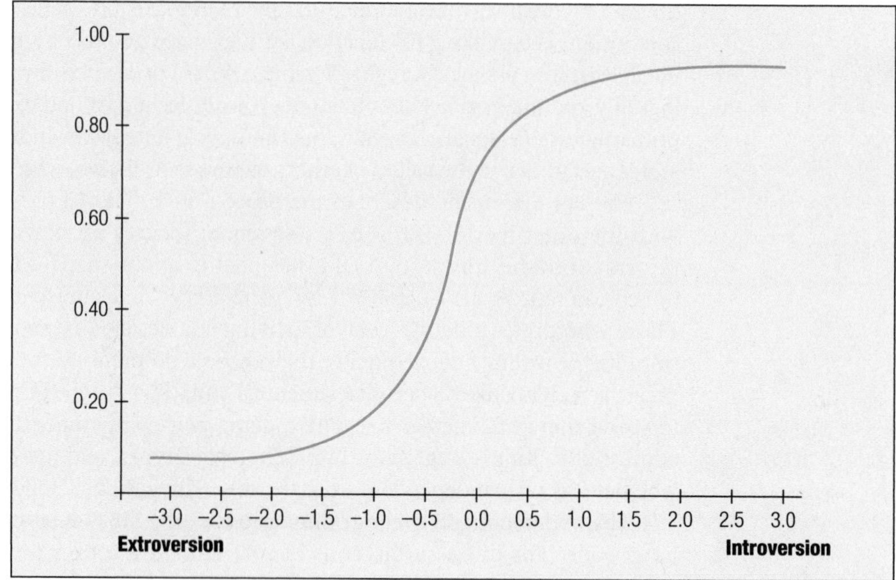

entire extroversion-introversion dichotomy. A score of −3.0 indicates a strong preference for extroversion, whereas a score of 3.0 reflects a strong preference for introversion. The developers look for an item, like the one in Figure 10.4, in which very few extroverts chose the introversion response but, on the other hand, the percentage of individuals who chose introversion dramatically rises as individuals' scores on the total measure of introversion increases. Particularly important for the MBTI are the midpoints for the four dichotomies, because the instrument separates people into types based on those midpoints. Previous editions of the MBTI had been criticized for claiming to measure dichotomies or bipolar discontinuous types (e.g., the client is either an E or an I) when the dimensions seemed to be more continuous variables that may even approximate a normal curve (Pittenger, 1993; Wiggins, 1989). Fleenor (2001) concluded that the IRT approach to item selection and scoring does reduce some of the scoring problems, specifically around the cutoff or midpoints of each of the four scales.

There is detailed reliability information on the MBTI that should be analyzed in depth by a clinician using it. The split-half reliability coefficients and the measures of internal consistency are mostly in the .90s, with some coefficients in the .80s. These coefficients, however, are based on continuous scoring of the dimensions rather than on the dichotomous types of scoring. Both Fleenor (2001) and Mastrangelo (2001) criticized the measures of internal consistency, citing research indicating that after four weeks, an average of only 65% of the sample had the same four-letter code that they had on the first testing. Using 70 reliability coefficients, in a reliability generalization study (see Chapter 3) by Capraro and Capraro (2002) found mean coefficients ranging from .76 to .84 for each of the four dimensions and an overall instrument average coefficient of .82.

In using the MBTI, a counselor needs to consider whether the use of Jungian theory is appropriate for the client and the situation because, unlike some personality instruments, this instrument is based on a theory. The Myers-Briggs Type Indicator assessment has been used in a wide variety of settings and for diverse reasons (e.g., family counseling, career counseling, team building). The widespread use of the MBTI is one of its major problems. As discussed in Chapter 4, an instrument is neither valid nor invalid; rather, validity concerns the support for specific interpretations and the uses of an instrument's results. A counselor who considers using the MBTI needs to be familiar with the validity evidence and determine if the validation evidence supports how the counselor is considering using the instrument. Mastrangelo (2001) criticized much of the research cited in the 1998 manual as mainly involving research in which the scoring is continuous on the four dimensions, concluding that research related to type scores (e.g., ENTJ) was ambiguous and wanting. Another area of criticism of the MBTI relates to the constructs being measured and whether they are sufficient to describe the complexities and important aspects of personality (Dahlstrom, 1995).

Other Standardized Personality Instruments

The three personality instruments previously discussed are commonly used standardized assessments in counseling and are examples of the different methods of constructing instruments. The empirical criterion keying method was used to construct the MMPI-2; the NEO-PI-R was constructed using factor analysis; and the MBTI is an example of an instrument based on personality theory. Another commonly used personality instrument is the *Sixteen Personality Factor Questionnaire* (Cattell, Cattell, & Cattell, 1993), which is commonly called the *16PF.* This instrument was constructed using factor analysis, which Cattell started by compiling personality adjectives. Cattell identified 17,953 adjectives that were reduced to 4,504 "real" traits. An examination of commonalties reduced this to 171 traits. Through a series of factor analyses, Cattell first identified 12 pure factors, and then 16 pure factors, of personality. The 16PF is now in its fifth edition and includes measures of 16 factors and 5 Global Factors: Extroversion, Anxiety, Tough-Mindedness, Independence, and Self-Control. Users of the 16PF should be aware that more current technical information and updated norms are available (Maraist & Russell, 2002). The 16PF is an instrument for adults, although a similar instrument, the 16PF Adolescent Personality Questionnaire (Schuerger, 2001), is available for adolescents.

Douglas Jackson influenced the area of personality assessment by constructing the *Jackson Personality Inventory—Revised* (JPI-R, Jackson, 1997), which contains 15 subscales organized in terms of the following five higher-order clusters: Analytical, Emotional, Extroverted, Opportunistic, and Dependable. The item selection procedures for the instrument were technically sophisticated. This instrument is easy to score by hand, and software is now available for generating computer reports. The Jackson instruments are psychometrically sound and well-researched instruments but are not used in counseling practice as often as some other instruments.

Limitations of Standardized Personality Inventories

One of the limitations of standardized personality inventories is that the majority of them are self-report instruments. Research has shown that when individuals are motivated to distort the results of a self-report personality inventory, they are quite adept at it (Strickler, 1969; Wiggins, 1966). However, outright lying on a self-report personality measure is not that common in counseling and hiring situations (Schwab & Packard, 1973). Some individuals may be motivated to "fake bad" as part of a trial defense, or some clients may attempt to "put the best foot forward" in order to present a more positive image to the counselor. Bornstein, Rossner, Hill, and Stephanian (1994) found that when a personality trait could be easily identified from the item (i.e., the item had high face validity), then that item was more likely to receive a socially desirable response. Although providing a socially desirable response is a common response set to personality instruments, it is not the only one. Some individuals who have a tendency toward acquiescence commonly select the "true" or "yes" response. Other individuals may have a tendency to select the uncommon or less socially desirable responses. Still others may have a tendency to select the extreme choices on almost all items.

As the previous discussion indicates, some instruments have validity scales that control for misrepresentation. Another method for controlling for faking and response set use is to inform the client of the inventory's purpose and how the results will be used (e.g., for the counselor to understand a client better or for a couple to have a better understanding of their different personalities). In addition, it is often helpful to instruct the client to answer each question honestly. Having clients focus on each question sometimes decreases the tendency to endorse items in a similar manner.

Projective Techniques

As indicated earlier, counselors often use a combination of informal and formal techniques in assessing personality. Within formal personality assessment, there are two major categories: standardized instruments and projective techniques. Projective techniques address some of the limitations of standardized instruments by providing clients with a relatively unstructured stimulus to which they respond. The intent of this technique is to make it more difficult for clients to fake their responses because they will be unsure what the unstructured stimuli are designed to measure. With projective techniques, there are no right or wrong answers because there are no specific questions. The client responds to the stimuli, and the examiner examines those responses and interprets their meanings.

Many individuals trace the use of projective assessments to the early 1900s and the rise of psychoanalytic theory. The psychoanalytic concept of projection concerns individuals' tendency to project their own drives, defenses, desires, and conflicts onto external situations and stimuli. Thus, projective techniques encourage clients to project their personality through their responses to the unstructured stimuli. Projective techniques are thought to uncover more of the client's unconscious and thus, provide an indication of covert or latent traits.

Projective techniques originated in clinical settings such as psychiatric hospitals and many remain in these settings. Some projective techniques, such as drawings and sentence completions, are also used in counseling settings. There is significant subjectivity in the interpretation of projective techniques, and extensive training is needed to use these instruments appropriately. In addition, there is no professional consensus on how any of these techniques should be specifically interpreted. Lindzey's (1959) categorization of projective techniques into five categories still provides a useful framework. The five categories of projective techniques are: *associations* (inkblots, word associations), *construction* (of stories or biographies), *completions* (of sentences or cartoons), *arrangement* or *selection* (toys or verbal options), and *expression* (drawing or dance).

Association Techniques

Rorschach Inkblot Test. The Rorschach Inkblot Test is a well-known association technique. The test consists of ten inkblots, with five cards in shades of black and gray; two in black and gray with additional touches of bright red; and the remaining three in several pastel colors. There are numerous methods or systems for using these ten cards, but typically the inkblots are presented in two phases. In the first phase, the association phase, the cards are presented and the examinee responds. In the second phase, the inquiry phase, the examiner goes back through the cards and, in a nondirective manner, questions the examinee on what prompted his or her responses. The information gathered in both phases is used in the scoring and interpretation of the responses.

One of the more widely used interpretation systems is Exner's Comprehensive System, which is based on research with the Rorschach Inkblots. In fact, this system is so detailed that some argue that the Rorschach is not a projective instrument when the interpretation is based on it. Exner's system takes into account the location, determinants, and content in terms of scoring and interpreting responses. *Location* refers to the section of the inkblot that the examinee's response focuses on. Some individuals will focus on the entire blot, whereas others will focus on common details, and still others will describe unusual details, white space, or some combination thereof. The *determinants* include the form, movement, color, and shading of the blot. For example, there is some evidence that the type of movement, whether it be human, animal, or inanimate, is associated with different psychological processes. The last scoring category is *content*, which looks at common popular responses as compared with other less common views concerning the content of the inkblot. Exner and his colleagues gathered considerable psychometric data on this interpretative system. The reliability coefficients of this system are significantly higher than those of other systems. There is also now better validity information than previously existed. No matter what scoring and interpretive system is used, however, the Rorschach Inkblots should never be used without extensive training and supervision. Furthermore, there is significant controversy associated with the Rorschach, with some researchers (Hunsley & Bailey, 1999) claiming, "There is currently no scientific basis for justifying the use of the Rorschach scales in psychological assessment" (p. 266). Others (e.g. Hiller, Rosenthal, Bornstein, Berry, & Brunell-Neuleib, 1999), however, concluded that the Rorschach is equally as valid as the MMPI for most professional uses. It should be noted that Maruish (2004) reported a decline in use of the Rorschach because it is extremely time-consuming.

Construction Techniques

Thematic Apperception Test. The Thematic Apperception Test (TAT) is an example of a constructive projective technique, in which examinees construct a story based on a picture shown to them by the examiner. Murray and his colleagues developed the TAT in 1938 as a measure of Murray's theory of needs and presses. The current version (Murray, 1943) has 31 cards—30 black-and-white pictures plus a blank card. Although the TAT is somewhat dated, Camara, Nathan, and Puente (2000) indicated that it is one of the 10 most frequently used instruments by psychologists, which is why counselors may see psychological reports that include the TAT. Depending on the examinee's age and gender, there are 20 specific cards that can be shown to them (19 pictures and 1 blank). The pictures primarily depict people in ambiguous situations (e.g., a young boy is staring at a violin that is placed on a table in front of him). The examinee then constructs a story based on each picture presented. Rarely does someone construct a story for each of the 20 pictures. The stories are recorded verbatim and then analyzed by the examiner.

Like the Rorschach Inkblot Test, numerous methods for scoring and interpreting the TAT have evolved over the years. Some quantitative scoring systems yield acceptable interrater reliability coefficients. These scoring systems, however, are somewhat time-consuming and are not used frequently. Although normative data exist on the TAT, clinicians often rely on clinical experience when interpreting the instrument. Relying on this experience can be problematic, however, because research indicates that conditions such as lack of sleep or hunger can influence performance. Another criticism of the TAT is that the pictures are somewhat out of date. However, some clinicians feel that the TAT provides a good method of entering the client's "world," while also providing a way for the client to open up to the counselor. Nevertheless, clinicians' interpretations of client responses are often quite diverse and can even contradict one another. Therefore, as with other projective techniques, counselors need to be cautious in interpreting the responses and to seek verification from other sources of information. Groth-Marnat (2003) recommended that TAT should not be used alone; rather, it should be used in conjunction with other instruments as part of an assessment battery.

Completion Techniques

Rotter Incomplete Sentences Blank. In completion techniques, examinees are provided an incomplete verbal stimulus that they must complete. For example, with sentence completion exercises, a frequently used projective technique, examinees are provided with incomplete sentences and asked to complete the sentence in their own words. Examples of sentences are "I hope . . . ," "People . . . ," "At home . . . ," and "I get upset when . . ." Some counselors have developed their own incomplete sentence assessments to address various types of issues and problems, including family conflict, transitional issues (such as going to middle/junior high school), career satisfaction, and self-concept.

A carefully constructed and standardized sentence-completion test is the *Rotter Incomplete Sentences Blank, Second Edition* (Rotter, Lah, & Rafferty, 1992). This instrument has three levels: high school, college, and adult. The client completes 40 sentences that are scored for conflict, positive responses, and neutral responses. An overall adjustment score can also be calculated from the responses. Boyle (1995) stated that the Rotter Incomplete Sentences Blank is often used in the early stages of counseling, where it is a useful quick screening device. Practitioners often do not score this instrument but, instead, clinically analyze the responses. The norms have recently been updated, and the manual provides new information on reliability and validity.

Rosenzweig Picture-Frustration Study. The *Rosenzweig Picture-Frustration Study* is derived from Rosenzweig's theory of frustration and aggression. The three forms of the instrument are based on age, with one form for adults, another for adolescents, and the third for children. An individual is presented with a series of cartoons that represent frustrating situations. In these cartoons, one of the character's speech bubbles is blank. The examinee fills in the empty cartoon bubble with a response to the frustrating situation. For example, one cartoon contains two people sitting in a car saying to the person standing beside the car, "I'm very sorry we splashed your clothing just now though we tried hard to avoid the puddle." The examinee would then fill in the empty cartoon bubble with the response for the person who was splashed. Considerable research has been done on the Rosenzweig. Clinicians must be familiar with this research when using this instrument, because there are cultural, developmental, and gender differences that must be taken into account when interpreting this instrument (Rosenzweig, 1977, 1978, 1988).

Arrangement or Selection Techniques

Assessment involving individuals selecting and arranging objects can avoid the difficulties associated with traditional assessment procedures. This is particularly true with young children as they often have difficulty answering questions or completing a paper-and-pencil exercise. Sandplay, or the use of sand trays, has become of some interest to counselors in the past 20 years. There is some disagreement about whether the sand tray should be used as a diagnostic or clinical assessment instrument or as a therapeutic tool. The International Society for Sandplay Therapy supports the psychotherapeutic application of the sand tray as compared with its diagnostic uses (Mitchell & Friedman, 1994). According to Mitchell and Friedman, the Sandplay literature indicates that five areas are predominantly considered when interpreting a sand tray: (1) how the sand tray is created, (2) the content of the tray, (3) the developmental perspective of a series of trays, (4) the Sandplay story, and (5) the therapist's feeling response.

Most research on Sandplay and the use of sand trays has been individual case studies, with very few empirical investigations. Because this technique has not been investigated extensively, it does not have the empirical base of other projective techniques. Without more research, its use as an assessment tool is questionable. Another problem with the use of sand trays is the lack of standardization. There is not a universal standard on the size of the tray, the amount of water available, or the number, size, or nature of the miniatures used. This lack of standardization severely hampers the research that can be performed or the ability to generalize from one sand tray to another. It may be easier to validate a projective technique such as the Scenotest (Straabs, 1991), which has uniformity in the figurines and materials.

Children's selection of, arrangement of, and play with toys have been used as a projective technique for many years. Because play allows for the natural expression of children's thoughts and affects, it lends itself to interpretation at multiple levels. The research on how to interpret play is not as extensive as that of other projective techniques, such as children's drawings. Schaefer, Gitlin, and Sandgrund (1991) included three of the more promising projective play assessments in their book. Interestingly, two of these projective techniques involve working with the entire family. In one of these techniques, the family engages in a collaborative drawing exercise that encourages participation of both adults and children. Each family member contributes to the drawing, which is used to aid in the understanding of the family's functioning. With the second technique, the family uses puppets for reenacting recent problematic situations. The third technique involves the use of puppets in diagnostic interviews with children and particularly focuses on analyzing the form and content of the child's play with the puppets.

Expression Techniques

Drawing techniques. It makes logical sense that the methods people use to express themselves may provide a window into their personalities. The method of self-expression that has received the most study in terms of being a projective technique is art or drawing. Oster and Crone (2004) asserted that many clients find drawing less threatening than other types of assessments. In particular, drawing techniques are often used with younger children to facilitate communication, as the clinician often asks questions as the child is drawing. One of the first formal techniques to incorporate drawing was Machover's (1949) *Draw-a-Person Test* (D-A-P). In the D-A-P, the client is first given a piece of paper and a pencil and told to draw a person. Once the first figure has been drawn, the examiner instructs the individual to draw a person of the opposite sex. After the drawing is completed, the examiner either asks the individual to tell a story about each figure or asks a series of questions concerning age, education, occupation, ambitions, and other pertinent details. Machover contended that individuals tended to project acceptable impulses on the same-sex figure and unacceptable impulses on the opposite-sex figure. In addition, certain characteristics of the drawing were thought to be indicative of certain personality traits. For example, hands behind the back were indicative of introversion; dark, heavy lines and shading suggested hostility and aggression; small drawings were related to low self-esteem; and disproportionately large heads indicated organic brain damage. However, Machover's interpretation of the D-A-P has been both questioned and criticized (Swenson, 1968).

There are a number of different approaches to interpreting human figure drawings. In general, interpretations examine pencil pressure, stroke and line quality, lack of detail, placement, erasures, shading, and distortions (Handler, 1996). Experts in this field stress that no single sign has only one fixed and absolute meaning. For example, a child drawing a face with a frown does not always indicate the child is depressed. It is also important to take into consideration the child's educational background and developmental level.

One of the outgrowths of the human figure drawings is the popular *House-Tree-Person* (H-T-P), which was originally published by Buck (1948), with the latest revision by Buck (1992) and revised by Warren. In H-T-P, the individual draws three separate drawings—one of a house, one of a tree, and one of a person. The individual is then given the opportunity to describe, define, and interpret each drawing. In general, Buck suggested that the house reflects the home situation of the client, the tree represents the self in relationship to the environment, and the person represents the self.

Burns is another influential name in projective drawing techniques. Burns (1987) adapted H-T-P into *Kinetic-House-Tree-Person*, in which the house, tree, and person in action are drawn on one sheet of paper. This technique incorporates the interconnections among the three figures and the person's action. Another technique that Burns (Burns, 1982; Burns & Kaufman, 1970, 1972) is known for is the *Kinetic Family Drawing* (K-F-D). A counselor using this technique asks the child "to draw the family doing something." The incorporation of action into the drawing, according to Burns, allows for a clearer picture of family dynamics. The child can depict the family as an active, functioning unit, which can provide indications of family interactional patterns. Figure 10.5 is an example of a 10-year-old boy's K-F-D. Burns (1982) suggested four major categories in interpreting a drawing: (1) Actions; (2) Distances, Barriers, and Positions; (3) Physical Characteristics of the Figures; and (4) Styles. *Actions* concern the overall content, theme, or activity

FIGURE 10.5 *Example of Kinetic-Family-Drawing*

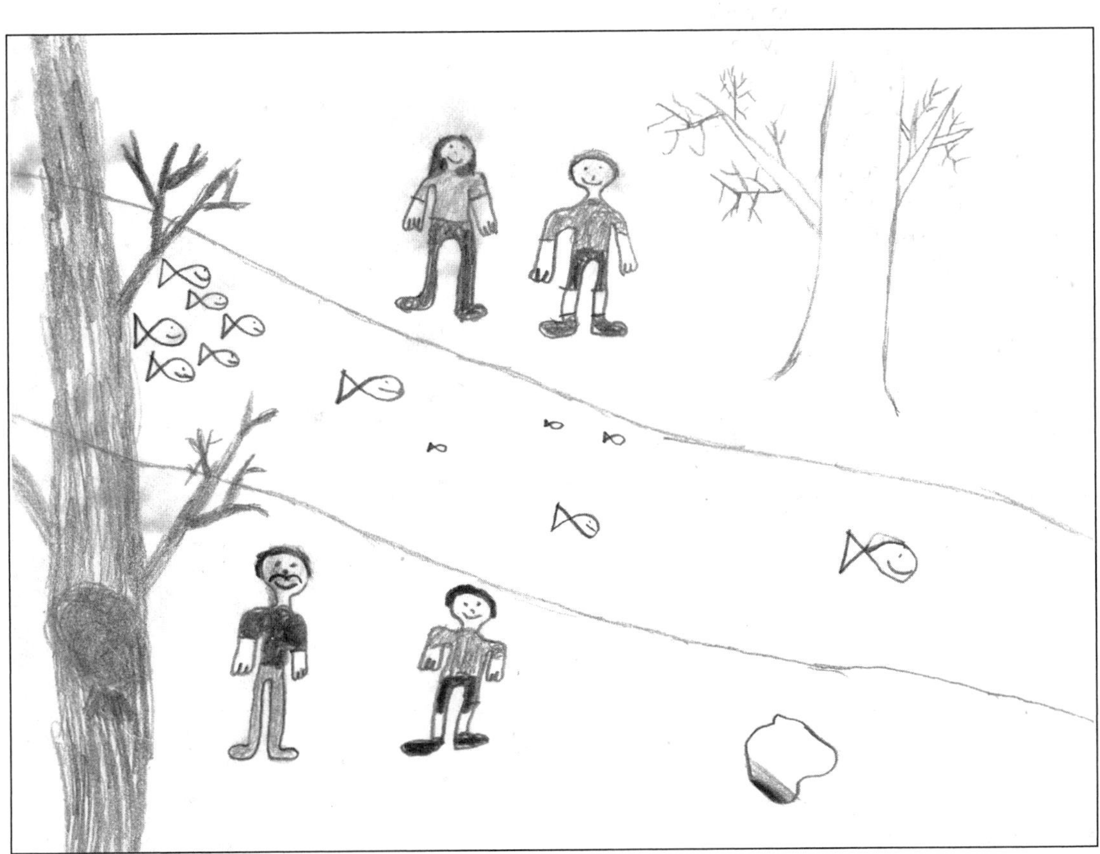

of the picture. *Distances, barriers, and positions* analyze how the family is arranged and what indicators of relationships are shown. *Physical characteristics* examine the formal aspects of the drawing (e.g., expressions, analysis of presentation of body parts, different sizes of the figures). *Style* variables are indicators of emotional problems or disturbance. Interested readers are directed to Burns' publications. A resource for counselors working with children, both in school and nonschool settings, is Knoff and Prout's (1993) *Kinetic Drawing Systems for Family and School: A Handbook,* which explores methods for examining children's difficulties both at home and in school.

Strengths and Limitations of Projective Techniques

Many projective techniques address some of the limitations of standardized personality instruments, in that the former are more difficult to fake. Projective techniques can also sometimes identify complex themes and multidimensional aspects of personality. With some clients, projective techniques can serve as an effective method of establishing rapport. In addition, with young children and nonverbal clients, some of the expressive techniques can provide an opening into the client's world that is difficult with other methods. On the other hand, projective techniques have some significant limitations. The reliability evidence for most of these techniques is quite low, which means there are higher proportions of error in these measures as compared with other measures. Because of these higher proportions of error, a counselor needs to regard the findings more cautiously. Certainly, the examiner and the situation need to be taken into consideration when interpreting the results of a projective technique, because both can have a significant influence on the process. The lack of normative data further compounds the problem. The central concern with the use of any instrument, however, is the validity of that instrument. The validation information on most projective techniques is often meager. In the wrong hands, a projective technique can be dangerous, as some clinicians might see every triangle any client draws as an indication that they were sexually abused. Anastasi and Urbina (1997) suggested that projective techniques should be viewed not as tests but rather as clinical tools. As clinical tools, these techniques inform practice by identifying possible hypotheses to be further investigated in the counseling process. Thus, these tools would not serve to confirm a clinical judgment but rather to generate hypotheses to be further explored and investigated.

Self-Concept Measures

Some counselors view self-concept as a construct closely related to personality, while others define it as a unique aspect of the individual. Self-concept is another area in which there is debate and differing opinions on definition and characteristics. When the topic of self-esteem is added to the discussion, the matter becomes more tumultuous, for self-esteem has become a social/political issue in the past 10 years. Leaving the debate over self-concept and self-esteem to other venues, this discussion addresses some of the prominent measures in this area. In some form, these measures are related to individuals' evaluation of their own performance or feelings about themselves. Counselors use self-concept or self-esteem measures primarily in two ways. First, counselors may want information on client attributes and may use these measures in the beginning of the counseling process to assess the client's level of self-esteem. Second, counselors may want to use these instruments to examine the effect of counseling interventions.

For example, counselors might examine whether a group counseling experience raised the self-esteem level of the participants. It should be noted that research has shown that counseling interventions have *not* been found to have a consistent effect on self-esteem (Kahne, 1996; Whiston & Sexton, 1998). This may be because of difficulties associated with measuring self-concept and self-esteem.

Piers-Harris Children Self-Concept Scale, Second Edition

The *Piers-Harris Children Self-Concept Scale, Second Edition* (Piers, Harris, & Herzberg, 2002) is a widely used measure of the self-perceptions of children and adolescents. The scale is composed of 60 items and is appropriate for individuals 7 to 18 years of age. The Piers-Harris provides one total score and six subscale scores that indicate the child's self-esteem in the areas of Physical Appearance and Attributes, Freedom from Anxiety, Intellectual and School Status, Behavioral Adjustment, Happiness and Satisfaction, and Popularity. Kelly (2005) considered the second edition of the Piers-Harris to be an improvement over the original scale and considered it to be one of the best current measures of self-concept. Conversely, Oswald (2005) expressed concern about the overlap of items in many of the different subscales and the essential unidimensionality of the instrument. The lack of a theoretical foundation was also noted by Oswald as a limitation of the *Piers-Harris Children Self-Concept Scale, Second Edition.*

Tennessee Self-Concept Scale

Another frequently used self-concept scales is the *Tennessee Self-Concept Scale—Second Edition* (TSCS-2) (Fitts & Warren, 1997). This instrument can be used with children, adolescents, and adults. The results provide two summary scores, with one being a measure of total self-concept and the other a general measure of conflict. There are six specific self-concept scores: Physical, Moral, Personal, Family, Social, and Academic/Work. Furthermore, there are three supplementary scores and validity scores that take into consideration inconsistent responses and faking. Hattie (1998) suggested that the TSCS-2 will continue to be a popular instrument but concluded that additional construct validation evidence would be beneficial.

Coopersmith Self-Esteem Inventories

The *Coopersmith Self-Esteem Inventories* (CSEI) consists of three forms: the School Form (for ages 8 through 15); the School Short Form (same ages); and the Adult Form (for ages 16 and above). The school forms both have 50 items, but the shorter form does not include the 8 Lie Scale items of the original School Form. The Adult Form is only 25 items and only provides a general measure of self-esteem. The School Forms provide measures of General Self, Social Self-Peers, Home-Parents, School Academic, Total Self, and Lie Scale. In reviewing these instruments, Adair (1984) found the standardization and normative data, reliability, and validity to be inadequate. In addition, the scoring provides percentile information but does not go any further in interpreting what the scores mean in terms of low to high self-esteem.

Summary

Assessing a client's personality is often part of the counseling process, because individuals' personalities are frequently intertwined with their problems and issues. In addition, clients' personalities should be considered when making treatment decisions and selecting interventions. Counselors often use both formal and informal personality assessment techniques. Observation is the most common technique in personality assessment. Counselors should attend to the reliability and validity of their observations because personal biases and attitudes can influence their abilities to be skilled observers. Interviewing is another personality assessment technique that counselors frequently use. The quality of the interviewing questions greatly influences the usefulness of the information gathered in an interview. Interviewing suffers from many of the same problems as observation; therefore, counselors need to evaluate the psychometric qualities of their interviews.

Within formal personality assessment, there are two major categories: standardized instruments and projective techniques. The most widely used standardized personality instrument is the MMPI-2. Individuals who are knowledgeable and well trained in the intricacies of this instrument should conduct the interpretation of MMPI-2 results. Other commonly used personality inventories are the Myers-Briggs Type Indicator, the NEO-PI-R, the 16PF, and the California Psychological Inventory. These self-report instruments do have some limitations, particularly concerning clients' abilities to manipulate the results and the tendency of clients to use a response set. Projective techniques are more difficult to fake or to be influenced by the client's response set. Projective techniques, however, usually have lower reliability coefficients than standardized instruments, and many are lacking in sufficient validation information. Furthermore, training is particularly needed in regards to interpreting projective assessments. Self-esteem or self-concept measures are sometimes considered part of personality assessment. However, the area of self-esteem or self-concept assessment has problems in that there is a lack of consensus on what precisely constitutes self-esteem and how to measure it.

CHAPTER 11

Assessment in Marriage and Family Counseling

Rebecca called and requested family counseling for herself and her two sons, Zack and Josh. Rebecca started the counseling session by explaining that her husband, Ben, had recently moved into an apartment; however, the reason she sought family counseling was to address Zack's hostility toward her and his younger brother, Josh. Rebecca explained that Zack is 15 years old and, in the past 6 months, has become sullen and withdrawn. Furthermore, according to Rebecca, when Zack is asked to complete any household duties or attend to his homework, he becomes openly hostile to her and refuses to do anything she asks him to do. Rebecca also indicated that Zack seems to provoke verbal arguments with Josh, which had escalated into two physical altercations between the brothers. Josh is 2 years younger than Zack, and Rebecca is concerned that Zack might hurt his younger brother if they continue to fight. As their counselor, you asked Zack, "What do you think about what your mother was saying?" He responded by saying, "I don't know." You then asked Josh to describe the fights between him and Zack, and he replied, "They were no big deal." Both Zack and Josh appeared to have little interest in talking and stared at their shoes during the entire initial session. You begin to sense some kind of undercurrent within this family, but it is difficult to assess because neither of the boys are willing to respond with more than a word or two to any comments or questions. Hence, you would like another way of gathering information about the dynamics of this family and issues that are related to their interactions.

Thus far, this section has focused on methods for assessing individuals; however, many counselors work with couples and families. Many marriage and family therapists or counselors use a systemic approach when working with couples or families.

A systemic approach is holistic with a focus on the interactions that occur and the belief that all members of the family interact and influence each other. According to this philosophical view, assessment would not be of individuals, but would focus on the dynamics or patterns that occur within the couple or family. Thus, testing each member within the family individually is not consistent with this systemic view.

Cierpka (2005a) extends this notion of clinical family assessment examining the family system and relational connections including the therapist's interactions within the family. Cierpka also stressed that family assessment is not done once to identify "the problem" but rather the assessment is of the current relational status and the assessment process is extended with attention to changes that may be occurring in the family.

Sometimes, counselors use instruments designed for individuals, such as personality instruments, when conducting marriage and family assessment. For example, some practitioners have used the Myers-Briggs Type Indicator to examine the differences in different family members' preferences. There are some difficulties, however, with using these tools because the assessment of individuals is essentially linear in concept—certain traits result in expected behaviors. Many marriage and family clinicians are grounded in systemic theories.

There are numerous measures for assessing couples and families, as evidenced by Touliatos, Perlmutter, and Straus (2001) compiling information on approximately 1,300 instruments. It does not appear that these instruments are being used in practice, however, because a survey of marriage and family therapists revealed that only 39% reported using standardized assessment instruments on a regular basis (Boughner, Hayes, Bubenzer, & West, 1994). This study also indicated that the marriage and family field does not use a specific battery of instruments, because no single assessment instrument was used by more than 8% of the sample. An inspection of the instruments used by marriage and family therapists reflects that the majority of these instruments were designed for individual counseling as compared to couples and family counseling. One reason for the dearth of instruments designed for assessing couples and families is that the field of family therapy or counseling is a comparatively recent development. Before the 1950s, the dominant paradigm was individual therapeutic approaches; only in the past 50 years have theories or approaches for working with families been developed. As therapeutic approaches designed for working with couples and families evolved, so did the beginnings of formal assessment instruments in this area. Hence, formal instruments designed specifically for couples and families do not have the long history that, for example, personality measures have. Another reason for the dearth of instruments designed for assessing couples and families concerns the difficulties associated with developing sound instruments in this area.

Difficulties with Assessment of Couples and Families

Numerous difficulties are associated with developing methods for assessing couples and families. One problem is in determining what should be assessed within families. Assuming a clinician adheres to a systemic approach, what then is meant by a family's or couple's dynamics? Even with specific terms, such as *interaction patterns*, there continue to be multiple views on what constitutes interaction patterns.

Some argue that it is impossible to assess family interaction patterns because every family is so unique that these elusive dynamics cannot be quantified. Assuming a clinician does identify some dynamic or characteristic of a family, how do we then determine what constitutes a well-functioning family as opposed to a dysfunctional one? Let us take, for example, family cohesion and determining the amount of cohesion that is considered appropriate. Not all family theorists maintain that low cohesion is detrimental and high cohesion is positive in families. The Olson Circumplex Model (Olson & DeFrain, 2002) suggests that cohesion should be viewed from a curvilinear perspective in which both too little and too much cohesion is problematic. In addition, what may be considered low cohesion for one family may function very well for another family. The difficulty in defining what constitutes functional as compared with dysfunctional becomes even more problematic when cultural differences are considered. Many differences exist between cultures regarding what are considered acceptable and unacceptable family behaviors. As an example, polygamy is accepted in some cultures and discouraged in others.

Family assessment is a broad term, because counselors might want very diverse information depending on the family's problems or issues. For example, a screening tool to determine if family counseling would be a suitable modality would be very different from an instrument to identify relational problems in a couple. Therefore, there is not just one area of focus in family assessment, because the focus could be on couples' satisfaction, the identification of communication patterns, perceptions of the family environment, self-reports of behaviors (e.g., battering), an analysis of relationships, the identification of problems, or many other familial aspects. A family assessment device or technique could be extremely helpful in identifying the issues in one family but not appropriate for another family. Another problem with family assessment is that many of the variables assessed are fluid and fluctuate as compared to the more stable traits or characteristics of individuals. As an example of how family dynamics may vacillate, consider the variation in the level of satisfaction a couple might report depending on whether they spent the night before dining at a wonderful French restaurant or completing their income tax forms. In addition to situational fluctuations, there are also developmental changes. As Carter and McGoldrick (1998) have documented, families go through developmental stages within a life cycle. Certainly, a couple has different developmental issues when they have been married for 4 months as compared with their issues when they have been married for 21 years and have two adolescent children. Furthermore, individuals who are technically in the same group may be at different developmental levels. For example, some newlyweds may be 17 years old, whereas others may be in their late 30s. Therefore, the assessment process needs to consider the developmental stage or level of both the family and the individual members within the family.

Another issue in couple or family assessment concerns getting multiple views rather than a single client's perspective. Members within a family often have divergent views on the problems and issues, which can lead to a problem in the scoring of family assessments. Olson, Portner, and Lavee (1985) found low correlations between husbands' and wives' perceptions of family adaptability and cohesion. Thus, if the husband's perceptions are highly positive and the wife's very negative, should the scores be added together and then averaged? Interpreting the results from the different family members' perspectives is more difficult than interpreting a single client's results. Another problem with gathering multiple perspectives concerns the confidentiality of the results of a family assessment. Sometimes problems arise when family members have access to each other's results. As an example, a child might be reluctant to disclose some information if the parents are going to see the results. Thus, the counselor needs to consider how the assessment information is going to be used and who will have access to the results.

The final problem with couple and family assessment concerns the difficulties associated with developing adequate norming samples. It is a time-consuming and arduous task to build adequate norms for instruments designed for individuals; however, that task is small compared with instruments for couples and families in which the norms need to be made up of couples and families. An instrument developer must assess entire families rather than single individuals. Gathering assessment information from each member of a family is complex and problematic. The instrument developer should also consider the ethnic makeup of the norming group. As Morris (1990) pointed out, many of the participants in family assessment norming groups are primarily Anglo Americans. This overrepresentation of Anglo Americans is problematic because not all ethnic groups share the same perspectives of family. Cultural values have a notable influence on what is considered functional and dysfunctional in families. Therefore, it may not be appropriate to evaluate a family who recently immigrated to the United States from Afghanistan with an instrument that has a norming group from one Midwestern state that is 90% Anglo Americans. Although problems with norming groups can be overcome, developing an instrument with a large and representative sample is difficult.

Even though numerous difficulties are associated with the development of marriage and family assessment tools, a number of assessment devices have evolved that are departures from traditional paper-and-pencil instruments. Many of these assessment techniques involve completing a task with the family or observing the family in an activity. The most widely known of these assessment tools is the genogram (Coupland, Serovic, & Glenn, 1995), which is discussed later in this chapter. Some types of family assessment are, in many ways, analogous to projective techniques in that there is a high degree of subjectivity in interpreting the results. Observation of family interactions is the predominant method of assessing families. In some cases the counselor will give the family a task to complete while in-session and observe the family members as they complete the task. A second area of assessment in marriage and family counseling involves instruments designed for use in individual counseling. Many counselors use instruments designed for individuals and administer these instruments to every member of the family. A majority of these individually oriented instruments measure personality, although there are examples in the literature of counselors using the Block Design subscale of the WAIS-III to examine differences in couples' task approach skills. The third area of assessment encompasses instruments designed specifically for assessment of couples and families. These instruments strive to assess the dynamics that occur among family members. The next three sections of this chapter address the multiple methods of assessing couples and families within the context of tasks and observation techniques, instruments designed for individual counseling, and instruments specifically developed for couples and family assessment.

The separation of these approaches is quite the antithesis of how assessment is viewed in family therapy because assessment is not considered a distinct phase or process because the therapist blends various methods in attempting to assess the family system.

Observational and Mapping Activities

In assessment with couples and families, therapists are typically interested in the interactional qualities among the members of the couple or family. Paper-and-pencil instruments that ask clients to report on their behavior toward other family members have some limitations. To illustrate this point, you might consider how individuals in your family might complete an instrument concerning family dynamics as compared with what a skilled observer may see when examining your family's interactions. With a paper-and-pencil instrument, it is nearly impossible to measure the changes in tone, facial expressions, and nonverbal messages that often accompany verbal communications in families. On the other hand, observational approaches also have problems, because counselors can misinterpret nonverbal expressions and inaccurately assess the family dynamics. To illustrate this point, let's examine the research related to differences in the amount of eye contact between distressed and nondistressed couples. Some clinicians might hypothesize that nondistressed couples are more likely to look into each other's eyes, but Haynes, Follingstad, and Sullivan (1979) found that distressed couples had a higher rate of eye contact than did nondistressed couples. Problems with observation are magnified as more clients are added to the process. A counselor cannot focus just on one individual in a couple or family. With this additional level of complexity, the reliability of the observations decreases. Furthermore, a counselor's biases and experiences both influence the inferences drawn from the family's behaviors. These inferences may be sound or distorted, depending on the counselor's ability to be objective.

According to Duffy and Chenail (2004), some of the historical leaders in family therapy (e.g., Salvador Minuchin and Jay Haley) suggested that therapists observe the structure, hierarchy, and interactions of the family. Table 11.1 on the following page reflects some concepts for counselors to consider when they are observing families to gain insight into dynamics within the family. Some researchers in the area of marriage and family assessment have attempted to address the limitations in observation by developing coding systems (Kerig & Lindhal, 2001).

Family assessment has a history of clinicians asking the family to perform a task and then observing familial interactions as they complete the assigned task. An example of these observational techniques is the *Family Task Interview* (Kinston, Loader, & Sullivan, 1985). In this assessment, the family is given seven tasks. The therapist observes the family completing the tasks and evaluates them by using a scale designed to measure family health. Examples of assigned tasks are planning something together that must take at least an hour, building a tower out of blocks, and discussing the likes and dislikes of each member of the family. Counselors can adapt this activity by identifying relevant tasks for the family to complete during counseling. While the family completes the tasks, the counselor can concentrate on observing the interactions. Using a predetermined system for recording observations improves the reliability of the observations.

TABLE 11.1 *Therapists' observations related to possible family structures, hierarchies, and interactional patterns (adapted from Duffy and Chenail, 2004)*

- Who sits close together and who sits way from whom
- Who initiates conversations and who remains quiet during discussions of family issues
- Who can interrupt or disagree and who appears unable to voice a differing opinion
- Who identifies problems or goals for therapy
- How are emotions expressed and responded to by family members
- Whose opinions seem to carry more weight and whose opinions are dismissed
- What topics seem to be off limits for family members to discuss
- Who attempts to solve problems and who is less involved
- Who seems to team up with whom regarding taking positions
- Who appears to be in charge of which activities and functions
- Who is in charge of discipline and who is in charge of fun
- Who has veto power over important decisions
- Who can make independent decisions and who must be consulted
- Who get nurtured by whom and who gets less nurturing

Some formal coding systems have been developed to assist practitioners in their observations. Most of these coding systems, however, are used in research and not typically by counselors. King (2001) provided a critique of coding systems used in the area of observing couples and his remarks also have applicability regarding coding of family interactions.

Genograms

Genograms offer an assessment technique often incorporated into counseling with couples and families (Timm & Blow, 2005) and are probably the most well-known assessment procedure in family counseling. Counselors work with families to help them draw a family tree that records information about family members and their relationships over at least three generations (McGoldrick, Gerson, & Shellenberger, 1999). Genograms are most closely associated with Bowen's family system theory (Bowen, 1978), although counselors with other theoretical orientations use them as well. Bowen contended that there are multigenerational transmissions of family patterns. Genograms can help identify which family patterns are being repeated by the family who is completing the genogram. With genograms, the clinician examines the previous generations and looks for patterns of functioning, relationships, and structure. A basic assumption with the use of genograms is that problems and symptoms reflect a system's adaptation and reaction to its context.

According to McGoldrick et al. (1999), gathering family information and constructing a genogram should be integrated into the more general process of joining, assessing, and helping a family. They suggested that creating a genogram involves three stages: (1) mapping the family structure, (2) recording family information, and (3) delineating family relationships. The first step involves mapping the family structure, which serves as the skeletal structure of the genogram. Typically, the counselor asks questions about family structure and maps the genogram for the past three generations.

FIGURE 11.1
Symbols used in a genogram

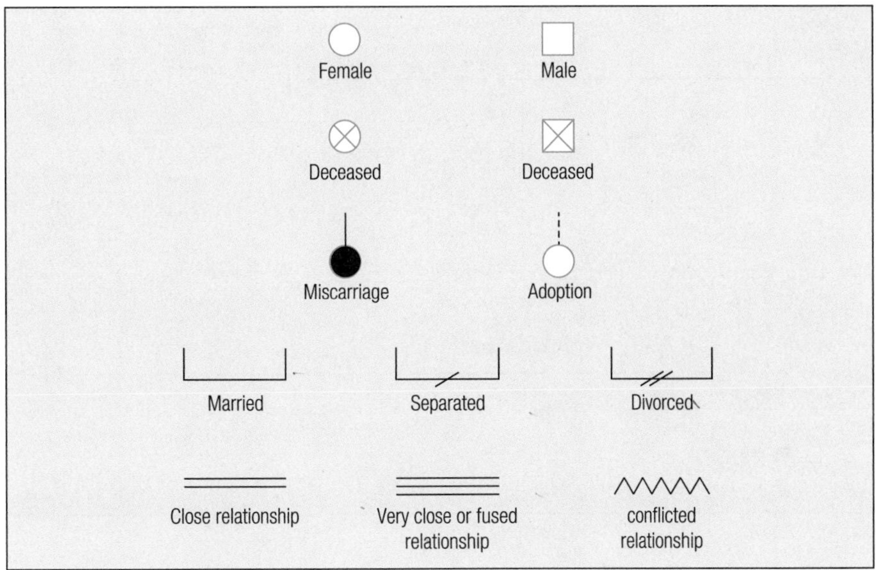

Circles represent female family members, and squares represent males. Figure 11.1 provides examples of many of the symbols used in a genogram, and Figure 11.2 on the following page is an example of an actual genogram. Horizontal lines connecting two symbols indicate married individuals. Separations are indicated by one slashed line, and divorce by two slashed lines. All pregnancies, stillbirths, miscarriages, and abortions are mapped. If an individual has died, then an X is drawn through the corresponding circle or square. In Figure 11.2, the genogram represents a couple, Richard and Judy, who sought counseling because of marital problems. As the genogram depicts, both Richard and Judy have been married before and both of those marriages ended in divorce. Richard and his first wife, Elizabeth, had two children, Hannah and Patrick. Judy also has two children, Lisa and Ivy, from her marriage to Lance. Richard is the only child of George and Betty. George's parents were Howard and Jane, and George had three sisters (Mary, Maureen, and Mabel) and one brother (Lowell). Betty's mother, Mary, died soon after she was born, and Betty's father, Martin, married Thelma two years after Betty's mother died. After their marriage, Betty's father and stepmother had three children (Ronald, Donna, and Daniel). Taking a look at Judy's side of the family, we see her parents are Stephen and Martha. Judy has one brother, Kip, and a sister, Mary Kay. Judy's father was raised primarily by his mother, Bridget, because his father left when he was a toddler. Judy's mother, Martha, was also an only child. As Figure 11.2 illustrates, Judy's mother's parents are Edward and Charlotte. Although in general, genograms trace three generations, neither Richard nor Judy could provide information on their great-grandparents.

Once the skeleton of the genogram is assembled, the next step is to record family information, which can include demographic information, functioning information, and critical family events (McGoldrick et al., 1999). Demographic information includes marking the year of each individual's birth (e.g., b. 1911) and the year of death (e.g., d. 1992). Dates of marriages and divorces are also recorded on the genogram.

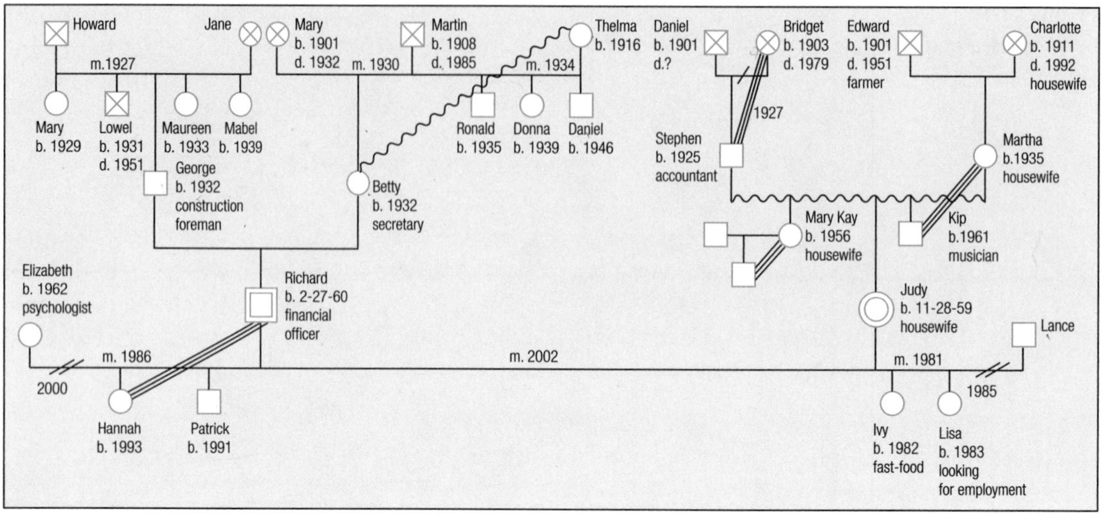

Howard Jane Mary b. 1901 d. 1932 Martin b. 1908 d. 1985 Thelma b. 1916 Daniel b. 1901 d.? Bridget b. 1903 d. 1979 Edward b. 1901 d. 1951 farmer Charlotte b. 1911 d. 1992 housewife

m.1927 m. 1930 m. 1934 1927

Mary b. 1929 Lowel b. 1931 d. 1951 Maureen b. 1933 Mabel b. 1939 George b. 1932 construction foreman Betty b. 1932 secretary Ronald b. 1935 Donna b. 1939 Daniel b. 1946 Stephen b. 1925 accountant Martha b.1935 housewife

Mary Kay b. 1956 housewife Kip b.1961 musician

Elizabeth b. 1962 psychologist Richard b. 2-27-60 financial officer Judy b. 11-28-59 housewife Lance

m. 1986 2000 m. 2002 m. 1981 1985

Hannah b. 1993 Patrick b. 1991 Ivy b. 1982 fast-food Lisa b. 1983 looking for employment

FIGURE 11.2
Example of a genogram

As Figure 11.2 shows, Richard and Judy were married in 2002, Richard was divorced from Elizabeth in 2000, and Judy was divorced from Lance in 1985. The genogram also indicates that Judy's grandparents, although they never divorced, separated in 1927. Often during this stage in the genogram construction, which McGoldrick et al. called "getting the facts," the clinician will also note information related to occupations, education, religious practices, or current situations. For example, as can be seen in Figure 11.2, Judy, her sister Mary Kay, and their mother are all homemakers. Judy's daughter, Lisa, has recently dropped out of a community college and is looking for work. Judy's younger daughter, Ivy, is working full-time in a fast-food restaurant. Richard's occupation of financial officer in a bank is more similar to Judy's father, who was an accountant, than to his father, who worked as a construction foreman.

After mapping the family's structure, the clinician begins to gather information related to patterns of functioning. Critical family events, such as losses, successes, or transitions, are also recorded. If an event is deemed particularly noteworthy, a counselor may map it in the genogram and note in again in the margins. The theoretical foundation of genograms is that family patterns are repeated; thus, the clinician gathers insights into current problems by examining previous family functioning. Included in Figure 11.1 are lines for mapping relational dimensions, such as close, very close or fused, and conflicted relationships. An examination of Figure 11.2 shows that there are a number of close or very close relationships. For example, Richard and his daughter, Hannah, have a close relationship. Richard also has a very close, possibly fused, relationship with his mother. In Judy's family, this same relational pattern also exists between Judy's mother and her youngest son and between Judy's father and his mother. Hence, there appears to be a pattern where one of the parents tends to have a very close or fused relationship with the youngest or only child in the family. Furthermore, these very close or fused relationships also appeared to have some negative influences on other familial relationships. In Judy's family, her father's enmeshed relationship with his mother was a significant contributor to the conflict between Judy's parents. Furthermore, Judy's mother's very close relationship with her youngest son, Kip, also caused friction between Judy's parents. Another past relational dimension that may be reemerging concerns the daughter/stepmother pattern. Richard's mother, Betty, had a very conflicted relationship with her stepmother, Thelma, and Judy reports she is beginning to feel conflict between herself and Richard's daughter, Hannah.

Watts-Jones (1997) advised clinicians to broaden the scope of the genogram when working with African American clients. She suggested that the practitioner should not restrict the genogram to biological relatives but should rather include "functional kinship," or non–biologically related individuals who play a significant role in the individual's life. Watts-Jones argued that the African proverb "It takes a village to raise a child" has relevance to the administration of genograms with African American clients. Not restricting the genogram to biological relatives may provide pertinent information to clinicians working with clients from other cultures. There are a number of cultures in which large, extended families are the norm, and restricting genograms to biological relatives may skew the information gathered. Readers interested in how to draw this sort of genogram are directed to Watts-Jones's article.

Interpreting the genogram involves constructing hypotheses that are later examined with the family. The counselor examines the relational structure and variables, such as whether the composition of the household is a nuclear family, the involvement of extended family, the order of the siblings, and any unusual family configurations. The family life cycle and stage should also be considered in the interpretation. As indicated earlier, genograms are based on the premise that family patterns can be transmitted from one generation to the next and by recognizing these patterns, the counselor can assist the family in avoiding ineffectual patterns. The genogram can also be used to analyze systemic connections among critical events that, at first, may not appear interrelated. Family therapists often focus on triangular relationships or triangles. The formation of triangles in families typically involves two people "triangling" or bringing a third member into their relationship, which usually serves to lessen the difficulties in the initial dyad. For example, two members of a family may join together to help a third member, or two members could join and gang up against a third. According to Bowen (1978), it is the collusion of the two in relation to the third that is the defining aspect of a triangle. In a general sense, the genogram is designed to provide information on the family structure, roles, level of functioning, and resources. However, the counselor works together with the family to create the genogram, and the clinician observes the family as the information is recorded. Both the observation and the recorded information are used in interpreting the genogram. The final form a genogram takes varies depending on how much detail is gathered and the patterns being identified. As an example, therapists would take more time examining a history of sexual abuse (Timm & Blow, 2005).

Some psychometric limitations need to be considered before using a genogram. Timm and Blow (2005) contended that there have been very few studies on the psychometrics of the genogram and contended there had been only study on its reliability (Coupland et al., 1995). Rohrbraugh, Rogers, and McGoldrick (1992) found poor interjudge reliability among practitioners in a medical setting. Coupland et al. found that doctoral students varied greatly in their accuracy in recording family information on genograms. This finding is even more disturbing because these advanced students had been trained in how to construct genograms. It also should be stressed that there is very little validation evidence for genograms. This lack of evidence is surprising given the popularity of genograms. Clinicians should be extremely cautious in the conclusions they reach based on genogram information. Similar to other observational techniques, genograms are particularly susceptible to counselor bias. Counselors need to view their interpretations of genograms as only hypotheses that need to be confirmed or invalidated by gathering additional information about the family.

Family Sculpting

Another mapping technique that has historically been associated with family therapy is family sculpting. Family sculpting emerged in the late 1960s as a method to assess and intervene with families (Bischof & Helmeke, 2005). The technique is associated with the work of Virginia Satir. Family sculpture involves positioning either family members or objects that represent the family in physical space that symbolizes the relations and roles within the family system. The steps in conducting a family sculpture are described in Table 11.2 are adapted from Bischof and

TABLE 11.2
Steps in conducting a family sculpture (adapted from Bischof & Helmet, 2005)

- **Introduction and Warm-up of Family**
  The counselor introduces the sculpting exercise, describes the process, and provides the rationale for using the sculpting technique.
- **Selecting a Sculptor**
  The therapist either specifically selects an individual to be the sculptor or asks for a volunteer.
- **Defining the Focus**
  The counselor helps focus the sculpture and may select a specific time in the family's history, a specific family situation or problem, or specific themes within the family (e.g., power, relationships).
- **Placing Family Members in the Sculpture**
  In this step, the family sculptor places family members physically as a representation of the focus. The therapist establishes that there should be little talking and family member may not challenge the instructions of the sculptor.
- **Detailing the Sculpture**
  Either after each person is placed or the entire sculpture is completed the counselor helps the sculptor express details about the placement. This is the period in which the therapist may explore clinical hypotheses about the interactions in the family.
- **Sculptor Adding Self**
  Once the family members are all placed and sculpture has been adequately explored, the sculptor adds her- or himself. Because this may influence the perspective of the sculptor, additional adjustments can be made. The counselor may also help sharpen the description of the sculpture.
- **Choice Point**
  At this point the therapist needs to make some clinical decisions regarding the therapeutic theme of the sculpture. The therapist might give the sculpture a name, describe the patterns that have emerged, or have different family members explore embedded patterns.
- **De-roling and Debriefing with the Sculptor and the Participants**
  In this step, the counselor carefully has the sculptor and the family members leave their roles in the sculpture and return to the present. Often the therapist's theoretical approach will influence this process.

Helmeke (2005). Sometimes after completing one family sculpture, the counselor will begin another with a different member of the family. This can facilitate an exploration of different perspectives within the family.

There is considerable subjectivity and inconsistence in family sculpture, but Cromwell, Fournier, and Kvebaek, (1980) developed the *Kvebaek Family Sculpture Technique,* which is more structured than most sculpting techniques. This technique uses a board that is similar to a chessboard except there are 100 squares. The family members are instructed first individually and then as a family to place figurines on the board depicting the relationships among the family. The family first represents the relationships as they currently exist and then sculpts the family again from an ideal perspective. The counselor assesses the sculptures by measuring the distances between the various placements of the figurines. Marriage and family therapists use sculpting techniques with a variety of objects, including family members arranging themselves in the room to depict their relationships. It is important to remember that sculpting techniques tend to be unreliable. Relationships within a family are fluid, and these techniques reflect only the clients' current perspectives. Therefore, counselors need to be cautious in interpreting this information and should not consider it a stable representation of the family.

Other Mapping Techniques

L'Abate (1994) suggested that the evaluation of a family should involve a battery of techniques, which might include a genogram and other mapping techniques. One of the mapping techniques described by L'Abate is the *ecomap*, which is used to gather information about the larger context of the family and the home. Gathering this information involves a collaborative process between the counselor and all members of the family. The process starts by positioning the home in the center of a piece of paper. Each family member then draws how far and where other resources are that are necessary for his or her "survival." The family members typically map schools, grocery stores, shopping, church, and recreational activities. The counselor can ask questions as the family creates the ecomap. The process the family uses to complete the ecomap may provide some indications of the dynamics in the family. (E.g., Does one member dominate? Does one member not participate?) The ecomap needs to be interpreted very cautiously, because there is little psychometric information for this technique. However, this technique can provide insight into how the family spends its time and what its priorities are. The ecomap also helps identify relational patterns and areas of social support.

Another mapping technique suggested by L'Abate (1994) is the *house floor plan.* As with the ecomap, the family, rather than the counselor, draws this map. The process begins with the counselor asking who wants to draw a plan of their house. The process requires the family to draw the floor plan of their home, indicating where each member sleeps and spends time. With this technique, the counselor needs to be skilled in facilitating the involvement of every family member. Different colored pencils can be used to add information on each family member. As the family draws the floor plan, the clinician should ask questions about who does what, who spends time together, what activities are typically performed where, and other questions relevant to the family. This technique can provide some indication of isolation or conflict among family members.

In conclusion, mapping and observation activities should not be used as the sole means of family assessment because of the problems with reliability and the limited validation information. When using a more subjective assessment tool, such as observation, the counselor needs to balance the process with other, more objective techniques. As is often repeated in this book, multiple forms of assessment are preferred because this provides a more thorough picture of the client or, in the case of couple and family assessment, the clients.

Use of Instruments Designed for Individuals

A number of instruments initially constructed for use in individual counseling have been adapted for use in couple and family assessment. Boughner et al. (1994) documented the prevalence of using an assessment instrument for individuals in marriage and family therapy. They found that the most frequently used assessment instruments in marriage and family therapy are the *Myers-Briggs Type Indicator*, the *Minnesota Multiphasic Personality Inventory-2* (MMPI-2), and the *Taylor-Johnson Temperament Analysis*. Given the interest in therapeutic interventions with couples and families, two new scales have been added to the scoring of the MMPI-2 (Nurse & Sperry, 2004). These scales are the Family Problem Scale (FAM) and the Marital Distress Scale (MDS). Other individually oriented instruments that marriage and family therapists reported using were the 16PF, the Millon Multiaxial Inventory, and the Beck Depression Inventory. In using these individually oriented instruments, the counselor, working with a family, often uses the information to identify how differences in personality or preferences may contribute to family issues. For counselors interested in using personality assessments with couples and families, Nurse (1999) provided some excellent examples and insights into the process.

Cierpka (2005b) proposed a three-level model of family assessment in which distinctions are made between the individual, the dyadic or triadic levels, and the system as a whole. In this case, an assessment of an individual could occur but the focus of gathering this information is on how the individual organizes himself or herself within the family. I will use the Myers-Briggs Type Indicator (MBTI) as an example of how an individually oriented assessment can be used to gain information on how the individual organizes herself or himself within the family. Rather than focusing on each individual's results, with a family, the focus would be on the interactions that occur using the framework of the Myer-Briggs Type Indicator. As an illustration, let's say that a counselor is conducting couples counseling and the wife's MBTI code is ENFP and the husband's code is ISTJ. The counselor could explain to the couple that in times of stress, the wife, who has the extroversion (E) preference, will seek others. The husband, on the other hand, with the introversion (I) preference, will desire time to himself. Hence, the interaction between them is difficult as they seek different methods for coping with stress. Furthermore, the couple's preferences on the second dimension, which concerns how they perceive information, may also contribute to relational difficulties. The husband prefers to use his senses (S), and he may become irritated that his wife misses what he considers important details. His wife, on the other hand, who prefers to use intuition (N) in perceiving information, may be annoyed because her husband does not perceive the "big picture" and is more interested in insignificant details.

This couple also varies on the third dimension, which concerns how they make sense of the information they perceive. The wife prefers to use her feelings (F), as compared to the husband, who prefers thinking (T). In this case, the husband may think the wife should be more rational and logical in her decision making, whereas the wife may perceive the husband to be cold and uncaring. The fourth dimension of the MBTI concerns differences in approaches to the outer world and whether individuals prefer to have their lives planned and organized or whether they prefer to be more spontaneous and respond to the moment. Once again, the couple's profiles indicate that there are differences. The wife prefers to react spontaneously, and the husband prefers to have activities arranged and organized. Thus, the marital difficulties are not related to one person's problem or flawed personality, but the focus of counseling is on the fact that each individual has different preferences in perceiving and processing information. One reason for the popularity of the MBTI with couples and families is it does not label preferences as right and wrong or good and bad. Instead the instrument is designed to understand and respect differences.

Another instrument originally designed for use in individual counseling that is now frequently used in counseling couples and families is the *Taylor-Johnson Temperament Analysis* (T-JTA). The T-JTA has new norms that were published in 2007 and a new manual that also was released in 2007. The Taylor-Johnson Temperament Analysis has been used for more than 40 years in individual, premarital, marriage, and family counseling. This tool was originally designed as a measure of an individual client's personality. The authors later developed a feature called "criss-cross" testing, which can be particularly useful in counseling couples. With the criss-cross technique, each individual first takes the instrument. The individuals then take it a second time, but this time they answer as they believe the other person would answer. Thus, the profile contains the individual's self-appraisal and the other person's perceptions of that individual. In marital and premarital counseling, the counselor then can use the criss-cross testing results to look at congruence in the couple's personalities as well as at congruence in how individuals view themselves and how their spouses view them.

Some clinicians, in the past, have objected to the profile sheets of the T-JTA because the sheets contained four shaded areas that corresponded to certain percentile scores. These shaded areas were labeled with the clinical designations of Excellent, Acceptable, Improvement Desirable, and Improvement Needed. Due to the complaints about the labels, it is now possible to purchase profile sheets with or without these clinical designations. Another previous problem with the T-JTA was an inadequate norming sample; however, the current version of the instrument was normed on 27,000 individuals.

Formalized Assessment Instruments Specific to Marriage and Family

Fredman and Sherman (1987) asserted that some of these well-known individually oriented instruments can provide therapists with insights into the family. These instruments do not, however, provide insight into level of satisfaction, qualities of the relationship, areas of conflict, or measures of parenting skill. During the past 50 years, researchers have studied marriages and families (Touliatos et al., 2001); however, this research on dynamics among couples and families is not reflected in instruments designed for individuals. Furthermore, many clinicians working with couples and families use a systemic approach, and although individually oriented instruments may describe the individuals within the system, these tools do not describe the family system. Hence, in the past 20 years, there has been significant interest in instruments designed specifically for assessing systemic family factors. This section focuses on assessment instruments designed specifically for use with couples and families. The first area addressed is measures designed expressly for premarital counseling, followed by couples' assessment, and, finally, instruments used to assess families.

Assessment in Premarital Counseling

In the area of premarital counseling, Boughner et al. (1994) found that practitioners reported using the *PREmarital Personal and Relationship Evaluation* (PREPARE) most often. In addition, PREPARE is one of the three premarital assessment questionnaires endorsed by the American Association of Marriage and Family Therapists (Larson, 2002). PREPARE is one of five instruments of the PREPARE/ENRICH program: (1) PREPARE for premarital couples, (2) PREPARE-MC for premarital couples with children, (3) PREPARE-CC for cohabiting premarital couples with or without children, (4) ENRICH for married couples, and (5) MATE for couples over the age of 50.

The entire program is designed to have the couples work with a trained counselor to (1) explore relationship strengths and limitations, (2) learn assertiveness and active listening skills, (3) learn how to resolve conflict using the 10-step model, (4) help the couple discuss their families of origin, and (5) help the couple with financial planning and budgeting. Couples are assessed in 20 areas, with 13 scales relating to significant couples issues (e.g., communication, conflict resolution, personality issues, financial management, marital satisfaction, and leisure activities). Another 4 scales measure personality in the areas of assertiveness, self-confidence, avoidance, and partner dominance, and 2 scales describe family of origin and the type of marriage/couple relationships in terms of closeness and flexibility.

In a recent study of PREPARE (Version 2000), Knutson and Olson (2003) found that those couples who participated in the PREPARE program and its feedback group reported greater couple satisfaction after participating than did couples who only completed PREPARE but received no feedback and a control group that did not take PREPARE. Although PREPARE was not designed to predict successful marriages, Fowers (1983) found that an earlier version of PREPARE was 86% accurate in predicting those who would divorce and 78% accurate in predicting those who would report being happily married. Druckman, Fournier, Robinson, and Olson (1980) found that PREPARE was rated as being more useful if the results were combined with counseling rather than only receiving feedback. Fitzpatrick (2001), however, voiced serious concerns about the lack of validation evidence and contended there was not sufficient information on the norming group.

Another assessment instrument for engaged couples endorsed by the American Association of Marriage and Family Therapists (Larson, 2002) is RELATE, which was developed by the Marriage Study Consortium at Brigham Young University. RELATE is available over the Internet (http://relate.byu.edu/), and clients can go directly to the website to take the instrument. According to Busby, Holman, and Taniguchi (2001), RELATE's conceptual model was drawn from more than 50 years of research regarding premarital predictors of later marital quality and stability. RELATE is comprised of 271 items that measure the 4 broad areas of personality characteristics, similarity of values, family background, and relationship experiences (e.g., communication skills and conflict resolution styles). Counselors can also set up accounts and have their clients take the assessments online. A limitation of the website, however, is that no psychometric information on the instrument is available. A study by Busby et al. (2001) does examine some of the basic psychometric qualities of the instrument.

Couples or Marital Assessment

The use of specific formal instruments in the area of marriage and family counseling is a comparatively recent addition to the field of assessment. One of the first widely used assessment instruments for couples was the *Marital Adjustment Test* (Locke & Wallace, 1959), which was often referred to as the Locke-Wallace. This instrument has been used for validating many of the later marital scales. As an indicator of where the field was at this point, the Marital Adjustment Test contained only 15 items, and the norming group was 118 husbands and 118 wives who were *not* necessarily married to each other.

Dyadic Adjustment Scale. The *Dyadic Adjustment Scale* (DAS, Spanier, 1976) is another instrument often used in marital counseling. It is intended to measure the adjustment quality of married couples or similar dyads. This 32-item instrument produces a total adjustment score plus scores on 4 subscales: Dyadic Consensus, Dyadic Satisfaction, Dyadic Cohesion, and Affectional Expression. The overall reliability of this instrument is quite high (.96), but the norming group consists of only 218 white married individuals from Pennsylvania. Graham, Liu, and Jeziorski (2006) contended that the DAS is probably the most widely used assessment of relationship quality. They found, using reliability generalization analyses, that the DAS total scores average reliability coefficient is .91 and the subscale averages range from .71 to .87. Supporting the contention that the DAS can be used with a wide range of couples, they found that reliability estimates did not differ based on sexual orientation, gender, marital status, or ethnicity of the samples.

Marital Satisfaction Inventory-Revised. One of the most widely used instrument in couples counseling is the *Marital Satisfaction Inventory-Revised* (MSI-R; Snyder, 1997), which was designed to assist couples in communicating about a broad range of relationship issues. In the revised edition, to be appropriate for both traditional and nontraditional couples, some of the items were changed to use terms such as *partner* and *relationship* rather than *spouse* and *marriage*. The items are scored on 13 scales (see Figure 11.3 on the following page). The first scale in Figure 11.3 is Inconsistency

FIGURE 11.3
Marital Satisfaction Inventory-Revised Profile Form
Copyright © 1997, 1998 by Western Psychological Services. Reprinted by permission. All rights reserved.

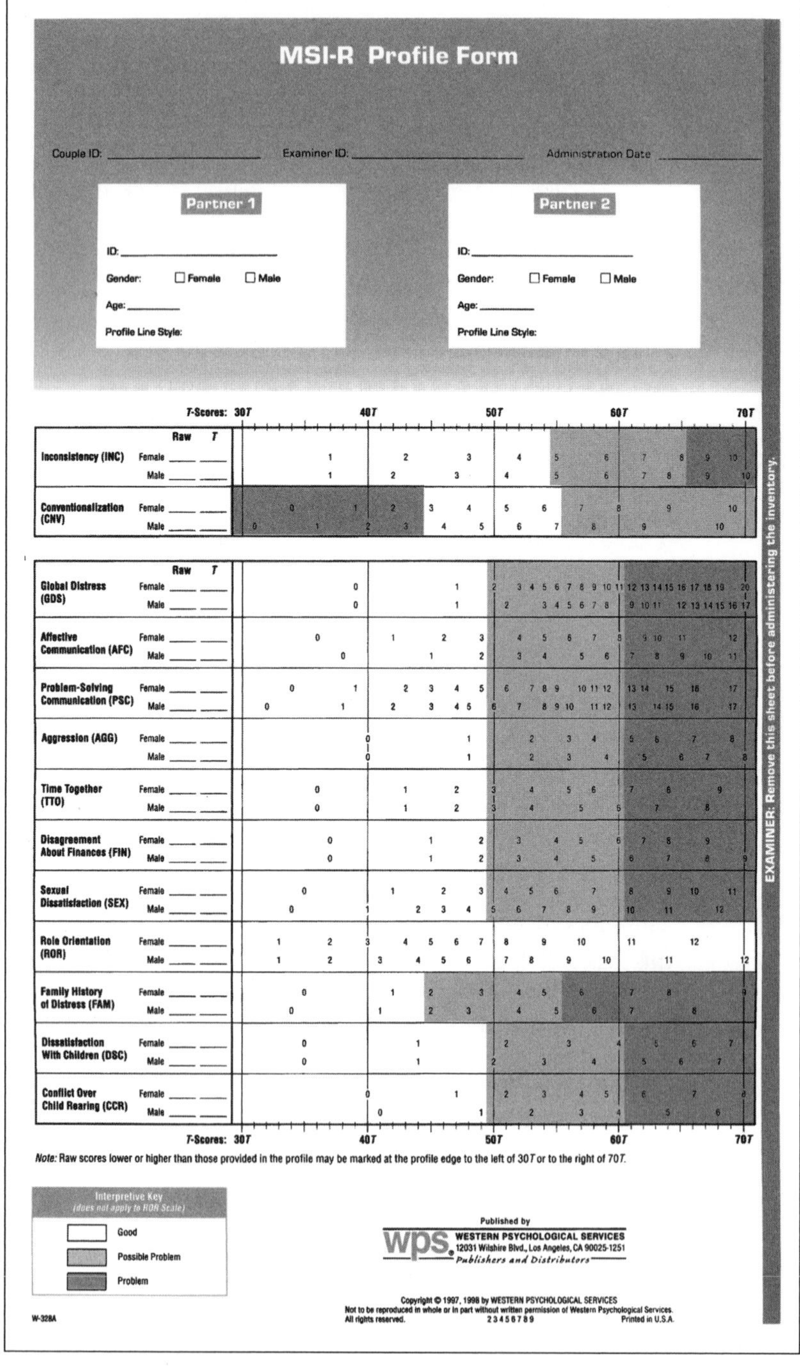

MSI-R Profile Form

Couple ID: ____________ Examiner ID: ____________ Administration Date ____________

Partner 1

ID: ____________
Gender: ☐ Female ☐ Male
Age: ______
Profile Line Style:

Partner 2

ID: ____________
Gender: ☐ Female ☐ Male
Age: ______
Profile Line Style:

T-Scores: 30*T* 40*T* 50*T* 60*T* 70*T*

Scale		Raw	*T*	Raw scores
Inconsistency (INC)	Female	___	___	1 2 3 4 5 6 7 8 9 10
	Male	___	___	1 2 3 4 5 6 7 8 9 10
Conventionalization (CNV)	Female	___	___	0 1 2 3 4 5 6 7 8 9 10
	Male	___	___	0 1 2 3 4 5 6 7 8 9 10

Scale		Raw	*T*	Raw scores
Global Distress (GDS)	Female	___	___	0 1 2 3 4 5 6 7 8 9 10 11 12 13 14 15 16 17 18 19 20
	Male	___	___	0 1 2 3 4 5 6 7 8 9 10 11 12 13 14 15 16 17
Affective Communication (AFC)	Female	___	___	0 1 2 3 4 5 6 7 8 9 10 11 12
	Male	___	___	0 1 2 3 4 5 6 7 8 9 10 11
Problem-Solving Communication (PSC)	Female	___	___	0 1 2 3 4 5 6 7 8 9 10 11 12 13 14 15 16 17
	Male	___	___	0 1 2 3 4 5 6 7 8 9 10 11 12 13 14 15 16 17
Aggression (AGG)	Female	___	___	0 1 2 3 4 5 6 7 8
	Male	___	___	0 1 2 3 4 5 6 7 8
Time Together (TTO)	Female	___	___	0 1 2 3 4 5 6 7 8 9
	Male	___	___	0 1 2 3 4 5 6 7 8
Disagreement About Finances (FIN)	Female	___	___	0 1 2 3 4 5 6 7 8 9
	Male	___	___	0 1 2 3 4 5 6 7 8 9
Sexual Dissatisfaction (SEX)	Female	___	___	0 1 2 3 4 5 6 7 8 9 10 11
	Male	___	___	0 1 2 3 4 5 6 7 8 9 10 11 12
Role Orientation (ROR)	Female	___	___	1 2 3 4 5 6 7 8 9 10 11 12
	Male	___	___	1 2 3 4 5 6 7 8 9 10 11 12
Family History of Distress (FAM)	Female	___	___	0 1 2 3 4 5 6 7 8 9
	Male	___	___	0 1 2 3 4 5 6 7 8
Dissatisfaction With Children (DSC)	Female	___	___	0 1 2 3 4 5 6 7
	Male	___	___	0 1 2 3 4 5 6 7
Conflict Over Child Rearing (CCR)	Female	___	___	0 1 2 3 4 5 6 7 8
	Male	___	___	0 1 2 3 4 5 6

T-Scores: 30*T* 40*T* 50*T* 60*T* 70*T*

Note: Raw scores lower or higher than those provided in the profile may be marked at the profile edge to the left of 30*T* or to the right of 70*T*.

Interpretive Key (*does not apply to ROR Scale*)
- Good
- Possible Problem
- Problem

EXAMINER: Remove this sheet before administering the inventory.

Published by
WPS WESTERN PSYCHOLOGICAL SERVICES
12031 Wilshire Blvd., Los Angeles, CA 90025-1251
Publishers and Distributors

W-328A

(INC), which indicates the accuracy of the profile by showing the degree to which the clients answered certain questions in a consistent manner. Conventionalization (CNV) is the validity scale and reflects an individual's tendency to distort the appraisal of the marriage in a socially desirable manner.

The Global Distress Scale (GDS) is an overall measure of dissatisfaction. High scores on the MSI-R indicate dissatisfaction. The other 10 scales measure specific sources of conflict: Affective Communication (AFC), Problem-Solving Communication (PSC), Aggression (AGG), Time Together (TTO), Disagreement About Finances (FIN), Sexual Dissatisfaction (SEX), Role Orientation (ROR), Family History of Distress (FAM), Dissatisfaction with Children (DSC), and Conflict Over Child Rearing (CCR). The items for the last two scales are answered only if the couple has children. The instrument was restandardized on 2,040 people (1,020 intact couples). The ages of the couples were from the late teens through the early 90s, and attempts were made to stratify the sample to approximate the U.S. population with regard to geographic region, education, and ethnicity. The reliability coefficients for the scales range between .80 and .97. The manual contains validity information, which is meager when compared with personality instruments but substantial when compared with other marital assessments. Bernt (2001) contended that the MSI-R is particularly well-suited to clinical settings and that the manual provides an extensive discussion on how to interpret the scales and use the information in counseling with couples.

Couples Pre-Counseling Inventory. Counselors who want to focus on marital counseling may want to explore Stuart and Jacobsen's (1987) *Couples Pre-Counseling Inventory, Revised Edition*. Both members of a couple complete this 16-page inventory before beginning counseling. In many of the sections of this detailed form, participants are asked to provide information about themselves and how they would expect their partners to answer. This inventory goes beyond evaluation of satisfaction and adjustment to include desired caring behaviors, violence, substance abuse, evaluation of sexual relationship, decision-making structure, and division of responsibilities. Computer scoring is available, and results are provided in 13 areas (e.g., Goals of Counseling, Communication Assessment, Conflict Management, Sexual Interaction, Child Management). The normative sample with this instrument was 60 couples, including nonmarried heterosexual couples and homosexual couples. Because the Couple's Pre-Counseling Inventory is 16 pages long, it takes time for clients to complete. The results, however, are quite detailed and can be useful to clinicians.

Family Assessment Instruments

Family Adaptability and Cohesion Evaluation Scale IV. The *Family Adaptability and Cohesion Evaluation Scale IV* (FACES IV; Olson, Gorall, Tiesel, 2004) is the latest version of a widely used measure of family dynamics (i.e., FACES-III). FACES IV was developed to measure the Circumplex Model of family functioning. The theorists asserted that the cohesion and flexibility dimensions are curvilinear with too little or too much being problematic. Family cohesion concerns the emotional bonding that couples and family members have toward one another. The definition of family flexibility is somewhat different from that given in earlier versions of

FACES. Olson and Gorall (2006) defined family flexibility as "the quality and expression of leadership and organization, role relationships, and relationships rules" (p. 6). Two scales on FACES IV measure the degree to which cohesion and flexibility are balanced (i.e., Balanced Cohesion and Balanced Flexibility), with higher scores reflecting a good balance and healthy functioning. There are also 4 "unbalanced" scales that measure more problematic family function. Two of these unbalanced scales concern problems with cohesion: Disengaged Scale and Enmeshed Scale. There are also two unbalanced scales related to problems with flexibility: Chaotic Scale and Rigid Scale. The scores on these scales result in a family being categorized into one of six family types. The six family types are on a continuum from the most healthy and happy to the least healthy and most problematic and they are: Balanced, Rigidly Cohesive, Midrange, Flexibly Unbalanced, Chaotically Disengaged, and Unbalanced. Individuals interested in a detailed discussion of these six types of families may go to http://www.facesiv.com.

Family Assessment Measure. An assessment that appears to be gaining recognition is the *Family Assessment Measure* (FAM-III) by Skinner, Steinhauer, and Santa-Barbara (1995). In fact, the National Institute on Drug Abuse used the FAM-III as part of its comprehensive assessment battery of problem adolescents. The FAM-III is designed to assess family functioning that integrates individual members and collective characteristics of the family. Spillane (2001) contended that it is particularly good at probing characteristics and processes of families. The FAM-III consists of three interrelated instruments. The first is the General Scale (50 items), which focuses on the family's general functioning. The second instrument, the Dyadic Relationship Scale (42 items), measures the quality of the relationship between two specific family members (e.g., mother and father). The third scale is the Self-Rating Scale (42 items), in which individuals evaluate their own level of functioning in the family unit.

Each of the three scales provides information on the following seven dimensions: Task Accomplishment, Role Performance, Communication, Affective Expression, Involvement, Control, and Values and Norms. The FAM-III is available in both paper-and-pencil and computer formats. Manges (2001) found the FAM-III to be a valuable, but time-consuming, tool. The reported Cronbach's alpha for each scale is comparatively high for both adults and children, with the range for adults being between .89 and .95 and that for children being from .86 to .94. The validity information is relatively limited but is growing rapidly. There is also a computerized version, in which the software scores and writes an interpretative report.

Family Environment Scale. The *Family Environment Scale* (FES; Moos & Moos, 1994) evolved out of Rudolf Moos's work on assessing social climates. Assessment of social climates is closely related to environmental assessment, which examines how environmental factors influence an individual's behavior. Moos (1973) contended that three dimensions provide insight into a social climate or environment: (1) a relationship dimension, (2) a personal development or personal growth dimension, and (3) a system maintenance and system change dimension. According to Moos, these dimensions provide insight into family environments as well as into other social climates or environments.

Table 11.3 describes the subscales related to each of the three dimensions in the FES. There are three forms of the FES: the Real Form (Form R) measures individuals' perception of their current family, the Ideal Form (Form I) measures preferences for an ideal family environment, and the Expectation Form (Form E) measures expectations about a family environment (e.g., prospective foster parents' expectations). Each form of the FES contains 90 items. These three forms can be used either individually or in combination in a variety of counseling interventions. Often, each family member's results are compared to examine differences in perceptions. For example, the counselor might want to explore discrepancies among the family members' perceptions of the environment. I once worked with a family in which the mother and the children rated the conflict high, but the father rated the conflict below average. Analysis of this discrepancy led to a useful discussion of the father's attempt to dismiss any opinion that varied from his stance on an issue. Another way to use the FES to explore family perceptions is to examine the differences between the results from the Real Form and those of the Ideal Form. Sometimes, a family will have amazing similarities among themselves on results from the Ideal Form, which can be an effective intervention for unifying the direction of the counseling.

The normative sample of the FES is 1,432 normal families and 788 distressed families. The manual does not provide very detailed information on the manner in which many of the normal families were selected. The internal consistency coefficients range from .61 to .78 on the nine subscales of the FES. There is also considerable validity information on this instrument, much of which concerns differences between normal and distressed families.

Other instruments. As indicated by Touliatos et al. (2001), hundreds of other family instruments are available to measure various familial aspects, such as family beliefs, the extent to which families celebrate, coping behaviors, and family empowerment.

TABLE 11.3
Dimensions and subscales of the Family Environment Scale

Relationship Dimension
Cohesion—the amount of commitment, help, and support family members provide for each other
Expressive—the degree to which members of the family are encouraged to express feelings and act in an open manner
Conflict—the amount of openly expressed conflict and anger in the family
Personal Growth Dimension
Independence—the extent to which members are assertive, self-sufficient, and able to make their own decisions
Achievement Orientation—the degree to which activities are framed in an achievement-oriented or competitive framework
Intellectual-Cultural Orientation—the extent to which the family is interested and participates in political, intellectual, and cultural activities
Active-Recreational Orientation—the level of the family's participation in social and recreational activities
Moral-Religious Emphasis—the amount of emphasis on values and religious and ethical issues
System Maintenance Dimension
Organization—the extent to which organization and structure are clear in responsibilities and planning family activities
Control—the degree to which set rules and procedures run family life

In selecting assessments to assess either couples or families, counselors need to examine the family constructs or dynamics that they are attempting to assess (e.g., hostility, communication patterns, domestic violence). Many of the instruments in the marriage and family area have very limited psychometric information; thus, clinicians should be cautious when using these instruments. As with any instrument, counselors need to carefully evaluate any instrument before using it with a couple or family and to understand the instrument's limitations. These instruments should be viewed more as a springboard for further discussion rather than as diagnostic tools.

Summary

In recent years, hundreds of instruments have been developed for assessing couples and families. These instruments are not as well-established as some of the instruments developed for use with individuals (e.g., the MMPI-2, WAIS-III). Developing instruments for use with couples and families is more difficult than developing instruments for individuals. This chapter addressed three areas of marriage and family assessment: tasks and observation techniques, instruments designed for individual counseling, and instruments specific to couple and family assessment.

Tasks and observation techniques can be helpful because they afford the counselor the opportunity to observe family interactions. There are many different tasks a counselor can initiate with a family to facilitate the gathering of relevant information. One of the most commonly used techniques is the genogram. Counselors and their clients construct a family tree that records information about family members and their relationships over at least three generations. Genograms are based on the premise that family patterns can be transmitted from one generation to the next and that by recognizing these patterns a counselor can assist the family in avoiding destructive patterns.

In addition, clinicians who are counseling couples and families sometimes use instruments designed for individuals. The instruments most commonly used by marriage and family therapists are the Myers-Briggs Type Indicator, the Minnesota Multiphasic Personality Inventory-2, and the Taylor-Johnson Temperament Analysis. The T-JTA uses a system that enables the practitioner to examine congruence in the couple's personality as well as congruence between how each client views himself or herself and how each client is viewed by the spouse or significant other.

Finally, there are instruments designed specifically for use with either couples or families. The most frequently used premarital instrument is PREPARE. In addition, a number of instruments exist that address marital satisfaction or issues after a couple is married. These instruments are typically used to identify areas in which the couple's perceptions may differ from one another. Assessment of families is probably one of the most difficult areas in counseling due to the complexities of family interactions. Some of the family assessment instruments are based on theory, and the clinician must have an understanding of the theoretical implications when using the instruments. Assessment in the area of marriage and family counseling does not have the extensive history of intelligence and personality assessments. Therefore, the instruments in this area are not as well researched, nor has the field had time to adequately address many of the limitations in current assessment devices.

SECTION III

Applications and Issues

CHAPTER 12

Assessment and Diagnosis

As we begin to explore the applications of assessment information, we need to consider that client assessment is performed for many different reasons and can have many different uses. All clinical decisions are actually built on a foundation of assessment—counselors make treatment decisions based on the information they gather through formal or informal assessment techniques. In many ways, making a treatment decision is a form of diagnosis. Although some may argue that diagnosis contradicts the developmental philosophy of counseling, Hohenshil (1993, 1996) maintained that client assessment and diagnosis are integral parts of the counseling process. He contended that thousands of counselors are in settings where their employers, licensing agencies, and insurance companies expect them to know how to formally diagnose mental disorders. Research tends to support Hohenshil's assertion; for example, Mead, Hohenshil, and Singh (1997) found in a survey of mental health counselors that 91% used the *Diagnostic and Statistical Manual of Mental Disorders (DSM)*. When developmentally oriented counselors determine that a client's problem is a normal developmental issue and not a psychopathology, this is essentially a form of diagnosis. Seligman (2004) argued that diagnosis has become increasingly germane to counselors over the past 20 years and that the importance of training in and understanding of diagnosis using the *DSM* will continue to grow and will be viewed as a necessity for all clinicians. Crew and Hill (2005) noted dilemmas faced by counselors who work with couples and families rather than one person because many third-party payers (e.g., insurance organizations) will not pay for counseling services without a diagnosis. Although school counselors are typically not required to provide a diagnosis, often they work with children and adolescents who have been diagnosed or they need to be familiar with diagnosis to refer a student to a certain agency, because in some agencies a student would not qualify for treatment unless that student is diagnosed with a mental disorder. Hence, it is important for various types of counselors to understand formal diagnostic procedures.

Another reason that counselors in diverse settings understand diagnosis is the prevalence of individuals with significant psychological difficulties. According to the National Institute for Mental Health (2007) an estimated 26.2% of American adults (ages 18 and older) suffer from a diagnosable mental disorder in a given year. This means that about one in four adults have a diagnosable problem. The New Freedom Commission on Mental Health (2003) found that, in a given year, around 5–7% of adults suffer from a serious mental illness. Furthermore, approximately 20.9 million adults in America per year suffer from a mood disorder. In a report from the Surgeon General (U.S. Department of Health and Human Services, 1999), it was estimated that around 20% of children 9 to 17 years old have either a mental health or a substance abuse disorder.

There are a number of diagnostic systems that mental health service providers might use; however, the American Psychiatric Association's (2000) *Diagnostic and Statistical Manual of Mental Disorders—Fourth Edition-Text Revision* (*DSM-IV-TR*) is the most widely used resource for diagnosis in mental health settings. Another diagnostic system is the *International Classification of Diseases* (9th ed., Clinical Modification; ICD-9-CM). In addition, in July 2007 the ICD-10-CM was officially released. Diagnostic systems are designed to provide a common language for professionals so that diagnostic terms have a unified meaning rather than individuals using their own unique definitions. For example, if I walked down the street and asked pedestrians for their definitions of *substance abuse*, the definitions would probably differ dramatically. Some people may not consider consumption of a six-pack of beer every night as an indication of substance abuse; others may consider one drink per night to be substance abuse. For effective communication within a profession, there needs to be uniformity in definitions. Diagnostic systems, such as the *DSM-IV-TR*, attempt to provide a nosology, or nomenclature, for counselors, psychiatrists, psychologists, social workers, and other health and mental health professionals. Diagnosis should not be viewed as providing a punitive label but rather as providing a description of the client's symptoms that others can understand.

Diagnostic systems can also be helpful in conceptualizing cases. Mead, Hohenshil, and Singh (1997) found that many mental health counselors used the *DSM* classification system to assist in case conceptualization. With the movement toward using empirically supported treatments (Wampold, Lichtenberg, & Waehler, 2002), it is important for the clinician to initially identify client concerns and then find the empirically supported treatments. Much of the literature related to empirically supported treatments is organized around *DSM-IV-TR* diagnoses, so it is imperative for counselors to have an understanding of diagnosis. In some settings (e.g., mental health clinics), knowledge and use of formal diagnostic systems is required of the counselor. In other settings (e.g., schools and career centers), counselors are not required to use the *DSM-IV-TR* or other formal diagnostic systems. However, even for counselors who do not use these diagnostic systems, having knowledge of the disorders does assist in the assessment and referral process. For example, when school counselors begin to hear some symptoms indicative of a particular disorder, they can explore further to get a more complete picture, which can then assist school counselors in making referrals that are more appropriate for the student. Furthermore, because school counselors are likely to have students with psychopathologies, counselors need to understand those disorders to assist schools in providing the best learning environments for those students. The likelihood of counselors in various settings having clients who suffer from mental disorders is quite high. In clients seeking assistance at university counseling centers, Pledge, Lapan, Heppner, Kivlighan, and Roehlke (1998) found consistent increases between 1989 and 1995 in the number of clients who had more serious concerns and psychopathology at college campuses. Essau, Conradt, and Petermann (2000) found that 17.9% of children between 12 and 17 years old met the criteria for having had a depressive mood disorder. Clinicians, particularly those who work with children, also need to have a comprehensive knowledge of diagnosis, as there is concern that certain disorders (e.g., Attention Deficit/Hyperactivity Disorder) are "over" diagnosed and that children are labeled based on faulty information (McClure, Kubiszyn, & Kaslow, 2002).

Diagnosis and assessment are intimately intertwined. Using one of the diagnostic systems requires a thorough appraisal of the client's problems, physical condition and symptoms, and environmental influences. A diagnosis typically is based on information about the client gathered through informal assessment tools, formal assessment instruments, or a combination of both techniques. Whether the diagnosis is formal or informal, assessment and appraisal skills are needed to make informed clinical decisions.

Using the DSM-IV-TR

Increasingly, insurance administrators and managed-care organizations are requiring that counselors determine if clients are experiencing specific problems (e.g., substance abuse, depression, anxiety disorders). In many counseling settings, counselors must diagnose client problems using criteria from the *Diagnostic and Statistical Manual of Mental Disorders—Fourth Edition-Text Revision* (*DSM-IV-TR*, APA, 2000). The *DSM-IV-TR* was produced to serve as a bridge between the *DSM-IV* and the *DSM-V*. The changes that were made in the *DSM-IV-TR*, as compared with the *DSM-IV*, were primarily in the text, which provides information to the clinician and not to the criteria sets. The process for developing the *DSM-V* has begun and interested readers are directed to http://www.dsm5.org/ to examine the progress being made toward developing the fifth edition of the *Diagnostic and Statistical Manual of Mental Disorders*.

Substantive training in diagnosis is beyond the scope of this chapter. Instead, this chapter provides readers with an introduction to diagnosis and an overview of disorders. For each diagnosis within the *DSM-IV-TR*, specific criteria must be met. Although this chapter provides an overview of many disorders, counselors are directed to the *Diagnostic and Statistical Manual of Mental Disorders—Fourth Edition-Text Revision* (*DSM-IV-TR*, American Psychiatric Association, 2000) to gain more precise knowledge of the specific criteria that must be met for each disorder. Counselors may also gain knowledge concerning the application of the *DSM-IV-TR* in Spitzer, Gibbon, Skodol, Williams, and First's (2002) casebook.

To understand the *Diagnostic and Statistical Manual of Mental Disorders*, counselors need to understand the term *mental disorder.* The definition of a mental disorder according to the *DSM-IV-TR* is

> a clinically significant behavioral or psychological syndrome or pattern that occurs in an individual and that is associated with present distress (e.g., a painful symptom) or disability (i.e., impairment in one or more important areas of functioning) or with a significantly increased risk of suffering death, pain, disability, or an important loss of freedom. (American Psychiatric Association, 2000, p. xxxi)

Mental disorders are categorically classified in the *DSM-IV-TR* based on the practitioner's evaluation of certain criteria. The *DSM-IV-TR* covers a wide array of diagnostic categories, with applications for clinicians in educational, clinical, and research settings. Counselors are not trained to intervene with all of the disorders in the *DSM-IV-TR*, but general knowledge of these disorders is expected of all professionals in the mental health field.

The *DSM-IV-TR* uses a multiaxial diagnostic system in which the practitioner uses five axes to ensure that information needed for treatment planning, prediction of outcome, and research is provided. Table 12.1 includes an overview of the five axes of the *DSM-IV-TR.* For appropriate treatment planning, Fong (1993) recommended that counselors determine a full five-axial diagnosis for all clients. Counselors use *Axis I* and *Axis II* to describe the client's current mental conditions. Axis I includes all clinical syndromes, except for Personality Disorders and Mental Retardation. For certain clients, counselors make multiple diagnoses on Axis I or diagnoses on both Axes I and II. *Axis III* is used to provide information on the client's general medical conditions. *Axis IV* is where information on psychosocial and environmental problems that influence treatment and prognosis of Axis I or II are listed. On *Axis V*, counselors estimate the client's current level of functioning. The Global Assessment of Functioning (GAF) scale contained in the *DSM-IV-TR* is the specific scale used for an Axis V diagnosis.

The client's current conditions and mental disorders are described on Axis I and Axis II. Most clients will seek treatment for clinical disorders and other clinical conditions that are classified in Axis I. Whether diagnosing on Axis I or Axis II, the clinician determines if the information about the client corresponds to a polythetic list of criteria (i.e., a set of many types of symptoms, emotions, cognitions, and behaviors). The *DSM-IV-TR* clearly stipulates the criteria that need to be present to meet

TABLE 12.1
DSM-IV-TR-TR five axial structure

Axis	Content
Axis I	Clinical Disorders and Other Clinical Conditions That May Be a Focus of Attention
Axis II	Personality Disorders and Mental Retardation
Axis III	General Medical Conditions
Axis IV	Psychosocial and Environmental Problems
Axis V	Global Assessment of Functioning (GAF)

the diagnostic conditions. For example, the diagnostic criteria for Conduct Disorder (312.8) are as follows:

A. A repetitive and persistent pattern of behavior in which the basic rights of others or major age-appropriate societal norms or rules are violated, as manifested by the presence of three (or more) of the following criteria in the past 12 months, with at least one criterion present in the past 6 months:

Aggression toward people and animals

(1) often bullies, threatens, or intimidates others
(2) often initiates physical fights
(3) has used a weapon that can cause serious physical harm to others (e.g., a bat, brick, broken bottle, knife, gun)
(4) has been physically cruel to people
(5) has been physically cruel to animals
(6) has stolen while confronting a victim (e.g., mugging, purse snatching, extortion, armed robbery)
(7) has forced someone into sexual activity

Destruction of property

(8) has deliberately engaged in fire setting with the intention of causing serious damage
(9) has deliberately destroyed others' property (other than fire setting)

Deceitfulness or theft

(10) has broken into someone else's house, building, or car
(11) often lies to obtain goods or favors or to avoid obligations (i.e., "cons" others)
(12) has stolen items of nontrivial value without confronting a victim (e.g., shoplifting, but without breaking and entering; forgery)

Serious violations of rules

(13) often stays out at night despite parental prohibitions, beginning before age 13 years
(14) has run away from home overnight at least twice while living in parental or parental surrogate home (or once without returning for a lengthy period)
(15) is often truant from school, beginning before age 13 years.

B. The disturbance in behavior causes clinically significant impairment in social, academic, or occupational functioning.

C. If the individual is age 18 years or older, criteria are not met for Antisocial Personality Disorder. (APA, 2000, pp. 98–99)

These systematic descriptions of the disorders provide diagnostic criteria that describe the frequency, duration, and severity of the symptoms. For a diagnosis to be given, the client must meet the specified criteria. Clinicians need to ensure that the criteria are truly met; an error in diagnosis can be harmful to clients, because diagnostic labels may not always be kept confidential by insurance companies and other organizations. Thus, a client could be irreparably harmed by an incorrect diagnosis. An incorrect diagnosis could also prevent a client from receiving the correct treatment and could prolong the suffering and the expense of treatment. Training on the appropriate uses of the *DSM-IV-TR* and supervised experience are important to accurate diagnosis.

Axis I

Axis I is for reporting clinical conditions, with the exception of the pervasive Personality Disorders and Mental Retardation. Table 12.2 lists the major groups of disorders included on Axis I. Counselors can list multiple diagnoses on Axis I, and comorbidity or dual diagnosis can be appropriate for some clients. If counselors use more than one diagnosis, they need to indicate which is the primary diagnosis. In an outpatient setting, counselors should write "reason for the visit" after the primary diagnosis; in an inpatient setting, they should write "principal diagnosis" after the diagnosis on which treatment should focus. Practitioners can also list **specifiers** (i.e., Mild, Moderate, Severe, In Partial Remission, In Full Remission, and Prior History) after the diagnoses. Because of the diversity of clinical disorders, it is impossible for any diagnostic system to contain every possible situation. For this reason, each diagnosis on Axis I has at least one Not Otherwise Specified (NOS) category.

Disorders Usually First Diagnosed in Infancy, Childhood, or Adolescence

In most cases, clients who meet the criteria for the diagnoses in this category will be identified in childhood or adolescence; however, some individuals will not be diagnosed until adulthood. Although the description of *Mental Retardation* is included

TABLE 12.2
Axis I: Clinical Disorders and Other Conditions That May Be a Focus of Clinical Attention

- Disorders Usually First Diagnosed in Infancy, Childhood, or Adolescence (excluding Mental Retardation, which is diagnosed on Axis II)
- Delirium, Dementia, and Amnestic and Other Cognitive Disorders
- Mental Disorders Due to a General Medical Condition
- Substance-Related Disorders
- Schizophrenia and Other Psychotic Disorders
- Mood Disorders
- Anxiety Disorders
- Somatoform Disorders
- Factitious Disorders
- Dissociative Disorders
- Sexual and Gender Identity Disorders
- Eating Disorders
- Sleep Disorders
- Impulse-Control Disorders Not Elsewhere Classified
- Adjustment Disorders
- Other Conditions That May Be a Focus of Clinical Attention

in this section of the *DSM-IV-TR,* the diagnosis is given on Axis II. According to the *DSM-IV-TR*, Mental Retardation is characterized by significantly subaverage intellectual functioning (typically an IQ of approximately 70 or below) with onset before the age of 18 years. The subaverage intelligence must be accompanied by concurrent deficits or impairments in adaptive functioning.

Learning Disorders are indicated when individuals' academic performance is substantially below what is expected for their age, schooling, and level of intelligence. The learning problems need to significantly interfere with academic achievement or daily activities in reading, mathematics, or writing skills to be classified as a learning disorder. There is debate within the field concerning what constitutes a substantial discrepancy between achievement and intellectual level. The *DSM-IV-TR* also addresses instances in which the discrepancy can be smaller (e.g., considering the individual's ethnic and cultural background).

Three other disorders that are usually first diagnosed in infancy, childhood, or adolescence concern developmental delays. *Motor Skills Disorders* includes the one diagnosis of Developmental Coordination Disorder, characterized by motor coordination substantially below that which is expected. Difficulties in speech and language are included in the *Communication Disorders. Pervasive Developmental Disorders* are characterized by pervasive and severe impairments in multiple development areas. Examples of these pervasive disorders are Autistic Disorder, Rett's Disorder, Childhood Disintegrative Disorder, and Asperger's Disorder. Autistic Disorder is manifested with marked impairments with social interactions and communication, and restricted repetitive and stereotyped patterns of behavior, interests, and activities. The onset of Autism is before the age of three and there are delays or abnormal functioning in either social interaction, language, or symbolic or imaginative play. Rett's Disorder is characterized be deceleration in head growth between the ages of 5 months and 48 months and accompanying impairments. Childhood Disintegrative Disorder is associated with normal development to age two and then significant loss of previously acquired skills. Asperger's Disorder is characterized by social impairments and restricted repetitive and stereotyped patterns of behavior, interest, and activities. Asperger's Disorder, however, is not characterized by a delay in language.

Attention-Deficit and *Disruptive Behavior Disorders* have received increased public attention in recent years. This category of disorders is characterized by socially disruptive behaviors that are often more distressing to others than to the client. The prominent symptoms for *Attention Deficit/Hyperactivity Disorder* are inattention and/or hyperactivity-impulsivity. The symptoms of inattention and/or hyperactive-impulsivity that cause impairment must be present before the age of seven. Furthermore, the impairment must be present in two or more settings (e.g., home and school). Subtypes are typically diagnosed in order to specify the predominant symptoms, and these include Predominantly Inattentive Type, Predominantly Hyperactive-Impulsive Type, and Combined. This section of the *DSM-IV-TR* also includes disorders that are disruptive in nature, such as *Conduct Disorder.* As indicated earlier, the essential characteristic of Conduct Disorder is a repetitive and persistent pattern of behavior that violates the basic rights of others or violates major age-appropriate societal norms or rules. *Oppositional Defiant Disorder*, similar to Conduct Disorder, involves the essential feature of a pattern of negativistic, defiant, disobedient, and hostile behavior. The symptoms of Oppositional Defiant Disorder, such as "often loses temper," "argues with adults," and "is angry and resentful," must be present for at least six months.

Feeding and Eating Disorders of Infancy or Early Childhood are included in this section but should not be confused with Anorexia Nervosa or Bulimia Nervosa, which are included in Eating Disorders. These infancy and early childhood disorders include Pica, Rumination Disorder, and a general Feeding and Eating Disorder of Infancy and Early Childhood. Another diagnostic area is *Tic Disorders*, which are characterized by vocal and/or motor tics (e.g., Tourette's Disorder). *Elimination Disorders* includes *Encopresis*, the repeated passage of feces into inappropriate places, and *Enuresis*, the repeated voiding of urine into inappropriate places. The final category is *Other Disorders of Infancy, Childhood, or Adolescence,* which includes disorders such as Separation Anxiety Disorder, not covered in the section.

Delirium, Dementia, and Amnestic and Other Cognitive Disorders

As reflected in Table 12.2, the second major category in Axis I is Delirium, Dementia, and Amnestic and Other Cognitive Disorders. Counselors are less likely to be involved with this diagnostic area as compared with others. This category is characterized by a clinically significant deficit in cognition or memory, which involves a substantial change from previous functioning. The disorders in this section are further subdivided depending on whether the etiology is a general medical condition, a result of substance use (or a combination of these factors). A *delirium* is described as a disturbance of consciousness and a change in cognition that develops over a short period of time. *Dementia* involves multiple cognitive deficits that include impairment in memory. Dementia Disorders are listed according to their presumed etiology (e.g., Alzheimer's Type, Vascular Dementia, Substance-Induced Persisting Dementia). An *Amnestic Disorder* also involves memory impairment but in the absence of other significant cognitive impairments.

Mental Disorders Due to a General Medical Condition

The third diagnostic section for Axis I involves mental disorders that are judged to be the direct consequence of a general medical condition. The term *general medical condition* is consistent with what is coded on Axis III and it refers to conditions that are not considered "mental disorders." This diagnostic section provides health care providers with a shorthand method of identifying the mental disturbances that are a direct physiological consequence of a general medical condition.

Substance-Related Disorders

In the *DSM-IV-TR*, the term *substance* includes drugs of abuse (including alcohol), the effects of prescribed and over-the-counter medications, or toxins. Therefore, these disorders are related to a wide range of substances. With these diagnoses, the substance class is identified and the substances are grouped into 11 classes (e.g., alcohol, amphetamine or similarly acting sympathomimetics, caffeine, cannabis, or cocaine).

Furthermore, the substance-related problem could be Polysubstance Dependence and Other or Unknown Substance-Related Disorders (which include most disorders related to medications or toxins). Clinicians often do not consider the possible problems associated with prescribed or over-the-counter medications. Examples of prescribed and over-the-counter medications that can cause Substance-Related Disorders are anesthetics and analgesics, anticonvulsants, antihistamines, corticosteroids, and muscle relaxants. Toxins could include heavy metals, rat poisons, pesticides, and carbon monoxide. The Substance-Related Disorders are separated into two major groups: *Substance-Use Disorders* and *Substance-Induced Disorders.*

When considering Substance-Use Disorders, counselors need to consider the difference between *Substance Dependence* and *Substance Abuse.* With **Substance Dependence,** regular substance use leads to the development of impaired control over that substance use and the continued use of the substance despite adverse consequences. Typically there is a pattern of self-administration of the substance that results in tolerance, withdrawal, and compulsive drug-taking behaviors. *Dependence* is defined as a cluster of three of the following symptoms occurring in the same 12-month period.

- Tolerance is either
  (a) a need for markedly increased amounts of the substance to attain intoxication or desired effect or
  (b) a markedly diminished effect with continued use of the substance at the same amount.
- Withdrawal is characterized by
  (a) the development of substance-specific syndrome due to the cessation or reduction of substance use, such as alcohol withdrawal that can involve hand tremors, nausea, or vomiting; psychomotor agitation;
  (b) the substance-specific syndrome causing significant distress or impairment with everyday functioning; and
  (c) the substance or something closely related being taken to relieve or avoid withdrawal symptoms.
- The substance is often taken in larger amounts or over a longer period than was intended.
- There is a persistent desire for the substance, or efforts to cut down or control use do not succeed.
- A great deal of time is devoted to activities necessary to obtain the substance, use the substance, or recover from its effect.
- Reduction or cessation of important social, occupational, or recreational activities is related to the use of the substance.
- Substance abuse continues despite the knowledge that it contributes to physical or psychological problems.

When a client meets the criteria for Substance Dependence, the actual diagnosis is for the substance he or she is dependent upon, using the categories listed earlier (e.g., 304.40 Amphetamine Dependence, 304.30 Cannabis Dependence).

The **Substance Abuse** diagnosis does not have the emphasis on dependency that Substance Dependency has. For Substance Abuse, the focus is on a maladaptive pattern of substance use leading to clinically significant impairments or distress. The substance use may result in repeated failure to fulfill major role obligations, repeated use in situations in which it is physically hazardous, multiple legal problems, and recurrent social and interpersonal problems. To warrant a diagnosis of Substance Abuse, these problems need to have occurred repeatedly over a 12-month period. Once again, the actual diagnosis of Substance Abuse is related to the specific substance abused (e.g., 305.00 Alcohol Abuse, 305.60 Cocaine Abuse).

Substance-Induced Disorders are the second major group of disorders under the general category of Substance-Related Disorders. As compared to Substance-Use Disorders, the concerns here are with *Substance Intoxication* and *Substance Withdrawal*. (As a note, other Substance-Induced Mental Disorders—such as Substance-Induced Delirium, Substance-Induced Psychotic Disorder, and Substance-Induced Mood Disorder—are included in other sections of the manual). When considering Substance Intoxication, we need to be aware that short-term, or acute, intoxication may have different signs and symptoms as compared with sustained, or chronic, intoxications. Intoxication requires recent use or exposure to a substance and the presence of maladaptive behaviors or psychological changes. Furthermore, these maladaptive behaviors or personality changes must be related to the substance's effect on the central nervous system. Substance Intoxication is often diagnosed in combination with Substance Abuse or Substance Dependency or with other diagnoses. To assist in differential diagnosis, the *DSM-IV-TR* provides diagnostic criteria for each of the major substances.

Substance Withdrawal diagnoses are also frequently accompanied by other diagnoses. With Substance Withdrawal, the practitioner must be familiar with the substance-specific withdrawal syndrome (i.e., the behavioral, physiological, and cognitive symptoms for withdrawal from specific substances). Not all of the common substances have a withdrawal diagnosis; for example, withdrawal from caffeine is not included in the *DSM-IV-TR*. With Substance Withdrawal diagnoses, the symptoms must develop as a result of the recent cessation or decreased intake of a substance after there has been prolonged and/or heavy use of the substance. Furthermore, significant impairment and distress are required.

Schizophrenia and Other Psychotic Disorders

All of the disorders in this section are characterized by having psychotic symptoms as the defining feature. Because counselors are primarily trained with a developmental approach, this area will be only briefly summarized. *Schizophrenia* is a disorder that lasts for at least six months and that includes at least one month of active-phase symptoms (i.e., the client must exhibit two or more of the following: delusions, hallucinations, disorganized speech, grossly disorganized or catatonic behavior, or other negative symptoms). The subtypes of Schizophrenia are Paranoid, Disorganized, Catatonic, Undifferentiated, and Residual. With *Schizophreniform Disorder,* the client also must exhibit two or more of the symptoms listed for Schizophrenia. The main difference between Schizophreniform and Schizophrenia is the duration of the disturbance; Schizophreniform can last from one to six months. There are also subtypes of Schizophreniform Disorder.

Mood Disorders

Before counselors can understand the criteria for diagnosing *Mood Disorders*, they first need to be familiar with the different Mood Episodes (Major Depressive Episode, Manic Episode, Mixed Episode, and Hypomanic Episode). Mood Episodes are *not* diagnosed as disorders; instead, they are the building blocks for the Mood Disorder diagnoses. A *Major Depressive Episode* is one in which the client is in a depressed mood or has lost interest or pleasure in nearly all activities for at least two weeks. In children and adolescents, the mood may be one more of irritability than of sadness. In addition, the client must experience five or more of the following symptoms, with at least one of the symptoms being either depressed mood or loss of interest or pleasure: (1) depressed mood most of the day, nearly every day; (2) markedly diminished interest or pleasure in all, or most all, activities most of the day, nearly every day; (3) significant changes in appetite or weight; (4) changes in sleep (insomnia or hypersomnia); (5) psychomotor agitation or retardation (observed by others); (6) fatigue or loss of energy; (7) feelings of worthlessness or guilt; (8) difficulty thinking, concentrating, or making decisions; or (9) recurrent thoughts of death or suicidal ideation, suicide plans, or attempts. These symptoms need to persist through most of the day and cannot be the direct result of a medical condition or bereavement.

A *Manic Episode* is characterized by abnormally elevated, expansive, or irritable moods. In addition, other symptoms that are present are grandiosity, decreased need for sleep, flight of ideas, distractibility, increased activity, and involvement in risky activities. These symptoms need to be obvious to an observer and last for at least a week. A Manic Episode is not a normal feeling good about oneself; rather, it is a feeling of becoming so driven that it causes marked impairments in occupational functioning, social activities, or relationships. A *Mixed Episode* is one in which the client has periods, on a daily basis, that meet the criteria for a Manic Episode and for a Major Depressive Episode. This rapid alternating of depressive and manic moods within a day must continue for at least a week. These mood alternations need to be severe and cause marked impairment in activities. A *Hypomanic Episode* is similar to a Manic Episode in that the individual needs to have a persistently elevated, expansive, or irritable mood; have a decreased need for sleep; be more talkative; exhibit flight of ideas; be distractible; engage in increased goal-directed activity or psychomotor agitation; and have excessive involvement in pleasurable activities having a high potential for painful consequences. The Hypomanic Episode, however, has to last only four days as compared with a week for the Manic Episode. Nevertheless, some of the same other symptoms need to be present (i.e., inflated self-esteem or grandiosity, decreased need for sleep, flight of ideas, distractibility, increased activity, and involvement in risky activities); however, these symptoms do not need to be so severe as to cause marked impairments.

The clinician then uses these four descriptions of episodes to diagnose Mood Disorders that can be categorized into three major areas: *Depressive Disorders, Bipolar Disorders,* and *Other Mood Disorders*. Within the Depressive Disorders, the first distinction is between the *Major Depressive Disorder* and the *Dysthymic Disorder.* Major Depressive Disorders are characterized by one or more Major Depressive Episodes without a history of Manic, Mixed, or Hypomanic Episodes. The Major Depressive

Disorders are further delineated by whether it is a single episode or a recurrent problem and the current state of the disturbance. Dysthymic Disorders differ from other depressive disorders in that clients do not suffer from a Major Depressive Episode but rather experience a chronically depressed mood for a long period of time (at least two years for adults and one year for children). Individuals usually describe themselves as being "down in the dumps," although children may seem more irritable than sad. Symptoms that are present with Dysthymic Disorders are poor appetite or overeating, insomnia or hypersomnia, low energy or fatigue, low self-esteem, poor concentration or difficulty making decisions, and feelings of helplessness.

A recent report from the National Institute of Health (2007) reported in the past decade there has been a dramatic increase in the diagnosis of bipolar disorders for children and adolescents. It should be noted that there is more than one diagnosis related to bipolar disorders. The essential feature of *Bipolar I* is that the client has had at least one Manic Episode or Mixed Episode. There are six separate criteria for Bipolar I Disorder: Single Manic Episode, Most Recent Episode Hypomanic, Most Recent Episode Manic, Most Recent Episode Mixed, Most Recent Episode Depressed, and Most Recent Episode Not Specified. Bipolar I Disorder, Single Manic Episode is when the individual is having his or her first manic episode. The other criteria sets are related to recurrent mood episodes with an identification of the current or most recent episode. *Bipolar II Disorders*, on the other hand, are characterized by one or more Major Depressive Episodes in conjunction with at least one Hypomanic Episode. Somewhat different from Bipolar I and Bipolar II is the *Cyclothymic Disorder*, in which a client needs to have had numerous periods of hypomanic symptoms that do not meet the criteria for Manic Episode and numerous periods of depressive symptoms that do not meet the criteria for a Major Depressive Episode.

Within the general categorization of Mood Disorder in the *DSM-IV-TR*, there is a third major section besides Depressive Disorders and Bipolar Disorders titled *Other Mood Disorders*. This section includes mood disorders related to a specific medical condition and ones that are induced by substances. Furthermore, in diagnosing Mood Disorders, counselors need to know about a number of specifiers (e.g., Mild, Moderate, Severe with Psychotic Features) that further delineate the diagnosis.

Anxiety Disorders

One or more of the following conditions may be diagnosed in clients whose prominent symptoms are anxiety-related. Morrison (2007) reported that most anxiety disorders begin when clients are relatively young. Similar to Mood Disorders, Anxiety Disorders have "building blocks" that are not codable diagnoses but are used to determine the precise Anxiety Disorder. The "building blocks" with Anxiety Disorders are *Panic Attacks* and *Agoraphobia*. A Panic Attack is a brief period during which the client feels intense apprehension, fearfulness, or terror. These feelings are often accompanied by a feeling of impending doom. During the attack, the client typically experiences physical symptoms such as shortness of breath, heart palpitations, chest discomfort, difficulty breathing, or a sense of losing control or "going crazy." With Agoraphobia, clients fear situations or places where they may have trouble coping or finding help if they become anxious or have a panic attack. Furthermore, this anxiety leads to avoidance of the places or situations in which the anxiety may occur. Agoraphobic fears often involve situations such as being outside of the home alone; being in a crowd or standing in line; being on a bridge; or traveling in automobiles, buses, or trains.

In terms of Panic Disorders, there are two diagnoses: *Panic Disorder with Agoraphobia* and *Panic Disorder without Agoraphobia*. With both of these diagnoses, there are recurrent and unexpected Panic Attacks. There is also a diagnosis of *Agoraphobia Without History of Panic Disorder*, in which the focus is on the Agoraphobia and the panic-like symptoms but without a history of unexpected Panic Attacks.

The Anxiety Disorder section also includes diagnoses related to phobias. A *Specific Phobia*, such as a phobia of spiders, is characterized by clinically significant anxiety induced by exposure to that specific feared object or situation. With a phobia, the fear of a specific object or situation leads to problematic avoidance behaviors. Within the *DSM-IV-TR*, there is a specific diagnosis for *Social Phobia*, which is associated with significant anxiety aroused by certain types of social or performance situations.

Another Anxiety Disorder is *Obsessive-Compulsive Disorder*, the characteristics of which are recurrent obsessions or compulsions severe enough to be time-consuming or to cause marked distress or impairment. Obsessions are defined as persistent ideas, thoughts, impulses, or images that interfere with normal activities. Compulsions are repetitive behaviors (e.g., checking the stove, hand-washing) or mental acts (e.g., counting, repeating certain words) with the goal being to reduce or prevent the anxiety. To meet the criteria for Obsessive-Compulsive Disorder, adults, at some point, must attempt to ignore, suppress, or neutralize the thoughts, impulses, or images and recognize that the obsessions or compulsions are excessive or unreasonable. This requirement of recognition does not apply to children because they may not have sufficient cognitive awareness to evaluate the situation. Simply checking the stove a couple of times will not meet the criteria for Obsessive-Compulsive Disorder because the obsessions or compulsions need to be problematic and/or time-consuming (at least an hour a day).

Posttraumatic Stress Disorder, another diagnosis contained within the Anxiety Disorders section, is characterized by the repeated reexperiencing of an extremely traumatic event. The reexperiencing can be in the form of distressing recollections, dreams, feeling as if the traumatic event were recurring, or other reactions to cues that might symbolize or resemble aspects of the traumatic event. Another criterion for Posttraumatic Stress Disorder is a persistent avoidance of stimuli associated with the trauma and a numbing of general responsiveness. Furthermore, the individual in question needs to have persistent symptoms of anxiety or increased arousal that were not present before the trauma (e.g., sleep problems related to nightmares, hypervigilance, exaggerated startle response, increased irritability or outbursts of anger, difficulty concentrating).

In addition, the posttraumatic symptoms are present not only immediately following the traumatic event but continue for more than a month. A similar diagnosis is *Acute Stress Disorder,* which has many of the same symptoms as Posttraumatic Stress Disorder except that additional symptoms are present in the first month after the traumatic event. In Acute Stress Disorder, the client experiences symptoms of dissociation during the event or immediately after the event.

Generalized Anxiety Disorder is somewhat different from the other Anxiety Disorders because it involves more generalized anxiety and worry that tends to persist for six months or more. An individual with this disorder finds it difficult to control the worry. In addition, the anxiety and worry result in symptoms such as restlessness, feeling keyed-up, being easily fatigued, difficulty concentrating, irritability, muscle tension, and sleep disturbance. Also in the Anxiety Disorder section of the *DSM-IV-TR* are diagnoses of Anxiety Disorder Due to General Medical Condition and Substance-Induced Anxiety Disorders.

Somatoform Disorders

All of the *Somatoform Disorders* have the unifying feature of the presence of physical symptoms that suggest a medical condition, yet these physical symptoms cannot be fully explained by a general medical condition. In contrast to Factitious Disorders and Malingering, these physical symptoms are not intentional. If counselors have a client for whom the somatic symptoms are the prominent reason for seeking counseling, then they should examine the different types of Somatoform Disorders in this section of the *DSM-IV-TR*.

Factitious Disorder

This section includes only one disorder, *Factitious Disorder*, and its subtypes. Factitious Disorder involves the intentional producing or feigning of physical or psychological symptoms. With Factitious Disorder, the motivation is to assume the sick role; however, the reasons are not for economic gain or for other incentives. The client is not trying to fool an insurance company or avoid responsibilities; rather, the individual is intentionally producing the symptoms to meet a psychological need.

Dissociative Disorders

Dissociation is the state in which one group of the normal mental processes becomes separated from other mental processes. In the *DSM-IV-TR*, a Dissociative Disorder is described as a disruption in the usually integrated functions of consciousness, memory, identity, or perceptions of the environment. The onset of the dissociation can be either sudden or gradual, and the dissociation can disappear or remain chronic. The *DSM-IV-TR* includes four Dissociative Disorders: Dissociative Amnesia, Dissociative Fugue, Dissociative Identity Disorder, and Depersonalization Disorder. There is also the common Not Otherwise Specified diagnosis. *Dissociative Amnesia* is characterized by the client's inability to recall important personal information. The information is usually of a traumatic or stressful nature and is too extensive to be explained by ordinary forgetfulness. With a *Dissociative Fugue*, the client unexpectedly and suddenly travels away from home or his or her work environment. This unexpected travel is accompanied by the inability to remember the past and confusion about identity. In some cases, the client will assume a new identity. *Dissociative Identity Disorder* (formerly Multiple Personality Disorder) involves the presence of two or more distinct identities or personality states that recurrently take control of the client's behavior.

These distinct identities or personalities are accompanied by the inability to recall important personal information that is too extensive to be explained by ordinary forgetfulness. Finally, in *Depersonalization Disorder* there is persistent depersonalization (i.e., a feeling of detachment or estrangement from oneself). Clients often have episodes during which they feel as if they were observing their actions from the outside. With Depersonalization Disorder, clients' abilities to test reality remain intact; they simply view their reality from an outsider's perspective.

Sexual and Gender Identity Disorders

The Sexual and Gender Identity Disorders involve three major areas: Sexual Dysfunction, Paraphilias, and Gender Identity Disorders. With *Sexual Dysfunction,* there is a disturbance in sexual desire and problems in the psychophysiological changes that characterize the sexual response cycle. The Sexual Dysfunction category is subdivided into disorders related to sexual desire, sexual arousal, orgasm, and sexual pain. The Sexual Dysfunction Disorders are often gender-specific because sexual difficulties typically differ between men and women. The term *paraphilia* means abnormal or unnatural attraction. In *Paraphilia Disorders,* the attraction or sexual-arousing fantasy has occurred over a period of at least six months and generally involves (1) objects or nonhuman animals; (2) humiliation or suffering of the individual or the partner; or (3) nonconsenting persons, including children. For Pedophilia, Voyeurism, Exhibitionism, Sexual Sadism, Sexual Masochism, and Frotteurism, the fantasies, urges, or behaviors do not need to be acted on to be diagnosed, but can be diagnosed if they cause clinically significant distress or impairment. Furthermore, for a diagnosis of Pedophilia, the paraphilia impulses and behaviors need to be the preferred methods of sexual excitement and expression, with the symptoms being present for at least six months. The third major category of disorders in this section is Sexual and Gender Identity Disorders. Clients with *Gender Identity Disorders* feel intensely uncomfortable with their biological gender. The diagnoses related to Gender Identity Disorder are not appropriate for clients who are questioning their own sexual orientation. Clients with Gender Identity Disorder have a strong and persistent cross-gender identification. They either see themselves as being of the opposite sex or they desire to become a member of the opposite sex. This cross-gender identification is not because of perceived advantages of being of the other sex; rather, the clients are intensely uncomfortable with their own assigned gender.

Eating Disorders

Eating Disorders involve severe disturbances in eating behavior. The *DSM-IV-TR* includes two specific diagnoses: Anorexia Nervosa and Bulimia Nervosa. The central feature of *Anorexia Nervosa* is the inability to maintain a minimal normal body weight. The client, even though underweight, is intensely afraid of gaining weight and exhibits a significant disturbance in the perception of her or his body. Some individuals feel globally overweight; others are concerned with certain parts of their body being "too fat." Amenorrhea (the absence of at least three consecutive menstrual cycles) is a sign of Anorexia Nervosa because severe dieting affects hormone levels. The mean age of onset for this disorder is 17, although some studies indicate that there are peaks around the age of 14 and around the age of 18. There are two subtypes, one in which the food intake is severely restricted and the other of the binge eating/purging type.

Bulimia Nervosa is an eating disorder characterized by binge eating and inappropriate compensatory behaviors to prevent weight gain. Clients with Bulimia Nervosa have recurrent episodes of binge eating during which, within two hours, they eat large amounts of food. These binges do not involve slight overeating; the amount of food is large and often consists of starches and sweets. Clients report a sense of lack of control over eating during these binge episodes. To prevent gaining weight, the person uses compensatory behaviors (e.g., self-induced vomiting, use of laxatives or diuretics, or excessive exercise). The Bulimia Nervosa diagnosis is given when the binging and purging occur at least twice a week for a three-month period. Similar to clients with Anorexia Nervosa, clients with Bulimia Nervosa have self-images that are unduly influenced by their body shape and weight. Clients with Bulimia Nervosa, however, are much more realistic in their perceptions of their own bodies as compared with anorexic clients. Bulimia Nervosa has two subtypes: Purging Types (those who vomit or use laxatives, diuretics, or enemas) and Nonpurging Types (those who use fasting or excessive exercise as the compensatory behaviors).

Sleep Disorders

In the *DSM-IV-TR*, the Sleep Disorders are organized into four sections according to the presumed etiology (cause or origin of the disorder): Primary Sleep Disorders, Sleep Disorders Related to Another Mental Disorder, Sleep Disorders Due to a General Medical Condition, and Substance-Induced Sleep Disorders. In *Primary Sleep Disorders*, the etiology is undetermined and not related to the other causes. These Primary Sleep Disorders are subdivided into Dyssomnias and Parasomnias. Dyssomnias involve abnormalities in the amount, quality, or timing of sleep. Parasomnias are characterized by abnormal behaviors while sleeping (e.g., sleepwalking) or physiological events that occur in conjunction with sleep, in specific sleep stages, or in the sleep-wake cycle. The diagnosis of Sleep Disorders is not simple and involves the systematic assessment of sleep complaints, physical condition of the client, and evaluation of substances and medications. Furthermore, the clinician must be knowledgeable of the sleep stages and methods for measuring these. Practitioners also need to understand the typical variations in sleep across the life span.

Impulse-Control Disorders Not Elsewhere Classified

The central characteristic of the disorders in this section is the individual's failure to resist an impulse, drive, or temptation to perform a harmful act. For most of the disorders in this section, the client feels an increasing sense of tension or pressure before committing the act. After committing the act, the person then feels a sense of relief, pleasure, or gratification. This feeling may later be followed with regret, guilt, or remorse.

Intermittent Explosive Disorder is associated with discrete episodes of failure to resist aggressive impulses that result in serious assaults or destruction of property.

These aggressive behaviors are markedly out of proportion to the situation or to any stressors. *Kleptomania* concerns the inability to resist impulses to steal objects that are not needed. The motivation for stealing is not anger or desiring the object; instead, it is to relieve the tension that mounts before the stealing behavior. With *Pyromania*, pleasure, gratification, or relief of tension is secured through a pattern of setting fires. *Pathological Gambling* is also classified as an Impulse Control Disorder and is characterized by persistent and frequent maladaptive gambling behaviors. The last disorder in this section is *Trichotillomania*, which involves the recurrent pulling out of one's hair for relief, pleasure, or gratification.

Adjustment Disorders

Adjustment Disorders involve the development of clinically significant symptoms in response to an identifiable psychosocial stressor(s). The significant symptoms must occur within three months of the beginning of the stress. Furthermore, for diagnosis, the symptoms need to be beyond what is considered a typical reaction, or there needs to be marked reaction that affects social or occupational functioning. The stressor can be a single effect (e.g., the ending of a significant relationship) or there can be multiple stressors (e.g., unemployment and marital discord). Stressors can be recurrent (e.g., seasonal business problems) or continuous. Stressors can also be a reaction to a developmental change (e.g., getting married, having a baby). A natural disaster could also be a stressor. In many ways, Adjustment Disorders are the focus of counselor training. The authors of the *DSM-IV-TR*, however, suggested that this diagnosis should not be used as a "catch-all."

Other Conditions That May Be a Focus of Clinical Attention

This category refers to conditions or problems, which are *not* considered to be a disorder but that may still be a focus of clinical attention. Because many of the conditions in this section are coded with a *V*, they are sometimes simply called "V-Codes." These conditions are coded on Axis I, except for the one related to borderline intellectual functioning. Because of the developmental and preventative focus of counseling, counselors are particularly prepared to counsel clients with these types of conditions and problems. Table 12.3 on the following page lists some of the common codes that counselors might use from this section.

Axis II

Axis II diagnoses are used to describe maladaptive Personality Disorders or forms of Mental Retardation. Diagnosis of the Axis II disorders uses the same approach as Axis I disorders, with a clinician examining a cluster of criteria around an essential feature. Personality Disorders are *enduring* patterns or personality traits that are inflexible and maladaptive and that cause significant functional impairment or distress. Thus, Axis II diagnoses differ from Axis I in that the diagnosed disorders are enduring and inflexible.

TABLE 12.3
Common V-Codes used in counseling

Relational Problems	
V61.9	Relational Problems Related to a Mental Disorder or General Medical Condition
V61.20	Parent-Child Relational Problem
V61.10	Partner Relational Problem
V61.8	Sibling Relational Problem
V62.81	Relational Problem Not Otherwise Specified
Problems Related to Abuse or Neglect	
V61.21	Physical Abuse of Child (995.54 for victim)
V61.21	Sexual Abuse of Child (995.53 for victim)
V61.21	Neglect of Child (995.52 for victim)
V61.12	Physical Abuse of Adult *(if focus of clinical attention is on the perpetrator and abuse is of partner)*
V62.83	Physical Abuse of Adult *(if focus of clinical attention is on the perpetrator and abuse is of person other than partner)*
V995.81	Physical Abuse of Adult *(if focus is on the victim)*
V61.12	Sexual Abuse of Adult *(if focus of clinical attention is on the perpetrator and abuse is of partner)*
V62.83	Sexual Abuse of Adult *(if focus of clinical attention is on the perpetrator and abuse is of person other than partner)*
995.83	Sexual Abuse of Adult *(if focus is on the victim)*
Additional Conditions That May Be a Focus of Clinical Attention	
V71.01	Adult Antisocial Behavior
V71.02	Child or Adolescent Antisocial Behavior
V62.82	Bereavement
V62.3	Academic Problem
V62.2	Occupational Problem
V62.89	Religious or Spiritual Problem
V62.4	Acculturation Problem
V62.89	Phase of Life Problem

Many clients seek treatment for an Axis I problem or a V-Code problem (not attributable to a mental disorder), but clients do not typically enter counseling with a clear awarenesss of their personality disorders. The Axis II Personality Disorders are, in many ways, difficult to diagnose because the criteria are somewhat less precise and because the client, as a function of the Personality Disorder, is less able to report symptoms accurately (Fong, 1995). With an Axis II disorder, the client often perceives that others are the ones with difficulties because their behavior and emotions are natural reactions to the situation. An Axis II diagnosis can be present with or without an Axis I diagnosis.

Because Personality Disorders are considered to be more difficult to diagnose, it is important for counselors to understand the general characteristics and early signs of these disorders. Clients with Personality Disorders will have long-term functioning difficulties; thus, these disorders are categorized by traits. The onset of the pattern of inflexibility and maladaption is typically first observed in adolescence or early adulthood. Although a client may seek counseling for difficulties in reaction to a specific stressor or event, a counselor should determine if there is a chronicity of maladaption. An Axis II diagnosis can be present with or without an Axis I diagnosis. Fong (1995) suggested that during the initial interview counselors should ask clients questions about the duration of the problems and whether the client can recall other such periods of distress or difficulties. These enduring patterns of inner experience and behavior are markedly different from the expectations of the culture and are manifested in two or more areas: cognition, affectivity, interpersonal functioning, or impulse control. A Personality Disorder is not something that appears over a few months, nor is it a reaction to something catastrophic (e.g., living in a war-torn country); rather, it is an enduring part of the personality.

Clients' perceptions of their Personality Disorders are *egosyntonic,* meaning that the disorder is an integral part of the self. Clients with an Axis I disorder, on the other hand, usually perceive the disorder as not part of themselves. In other words, clients with a Mood Disorder will not see the Mood Disorder as a part of who they are; but rather, symptoms of their problems. Clients with a Personality Disorder, however, will see the maladaption as a part of themselves and view the situation as just being the way it is. Therefore, clients with Personality Disorders think counseling has a low probability of changing their situations because the problems are immutable.

Another important feature of Personality Disorders is significant impairment in social and/or occupational functioning. Although clients occasionally experience anxiety or depression, the most dominant features of Personality Disorders are impairments in occupational and social functioning (Fong, 1995). Because Personality Disorders are related to enduring traits, difficulties will arise across many different situations. One way the tendency toward inflexibility is manifested is that clients with Personality Disorders continue to use the same maladaptive strategies over and over again.

A Personality Disorder may not be evident to a practitioner in the first counseling session, in which the focus is typically on the immediate or acute client difficulties. Fong (1995) proposed looking for the following signs that may be indicative of a possible Personality Disorder: (1) the counseling seems to suddenly stall or stop after making initial progress, (2) the client does not seem to be aware of the effect of his or her behaviors on others, (3) the client seems to accept the problems, (4) the client is underresponsive or noncompliant with the counseling regimen, and (5) the client is often involved with intense conflictual relationships with institutional or employment systems.

In the *DSM-IV-TR*, there are 10 personality disorders that are organized within three clusters (see Table 12.4 on the following page). The clusters are atheoretical and are grouped together because of shared features. *Cluster A* concerns the disorders with odd and eccentric dimensions, whereas *Cluster B* includes disorders characterized by dramatic-emotional features. *Cluster C* contains the disorders with anxious-fearful characteristics.

Cluster A

Cluster A disorders are characterized by a client's lack of relationships, aloof behaviors, restricted affect, and peculiar ideas. There are three disorders within this cluster: Paranoid Personality Disorder, Schizoid Personality Disorder, and Schizotypal Personality Disorder. The essential feature of *Paranoid Personality Disorder* is a pattern of pervasive distrust and suspicion of others, such that others' behavior is considered

TABLE 12.4 *DSM-IV-TR clusters of personality disorders and diagnoses*

Cluster DSM-IV-TR	Diagnosis
Cluster A	Paranoid Personality Disorder
	Schizoid Personality Disorder
	Schizotypal Personality Disorder
Cluster B	Antisocial Personality Disorder
	Borderline Personality Disorder
	Histrionic Personality Disorder
	Narcissistic Personality Disorder
Cluster C	Avoidant Personality Disorder
	Dependent Personality Disorder
	Obsessive-Compulsive Personality Disorder

threatening or malevolent. Clients with this disorder will expect other people (including the counselor) to exploit, harm, or deceive them. They do not trust others and have great difficulty with interpersonal relationships. These clients feel they have been deeply and irreversibly injured and are preoccupied with doubts about the loyalty or trustworthiness of friends and associates. They are continually looking for confirmation of their paranoid beliefs. Because they are constantly wary of harmful intentions, these individuals are often quick to identify any slight as an attack on their character or reputation. Furthermore, they often react with intense anger to any perceived insults.

The central feature of *Schizoid Personality Disorder* is a pervasive pattern of detachment from social relationships and a restricted range of emotions. These individuals prefer to be alone and have little desire for personal relationships. They appear indifferent to the approval or criticism of others and are not particularly concerned about what other people may think of them. These individuals do not have close friends or confidants, except, possibly, a first-degree relative. They tend to have flattened affect or appear to be emotionally cold and detached. They are not likely to seek counseling because they see little purpose in talking with someone else or seeking assistance from another person.

The essential feature of the *Schizotypal Personality Disorder* is a pervasive pattern of peculiar ideation and behavior with deficits in social and interpersonal relationships. These individuals incorrectly interpret casual incidents as having particular and unusual meanings to the individual. They have odd beliefs or magical thinking that is inconsistent with the subcultural norms (e.g., superstitions, belief in clairvoyance). Paranoia, unusual perceptions, and odd beliefs are evident, but they do not reach the level of chronic delusional proportions. They also have difficulties forming relationships with other people because their ideas and interpretations of current events often seem strange.

Cluster B

Individuals with Cluster B disorders are very different from Cluster A clients, because the former are quite emotional and often try to impress the counselor. The behavior of individuals in this group tends to be erratic and unstable, with affect that is quite changeable and heightened. The first of the four disorders in this cluster is the *Antisocial Personality*

Disorder. The central characteristic of the Antisocial Personality Disorder is a pervasive pattern of disregard for and violation of others' rights, which begins in childhood or adolescence and continues into adulthood. This diagnosis, however, cannot be given until the person is at least 18 years of age and has a history of some of the symptoms of Conduct Disorder before the age of 15. After the age of 15, the individual's disregard for others is a pattern reflected in the following: (1) repeated involvement in illegal behaviors; (2) deceitfulness, lying, or conning others; (3) being impulsive and not planning; (4) aggressiveness and repeated physical fights or assaults; (5) reckless disregard for the safety of self and others; (6) being consistently irresponsible; and (7) a lack of remorse.

Borderline Personality Disorder is characterized by a pervasive pattern of instability in interpersonal relationships, self-image, and mood. This instability is also accompanied by impulsivity. Borderline clients may display frantic efforts to avoid real or imagined abandonment. Often their relationships are unstable and intense, fluctuating between idealizing and devaluing the other person. There is usually a marked and persistent disturbance of identity. There may be self-damaging behaviors and recurrent suicidal gestures or threats. These clients often have intense feelings, and there is considerable emotional instability. Others may perceive these individuals as overreacting with brief, but intense, episodes of depression, irritability, or anxiety. These individuals also have a tendency to feel chronically empty and have anger control problems. Furthermore, the basic dysphoric mood is often disrupted by feelings of anger, panic, or despair but is rarely interrupted by feelings of well-being or satisfaction. According to the American Psychiatric Association (2000), clients with Borderline Personality Disorder make up about 10% of the individuals seen in outpatient mental health clinics; hence, there is a high probability that mental health counselors will work with clients that have a Borderline Personality Disorder.

The essential features of the *Histrionic Personality Disorder* are an excessive and pervasive emotionality and attention-seeking behaviors. These individuals are dissatisfied unless they are the center of attention. Their interactions with others may be inappropriately sexual or provocative. Emotions change rapidly, and their behavior is often considered inappropriately exaggerated, sometimes to the point of being theatrical. Their speech is dramatic and impressionistic but also tends to lack detail. They are often quite suggestible and perceive relationships to be more intimate than the relationships actually are. They often have difficulty maintaining work because they become easily bored and co-workers have difficulty with their emotionality and attention-seeking behavior.

With *Narcissistic Personality Disorder,* there is a pattern of grandiosity, a need for admiration, and a lack of empathy. These individuals have a grandiose sense of self-importance and are preoccupied with their fantasies of success, brilliance, beauty, or ideal love. Narcissistic clients expect special regard from others but often devalue others' achievements and abilities. They require excessive admiration and expect to be catered to. They often exploit people and lack any empathy toward others. They feel entitled and expect to receive acknowledgement for a job well done even though they may have contributed very little to project. Narcissistic clients are often envious of other people and expect that others are envious of them in return. They typically appear arrogant and seem to have haughty attitudes and behaviors. They are unlikely to seek counseling because any problematic situation is not related to their behavior, which is beyond reproach.

Cluster C

The disorders in this cluster are characterized by the client's anxiety and avoidant behaviors. Clients with these disorders rigidly respond to demands by passively enduring, changing self, or withdrawing. The three disorders are the Avoidant Personality Disorder, the Dependent Personality Disorder, and the Obsessive-Compulsive Personality Disorder. The essential feature of the *Avoidant Personality Disorder* is a pervasive pattern of social inhibition, feelings of inadequacy, and a fear of negative evaluation. These individuals avoid work, school, or even promotion opportunities because of these fears. They are unlikely to enter into relationships without strong guarantees of unrelenting acceptance. Because they are preoccupied with being criticized or rejected, they have a markedly low threshold for detecting such behaviors. They often view themselves as being socially inept, personally unappealing, or inferior to others. They show restraint in both relationships and activities because of fear that they may be ridiculed or embarrassed.

Dependent Personality Disorder is characterized by a pervasive and excessive need to be taken care of. This need leads to submissive and clinging behaviors accompanied by fears of separation. These individuals have great difficulty making decisions. They want others to take the lead and are fearful of disagreeing with them. Individuals with Dependent Personality Disorder are fearful of being alone and will go to excessive lengths to obtain nurturance and support from others. If a relationship ends, they frantically seek another relationship as a source of care and support. They can go to excessive lengths to obtain nurturance and support from others.

The central feature of *Obsessive-Compulsive Personality Disorder* is a preoccupation with orderliness, perfectionism, and interpersonal and mental control. The person's overly stringent standards continually interfere with his or her ability to complete tasks or projects. Individuals with this disorder strive to make every detail perfect and display excessive devotion to work and productivity. They rarely take time for leisure, and when they do, the focus is on performing the leisure activity perfectly. Harsh judgments of oneself and others are common. Some people will have difficulty discarding even unimportant objects and may be frugal in their spending in order to be prepared for a future disaster. These individuals tend to be rigid and stubborn and contend that there is only a single "right" way to perform.

Axis III

Axis III is used for reporting the client's current medical conditions, which may be relevant to the individual's mental condition or disorder. Medical conditions that cause the disorder should not be coded here; rather, the appropriate code should be selected from the Axis I Disorders (e.g., 310.1 Personality Change Due to a General Medical Condition). Axis III is used to describe medical conditions that should be considered in treatment decisions but that are not a direct cause of the disorder. Another reason for including Axis III information is that, in some circumstances, the reporting of Axis III conditions may affect the number of treatment sessions allowed by a managed care organization.

Axis IV

As indicated in Table 12.1, Axis IV is for reporting psychosocial and environmental problems that may influence the diagnosis, treatment, and prognosis of the disorder. This axis is where counselors report psychosocial or environmental issues that affect the Axis I or Axis II diagnosis. Examples of these problems are death of a family member, divorce, inadequate social support, unemployment, or extreme poverty. Typical problems are grouped together in this section of the *DSM-IV-TR* for convenient reference and are:

- Problems with primary support group
- Problems related to the social environment
- Educational problems
- Occupational problems
- Housing problems
- Economic problems
- Problems with access to health care services
- Problems related to interaction with the legal system/crime
- Other psychosocial and environmental problems

If psychosocial or environmental issues are the primary reason for a client seeking services, then the counselor should record these issues in Axis I, using the "Other Conditions That May Be a Focus of Clinical Attention."

Axis V

On Axis V, the clinician reports his or her professional judgment concerning the client's overall level of functioning. This information can be used in treatment planning and also to later assess the outcome of the counseling. The Global Assessment of Functioning (GAF) is typically used to report the client's level of functioning. With the GAF, the practitioner provides a single indicator from 0 to 100, reflecting the global functioning. The GAF scale is reported on Axis V by "GAF = [insert number]." The GAF should reflect only psychological, social, or occupational functioning and should not include physical (or environmental) limitations. Furthermore, the GAF reflects only the client's *current* level of functioning unless otherwise noted. For example, there may be times when a clinician will want to report the highest level of functioning over the past three months. On page 34 of the *DSM-IV-TR*, practitioners will find an easy-to-use scale indicating the appropriate GAF codes. There are other components of functioning that can be included such as the Social and Occupational Functioning Assessment Scale (SOFAS), a Global Assessment of Relational Functioning (GARF), and a Defensive Functioning Scale (DFS).

Multiaxial Evaluation

The reporting of the multiaxial system of diagnosis will vary somewhat depending on the setting. Some agencies require a full five-axial diagnosis for all clients, whereas other agencies or organizations do not. Fong (1995) suggested that counselors should always provide a full five-axial diagnosis because of the information's relevance to treatment. Table 12.5 provides some examples of how to record *DSM-IV-TR* multiaxial evaluations.

Considering the multitude of possibilities, diagnosis can be an overwhelming endeavor to the novice clinician. This selection process becomes even more taxing when the consequences of diagnostic decisions are considered. Therefore, practitioners often need tools to guide them through the process of using the *DSM-IV-TR.* The DSM-IV-TR is a differential diagnostic system in which the clinician uses a hierarchical and

TABLE 12.5 *Examples of how to record DSM-IV-TR diagnoses*

Example 1		
Axis I	309.81	Posttraumatic Stress Disorder, Acute
	305.00	Alcohol Abuse
Axis II	V71.09	No diagnosis
Axis III	446.0	Bronchitis, Acute
Axis IV		Lives Alone
Axis V	GAF = 45	(current)
Example 2		
Axis I	315.00	Reading Disorder
Axis II	301.6	Avoidant Personality Disorder
Axis III		None
Axis IV		Unemployed
Axis V	GAF = 57	(current)
Example 3		
Axis I	V61.10	Partner Relational Problem
Axis II	V71.09	No diagnosis
Axis III	50.00	Diabetes mellitus,Type II/noninsulin-dependent
Axis IV		Discord with boss
Axis V	GAF = 62	(current)
Example 4		
Axis I	312.81	Conduct Disorder, Childhood-Onset, Moderate
Axis II	V71.09	No diagnosis
Axis III		None
Axis IV		Death of brother, Discord with teacher and principal
Axis V	GAF = 50	(current)
	GAF = 72	(highest level in past 6 months)

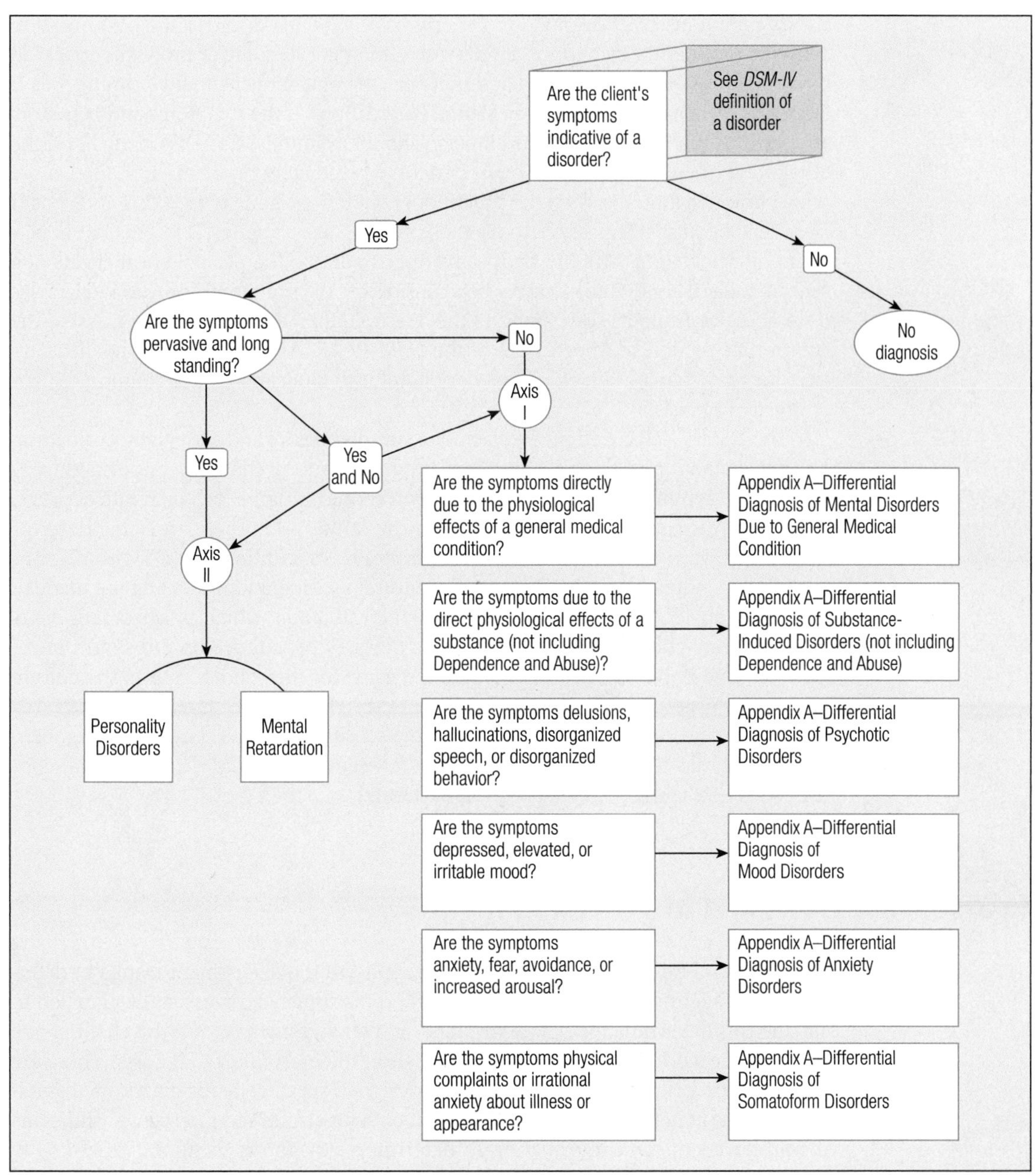

FIGURE 12.1 *Decision tree for DSM-IV-TR*

systemic approach to differentiate among criteria to identify the appropriate diagnosis. Figure 12.1 provides an initial framework for using the *DSM-IV-TR* for Axis I and Axis II diagnoses. In using the *DSM-IV-TR*, the first question a counselor should consider is whether the client's symptoms and behaviors are indicative of a mental disorder according to the *DSM-IV-TR* definition. If the answer is "no," then the counselor should not go any further because the *DSM-IV-TR* is only for diagnosing disorders. If the client's symptoms do correspond to the criteria of a mental disorder, the next question concerns whether the symptoms are pervasive and long standing. If problems appear to be more pervasive, long standing, and trait-like, the practitioner should examine Axis II Disorders (Personality Disorders or Mental Retardation). If the symptoms and behaviors appear to be more acute, then the clinician should examine Axis I Disorders. If, on the other hand, there is a combination of pervasive personality problems and other more acute clinical symptoms, then the practitioner should examine both Axis I and Axis II Disorders, because it is possible to diagnose on both axes. Figure 12.1 contains six pertinent questions (e.g., Are the symptoms directly due to the physiological effects of a general medical condition?) to ask when considering the symptoms for Axis I diagnosis. If the client's symptoms correspond to the question, then the clinician is referred to the appropriate section of Appendix A of the *DSM-IV-TR*. Appendix A contains decision trees for the six areas, which can be very helpful to clinicians in determining the appropriate diagnosis.

The *DSM-IV-TR* is designed to facilitate comprehensive and systematic evaluation. The determination of these diagnoses is important and needs to be performed carefully and with training. Cultural consideration should certainly be taken into account. Within the discussions of the disorders in the *DSM-IV-TR*, there are some descriptions of the ways culture may affect the symptoms. In addition, the *DSM-IV-TR* contains an appendix (Appendix I) related to cultural considerations in using the manual. This appendix includes an outline for cultural formulation, which assists practitioners in considering cultural factors, as well as a glossary of "culture-bound syndromes." These culture-bound syndromes include the name for the condition from the culture in which it was first described and a brief description of the psychopathology. Although the developers of the *DSM-IV-TR* were sensitive to cultural issues in diagnosis, the clinician has the ultimate responsibility to keep in mind the client's cultural context when determining if a diagnosis is warranted.

Instruments Designed to Provide Diagnosis

This section of the chapter is related to the application of assessment results in determining a diagnosis. Many assessment tools and instruments can assist the clinician in making this determination. Certainly, talking with and interviewing the client is one of the major methods for gathering information to determine a diagnosis. There are also structured clinical interviews that are designed specifically for diagnostic assessment. At the conclusion of these structured or semi-structured interviews, clinicians should have sufficient information to determine a diagnosis using the *DSM-IV-TR*. Vacc and Juhnke (1997) found that, for adults, two published structured interviews were noteworthy: the Diagnostic Interview Schedule (DIS) and the Composite International Diagnostic Interview: Authorized Core Version 1.0 (CIDI-Core). According to Kessler and Unstün (2004), the CIDI was an expansion of the DIS. Furthermore, they described the process by which the World Health Organization (WHO) Composite International Diagnostic Interview Survey was examined so that it could be used in the World Mental Health Survey. It is now called the World Mental Health-Composite

International Diagnostic Interview (WMH-CIDI). The entire WMH-CIDI takes an average of 2 hours to administer in most populations. In total, there are 41 sections of the WMH-CIDI that not only address disorders, but also functioning and physical disorders, current treatments, risk factors, and socio-demographics. The developers of the WMH-CIDI also developed elaborate training materials to teach interviewers how to administer this structured interview. As mental health services are needed throughout the world, it is important for counselors to be acquainted with instruments such as the WMH-CIDI that were developed to be used with international populations.

In terms of semi-structured interviews, Vacc and Juhnke (1997) found the Psychiatric Research Interview for Substance and Mental Disorders (PRISM) and the Structured Clinical Interview for Axis I *DSM-IV-TR* Disorders (SCID-I) to be psychometrically sound. They found that the interrater reliability coefficients are good to excellent, and both instruments have been well researched. The PRISM assesses Axis I disorders and antisocial and borderline personality disorders. Trained clinicians are usually the ones to conduct this semi-structured interview, and the amount of time it takes to administer it varies depending on the psychopathology. The SCID-I (First, Spitzer, Gibbon, & Williams, 1997) can be administered only by clinicians and is designed to assess Axis I. There is also an SCID-II (First, Gibbon, Spitzer, Williams, & Benjamin, 1997), which is structured to diagnose Axis II disorders. Beutler and Harwood (2000) concluded that the SCID interviews are the current standard in the field. According to these well-known researchers, the SCID interviews are helpful in both determining a diagnosis and ascertaining the level of impairment or severity of symptoms. With the SCID-I, clinicians use a reusable booklet, which contains the interview questions and diagnostic criteria, and a one-time answer sheet, which contains abridged diagnostic criteria and places for clinicians to record diagnostic decisions. Before starting the systematic questions about the presence or absence of particular *DSM-IV-TR* criteria, the clinician begins with an open-ended overview of the presenting concerns and past episodes of psychopathology. The sequencing of questions in the SCID-I is designed to approximate the differential diagnostic process of an experienced clinician. Module A begins with ratings for Major Depressive Episode, Manic Episode, and Hypomanic Episode. The clinician then proceeds through five other modules. It typically takes between 45 and 90 minutes to administer the SCID-I, and it provides documentation of the diagnostic decision-making process.

Although there are fewer clinical interviews published for children, it appears that clinicians are increasingly using these tools. Vacc and Juhnke (1997) recommended two structured interviews for children: the Diagnostic Interview for Children and Adolescents (DICA) and the Diagnostic Interview Schedule for Children (DISC-IV). Both of these are structured interviews that can be performed by a clinician or a trained layperson. The DICA assesses a wide range of child and adolescent psychopathology, and the DISC-IV assesses Axis I disorders.

Millon Clinical Multiaxial Inventory. There are also standardized instruments developed for the specific purpose of assisting in the diagnostic process. One instrument, the *Millon Clinical Multiaxial Inventory* (MCMI-III; Millon, Davis, & Millon, 1997; Millon, 2006), is an interesting combination of a measure based on theory and a measure designed to correspond with the *DSM-IV.* The MCMI-III is based on

Millon's theory of personality, in which he suggested that psychopathology could be described by using two dimensions. The first dimension pertains to the primary source from which individuals gain positive reinforcement or avoid negative reinforcement, and the types are Detached, Discordant, Dependent, Independent, and Ambivalent. The second dimension concerns the client's coping behaviors, which can be either active or passive. These two dimensions produce 10 personality disorders (5 × 2), which are listed under Clinical Personality Patterns in Figure 12.2. The Severe Personality Patterns are a combination of types within the theory. These two categories also are consistent with the diagnoses in Axis II of the *DSM-IV-TR*. The Clinical Syndromes and the Severe Syndromes, on the other hand, include many of the disorders coded on Axis I (see Table 12.2). The MCMI-III also includes indices of the examinee's attitudes in the Modifying Indices, which are similar to the Validity Scales of the MMPI-2.

The primary use of the MCMI-III is to differentiate psychiatric disorders, and this focus on differentiation is reflected in the scoring process. The scoring system uses what are called *base rates,* which calculate the probability that the client is or is not a member of a particular diagnostic group. The scoring of the MCMI-III is quite complex and can be done only by computer. Rather than using indicators such as two standard deviations above the mean to indicate psychopathology, the MCMI-III considers the actual prevalence of disorders in the clinical population. Prevalence rates do vary among settings, and some adjustments can be made in the scoring, depending on the setting. It is important to note, however, that an individual's responses on the MCMI-III are compared with the responses of psychiatric clients.

New to the interpretation of the MCMI-III are the Grossman Facet Scales. Grossman factor-analyzed the items of the MCMI-III and identified subcategories within each of the Clinical Personality Patterns and Severe Personality Pathology scales of the MCMI-III. Using these fact scales, trained clinicians can better pinpoint processes within the scales. For example, the Grossman Facet Scales for the Narcissitic scale are Admirable Self-Image, Cognitively Expansive, and Interpersonally Exploitive.

Counselors, therefore, should consider some important factors when using the MCMI-III. This instrument is *not* designed for normal functioning adults and should not be used as a general personality inventory. The MCMI-III should be used for diagnostic screening or clinical assessment. In addition, the computer-generated reports are written toward clients with moderate levels of pathology. Hence, for clients with lower ranges of psychological disturbance, the reports will probably overestimate their degree of difficulty. On the other hand, Fong (1995) recommended the use of the MCMI-III over other instruments with clients who may have symptoms of a personality disorder. There is empirical support for using the MCMI-III in diagnosing personality disorders (Craig, 1993). Millon's (1969) theory of personality functioning and psychopathology influenced the original formulation of Axis II personality disorders in earlier versions of the *DSM*. Most master's-level practitioners cannot use the MCMI-III unless supervised by someone with the appropriate qualifications.

Two other instruments have emerged from Millon's work. The first is the Millon Adolescent Clinical Inventory (MACI; Millon, Millon, & Davis, 1994), which also is aligned with the *DSM-IV-TR* diagnostic system. This instrument is appropriate for adolescents ages 13 through 19. The second instrument, the Millon Index of Personality

MCMI-III™ Corrections Report **MCMI-III Sample**
Page 3 **ID: 12566 Administration Date: 1/23/2004**

MILLON CLINICAL MULTIAXIAL INVENTORY - III
CONFIDENTIAL INFORMATION FOR PROFESSIONAL USE ONLY

Valid Profile

PERSONALITY CODE: 8A 3 2A 2B ** 6B * 8B 6A 1 + 5 " 4 7 ' ' // C ** - * //
SYNDROME CODE: A ** T H D R * // CC ** - * //
DEMOGRAPHIC: 12566/ON/F/44/W/D/--/--/--/-----/--/-----/

CATEGORY		SCORE RAW	BR	PROFILE OF BR SCORES (0 – 60 – 75 – 85 – 115)	DIAGNOSTIC SCALES
MODIFYING INDICES	X	163	93		DISCLOSURE
	Y	4	20		DESIRABILITY
	Z	28	91		DEBASEMENT
CLINICAL PERSONALITY PATTERNS	1	13	64		SCHIZOID
	2A	20	87		AVOIDANT
	2B	20	87		DEPRESSIVE
	3	22	94		DEPENDENT
	4	7	16		HISTRIONIC
	5	12	46		NARCISSISTIC
	6A	14	66		ANTISOCIAL
	6B	14	75		SADISTIC
	7	8	16		COMPULSIVE
	8A	24	97		NEGATIVISTIC
	8B	13	71		MASOCHISTIC
SEVERE PERSONALITY PATHOLOGY	S	16	64		SCHIZOTYPAL
	C	23	95		BORDERLINE
	P	15	70		PARANOID
CLINICAL SYNDROMES	A	17	95		ANXIETY
	H	13	76		SOMATOFORM
	N	11	63		BIPOLAR: MANIC
	D	17	76		DYSTHYMIA
	B	8	61		ALCOHOL DEPENDENCE
	T	14	82		DRUG DEPENDENCE
	R	18	76		POST-TRAUMATIC STRESS
SEVERE CLINICAL SYNDROMES	SS	17	66		THOUGHT DISORDER
	CC	21	99		MAJOR DEPRESSION
	PP	7	66		DELUSIONAL DISORDER

Note. Base rate transformations for the Clinical Personality Patterns scales are based on a sample of female correctional offenders.

FIGURE 12.2

Profile of the Millon Clinical Multiaxial Inventory

Styles (MIPS; Millon, 1994), is not for diagnosis or clinical assessment; instead, it is intended for use with normal adults. This instrument incorporates Millon's theory with Jungian theory in an assessment of personality styles.

Summary

When counselors assess clients, their primary purpose is to gather information to effectively counsel clients. In determining the issues and problems that exist, the counselor will often, either formally or informally, diagnose the client. Hence, assessment, diagnosis, and treatment are often closely connected. Sound assessment information is the precursor to sound diagnostic decision making. This chapter focused on the most widely used diagnostic system in mental health settings, the *Diagnostic and Statistical Manual of Mental Disorders—Fourth Edition-Text Revision (DSM-IV-TR)*. The *DSM-IV-TR* is a multiaxial system, where the practitioner provides information about the client on five axes. Axis I and Axis II are for recording the mental disorders, with Axis I for clinical disorders and Axis II for personality disorders or mental retardation. Axis III is where counselors report any medical conditions that need to be considered in treatment. Psychosocial and environmental problems, which are also important to consider in counseling, are listed on Axis IV. The last axis, Axis V, concerns the client's overall level of functioning and is where the counselor provides a score on the Global Assessment of Functioning scale. A client's diagnosis may not always remain within the confines of a counselor's office (e.g., reporting it on an insurance form); therefore, clinicians need to be extremely cautious and careful in the diagnostic process. Social and cultural factors also need to be examined and considered in this process. Counselors need to thoughtfully examine both information about clients' behaviors and symptoms and the diagnostic criteria to determine appropriate diagnoses.

CHAPTER 13

Using Assessment in Counseling

Thus far in this book, the focus has been on measurement concepts (e.g., reliability and validity), specific types of assessments (initial interview, achievement testing), and diagnosis. This chapter is somewhat different in that the focus is on *using* assessments. Assessment procedures often are used throughout the counseling process and skilled counselors know how and when to either gather more assessment information or apply the information they gathered previously. Turner et al. (2001) categorized the uses of psychological assessments based on purpose, arguing that assessments are used for classification, description, prediction, intervention, planning, and tracking.

In considering psychological assessment, Mariush (2004) argued that many practitioners consider assessment to be an activity that occurs only in the initial session. Counselors do not simply use assessments to make a diagnosis and stop there. This would be like a physician using test results (e.g., MRI images) only diagnostically and then ignoring the test results in deciding on the best course of treatment. In addition, physicians often, during the course of treatment, have additional tests conducted to determine if the treatment is working. Using assessment techniques to monitor the effects of counseling is another way in which assessment is intertwined with counseling. This analogy to medical tests should not be taken as an endorsement of the medical model. The medical model assumes there is an illness, which is incongruent with counseling's philosophical foundation that prevention is critical in avoiding pathology and that normal individuals also have developmental issues with which counseling can help. Counselors' endorsement of the developmental-preventative model, however, does not mean that assessment is seen as obsolete. Informal and formal assessments often play a role in (1) treatment planning, (2) monitoring client change, and (3) evaluating the effectiveness of the counseling. This chapter will discuss using assessment in each of these three areas.

Treatment Planning

Counseling is not a process in which every client gets the exact same service. In counseling, the practitioner varies the therapeutic interventions depending on the needs of the individual client. According to Goodyear and Lichtenberg (1999), while working with clients, any mental health professional will make, formally or informally, an assessment of the client's level of functioning. Therefore, counselors need to have sound information about the client or clients to select treatment approaches that have the best probability of succeeding. Beutler and Harwood (2000) argued that it is professionally irresponsible to counsel clients without considering their unique characteristics. Understanding clients' pretreatment characteristics does not apply only to individual counseling; these factors also apply to group counseling and classroom guidance interventions. For example, school counselors will facilitate a group more effectively if they have accurately assessed the students within the group.

Research has continually indicated that statistical or actuarial methods are much better predictors than clinician judgment (Ben-Porath, 1997; Dawes, Faust, & Meehl, 1989; Meehl, 1956). In a recent comprehensive meta-analysis, Æquisdóttir et al. (2006) found that statistical methods were more effective than clinical methods when making clinical predictions. In fact, their findings that statistical models were better than clinical models was strikingly similar to Grove et al.'s (2000) findings concerning the degree to which statistical models were better predicators. Æquisdóttir and her colleagues found that statistical methods increased the likelihood of an accurate clinical decision by 13%.They also found, unexpectedly, that clinicians seemed to be more accurate when they were working with less familiar or novel information. Some researchers have responded to these findings (i.e., regression methods are better than clinical judgment) by suggesting that clinical judgment needs to be more objective (Tracey & Rounds, 1999). Hummel (1999) presented compelling evidence supporting the value of using tests in clinical decision making. He further documented that tests can lead to a better understandings of clients, which has a direct influence on the effectiveness of the treatment. Although assessment instruments may contribute to more objectivity in clinical decision making, clinicians should continue to use informal assessment procedures to gather thorough information. What is important in clinical decision making and treatment planning is to gather *quality* information and evaluate it with a scientific approach.

Although diagnosis does have a significant influence on treatment planning, Beutler and Harwood argued that treatment planning involves more than just determining a diagnosis. For treatment planning to be effective, counselors need to assess the following: To what degree are the problems affecting the client? What environmental or social factors are contributing to the client's issues? What are the client's strengths? Are there cultural issues that need to be considered? What is the prognosis? Many of the assessment techniques discussed in earlier chapters of this book can assist in providing insights related to these questions.

Treatment Matching

Many sages in the counseling field would say matching the treatment to the client has a long historical tradition in counseling. Matching the treatment to the client's problem has always been a common practice, but this philosophical approach has gained momentum with the rise of empirically supported treatments (Sanderson, 2003). Beutler and his colleagues (Beutler & Clarkin, 1990; Beutler & Harwood, 2000) supported treatment matching, citing research indicating that client-counselor match was one of the strongest predictors of outcome. In particular, a significant amount of the variance in counseling outcome is predicted when client characteristics are matched with appropriate treatment and there is a strong therapeutic relationship (Beutler et al., 1999). Before appropriate treatment matching can occur, however, the counselor must gather reliable client information.

Beutler and Harwood stressed that the matching of treatment to client characteristics involves more than determining an appropriate diagnosis. They argued that variations in nondiagnostic qualities, including enduring traits and situation-related states, should be used to select interventions that can be applied in similar ways to individuals with different problems and diagnoses. Table 13.1 includes client characteristics that Beutler, Malik, Talebi, Fleming, and Moleiro (2004) suggested clinicians consider when planning treatments to match client characteristics. Concerning functional impairment, counselors need to ensure that they do not under- or over-estimate client's level of impairment. Mohr (1995) found that clients who get worse during treatment are often individuals who are working with therapists who have underestimated the level of impairment. In certain cases, such as schools and some agencies, a client may need to be referred to another organization to receive the type of treatment warranted by their level of functional impairment. The second client characteristic, Beutler et al. suggested considering in treatment matching is subjective distress. Although reports of distress are inconsistent and subject to change, they also suggest that subjective stress should be assessed and treatment should be selected accordingly. In addition to assessing problem severity, these authors also suggested gathering information related to problem complexity. In some cases, the complexity of the problems may be best treated by a multi-disciplinary treatment team. There

TABLE 13.1
Beutler, Malik, Talebi, Fleming, and Moleiro's (2004) suggested client characteristics to consider in treatment selection

- Functional impairment
- Subjective distress
- Problem complexity
- Readiness for change
- Reactant/Resistance Tendencies
- Social support
- Coping style
- Attachment style

is substantial research (see Prochaska & Norcross, 2002) demonstrating that client progress in treatment is a function of how well counselors match the treatment to the client's readiness for change. To ensure quality information gathering, they recommended also assessing client reactant/resistance tendencies. An instrument specifically designed to predict resistance to therapy is the Therapeutic Reactance Scale (Dowd, Milne, & Wise, 1991). Beutler et al. also recommended assessing factors that might facilitate counseling and assessing clients' social support systems. Another client characteristic they suggested assessing as a part of treatment planning is client coping styles because people typically have patterns in how they respond to distress. Similar to client coping styles, and to some extent social support, are clients' attachment styles. Clients' attachment styles may be contributing to their current issues, but should also be considered, because the counseling relationship is one of the best, if not the best, predictor of positive outcome.

Sometimes counselors have a narrow view of assessment and believe that the term only applies when they are responsible for selecting, administering, scoring, and interpreting the results. This narrow view may restrict counselors' effectiveness, because they may be eliminating a wealth of assessment information. Oftentimes, there is existing testing or assessment information that a counselor could use in effective treatment planning. As indicated earlier, school counselors can easily access achievement test results, and many students' files will also contain general ability or group intelligence test results. This information can be used in making counseling decisions, such as whether a student might feel out of place with other students in a group because of his or her lower academic performance. Sometimes practitioners ignore existing assessment information and rely almost exclusively on information gained from the counseling sessions. This seems like an unwise use of time and resources.

Assessment procedures should focus on more than simply identifying client deficits, because counseling also often involves building and expanding client strengths. Lopez, Snyder, and Rasmussen (2003) argued that counselors and psychologists have been biased toward identifying client problems and psychopathology and have neglected the anatomy of optimal functioning and enhancing human strengths. *Positive psychology* is a term often associated with developing strengths and enhancements of well-being, while at the same time, not ignoring weakness. Lopez et al. recommended that practitioners should abide by the rule of giving equal space and equal time to the assessment of both client strengths and client weaknesses.

One area to consider when assessing strengths is level of optimism (Reivich & Gillham, 2003). Optimism usually concerns hopeful expectation and a general expectancy that the future will be positive. Dispositional optimism is associated with fewer depressive episodes, coping strategies that are more effective, and fewer physical symptoms than a pessimistic outlook. There are formal assessments of optimism, but informal assessments, such as asking people to report their expectancies, can also provide an indication of optimism. Other constructs typically associated with positive psychology are hope, subjective well-being, problem-solving ability, coping skills, forgiveness, and gratitude. In their book *Positive Psychological Assessment: A Handbook of Models and Measures*, Lopez and Snyder (2003) highlighted the assessment of

20 human strengths. In treatment planning, the importance of assessing strengths, resources, and healthy processes cannot be overstated.

Case Conceptualization and Assessment

Clark (1999) argued that failure to completely conceptualize a client situation can lead to treatment failure. Because most counselors assist clients with diverse issues and problems, they must be able to gather complex information and organize and analyze that massive amount of information to make sound clinical decisions. Needleman (1999) argued that case conceptualization skills can help counselors make sense of the overwhelming amount of details presented in any case. Meir (2003) provided the following model for case conceptualization:

Step 1: Identify the initial process and outcome elements. This step should not be confused with identifying process and outcome factors within the counseling process; rather, the focus is on the client's problems and the processes that lead to the problematic outcomes.

Step 2: Learn etiology of client problem. Etiology refers to the causes, precipitants, and maintaining influences of a client's problems (Eells, 1997). Naturally, a clinician's theoretical perspective will influence his or her perspective on etiology; therefore, Meir suggests considering other theoretical approaches when contemplating issues of etiology.

Step 3: Choose interventions for selected problems. In selecting specific interventions for particular problems, the clinician should rely primarily on theory and research. In particular, a clinician should consider an empirically supported intervention when there is sufficient research related to that client problem.

Step 4: Consider the time frame of interventions and outcomes. The clinician needs to identify the short-term, intermediate, and long-term outcomes of counseling. These outcomes refer to the sequencing of events or processes that must occur before a desired long-term outcome is achieved.

Step 5: Represent the conceptualization explicitly. When the conceptualization is explicit, it is easier for the counselor to test, modify, and act on that conceptualization. The clinician needs to verbalize the process of counseling and the expected outcomes. Three methods for making the conceptualization explicit are to (1) represent it graphically, (2) write a concise overview, or (3) explain in detail to a supervisor or colleague.

Step 6: Include at least one alternative explanation. Clinicians, like all humans, are biased observers. Thus, it is important to consider at least one alternative explanation. For example, when a clinician hypothesizes that a client's depression results from faulty cognitions, it is important for that clinician to also consider other potential causes of the depression.

Step 7: Consider the model's balance between parsimony and comprehensiveness. Parsimony concerns whether the clinician has identified the simplest and most workable model; however, the model must also be comprehensive and include all pertinent factors. Thus, case conceptualization involves a need to balance parsimony and comprehensiveness.

Case conceptualization is not just done once and then forgotten; counselors need to continually conceptualize client issues and, correspondingly, adjust and change the counseling process. Furthermore, case conceptualization involves more than the selection of specific strategies and techniques; factors such as the therapeutic relationship are also critical to the counseling's effectiveness. Assessment information can be very helpful in determining how to structure the therapeutic relationship. Because there are no universal guidelines for developing a therapeutic relationship, counselors need to adapt their style to the individual client. Both formal and informal assessment measures can provide information useful in determining methods for enhancing the therapeutic relationship.

Although case conceptualization and treatment planning should never be based on one instrument, the *Butcher Treatment Planning Inventory* (BTPI, Butcher, 1998) was published to assist clinicians in treatment planning. The BTPI is a 210-item instrument designed to assess client characteristics that may either facilitate or interfere with counseling progress. This instrument is unique in that it focuses on 14 "process portraits," such Consistency of Self-Description, Honesty of Self-Description, Closed-Mindedness, and Low Expectation of Therapeutic Benefit. The BTPI has two composite scores, General Pathology Composite and Treatment Difficulty Composite, which may be particularly useful for counselors in mental health settings. There are also three briefer forms (i.e., the 80-item Symptom Monitoring Form, the 171-item Treatment Process/Symptom Form, and the 174-item Treatment Issues Form). Normative information is available for three separate samples: a college sample; an adult nonclient or "normal" sample; and an adult clinical sample. Not only can the BTPI be useful in treatment planning but the full scale or the three briefer scales can also be used for monitoring clients' progress (Hanson, 2001). Although these instruments are comparatively new, the merging of assessing client information with treatment planning could prove to be very helpful in numerous clinical settings.

In conclusion, information gained from sound assessments can often assist counselors in making effective clinical decisions and in determining effective treatments. With the field changing from the matching of client characteristics to the use of empirically supported interventions, the accurate identification of client issues becomes crucial. There is evidence that relying only on an interview may not be enough, and counselors should consider multiple assessment approaches. Clinicians can generate more comprehensive client information by supplementing subjective measures with instruments that are more objective. Using assessment information for treatment planning is, by far, the most common way in which practitioners use assessment results.

Monitoring Treatment Progress

The premise of this chapter is that assessment results can be used in counseling in three ways: (1) for treatment planning, (2) monitoring treatment progress, and (3) for evaluating counseling. Outcome research or measuring outcome has come to connote an evaluation of the effects or effectiveness of counseling or psychotherapy. In the past, outcome assessment was rarely conducted outside of the research setting, and practitioners who did employ outcome assessments typically did so only at the conclusion of the counseling services. Assessing outcome, however, should not be a "one-time event," because counselors have a responsibility to monitor clients' progress during treatment and to determine if clients are making positive gains. The landscape of mental health practice is changing, and counselors are being required to evaluate their services and provide documentation of their effectiveness.

As we discuss evaluating counseling services, it is probably useful to discuss the distinctions typically made between the two major types of evaluation: formative evaluation and summative evaluation. **Formative evaluation** is the continuous or intermediate evaluation typically performed to examine the process. **Summative evaluation**, which is more cumulative than formative evaluation, concerns an endpoint or final evaluation. Sometimes the difference between the two is explained by the distinction that the focus of formative evaluation is on the *process*; whereas, the focus of summative evaluation is on the *product*. The evaluation of counseling services for accountability reasons, which is more related to summative evaluation, is discussed later in this chapter. This section of the chapter focuses on monitoring client progress, which is a continuous process that informs formative evaluation. Although many of the same concepts discussed in the last section about selecting outcome measures apply to monitoring client progress, this discussion will be postponed and considered when the focus is on more comprehensive and elaborate evaluation activities. In monitoring client progress, the counselor will have clients continually assess the effectiveness of the counseling services; therefore, counselors will want to select one or two measures, as it is time consuming (and often very expensive) to have clients take a battery of outcome assessments on a repeated basis. Furthermore, as will be discussed later, monitoring clinical progress does not necessitate the use of a formal instrument.

It is important for counselors to continually monitor the progress that clients make during counseling. If clinicians wait until the end of counseling to do this assessment, they may discover too late that the client has made little improvement. Interesting new research indicates that when clinicians receive feedback about client progress during psychotherapy, the clients have better outcomes than clients whose clinicians do not receive feedback (Whipple et al., 2003). Lambert, Hansen and Finch (2001) used the Outcome Questionnaire-45 to monitor clients' weekly progress. By providing this simple feedback to clinicians, their clients improved significantly as compared to the clients whose therapist did not receive weekly monitoring information. The efficacy of providing counselors feedback was further substantiated by Lambert and colleagues (2003), which summarized the results from three large-scale studies. They found when clients were not improving and the counselor was given feedback regarding the lack of progress, the client started to make progress once the counselor received feedback. On the other hand, if clients were not making progress and business was carried out as usual, with counselors receiving no feedback, the clients often stayed the same. Their results indicated that feedback to the therapist makes an appreciable difference when clients are responding poorly to the counseling.

Even though client feedback, particularly when clients are not making progress, seems to have a positive influence on outcome, not all therapists appear to be open to receiving information about client progress. Bickman et al. (2000) found that only 23% of helping professionals wanted to receive outcome information more frequently than every fourth session. Lambert (2007) asserted that even good clinicians have better outcomes when information is shared that their clients are "off-track." Lambert has been able to build a statistical model that charts clients' expected progress and when clients are not progressing in the expected manner, simply informing the clinician of this has a significant influence on final client outcome. Lambert made a compelling case for mental health organizations to institute a system in which clients would quickly complete an outcome assessment after each session. Although some professionals might contend that completing assessments after every session is too cumbersome, Lambert articulately asserted that there are practical methods for gathering this information and that the benefits to clients outweigh the inconvenience.

When starting to monitor clients' therapeutic changes, it is important to consider what information can be gathered at the beginning and throughout the process. Baseline information can be gathered using different approaches, some of which were addressed in Chapter 6 and in the discussion of issues related to making an initial assessment of a client. Some mental health organizations will use the Symptom Checklist-90-Revised (SCL-90-R, Derogatis, 1994) or the Brief Symptoms Inventory (BSI, Derogatis, 1993), but these instruments have 90 and 53 items, respectively. This would be a quite cumbersome task for each session. An alternative might be the Brief Symptoms Inventory 18 (BSI-18), which has only 18 items and can be completed relatively quickly after every session. The OQ-45.2 (Outcome Questionnaire) has been used in a number of the studies that have examined the effects of clinicians receiving feedback; one finding was that having clients complete this 45-item questionnaire was not overly cumbersome. There is also a 10 item version, which is the OQ-10.2 (A Brief Screening & Outcome Questionnaire).

Bickman et al. (2000) recommended that clinicians should be assertive in advocating what information is gathered, how often it is gathered, and in what format the information will be provided back to the clinician. With the advent of computers and scanners, assessment results from many commercially available instruments are now readily accessible to clinicians, whereas in the past, clinicians would need to wait for results to be mailed in, scored, and returned. Callaghan (2001) stressed the importance of talking with the client about why this data is being gathered over the course of counseling. Filling out assessment forms can be tedious, and clients who are unsure of the benefits of such activities are much less likely to comply. Moreover, it is important to share the results with the client, even when the results indicate that little progress is being made. This type of data can facilitate discussion of being "stuck" and consideration of what aspects of counseling are less productive for the client.

Many counselors only think of assessing outcomes by using detailed surveys or formal outcome assessments. This narrow view ignores an important source of information, which is client self-report. For example, clinicians can systematically ask clients at the beginning of each to session to rate their level of depression, anxiety, or other feelings on a scale of 1 to 10. Meir (2003) recommended that counselors graph these types of assessment to assist them in identifying trends and/or lack of progress. Figure 13.1 provides an example of charting a client's self-report on levels of depression on a scale of 1 to 10 over the course of 10 counseling sessions. In this case, the counselor could clearly see that progress was being made, and the client's level of depression was abating. Crucial to gathering a client's self-report of progress is a clear understanding by both the client and the counselor, of what is being measured. For example, a counselor may have a client who has difficulties with insomnia analyze the level of anxiety. Although the counselor may see the direct link between the client's level of anxiety and insomnia, the client needs to understand the pertinence of

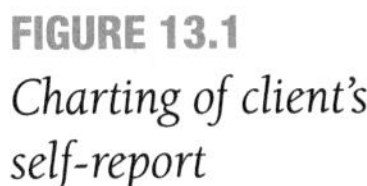

FIGURE 13.1
Charting of client's self-report

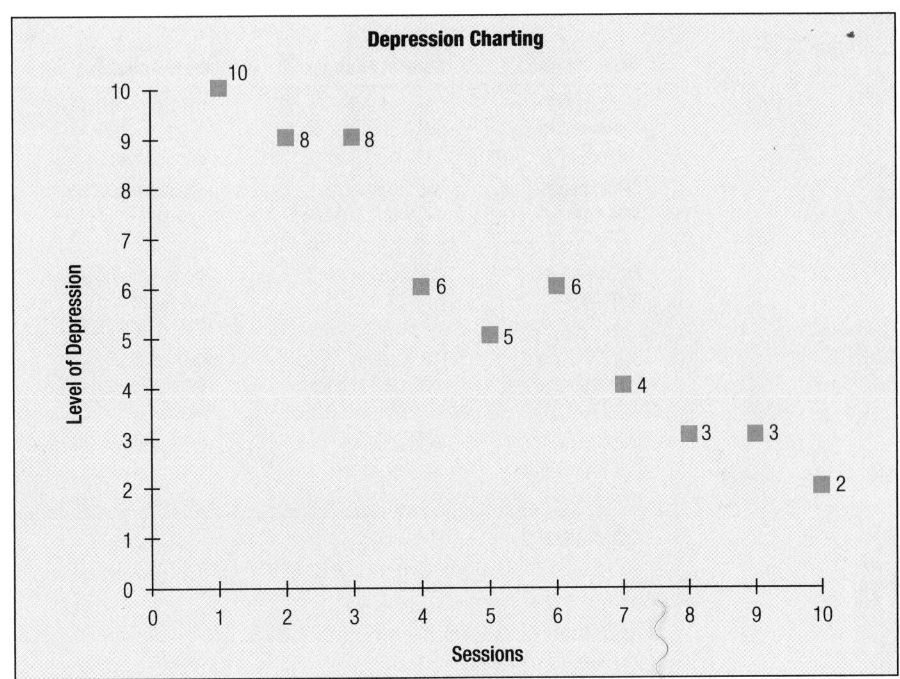

the construct being assessed. Furthermore, with these types of self-assessments, there needs to be a clear definition of what the client is attempting to measure (e.g., what constitutes depression).

If counselors want to make the continuous outcome assessment a little more formal, yet still keep its individual or idiographic character, then they may want to consider *Goal Attainment Scaling* (GAS, Kiresuk, Smith, & Cardillo, 1994). The GAS has been used with a number of different client issues. The first step of this technique involves identifying a target area or complaint (e.g., level of depression). With GAS, the client and counselor need to select an indicator for each therapeutic goal. The indicator is the behavior, affective state, or process that most clearly represents the goal and can be used to indicate progress in reaching the goal. For example, with a goal of decreasing level of depression, the indicator could be a depression scale or a record of the number of times in a week that the client feels "down." Avoid outcomes that are too vague or that could not be evaluated by an outside observer. Outcomes such as "better than when counseling began" are not specific enough. The next step is for the counselor and client to specify an expected level of outcome that is an accurate prediction of the client's status at the conclusion of treatment (e.g., feeling down only once or twice during a week). In Table 13.2 on the following page, these expected levels of outcome are associated with the numerical value of zero. Once the expected level of outcome has been determined, then the client and counselor determine levels for greater-than-expected outcomes and less-than expected outcomes. In GAS, numerical ratings are associated with less-than-expected and greater-than-expected outcomes on

TABLE 13.2
Example of Goal Attainment Scaling

Level of Attainment	Scale 1 Control of anger	Scale 2 Career planning	Scale 3 Insomnia
Much less than expected −2	Has an angry outburst once a day	Has done nothing	Within a week, has 4 nights with less than 8 hours sleep
Somewhat less than expected −1	Has an angry outburst 2 to 6 times a week	Has begun to look into other careers	
Expected level of outcome 0	Has an angry outburst once a week	Has determined a new career and a plan for entering it	Within a week, has 1 night with less than 8 hours of sleep
Somewhat more than expected 1	Has an angry outburst 2 to 5 times a month	Has sent out résumés for a new job	
Much more than expected 2	Has an angry outburst once a month	Has a new job	Sleeps 8 hours every night for 2 weeks

COMMENTS

a scale from -2 to +2 (see Table 13.2 for examples). There also are ways to combine scores across goals and convert them to standard scores if a clinician is doing research or wants group data (e.g., comparing effectiveness of different counselors).

One of the concerns with tracking client changes is the accuracy or validity of using self-report data (Callaghan, 2001). As repeated throughout this book, decisions should not be made based on one source of information, and self-reports of client change should be supplemented with other clinical information, including the counselor's assessment of client change. It is also important that the monitoring of progress become systemized, as some clients may feel somewhat uncomfortable expressing their disappointment with the counseling unless they are frequently and directly asked about their progress.

Using Assessment for Evaluation and Accountability

The complexion of mental health services changed dramatically in the 1990s because of various changes in healthcare. One of the major changes was the emergence of managed health care and the corresponding demands for accountability information from clinicians. Some managed-care organizations will not approve counseling services unless clinicians can show that that they are effective with clients. Therefore, many practitioners are examining methods that evaluate their own counseling effectiveness. This is also true in school counseling, for the American School Counselor Association's (2003)

National Model specifically encourages school counselors to gather accountability data that is measureable and linked to the school counseling program. Counselors can never be quite sure when parents, administrators, oversight boards, or governmental agencies may want documentation that the services counselors provide are worth the monetary investment. Therefore, counselors need to understand the methods for gathering and analyzing accountability information.

Whiston (1996) advocated that practitioners provide accountability information by adapting the methodologies and measures developed in research of counseling outcomes. As stated earlier, outcome researchers conduct studies that indicate the degree to which counseling is effective. Often our interest in outcome research is determined by whether clients change (e.g., stop drinking or become less depressed) in a positive manner. A related concept is process research, which involves identifying factors or approaches that contribute to the outcome. Researchers have actively scrutinized the research methods for investigating the outcome of counseling for more than 60 years. This scrutiny has resulted in a wealth of information that counselors can use in evaluating their own effectiveness.

In developing evaluation or accountability information, clinicians first need to consider what they are attempting to evaluate. Sometimes, a counseling organization will seek one method of developing accountability information on all of the different services they provide. Identifying one method of developing accountability information may be difficult, however, because the services vary (e.g., individual counseling, group counseling, substance abuse services, parenting classes, brief crisis interventions). Thus, practitioners need to determine what services they want to evaluate. As an example, an elementary school counselor may decide to focus first on evaluating a series of classroom guidance activities performed with fifth graders to ease the transition into middle school, rather than evaluating all the services the counselor provides to the children in that school. Because there needs to be a direct connection between the services provided and the outcome measures used, better accountability information can often be gathered by examining different types of counseling services separately.

The selection of outcome measures is, however, more intricate than simply selecting one measure that appears to be appropriate. Humans are complex and it is often difficult to assess the changes that may be occurring internally as a result of the counseling. Counseling is complex and multidimensional; therefore, simple outcome measures may fail to adequately evaluate the therapeutic services provided. In addition, whose perspective should we use in determining outcome? Although we often ask the client if they are getting better, there may be times when a better indicator of actual change might come from a teacher or a parent. Interestingly, research has consistently shown that the effectiveness of counseling varies depending on whether the client, the counselor, or an outside observer completes the outcome measure (Orlinsky, Ronnestad, & Willutzki, 2004). Hence, measuring counseling outcome is not a simple enterprise; however, counselors can learn from the results of many years of substantial research on counseling outcomes. Two premier process and outcome researchers are Hill and Lambert (2004), who state that the best strategies in assessing outcome involve (1) clearly specifying what is being measured; (2) measuring change from multiple perspectives (client, counselor, and outside observer); (3) using diverse types of assessments (e.g., rating scales, checklists); (4) using symptom-based and atheoretical measures; and (5) examining, as much as possible, patterns of change over time.

It is often difficult to select outcome measures and counselors do not want to waste clients' time by having them complete two instruments that measure the same construct. Ogles, Lambert, and Fields (2002) developed a model for clinicians and researchers to use to gather outcome data from a variety of viewpoints and domains (see Table 13.3). The first dimension in Ogles et al.'s model is *content* and the subcategories are cognition, affect, and behavior. This would mean that if one outcome assessment measures feeling or affect, the clinician might want to consider another one that focuses on thinking or a behavioral rating scale. The second major category in the model is social level, which includes the categories of intrapersonal, interpersonal, and social role performance. In relation to this dimension, a practitioner may want to select instruments that have clients examine themselves (intrapersonal), their relationships with others (interpersonal), and how well they function in certain roles (social role).

The third dimension in the model is source, which includes self (i.e., the client), therapist, trained observer, and relevant other (e.g., parent or institution). An example of outcome that would fall under the institutional category is grade point average in which the outcome measure is retrieved from an institution (i.e., school). The fourth dimension is technology, or the type of assessment. The technology dimension includes the subcategories of global, specific observation, or status. Some outcome assessments measure an overall level of functioning and would be categorized as global; whereas, other measures may only assess level of anxiety and would be considered more specific. An observational assessment would be where the client is observed

TABLE 13.3
Ogles, Lambert, and Fields' (2002) Scheme for Selecting Outcome Measures

Content	Social Level	Source	Technology	Time Orientation
Cognition	Interpersonal	Self	Global	Trait
a	*a*	*a*	*a*	*a*
b	*b*	*b*	*b*	*b*
Affect	Intrapersonal	Therapist	Specific	State
a	*a*	*a*	*a*	*a*
b	*b*	*b*	*b*	*b*
Behavior	Social Role	Trained Observer	Observation	
a	*a*	*a*	*a*	*a*
b	*b*	*b*	*b*	*b*
		Relevant Other	Status	
		a	*a*	
		b	*b*	
		Institutional		
		a		
		b		

performing a desired outcome, such as a client with fear of flying being observed taking a flight. Status concerns a state or position and includes measures such as recidivism, expulsion from school, becoming divorced, or employment. The last dimension in Ogles et al.'s (2002) model is time orientation, which concerns whether the outcome measure is assessing a trait or a client state.

In using Ogles et al.'s (2002) model, a counselor does not need to find an outcome measure for each dimension or subcategory, as the goal is to consider comprehensive outcome assessment. Let us consider marital counseling and how a clinician may use the scheme to select outcome assessments. In terms of content, the counselor might consider the Marital Satisfaction Inventory—Revised, which in terms of content would be measuring affect. Hence, the clinician would consider other content areas such as behavior and possibly have the couple keep track of their arguments. The counselor might also consider having the couple complete a communication exercise at the beginning of counseling and at the end of counseling and observe different behaviors, which would include another source (i.e., therapist) and a different technology (i.e., observation). The Marital Satisfaction Inventory—Revised is a global measure, so the clinician may want to consider other types of technology (e.g., specific measures). An example of another technology measure could be status, such as documenting a couple's marital status at the end of the counseling (i.e., married, separated, or divorced).

As another example of considering multiple measures of outcome, let's consider a facilitator of a group for mildly depressed clients. To gain comprehensive information, the facilitator may begin by looking at the content subcategories of cognition, affect, and behavior. The clinician might consider using the Beck Depression Inventory-II (BDI-II), which would measure affect, by having the clients chart behavioral aspects of depression (e.g., sleep, eating, exercise). As the BDI-II measures intrapersonal affect, the clinician may want to consider some measure of interpersonal functioning. Social role might include developing a simple instrument to have clients evaluate their functioning at work. In terms of source, since the group members are completing the Beck Depression Inventory-II (BDI-II), the facilitator could complete the Hamilton Rating Scale for Depression (HRSD). The HRSD is designed for therapists to complete. In terms of technology, the BDI-II and the HRSD are specific to depression; the facilitator might want to consider a more global measure of outcome, such as the Outcome Questionnaire-45. In addition, the facilitator may want to consider a measure of satisfaction with the counseling.

In assessing outcome, multiple measures that draw relevant information from diverse sources often provide the best measures. Therefore, clinicians need to consider a variety of factors when selecting measures to use so they can gather sound accountability information.

Outcome Assessment in Mental Health Settings

As indicated earlier, providing mental health services to clients has been significantly influenced by the rise of managed care (Brown, Dreis, & Nace, 1999). Managed care agencies or third-party payers are interested in reimbursement for mental health services that are effective. They want to work with clinicians who can show that the counseling they provide results in clients getting better. Furthermore, many clients would respond positively if counselors could provide data showing that the majority of their clients do make significant improvements. In addition, clinicians need to continually analyze their own work to identify ways of providing the best possible service to clients. Hence, outcome data can provide critical information that serves clinicians in a variety of ways.

There are movements toward identifying core batteries of outcome assessment for mood, anxiety, and personality disorders (Strupp, Horowitz, & Lambert, 1997). At this point, however, there are no established batteries, and different agencies use a variety of different instruments. Thus, clinicians are often faced with the important duty of selecting outcome measures themselves. Commonly used instruments in research are the Beck Depression Inventory, author-created scales, diaries of behaviors or thoughts, State-Trait Anxiety Inventory, Symptom Checklist-90—Revised, Minnesota Multiphasic Personality Inventory II, Dysfunctional Attitude Scale, Hassles Scale, and the Schedule for Affective Disorders and Schizophrenia (Hill & Lambert, 2004). There are also other assessments that mental health counselors may want to consider. An instrument that is increasingly being used is the *Outcome Questionnaire* (OQ-45.2, Lambert & Burlingame, 1996). The OQ-45 was designed to measure three areas of client functioning: symptomatic distress, interpersonal problems, and social role adjustment. Furthermore, as discussed by Lambert, Okiishi, Finch, and Johnson (1998), the OQ-45 is intended to provide an indication of where *clinically* significant change has occurred, not just statistical or numerical change. One of the methods used to develop this type of information is an examination of the score differences between normal and dysfunctional samples. There are other OQ assessments (e.g., shortened versions and ones for youth); to use of any of these instruments, the individual or agency must submit an application for a license. Another instrument that mental health clinicians might consider is the *Quality of Life Inventory* (Frisch, 1994), which measures satisfaction with 16 areas of life, such as work, love, and recreation. There also are a number of formal and informal measures of client satisfaction, such as the *Client Satisfaction Questionnaire 8* (Nguyen, Attkisson, & Stegner, 1983).

Outcome Assessment in Career Counseling

Similar to mental health counseling, there have been calls for a standard battery of instruments to be used in career counseling (Oliver & Spokane, 1988; Whiston et al., 1998); however, this has not yet occurred. Many of the research studies that have examined the efficacy of career counseling involved measures of career maturity and career decidedness (Whiston, 2002), which were discussed in Chapter 9. Although these measures indicate some level of effectiveness, there are limitations, because many external agencies are more interested in concrete career outcomes (e.g., gaining employment) than in increases in career maturity or in becoming more decided in one's career choice. Whiston et al. (1998) also found variation among career outcome measures. They contended that measures of career decidedness typically showed little difference between those who received career counseling and those who did not. Hence, practitioners may want to consider measures of effectiveness of career counseling other than career maturity and career decidedness. Some noteworthy examples of career outcomes are employment, job satisfaction, and quality of life. In high school settings, counselors may want to consider academic measures and indicators of post-secondary planning. Lapan and Kosciulek (2001) presented a framework for identifying postsecondary placements for high school students and a procedure for creating career counseling programs with sensitivity to the needs of diverse communities.

With college students, there are issues related to how many times a student changes his or her major, time spent completing a degree, and grade point average, among others. Although Goal Attainment Scaling has rarely been used in career counseling research (Hoffman, Spokane, & Magoon, 1981), it has many advantages and is applicable in many career counseling situations. To assist counselors in selecting multiple measures from multiple perspectives, Whiston (2001) developed an outcome scheme specifically for selecting outcome measures for career counseling interventions.

Outcome Assessment in School Counseling

The American School Counselor Association's (ASCA, 2003) National Model, a document designed to guide school counseling programs, clearly states that school counseling programs are data driven. The ASCA National Model urges school counselors to move beyond simply gathering data on services that are provided to students, to gathering data on the impact of these programs. According to the ASCA National Model, "Counselors analyze student achievement and counseling-program-related data to evaluate the counseling program, conduct research on activity outcomes, and discover gaps that exist between different groups of students that need to be addressed" (p. 44). In school counseling, as compared with other counseling areas, there has been significantly less outcome research (Sexton, 1996). Furthermore, as noted by Whiston and Sexton (1998), the outcome instruments used in research are often author-developed for that particular study. Hence, the school counselor does not have the same supply of researched instruments to use in evaluating school counseling programs as mental health and career counselors have to evaluate their activities. This does not mean that there are no readily available outcome assessments for school counselors. School counselors do have access to many important outcome assessments, such as measures of academic achievement (e.g., achievement test scores). Lapan (2001) provided a framework for planning and evaluating a comprehensive guidance and counseling program.

In selecting outcome instruments, school counselors should also consider the general guidelines of using multiple measures from multiple perspectives. Table 13.4 on the following page contains a number of different strategies for evaluating school counseling interventions and programs, and also shows that school counselors should consider gathering evaluative information from students, teachers, parents, and other members of the community. Another instrument to consider is the recently developed School Counseling Program Evaluation Scale (SCoPES) (Whiston & Aricak, in press). This instrument is based on the student competencies in the National Standards for School Counseling Programs (Campbell & Dahir, 1997).

TABLE 13.4
School counseling outcome measures

Measures of students' performance/attitudes
Grades or grade point average
Achievement test scores
Pursuing postsecondary training
Dropout rates
Credit completion rates
Behavioral ratings
Disciplinary referrals
Symptomologies/adjustment measures
Career measures (e.g., career maturity)
Satisfaction with school counseling program/interventions
Measures of teachers' behavior/attitudes
Satisfaction with school counseling program/interventions
Referral rate to school counselor
Ratings of student behaviors
Measures of parents' behavior/attitudes
Satisfaction with school counseling program/interventions
Parenting measures
Ratings of student behaviors (e.g., homework time)
School involvement measures
Measures of community members' behavior/attitudes
Satisfaction with school counseling program/interventions
School involvement measures

As an example of the importance of continuing to gather accountability data, let's consider a school district that is experiencing some financial problems because the state has cut its budgetary allocations to education. This school district has four elementary schools, and each of these schools has a school counselor. However, because elementary school counselors are not mandated in this state, the school board is seriously considering eliminating these elementary school counseling programs. If these school counselors do not have compelling data indicating that their activities make a positive difference, then they can probably expect to lose their jobs. They would be more likely to retain their jobs if they have data indicating that their students have better achievement test scores, attend more school days, and have fewer discipline problems when compared with students in elementary schools that do not have elementary school counselors. Furthermore, if these school counselors had instituted a bullying or peer mediation program, then the school board might be more favorably disposed toward that program if reports existed showing that fights on the playground had decreased. Counselors often procrastinate in gathering accountability information because they are committed to and engaged in helping others. This commitment to others, however, needs to include gathering accountability information to ensure that needed counseling services for individuals and groups continue to be available to them.

Data Analysis

Some counseling practitioners shy away from gathering accountability information because they are unsure of how to analyze the data. New computerized statistical packages make data analysis less difficult and more user friendly than they have been in the past. Sometimes, descriptive information, rather than statistical analysis, is sufficient, with practitioners describing the changes in the outcome measures. Thompson and Snyder (1998) advocated that researchers should use effect size more often because of its practical applications. Effect size is traditionally calculated by subtracting the control group's mean from the experimental group's mean and dividing by the standard deviation of the experimental group (Glass, McGaw, & Smith, 1981), although there are other methods of calculating effect size (see Hedges & Olkin, 1985; Rosenthal, 1991). Many times, practitioners in the field do not have a control group. If this is the case, they can calculate average effect size by subtracting the posttest score from the pretest score and dividing by the posttest standard deviation. Practitioners should also be aware that many researchers are often willing to consult with practitioners on methodological and statistical questions. Therefore, if clinicians are unsure of the correct methods for analyzing the data, they should consult with someone who has expertise in that area.

In conclusion, there appears to be increased pressure for counselors to provide accountability information on their own effectiveness. Meeting the needs of third-party payers or administrators is not the only reason to gather accountability information. Providing outcome assessment results to clients can also have a therapeutic effect. Duckworth (1990) contended that graphically showing clients the progress they have made in counseling can often confirm their progress. Perhaps the most important reason for gathering accountability information is so that counselors can analyze factors that may contribute to or lessen their effectiveness. Thus, professional development and better services to clients can be promoted through the process of gathering outcome information.

Summary

In this chapter, the discussion focused on moving beyond diagnosis to using assessment results in three primary ways: in treatment planning, in monitoring client progress, and for evaluation purposes. Information gained from both formal and informal assessment strategies is often used in treatment planning. Counselors need information about their clients to structure the counseling to meet the client's needs. Research, however, indicates that clinicians are often biased in their clinical judgments. Incorporating quality assessment information into the clinical decision-making process may assist clinicians in making better treatment decisions. For many clients, there is assessment information that already exists (e.g., scholastic aptitude tests) that counselors can use.

Assessment results can also be used to monitor client progress. Because early gains in counseling are particularly predictive of positive outcome, it is important to monitor changes from the beginning and identify clients who are not making progress. Monitoring client progress requires a delicate balance between gathering sound and comprehensive information and having procedures that are realistic and "doable." Furthermore, monitoring information must be readily available to the clinician and provided in a format that facilitates the identification of client progress or lack of improvement. Although monitoring client progress can be somewhat time consuming, the information provided is usually worth the time invested.

The third area in which assessment results play a crucial role in counseling is in evaluating the services provided to clients. Because of increasing demands for counselors to provide accountability information, many practitioners use assessment instruments to produce that information. Counselors need to use sound outcome measures and evaluate their services from multiple perspectives. There are also various methods that practitioners can use to analyze the data and convey results to managed-care organizations, administrators, or other groups.

CHAPTER 14

Ethical and Legal Issues in Assessment

This chapter addresses some of the possible misuses of assessment and methods for ensuring that client appraisals are performed in an ethical and legal manner. Many times, misuses of assessments do not result from malicious behaviors; rather, these problems arise from ill-informed practitioners assessing and interpreting results in a careless manner. Counselors need to understand both ethical and legal guidelines to practice in a professional and competent manner. Before discussing ethical and legal issues, it is important to ensure that counselors understand the differences between these two entities. Laws are related to a body of *rules,* whereas ethics are a body of *principles* that address proper conduct. Therefore, ethics and laws sometimes focus on different aspects or issues in assessment. The intent of both, however, is to protect people from the possible harm caused by misuse of assessments.

Ethics

Sources for Ethical Decisions

Due to the complexities of appraisal issues in counseling, a number of sources are available to aid practitioners in practicing in an ethical manner. Table 14.1 on the following page includes a listing of some of the primary resources related to making ethical decisions. The ethical standards of professional organizations related to counseling and assessment are the foundational source for these materials. In the American Counseling Association's (2005a) *Code of Ethics,* an entire section is devoted to evaluation, assessment, and interpretation (this section is reproduced in Appendix C

TABLE 14.1 *Resources for ethical practices in counseling assessment*

- American Counseling Association (2005). *ACA code of ethics.* Alexandria, VA: Author.
- American Counseling Association (2003). *Standards for qualifications of test users.* Alexandria, VA: Author.
- American Educational Research Association, American Psychological Association, & National Council on Measurement in Education (1999). *Standards for educational and psychological testing.* Washington, DC: American Educational Research Association.
- American Psychological Association (2002). Ethical principles of psychologists and code of conduct. *American Psychologist, 57,* 1060–1073.
- Association for Assessment in Counseling (2003a). *Responsibilities of users of standardized tests (RUST)* (3rd ed.) Alexandria, VA: Author.
- Association for Assessment in Counseling. (2003b). *Standards for multicultural assessment.* Alexandria, VA: American Counseling Association.
- Commission of Rehabilitation Counselor Certification (2001). *Code of professional ethics for rehabilitation counselors.* Rolling Meadows, IL: Author.
- Eyde, L. D., Robertson, G. J., Moreland, K. L., Robertson, A. G., Shewan, C. M., Harrison, P. L., Porch, B. E., Hammer, A. L., & Primoff, E. S. (1993). *Responsible test use: Case studies for assessing human behavior.* Washington, DC: American Psychological Association.
- Joint Committee on Testing Practices (2003). *Code of Fair Testing Practices in Education.* Washington, DC: Author. (Mailing address: Joint Committee on Testing Practices, American Psychological Association, 750 First Avenue, NE, Washington, DC, 20002–4242.)

of this book). There are also ethical guidelines specific to school counseling (American School Counselor Association, 2004) and career counseling (National Career Development Association, 2007). Other professional organizations have standards that address assessment issues, such as the American Psychological Association's (2002) *Ethical Principles of Psychologists and Code of Conduct* and the Commission of Rehabilitation Counselor Certification's (2001) *Code of Professional Ethics for Rehabilitation Counselors.* These ethical standards and codes establish principles and define ethical conduct for members of the organizations. Members of these organizations are required to adhere to their ethical standards, which have arisen out of clients being harmed or the potential for clients to be harmed.

Another major resource regarding both ethical and legal questions is the *Standards for Educational and Psychological Testing* (AERA, APA, & NCME, 1999), which is often referred to as the *Standards.* The *Standards* serves as a technical guide for testing practices and concerns the appropriate uses of tests with a focus on standards for the following: (1) test construction, evaluation, and documentation; (2) fairness in testing; and (3) testing applications. The *Standards* provides expectations of professional services and should be reviewed by every practitioner who is involved in any type of assessment. The *Standards* has also been used in legal cases as an indicator of standards of practice related to assessment in counseling. The process of revising the *Standards* has begun and counselors should become acquainted with this new edition as soon as it is published. Another source currently available is the *Standards for the Qualification of Test Users* (American Counseling Association, 2003), which synthesizes the professional qualifications essential when using tests in counseling.

A third resource counselors can use to find out more about ethical behavior is the *Code of Fair Testing Practices in Education* (Joint Committee on Testing Practices, 2003), which is also related to the *Standards*. This set of standards is designed "to represent the spirit of selected portions of the *Standards* in a way that is relevant and meaningful to developers and users of tests, as well as to test takers and/or their parents or guardians" (p. 2). The *Code* addresses four areas: (1) developing and selecting appropriate tests, (2) administering and scoring tests, (3) reporting and interpreting test results, and (4) informing test takers. This document is not copyrighted and may be duplicated for clients, parents, or others who might benefit from this knowledge. In 1995, the Joint Committee on Testing Practices (JCTP) developed a videotape called *The ABC's of Schools Testing*, which is designed to help parents understand the many uses of testing in schools. A *Leader's Guide* is a manual available with this tape to assist counselors who are working with parents on testing issues.

Another excellent resource related to ethical issues in assessment is the *Responsibilities of Users of Standardized Tests* (Association for Assessment in Counseling, 2003a), which is often referred to as the *RUST Statement*. The *RUST Statement* is intended to address the needs of members of the American Counseling Association and to promote accurate, fair, and responsible use of standardized tests. The focus of this document is not on the development of instruments but rather on the proper use of tests and methods for safeguarding against the misuse of tests. As can be seen in Appendix D of this book, the *RUST Statement* includes discussion of the test user's responsibilities concerning qualifications of test users, technical knowledge, test selection, test administration, test scoring, interpreting test results, and communicating test results.

A fifth resource that practitioners find extremely helpful is the casebook entitled *Responsible Test Use: Case Studies for Assessing Human Behavior* (Eyde et al., 1993), which was also developed by a working group of the JCTP. This resource includes 78 cases illustrating both proper and improper test usages. Examples relate to such topics as testing special populations, individuals with disabilities, test translations, and reasonable accommodations. This resource is particularly useful in describing real-world situations and applying ethical principles to these actual incidents. The casebook's major emphasis is on the application of basic principles of sound test selection, use, and interpretation.

There are a number of other helpful resources for counselors involved in assessment. A resource designed to inform and educate test takers, which was developed by the Joint Committee on Testing Practices (1998), is the *Rights and Responsibilities of Test Takers: Guidelines and Expectations*. This document was developed so that test takers would understand their rights before taking an assessment and to provide test takers with descriptions of responsible behaviors that will make the test results more meaningful. For school counselors, there is specific guide, *Standards for School Counselor Competence in Assessment and Evaluation*, which was developed by a committee from the Association for Assessment in Counseling and the American School Counselor Association. This document is available through the Association for Assessment in Counseling website (http://aac.ncat.edu/resources.html). Because other resources are being developed that will shed even more light on the complicated issues related to assessment, counselors need to be involved professionals to be aware of new resources and guidelines as they become available.

Who Is Responsible for Appropriate Use?

In ethics, there often are gray areas; however, the responsibility for test or instrument usage is *not* an equivocal area. It is clear from many ethical sources that the *clinician* is responsible for appropriate use. The *ACA Code of Ethics* in section E.2.b states, "Counselors are responsible for the appropriate application, scoring, interpretation, and use of assessment instruments relevant to the needs of the client, whether they score and interpret such tests themselves or use technology or other services" (p. 12). Test publishers are responsible for publishing the needed information, but the ultimate responsibility for the ethical use of an assessment lies with the counselor. As the *Standards* indicate, this responsibility also includes scoring and interpretation performed by computers. Thus, practitioners must ensure that the computer programs or other scoring services used are reliable, valid, and appropriate.

Part of being a responsible user of tests or other assessment instruments is practicing within one's limits. Instruments can easily be misused by inadequately trained practitioners. Once again, the ACA's (2005a) *Code of Ethics and Standards of Practice* provides assistance in section E.2.a:

> *Limits of Competence.* Counselors utilize only those testing and assessment services for which they have been trained and are competent. Counselors using technology assisted test interpretations are trained in the construct being measured and the specific instrument being used prior to using its technology based application. Counselors take reasonable measures to ensure the proper use of psychological and career assessment techniques by persons under their supervision. *(See A.12.)*

In other words, counselors must be knowledgeable about the specific instrument before they can give it to a client. Instruments vary in the amount of training and experience required before counselors can be considered competent. Although some publishers require that user qualifications be documented before they will sell an instrument to an individual, the ultimate responsibility still rests with the individual counselor. The traditional three levels (i.e., Level A, Level B, and Level C) serve as a guideline to practitioners on the types of instruments they may use. The *RUST Statement* (AAC, 2003) indicates that the qualifications of test users depend on at least four factors: (1) purposes of testing; (2) characteristics of tests; (3) settings and conditions of tests; and (4) roles of test selectors, administrators, scorers, and interpreters. Turner et al. (2001) described two types of test user qualifications: "(a) generic psychometric knowledge and skills that serve as a basis for most of the typical uses of tests, and (b) specific qualifications for the responsible use of tests in particular settings or for particular purposes (e.g., health care settings or forensic or educational decision making)" (p. 1100).

In the past 10 years, some efforts have been made to restrict counselors from using psychological assessments. Therefore, it is imperative for counselors to ensure they have the proper training and background when using psychological assessments (Clawson, 1997). The American Counseling Association (2003) approved the *Standards for Qualifications of Test Users,* and Table 14.2 list the major areas of knowledge related to assessment. Counselors must have technical knowledge

TABLE 14.2
Major areas within the Standards for Qualification of Test Users (ACA, 2003)

1. Skill in practice and knowledge of theory relevant to the testing context and type of counseling specialty.
2. A thorough understanding of testing theory, techniques of test construction, and test reliability and validity.
3. A working knowledge of sampling techniques, norms, and descriptive, correlational, and predictive statistics.
4. Ability to review, select, and administer tests appropriate for clients or students and the context of the counseling practice.
5. Skill in administration of tests and interpretation of test scores.
6. Knowledge of the impact of diversity on testing accuracy, including age, gender, ethnicity, race, disability, and linguistic differences.
7. Knowledge and skill in the professionally responsible use of assessment and evaluation practice.

related to assessment and be conversant and competent in aspects of testing, such as validity of test results, reliability, errors of measurement, and scores and norms (Association for Assessment in Counseling, 2003a). Qualified and competent use requires more than having the necessary training; the practitioner must also be knowledgeable about the specific instrument being used. Sufficient knowledge of an instrument is gained only by thorough examination of the manual and accompanying materials. The counselor must know the instrument's limitations and for what purposes it is valid.

Counselors are responsible for monitoring their own practice and use of assessment. In addition, counselors are professionals, and, as such, they are responsible for monitoring their profession. This means counselors are responsible for monitoring not only their own competencies in test usage but also the use of assessment instruments by others. If a counselor becomes aware of another practitioner who is misusing an assessment measure, the counselor is bound, first, to discuss the misuse with the other practitioner. If the situation is not remedied at that point, the counselor should then pursue appropriate actions with appropriate professional organizations. For example, if you discover that another counselor is conducting neuropsychological testing without the proper training and background, you should first approach the clinician conducting the neuropsychological testing and discuss the ethical (and probably legal) implications of this practice. If the other clinician continues this unethical practice, then you should contact the American Counseling Association (2005b) and, possibly, a state licensing board.

Because assessment can have a profound effect on clients' lives, counselors need to consider clients' rights in this process. The importance of test takers' rights, which are listed in Table 14.3 on the following page, is clarified in the *Rights and Responsibilities of Test Takers: Guidelines and Expectations* (Joint Committee on Testing Practices, 1998). This document, which is available on-line (http://www.apa.org/science/ttrr.html), is given to clients to inform them of their rights and responsibilities regarding tests. This document is often given to clients prior to testing. Appropriate and ethical assessment considers what is in the client's best interest. In terms of assessment, it is particularly critical that clinicians attend to issues related to the rights to privacy, to results, to confidentiality, and to the least stigmatizing label.

TABLE 14.3
Rights and Responsibilities of Test Takers

As a test taker, you have the right to:

1. Be informed of your rights and responsibilities as a test taker.
2. Be treated with courtesy, respect, and impartiality, regardless of your age, disability, ethnicity, gender, national origin, religion, sexual orientation, or other personal characteristics.
3. Be tested with measures that meet professional standards and that are appropriate, given the manner in which the test results will be used.
4. Receive a brief oral or written explanation prior to testing about the purpose(s) for testing, the kind(s) of tests to be used, if the results will be reported to you or to others, and the planned use(s) of the results. If you have a disability, you have the right to inquire and receive information about testing accommodations. If you have difficulty in comprehending the language of the test, you have a right to know in advance of testing whether any accommodations may be available to you.
5. Know in advance of testing when the test will be administered, if and when test results will be available to you, and if there is a fee for testing services that you are expected to pay.
6. Have your test administered and your test results interpreted by appropriately trained individuals who follow professional codes of ethics.
7. Know if a test is optional and learn of the consequences of taking or not taking the test, fully completing the test, or canceling the scores. You may need to ask questions to learn these consequences.
8. Receive a written or oral explanation of your test results within a reasonable amount of time after testing and in commonly understood terms.
9. Have your test results kept confidential to the extent allowed by law.
10. Present concerns about the testing process or your results and receive information about procedures that will be used to address such concerns.

From *Test Taker Rights and Responsibilities* by the Working Group of the Joint Committee on Testing Practices (1998). Used by permission.

Invasion of Privacy

When clients enter counseling, they retain the right to decide what information to disclose and what information to keep private. In assessment, however, that choice can sometimes be blurred because of the subtleties involved in assessment. An example of how a client's privacy could be unintentionally invaded is illustrated through the case of a client named Claire. Claire's company is paying for career counseling for employees who are being permanently laid off because of downsizing. The counselor's procedure for all of his clients in this situation is to have them take an interest inventory, an abilities assessment, and a values inventory before he meets with the clients. The counselor believes this procedure expedites the process because it enables him and the clients to begin counseling with meaningful information already available. Although there are three distinct inventories, the instruments are packaged as one, with a generic career exploration title, for easy administration. Claire felt some discomfort with many of the questions, but felt compelled to answer; she was unsure of the consequences of not answering all of the questions because the company had arranged the counseling as part of the termination process. Claire was receiving some severance pay and was concerned that being seen as uncooperative with the counseling process could affect that agreement. As the clinician interpreted the results to Claire during the first session, Claire became upset and began to feel as though her privacy had been invaded. Claire is a very spiritual and private woman who believes her values are a private and intensely personal matter. The counselor, in this case, inadvertently impinged on Claire's right to privacy.

Clinicians need to consider two major points in assessment to avoid invading an individual's privacy: informed consent and relevance. *Informed consent* involves letting the client know about both the nature of the information being collected and the purpose(s) for which the results will be used. Informed consent is clearly stated in the ACA's *Code of Ethics* (see E.3.a in Appendix C). The counselor in Claire's case was not in accordance with these standards. First, Claire was never informed about the nature of the instruments she was taking nor how the information would be used. The instrument that assessed values had a generic career exploration title, so even that did not indicate to Claire what types of questions she was answering. Second, Claire was never given the opportunity to consent to or decline taking the assessments. She might have declined to take the values inventory if she had been given previous information on what it measured and how the information was going to be used. The counselor could probably make a case as to the relevance of the values inventory, but he invaded her privacy by not obtaining informed consent prior to her taking the assessments.

Clients need to be informed about any assessment in language that they can understand. Clients also must be given the opportunity to consent to the assessments. There are, however, some exceptions to this as covered by the *Standards for Educational and Psychological Testing* (AERA, APA, & NCME, 1999): "Informed consent should be obtained from test takers, or their legal representative when appropriate, before testing is done except: (a) when testing without consent is mandated by law or governmental regulation, (b) when testing is conducted as a regular part of school activities, or (c) when consent is clearly implied" (p. 87). Even when consent is not required, the individual should still be informed about the assessment process. If the client is a minor, a parent or guardian must provide the informed consent.

In general, a written informed consent is better; however, if this is taken to an extreme, it could affect the counseling process. The decision between written or oral informed consent mainly depends on the significance of the assessment situation. If the assessment process and results could have a significant impact on the client, then a written informed consent is wise. On the other hand, there may be times when oral consent is acceptable (e.g., the use of a self-exploration inventory). Many practitioners have general written informed consent forms explaining the counseling process, which the client (or the client's parent or guardian) signs before counseling begins. If counselors have standard instruments that they typically use (e.g., instruments given during the intake process), then the nature of those assessments and how the information is to be used should be covered in the general informed consent materials. Often, practitioners will also cover the possibility of future formal and informal assessment procedures (e.g., interviewing, exercises) in their general informed consent form that clients sign.

As was mentioned earlier, informed consent is only one part of the invasion of privacy issue. The second major concept is *relevance*. With some instruments, particularly personality instruments, clients may not be aware of the variables or characteristics being measured and, thus, may unintentionally disclose information about themselves. Many of us have limitations or weaknesses that we would rather others did not have information about. One of the critical questions related to invasion of privacy is whether the assessment is relevant to the counseling. If the assessment is not relevant to the counseling, then no purpose is served by uncovering this information. Therefore, the clinician should be able to clearly state to the client or the client's parent or guardian the purpose of the assessment and the benefits gained from the process. The practitioner is responsible for identifying and using assessment tools that do, indeed, match that purpose. In selecting a relevant measure, the clinician needs to consider the reliability, validity, psychometric limitation, and appropriateness of the instrument.

The concept of relevance is certainly logical, but it is occasionally unheeded. For example, some practitioners become quite enthralled with an instrument and will give it to all of their clients, regardless of its relevance to their issues. Another more common example of neglecting the concept of relevance is a counselor interviewing a client on an area that is of interest to the counselor but is not relevant to the counseling. Because counselors are responsible for respecting the client's privacy when using any assessment technique, the concepts of informed consent and relevance apply to both formal assessment instruments and informal techniques, such as interviewing.

The Right to Results

Not only do clients have the right to have the assessment process explained to them, they also have the right to an explanation of the results. In section E.1.b (Client welfare), the *ACA Code of Ethics* contains the statement, "They [counselors] respect the client's right to know the results, the interpretations made, and the bases for counselors' conclusions and recommendations" (p. 12). This does not mean that the client has to be told every result and conclusion; the client's welfare dictates the interpretation of the results. In section E.3.b (Recipients of results), the *ACA Code of Ethics* indicates, "Counselors consider the examinee's welfare, explicit understandings, and prior agreements in determining who receives the assessment results." As an example, if a certain diagnostic conclusion would probably increase the anxiety level of a client, then the practitioner may decide it is in the best interest of that client not to disclose the information at that time. The informed consent will also determine if anyone else can have access to the results (e.g., other family members in a family counseling situation or teachers). In terms of releasing information, counselors need to comply with section E.4 of the *ACA Code of Ethics*.

Clients also deserve an interpretation of their assessment results in terms that they can understand. Misinterpretation of the results can be enormously painful to individuals. An 11-year-old child may hear 60%, when the result is actually the 60th percentile. In fact, even some well-educated adults have been known to confuse *percentile* and *percentage*. Interpreting results requires well-developed counseling skills. The misinterpretation of results often occurs when an individual is given the results without a thorough explanation. As was stated in the discussion concerning the interpretation of results in Chapter 5, a counselor should prepare different methods for explaining the results in case the client does not understand the initial explanation.

The Right to Confidentiality

As a part of any assessment, clients have the right to have their results kept confidential. Confidentiality means that only the counselor and the client (or parents/guardians in the case of a minor) have access to the results. The results can only be released to a third party with the client's consent. In addition, the release of information needs to be to individuals who have the expertise to competently interpret the information. Exceptions to this are institutions (e.g., schools, court systems), where a number of people may have legitimate reasons for examining the assessment results. In these cases, the informed consent should address the question of who may have access to the results and how those individuals will use the results. As is discussed later in this chapter, there are laws that govern who can have access to the assessment results in schools.

Counselors often fail to keep assessment results confidential through acts of carelessness. For example, a school counselor who allows a student aide to file papers that contain the achievement results of other students is breaking confidentiality. A marriage and family counselor who provides a summary of the wife's scores on a marital satisfaction inventory to the husband without consent from the wife to release the information is breaking confidentiality. A counselor in a college counseling center who allows an unmonitored, computerized career assessment and information system in the waiting room of the center might also be breaking confidentiality, because some students may have the computer sophistication to retrieve other students' confidential information. Counselors are responsible for securing assessment information, and any limits to confidentiality should be communicated to the client beforehand. This includes ensuring that test data transmitted electronically (e.g., by email or facsimile) are truly secure and confidential.

Clinicians also need to understand that client records, including assessment results, could be subpoenaed. Therefore, clinicians should ensure that assessment records are retained and maintained in a professional manner. Counselors cannot predict future court action that may occur and, hence, attendance to detail is important. The case of Carole illustrates this point. Carole entered counseling when her husband requested a divorce. During this period, Carole was saddened and upset by the end of her marriage. The counselor decided to have Carole take a depression inventory to assess her level of depression, the results of which indicated Carole was slightly depressed. The results of this inventory were kept in her file, but the counselor did not record in the case notes why the inventory was given. Three years later, Carole was in a car accident, which resulted in Carole requiring extensive medical care. When Carole sued the driver who caused the accident, the other driver's attorney had Carole's counseling records subpoenaed. This attorney attempted to make the case that Carole's depression, as documented by the assessment results, was at the root of her medical problems. If the counselor had documented that the reason for the depression assessment was because of the divorce, Carole's case in court would have been considerably easier.

Counselors are responsible not only for keeping assessment results secure but also for keeping the assessment questions or content secure. Securing test content is particularly important in the areas of intelligence or general ability, achievement, and aptitude assessment. It is also important when personality instruments are used for decision making (e.g., employment). Sometimes parents will have concerns about an assessment and want to preview that instrument before it is administered to their child. In this case, the counselor should keep the exact content of the instrument secure and should talk about what the test measures in general. The parents should not be shown the specific test questions. Counselors need to be familiar with the instrument's manual in order to know the procedures for keeping an instrument secure. For example, in some states, the achievement tests used to comply with *No Child Left Behind* legislation have quite elaborate procedures for ensuring the security of the tests.

The Right to the Least Stigmatizing Label

Sometimes in counseling, the purpose of the assessment is diagnosis, which, in many ways, means applying a label to an individual. Standard 8.8 of the *Standards for Education and Psychological Testing* states, "When score reporting includes assigning individuals to categories, the categories should be chosen carefully and described precisely. The least stigmatizing labels, consistent with accurate representation, should always be assigned" (p. 88). The least stigmatizing label does not mean that clinicians should always use less or nonstigmatizing diagnostic codes, because a less stigmatizing code that is inaccurate could prevent the client from receiving the appropriate treatment. Ethical standards also reinforce the importance of proper diagnosis of mental disorders. When clinicians consider diagnostic categories, they need to incorporate contextual factors, such as the clients' cultural and socioeconomic experiences. A diagnostic label, however, can have a significant impact, and, therefore, practitioners need to carefully reflect on these professional decisions. The decisions related to diagnosis are further complicated because, in some situations, the determination of whether an individual should receive treatment is connected to the diagnosis. For example, some managed-care organizations will not pay for treatment for certain diagnoses, such as V-Codes, and individuals may not be able to afford treatment unless their insurance company covers it. This ethical issue seems to be problematic: Danzinger and Welfel (2001) found that 44% of the mental health counselors who participated in their study indicated that they had changed or would change a client's diagnosis to receive additional managed-care reimbursement.

In conclusion, the ethical use of assessment interventions is a professional responsibility. Counselors are responsible not only for their own professional conduct but counselors are also responsible for taking reasonable steps to prevent other professionals from misusing assessment procedures or results. Certainly, there have been misuses of assessment devices in the past; however, if professionals monitor their own and others' use of assessments, then future misuses should be significantly reduced.

Legal Issues in Assessment

As mentioned earlier, principles and ethical standards direct professional behavior in assessment. There are also *laws* to which professionals need to adhere. Laws emanate from two sources: legislation and litigation. *Legislation* concerns governmental bodies passing laws. For example, many state legislatures have passed bills related to the licensing of Licensed Professional Counselors. *Litigation* is the other way that laws are formed by "rules of law." In this case, courts interpret the U.S. Constitution, federal law, state law, and common law in a particular case, and their ruling then influences the interpretation of the relevant laws. Both legislation and litigation have had an effect on assessment. In the past, most of the legislation and litigation that influenced assessment concerned employment testing and educational testing. This area, however, is always evolving and changing—a new law could be passed tomorrow or a court could make an influential decision next week. Therefore, counselors must continually strive to keep abreast of these evolving legal issues.

Legislation

The U.S. Congress has passed a number of influential legislative acts related to assessment. Most of these laws were not written for the specific purpose of controlling assessment practice, but they do contain content and language that are related to testing practice. Because these are federal laws, rather than state laws, these acts affect the entire country.

Civil Rights Act of 1991. Title VII of the Civil Rights Acts of 1964 and the 1972 and 1978 amendments of this act outlawed discrimination in employment based on race, color, religion, sex, or national origin. The original legislation created the Equal Employment Opportunity Commission (EEOC), which was charged with developing guidelines to regulate equal employment. In the 1970s, the EEOC developed very strict guidelines related to the use of employment tests, addressing the type of reliability and validity evidence that needed to be present. During the 1980s, there was considerable controversy about the EEOC. This controversy is partly what led to the passing of the Civil Rights Act of 1991.

Several controversial court decisions that certain civil rights advocates found disturbing also may have influenced the passage of the Civil Rights Act of 1991. These decisions, during the 1980s, were changes that resulted from the landmark case *Griggs v. Duke Power Company* (1971). This case involved African American employees of a private power company. The employees filed suit against the power company, claiming that the criteria for promotion, such as requiring a high school diploma and passing scores on the Wonderlic Personnel Test and the Bennett Mechanical Comprehension Test, were discriminatory. The Supreme Court ruled in favor of the employees and found that although an instrument may not appear biased, it may discriminate if it has a disparate or adverse impact. The Court also ruled that if there is disparate impact, the employer must show that the hiring procedures are job-related and a reasonable measure of job performance. Because the validity of the two instruments was an issue in this decision, this case spurred a stronger focus on the validity of employment tests in making employment decisions.

One of the first cases that diverged somewhat from the *Griggs* case was *Watson v. Fort Worth Bank and Trust* (1988). In this case, the Supreme Court did not rule on behalf of the African American woman who had been passed over for a supervisory position. This ruling raised questions about employment selection procedures for supervisory positions. The findings indicated that, for supervisory positions, employment testing procedures do not need strong validity evidence and that subjectivity can enter into these decisions. In *Wards Cove Packing Company v. Antonio* (1989), the Supreme Court ruled on the concept of adverse or disparate impact that some employers thought the Court would rule on in the *Watson* case. In *Wards Cove*, most of the cannery jobs were held by Eskimos and Filipinos, whereas the company's noncannery jobs were held by European Americans. The judicial decision in this case shifted the burden to the plaintiff to show that there are problems with the selection procedures. Based on this case, plaintiffs would need to show that the instruments were not job-related, which is difficult to do with limited access to human resources or personnel information and records.

In many ways, the Civil Rights Act of 1991 codified the principles of *Griggs v. Duke Power Company.* The plaintiff must show that there is an adverse or disparate impact. Then the burden shifts to the employer to show that discriminatory hiring procedures are needed because of business necessity and job relatedness (Hagen & Hagen, 1995). Therefore, the Civil Rights Act shifts more of the burden back to the employer and requires that hiring procedures and employment tests be connected to the duties of the job.

Another feature of the Civil Rights Act of 1991 is the ban on separate norms in employment tests. The act specifically states that it is unlawful to adjust the scores of, use different cutoff scores for, or otherwise alter the results of employment-related tests because of race, color, religion, sex, or national origin. Some individuals in the assessment field believe that this portion of the act may have untold ramifications. The focus of the ban was on separate norms used by the U.S. Employment Services (USES) for minority and nonminority job applicants. In the 1980s, the USES sent potential employees' General Aptitude Test Battery (GATB) percentile scores to employers for them to use in hiring decisions. A problem with this procedure was that African Americans and Hispanics tended to have lower average scores on the GATB, and, thus, their percentile scores were not competitive. The USES decided to use separate norms so that African Americans would be compared with other African Americans. The public outcries, however, led to the ban of separate norms in 1991 (Sackett & Wilk, 1994). In addition to issues of race, there are other concerns about whether to use separate norms, such as for men and women on personality tests. Some findings indicate that women are more likely to disclose negative information about themselves, which may be problematic when personality instruments are used for hiring. Certainly, tests that involve muscular strength or cardiovascular endurance also favor men. The debate surrounding the advantages and disadvantages of separate norms will most likely continue in the coming years. Racial differences in hiring and performance on employment tests are complex and multidimensional issues. Gottfredson (1994) suggested that the approach to these issues needs to be broadened. She contended that employment tests did not cause the racial differences, and we cannot expect that adjusting or not adjusting the scores will solve these complex problems.

Americans with Disabilities Act of 1990. The Americans with Disabilities Act (ADA) bans discrimination in employment and in access to public services, transportation, and telecommunications on the basis of physical and mental disabilities. A disability is defined firstly as a physical or mental impairment that substantially limits one or more life activities and, secondly, there must be a record of such impairment. ADA came to address testing through the focus on employment and employment testing. The language of the bill, however, is broad and covers multiple testing situations. Under ADA, individuals with disabilities must have tests administered to them with reasonable and appropriate accommodations (Geisinger, 1994). This language raises some troublesome questions related to assessment. First, how are reasonable and appropriate accommodations defined? As of yet, there is still some ambiguity related to what constitutes reasonable and appropriate accommodation. In addition, there are thousands of disabilities, and, therefore, it is difficult for counselors to know precisely how to make accommodations that are reasonable for all possible situations. A counselor must be careful with any nonstandard administration of a standardized instrument because standardized instruments are designed to be administered in a uniform manner. As indicated earlier in the discussion of ethics, the ultimate responsibility for the appropriate use of an instrument rests with the user, so clinicians have a responsibility to investigate what are appropriate accommodations. In addition, more materials are being developed to assist practitioners in appropriately adapting assessments. For example, CBT/McGraw-Hill (2004) published a document designed to assist school personnel in administering standardized achievement in an inclusive manner, which is a resource that many school counselors might find helpful. The nonstandard administration of a standardized test leads to another major issue related to using and interpreting the results of a nonstandard administration. It is often difficult to determine whether the accommodations that were made met the intent of ADA, which is to make accommodations so that instruments measure the intended construct and not the disability. Interpreting the results of clients with disabilities involves determining if the accommodations were sufficient or if the results still may be unfairly influenced by the disability. There is also an opposite risk in which the accommodations provide an advantage to the examinee with the disability as compared with those without the disability. Geisinger suggested that the assessment field should consider new ways of assessing individuals with disabilities in order to develop fair measures and assessment procedures.

Individuals with Disabilities Education Act of 2004. Another piece of legislation affecting assessment and testing of individuals with disabilities is the Individuals with Disabilities Education Act (IDEA), which was last reauthorized in 2004. IDEA is a law ensuring services to children with disabilities. Services and early interventions for infant and toddlers with disabilities (birth to age 2) and their families is addressed in Part C. Part B of IDEA address services for children with disabilities ages 3 to 21. The regulations were published in the *Federal Register on* August 14, 2006 (Volume 71,

Number 156) and can be found at www.nichy.org/reauth/IDEA2004regulations.pdf. Many different aspects of IDEA are pertinent to counselors, particularly school counselors. However, the focus of this discussion will be on assessment. IDEA legislates that each state must have a comprehensive system that can identify, locate, and evaluate children ages birth through 21 who may have a disability (Kupper, 2007). The request for evaluation can come from either the parent or a public agency (e.g., the child's school) when there is a suspicion that there may be some sort of disability. If a public agency suspects there is a disability, the agency must provide prior written notice to the parents explaining why they wish to conduct the evaluation, a description of each assessment, and a description of procedural safeguards (e.g., where parents can go to receive more information about the process). Once the parents have consented to the evaluation, the evaluation must be conducted within 60 days unless there is other timeframe legislation at the state level. A parent's request for an evaluation can be refused by the public agency if they believe there is not a disability and there is a system for parents to appeal this decision. The intent of the evaluation is not just to identify whether a child has a disability; rather, the evaluation is designed to *fully learn* the nature and extent of the special education and related services the child needs. If a child has a disability, then the public agency must develop an **Individualized Education Plan (IEP),** which is developed by a team of educators and the parents. The evaluation must be conducted individually. Table 14.4 includes specifics about how the evaluation must be conducted.

Often these evaluations will be conducted by school psychologists, but school counselors are often on an IEP team, which will have input into the evaluation and subsequent decisions about the appropriate educational plan. In some cases, mental health counselors may be working with children or adolescents who have been assessed, and these professionals may ask the parents to have the results released to them. If you examine Table 14.4, you will notice that a significant portion of the federal regulations are consistent with best practices in assessment. For example, as has been emphasized in this book, the evaluation should not be based on one test but should include a variety of assessment tools. Typically information is gathered using a variety of techniques (e.g., observation, interviews) and from a variety of sources (e.g., the student, parents, and teachers). The evaluation should also include instruments that are technically sound in all areas in which there is a suspected disability. As also can be seen from Table 14.4, there is considerable focus on issues of race, culture, and language so that the assessments are not discriminatory. The assessments should be given in the child's native language or in another mode or form that is likely to yield accurate information on what the child knows and can do academically, developmentally, and functionally. If this is not possible, then the public agency needs to be cautious in interpreting the assessment results. The focus of this section of the law is to ensure that children are assessed fairly. The team must ensure that the evaluation is comprehensive and also sensitive to the child's impairment. For example, if a child has a reading disability and one of the assessments is of mathematics, then the assessment should be related to mathematics and not include the child's ability to read math story problems. Furthermore, these individual assessments must be conducted by trained individuals who are knowledgeable about the specific instrument and techniques used in this comprehensive evaluation. After the evaluation, if a child

TABLE 14.4
Section 300.304 Evaluation procedure from the Individuals with Disabilities Education Act of 2004

(a) Notice. The public agency must provide notice to the parents of a child with a disability, in accordance with Sec. 300.503, that describes any evaluation procedures the agency proposes to conduct.

(b) Conduct of evaluation. In conducting the evaluation, the public agency must—

(1) Use a variety of assessment tools and strategies to gather relevant functional, developmental, and academic information about the child, including information provided by the parent, that may assist in determining—

(i) Whether the child is a child with a disability under Sec. 300.8; and

(ii) The content of the child's IEP, including information related to enabling the child to be involved in and progress in the general education curriculum (or for a preschool child, to participate in appropriate activities).

(2) Not use any single measure or assessment as the sole criterion for determining whether a child is a child with a disability and for determining an appropriate educational program for the child; and

(3) Use technically sound instruments that may assess the relative contribution of cognitive and behavioral factors, in addition to physical or developmental factors.

(c) Other evaluation procedures. Each public agency must ensure that—

(1) Assessments and other evaluation materials used to assess a child under this part—

(i) Are selected and administered so as not to be discriminatory on a racial or cultural basis;

(ii) Are provided and administered in the child's native language or other mode of communication and in the form most likely to yield accurate information on what the child knows and can do academically, developmentally, and functionally, unless it is clearly not feasible to so provide or administer;

(iii) Are used for the purposes for which the assessments or measures are valid and reliable;

(iv) Are administered by trained and knowledgeable personnel; and

(v) Are administered in accordance with any instructions provided by the producer of the assessments.

(2) Assessments and other evaluation materials include those tailored to assess specific areas of educational need and not merely those that are designed to provide a single general intelligence quotient.

(3) Assessments are selected and administered so as best to ensure that if an assessment is administered to a child with impaired sensory, manual, or speaking skills, the assessment results accurately reflect the child's aptitude or achievement level or whatever other factors the test purports to measure, rather than reflecting the child's impaired sensory, manual, or speaking skills (unless those skills are the factors that the test purports to measure).

(4) The child is assessed in all areas related to the suspected disability, including, if appropriate, health, vision, hearing, social and emotional status, general intelligence, academic performance, communicative status, and motor abilities;

(5) Assessments of children with disabilities who transfer from one public agency to another public agency in the same school year are coordinated with those children's prior and subsequent schools, as necessary and as expeditiously as possible, consistent with Sec. 300.301(d)(2) and (e), to ensure prompt completion of full evaluations.

(6) In evaluating each child with a disability under Sec. Sec. 300.304 through 300.306, the evaluation is sufficiently comprehensive to identify all of the child's special education and related services needs, whether or not commonly linked to the disability category in which the child has been classified.

(7) Assessment tools and strategies that provide relevant information that directly assists persons in determining the educational needs of the child are provided.

(Authority: 20 U.S.C. 1414(b)(1)-(3), 1412(a)(6)(B))

is found eligible for services, then an IEP meeting is scheduled that includes the parents. The meeting is held and an IEP is written for the student that includes stated and measureable goals. At least once per year, the student's IEP is reviewed to examine progress toward those goals. As students age and mature, it is expected that there will be changes and a comprehensive reevaluation can occur after a year and should occur at least once every three years.

Family Educational Rights and Privacy Act of 1974. The next piece of legislation in this discussion also concerns education but includes both individuals with disabilities and those without. The Family Educational Rights and Privacy Act (FERPA) provides parents and "eligible students" (those older than 18) with certain rights regarding the inspection and dissemination of educational records. This law was designed to protect student privacy and applies to all school districts and schools that receive funds from the U.S. Department of Education. FERPA, which mainly concerns the access of educational records, provides parents with access to their children's educational record. Students over 18 also have access to their own records. The law further specifies that an educational record cannot be released, without parental permission, to anyone other than those who have a *legitimate* educational interest. The contents of the educational record will vary somewhat from school district to school district, but group achievement tests, student grades, and attendance records are routinely considered part of a student's educational records. Although counseling records kept in a separate locked cabinet and accessible only to the counselor are not considered part of the educational record, bills have been introduced in the U.S. House of Representatives that would require counselors to provide those records to parents.

Another provision in FERPA concerns assessment in the schools. FERPA includes language stating that no student shall be required, without parental permission, to submit to psychological examination, testing, or treatment that may reveal information concerning mental and psychological problems potentially embarrassing to the student or the student's family. This issue was addressed in an amendment to the Goals 2000: Educate America Act of 1994. This amendment, which is titled the Protection of Pupil Rights Amendment and which is often called the Grassley Amendment, has language similar to FERPA, but it specifies written parental consent before minor students are required to participate in any survey, analysis, or evaluation that reveals any information concerning mental and psychological problems potentially embarrassing to the student or the student's family. Some educational administrators have interpreted this to include self-esteem measures or any exercise that involves self-analysis. Many school districts have adopted the policy that any type of assessment, except routine achievement tests, requires written parental consent before the assessment. Therefore, school counselors are encouraged to discuss with an administrator the school district's policy concerning any assessment they may want to initiate. This does not mean that counselors cannot use assessment tools, but in many instances, they are advised to secure written parental permission beforehand.

After some of the recent violent episodes at schools and universities, there has been debate about balancing students' privacy and school safety. Particularly in response to the episode at Virginia Tech in April of 2007, U.S. Secretary of Education Margaret Spelling sent a letter on October 30, 2007, along with a brochure that specifically addressed issues concerning FERPA and disclosing information in cases of health or safety emergency. The brochure is available at http://www.ed.gov/policy/gen/guid/fpco/brochures/elsec.pdf. Secretary Spelling stipulated that though the Family Educational Rights and Privacy Act (FERPA) generally requires schools to ask for written consent from the student's parents before disclosing a student's personally identifiable information to individuals, it also enables school officials to take necessary precautions to maintain school safety. In an emergency, FERPA does enable schools without consent to disclose education records that include personally identifiable information to protect the health or safety of students or other individuals. The release of information, however, is limited to the period of the emergency and it does not allow for unlimited release. Schools are increasingly using law enforcement units or security videos and these reports are not considered part of the student record and should be kept separately. Also, FERPA does not prohibit a school official from disclosing information about a student if the information is obtained through the school official's personal knowledge or observation, and not from the student's education records. For example, if a teacher overhears a student making threatening remarks to other students, this is not considered part of the student's educational record and the teacher may disclose what she overheard to appropriate authorities. If a student discloses to a counselor that he is going to harm himself or someone else, then the counselor is required to report this and students need to be aware of this exception in terms of confidentiality. If school personnel have questions about FERPA and releasing information, they can contact the U.S. Department of Education Family Policy Compliance Office.

Health Insurance Portability and Accountability Act of 1996. The Health Insurance Portability and Accountability Act (HIPAA) is applicable to counselors working in community agencies and requires that all clients be provided with notification describing how psychological and medical information may be used and disclosed as well as how the agencies can get access to that information. HIPAA requires the U.S. Department of Health and Human Services to establish national standards for electronic health care transactions and national identifiers for providers, health plans, and employers. Occasionally, these regulations apply to counselors who may be electronically transmitting mental health information. In addition, HIPAA concerns the security and privacy of health information that is sometimes related to psychological assessment information. HIPAA is quite complicated and beyond the scope of this book; furthermore, provisions of state law, which are more strict about protecting a patient's health information, take precedence over related provisions of the HIPAA privacy rule. Although it is difficult to interpret the HIPAA regulations and identify which specific counseling agencies they apply to, many of the regulations are good practices. These practices include safeguarding clients' privacy and informing clients during the initial meeting of the agency's privacy practices. Clearly, if a counselor is involved with any third-party source (e.g., insurance company), HIPAA regulations apply. According to Rada (2003), health care providers must supply a privacy notice to patients or clients, and health care providers must make a good-faith effort to obtain the patients' or clients' written acknowledgment of receipt of this notice. The notice should be in plain language and should outline the individual's privacy rights in a manner that clients will understand. The notice should describe the uses and disclosures of client information, include information on client rights, provide an overview of the counselor's responsibilities concerning privacy, indicate that clients will be informed if privacy policies change, and identify who clients can contact if they believe their privacy has been violated. Some counselors will specifically note exceptions to the authorized disclosures, such as child abuse, adult and domestic abuse, judicial or administrative proceedings, serious threats to health or safety, and worker's compensation situations. Pertinent to assessment results are the rights of clients, which include (1) the right to request restrictions on certain uses and disclosures, including a statement that the covered entity is not required to agree to a requested restriction; (2) the right to receive confidential communications of protected health information; (3) the right to inspect and copy protected health information; (4) the right to amend protected health information; and (5) the right to an accounting of disclosures of protected health information (Rada, 2003). Counselors are also responsible for developing, maintaining, and accounting disclosures of private client information that clients can access for a period of six years.

Truth in Testing. This last piece of legislation that we will discuss here, which was passed by the New York State legislature, does not apply nationally. New York passed a Truth in Testing law mainly in reaction to attacks on Educational Testing Service by Ralph Nader and others. A report by one of Nader's associates, Allan Nairn (1980), criticized the SAT in many areas, alleging it had a propensity to rank people by social class rather than by aptitude. Nairn's report further purported that the SAT was a poor predictor of college grades and called for a full disclosure of the questions and answers on each SAT. The New York Truth in Testing law requires that testing companies (1) make public their studies on validity, (2) provide a complete disclosure to students about what scores mean and how they were calculated, and (3) upon student request, provide a copy of the questions and the correct answers to the student. Most test publishers did not object to the first two regulations but argued that the third posed a hardship due to the difficulty of compiling new questions after each testing. According to Thorndike (2005a), there have been very few requests for the copies of the tests. *Sharif v. New York State Department of Education* (1989) is a court case somewhat related to the Truth in Testing legislation. In *Sharif*, the judge ruled that the SAT could not be used as the sole criterion for scholarship awards. This ruling, however, is consistent with what the College Entrance Examination Board (2002) suggested should be done when using the SAT.

In concluding this section on legislation related to assessment, it is also important to remember the No Child Left Behind Act (NCLB) of 2001, which was discussed in Chapter 8. This controversial act of legislation is being reauthorized at the writing of this book and counselors are encouraged to follow this debate and be aware of changes that may occur during the reauthorization process.

Litigation

In the discussion of the second manner by which laws are established, litigation, the approach is somewhat different. Rather than discussing the information court case by court case, the focus is on areas in appraisal where judicial decisions have been influential.

Test bias and placement. There have been some controversial decisions related to the use of intelligence tests for permanently assigning African American children to classes for the mentally retarded (Fisher & Sorenson, 1996). In California, because classrooms for the mentally retarded had a substantial overrepresentation of African American students, there were concerns that testing procedures were discriminatory. In the Federal District Court of San Francisco, Judge Peckham found in the case of *Larry P. v. Riles* (1979) that because intelligence tests discriminated against African American children, these tests could not be used to test for placement in educable mentally retarded classrooms in California. Less than a year later, Judge Grady in Illinois—who had a similar case, *Parents in Action on Special Education (PASE) v. Hannon* (1980)—ruled the opposite way, declaring that intelligence tests could be used when used in conjunction with other criteria. In both cases, the rulings affected only those states. There was confusion in other states as well as about the legality of using intelligence tests with minority children. In a similar case in Georgia, *Georgia NAACP v. State of Georgia* (1985), the ruling was once again that intelligence tests did not discriminate. In 1986, Judge Peckham in California reissued his ban on intelligence tests. Therefore, in the mid-1980s, personnel in other states questioned the use of intelligence tests with minority students. However, in 1992, Judge Peckham lifted the ban on intelligence tests after African American parents sought to have their children assessed with intelligence tests to identify possible learning disabilities. Nevertheless, all of these cases resulted in the practice of using other criteria, along with intelligence tests, to determine whether a child has a mental disability.

Minimum competency. During the 1980s, there was an upsurge of interest in competency testing or minimum competency testing. Considerable focus was on the lack of academic skills that some students had when graduating from high school. Fisher and Sorenson (1996) indicated that courts have consistently ruled that it is within the scope of the U.S. Constitution for states to require competency examinations for high school graduation. As with the example of intelligence tests, a judicial controversy in the area of minimum competency centered on discrimination. Although other cases were filed in Florida related to the institution of a minimum competency examination for high school graduation, the case of *Debra P. v. Turlington* (1981) was the most influential. A minimum competency examination was instituted in Florida in 1978, and a challenge was filed that year on behalf of all Florida seniors and on behalf of African American Florida seniors. A federal district court ruled that the exam violated all students' rights to procedural due process and violated African American students' right to equal protection. The court postponed the use of the examination until the 1982–1983 school year. The reason for the postponement was that Florida schools were segregated until 1971, and the court ruled that the African American students had not received an equal education. Starting in the 1982–1983 school year, all seniors would have received all of their education in desegregated schools and, thus, had equal educational opportunities. This case is also important because it raised the question of instructional validity. Instructional validity concerns the evidence that students were taught the material covered on the test. The court ruled that if the test covers material not taught to the students, then the test is unfair and violates the equal protection and due process clauses of the U.S. Constitution. This ruling set a precedent concerning the need for a relationship between the curriculum and the minimum competency examination in each state. Most states do not have a standardized curriculum, which confounds the development of a high school competency examination.

In a related case, *GI Forum v. Texas Education Agency* (1997), the plaintiffs argued that the Texas graduation test unfairly discriminates against minority students because the percentage of Hispanic and African American students passing this test was lower than white students. In particular, they asserted that tests administered to nonnative English speakers should be designed to minimize threats to reliability and validity related to English language proficiency. In reviewing the evidence from *Debra P.*, the judge in *GI Forum v. Texas Education Agency* found that the graduation test was reliable and did assess the state mandated curriculum. The court in this case also considered court cases related to employment testing. For employment testing, a guideline that has been supported in the court is that adverse impact occurs when the passing rate for the minority groups is less than 80% of the passing rate for the majority group. In this case, there were a few years in which the percentage of Hispanic and African Americans was less than 80% of whites, but the court ruled that cumulative records can be used in determining if a graduation test is having an adverse impact. This case is noteworthy because it supported the 80% rule in educational testing. For more information on this case, interested readers are directed to Phillips (2000).

Diversity in education. In *Regents of the University of California v. Bakke* (1978), Alan Bakke was a white male in his 30s who applied to medical school at the University of California–Davis and was denied. Mr. Bakke investigated his denial and found minority students who had lower MCAT scores were admitted. He then sued, saying that he was discriminated against, and the case went to the U.S. Supreme Court. The Supreme Court did not rule specifically about the use of tests but did rule that Mr. Bakke should be admitted. The ruling indicated that admissions programs should allow for truly individualized admissions and there should not be quotas for minority applicants, but race could be considered in a flexible and nonmechanical way.

Almost 25 years later the U.S. Supreme Court ruled on a similar case in *Grutter v. Bollinger et al.* (2003). Barbara Grutter, a white resident of Michigan, applied to the University of Michigan Law School and was denied admission. She sued the then dean of the law school (Lee Bollinger) and others, alleging that they had discriminated against her based on race. As this case progressed through the courts, there were different rulings and the U.S. Supreme Court decided to hear the case. Bollinger and others argued that the University of Michigan Law School strove to admit a "critical mass" of underrepresented minority groups. This critical mass was not a specific number, but rather a sufficient number so that there were not just token members of a minority group that could represent a variety of viewpoints. The University of Michigan faculty argued that the quality of education was improved by the diversity of students accepted. The Supreme Court ruled that race-conscious admissions programs are time-limited; however, race can be considered in admissions in order to obtain the educational benefits of a diverse student body.

Right to privacy. One case that has been controversial within the field of assessment is *Soroka et al. v. Dayton-Hudson Company* (1991), which is also known as the Target case. The Target case involved the use of a personality inventory as an employment screening device for security officer positions at Target department stores. The plaintiffs asserted that the required psychological inventory was not job-related and, furthermore, it was offensive and intrusive to the point that it invaded their privacy. Many of the items on the assessment device in question were developed from the original version of the Minnesota Multiphasic Personality Inventory (MMPI). The case, which was scheduled to go the California Supreme Court, was settled out of court. The appellate court concluded that the Target preemployment psychological screening instrument violated the plaintiffs' constitutional right to privacy and the statutory prohibition against improper inquiries and discriminatory conduct by inquiring into religious beliefs and sexual orientation. According to Merenda (1995), many in the testing field reacted negatively to this ruling, believing that it indicated that every question on a personality inventory could be challenged in terms of its relationship to job performance. Merenda argued that the ruling was the result of the instrument not being developed, scored, or interpreted in accordance with professional standards. He concluded that this ruling did *not* mean that offensive items must be stricken from every employment test. There may, however, be other court cases that are similar to *Soroka et al. v. Dayton-Hudson Company* or the Target case, because the appellate court's ruling left some question as to whether using personality inventories as employment hiring tools is an invasion of privacy.

Summary

This chapter discussed ethical and legal issues in assessment. Ethics concerns the principles that guide professionals in their performance of duties. Laws are legal rules enforced by governmental entities. A number of resources, including the *Standards for Educational and Psychological Testing*, are available to assist counselors when faced with ethical dilemmas regarding assessment. In terms of ethical responsibility, a clinician bears the ultimate responsibility for the appropriate use of any instrument. Although test publishers may attempt to restrict the sale of instruments to untrained individuals, ethical standards clearly indicate that a practitioner must practice within his or her level of competency. Because instruments vary in the amount of training and experience that is necessary in order to be competent, counselors need to ensure that they have been adequately trained before giving an instrument to a client. Being competently trained also means having thorough knowledge about the specific instrument being used.

Clients retain the right to privacy when they enter a counseling relationship. Assessments, however, are sometimes subtle, and there is a chance that a client's privacy could be intentionally or unintentionally invaded. The two keys to avoiding invasion of a client's privacy are informed consent and relevance. Not only do clients have the right to be informed about the assessment process, they also have the right to an explanation of the results. Clients also have the right to have their results kept confidential. Confidentiality means that only the counselor and the client (or parents/guardians in the case of a minor) have access to the results without written permission to release the results. In terms of diagnosis, the least stigmatizing labels consistent with accurate reporting should be assigned.

Laws related to assessment have emerged from both legislation and litigation. Concerning legislation, the Civil Rights Act of 1991, the Americans with Disabilities Act, and the Individuals with Disabilities Education Act have all influenced the practice of assessment. The crux of all of these laws is the use of sound and appropriate instruments with individuals in a manner that is fair and equitable. The Family Educational Rights and Privacy Act governs who has access to educational records and assessments in the schools. Legal cases that have significantly influenced assessment have often focused on discrimination issues. The Health Insurance Portability and Accountability Act (HIPAA) also governs the privacy of health information, which could include psychological assessments in some counseling settings. Litigation has primarily involved test bias, minimum competency examinations, and invasion of privacy. It is important for counselors to stay informed about pending legislation and litigation that have the potential to affect assessment in counseling. Because social factors influence litigation and legislation, there will be changes in the laws governing appraisal as our society changes in the coming years.

CHAPTER 15

Issues Related to Assessment with Diverse Populations

You are working as an elementary school counselor. A kindergarten teacher has requested your advice about a student named Maria, who, with her parents, immigrated to the United States from Costa Rica within the past month. Maria does not speak any English. In this small school district, the kindergarten teachers do an informal kindergarten readiness assessment, but Maria's teacher only feels comfortable in conducting these assessments in English. She did not assess Maria, but she is concerned about whether Maria is ready for kindergarten, because Maria's birthday is only two weeks before the cutoff date for matriculation. Furthermore, Maria whimpers through most of the school day and does not interact with any of the children on the playground. The teacher wants your advice on how to assess Maria's level of academic and emotional development.

In appraisal, there is the assumption that everyone has an equal opportunity to perform. The assumption may not always be correct, for there may be a variety of reasons why an assessment may be fair to some individuals but not fair to others. Individuals' backgrounds may vary, and they may have different experiences and knowledge to draw from while being assessed. For example, let's say that only people who could sing the Indiana University fight song (i.e., *Indiana, Our Indiana*) could be hired as counselors in a counseling agency. Many counselors would be able to learn this song but were probably not exposed to it during their counseling classes. When it comes to assessment, questions related to equal opportunity to learn or to be exposed to material can often be an issue. In the case of the Indiana University fight song being used as an employment test, it might be slightly unfair because those who attended Indiana University may have an advantage. In many testing situations, the influences of background and culture are not as blatant as in the Indiana University example. Culture has a significant influence on all aspects of the individual, and problems can occur with instruments that do not consider cultural differences. In pondering the ludicrous example of the fight song, we might also question its fairness for individuals who, for some reason, are physically unable to sing. Once again, although this example is somewhat asinine, it is raised in the hopes that readers of this book will begin to reflect on the importance of considering background, opportunities, and physical and emotional disabilities in the area of assessment.

Knowledge of using appropriate appraisal techniques with diverse populations is crucial. Some of the instruments discussed in this book were originally developed for white or European Americans, and the norming groups are primarily made up of European Americans. There is concern about the misuses of assessment instruments with women, ethnic and racial minorities, limited-standard-English speakers, and the physically challenged (Padilla, 2001). Many counseling-related ethical standards (e.g., those of the American Counseling Association, the American Psychological Association, and the American Association of Marriage and Family Therapists) contain specific information about assessment with special populations.

Individuals from different cultures vary in many aspects, including how they view the world. According to Dana (2005), *worldview* involves group identity, individual identity, beliefs, values, and language. Worldview influences all perceptions and, thus, influences not only what is learned but also how people learn. Therefore, clients' culture and worldview can affect their performance on traditional achievement, aptitude, and ability tests. Assessment in the affective domain may also be influenced, because clients' worldviews influence responses to questions, nonverbal behaviors, and communication styles. To work effectively with diverse clients, counselors need to understand differences in worldview. Furthermore, counselors need to recognize that their own worldview is influenced by their own culture, which can have a detrimental effect on their perceptions of individuals who are ethnically or racially different from them.

One of the factors to consider in multicultural assessment is the influence of culture and language. *Culture* is defined as the belief systems and value orientation, including customs, norms, practices, and social institutions (Fiske, Kitayama, Markus, & Nisbett, 1998). A postmodern perspective would suggest that language has a pervasive influence affecting perceptions of reality. The influence of language needs to be considered in the assessment techniques most commonly used by counselors, which are primarily verbal techniques such as questioning, clarifying, and reflecting. For example, cultures differ in terms of the degree to which self-disclosure, particularly to a nonfamily member, is encouraged. An insensitive counselor may perceive the client's reticence to open up as resistance rather than seeing that it is due to cultural differences. This perception could encourage misunderstandings and problems in the client-counselor relationship. Because counseling is predominantly a verbal process, the subtle influences of culture on language need to be considered by a multiculturally competent practitioner.

Multicultural Assessment

Today, counselors need to be prepared to work with clients from diverse backgrounds. Nearly one in every 10 counties in the United States has a population that is more than 50% minority (Bernstein, 2007). According to the U.S. Census of 2001, 69% of the U.S. population indicated that they were white or European Americans, and the other 31% indicated that they were of another racial group or a combination of racial groups. Brewer and Suchan (2001) found that the populations in all 50 states had become more diverse. Some projections indicate that white or European Americans will constitute 50% or less of the population by the year 2050 (U.S. Bureau of Census, 2004).

Many researchers have proposed that there have been four major influences, or four major forces, in the field of counseling and psychotherapy (Ivey, Ivey, & Simek-Morgan, 1993). The first three relate to the theoretical approaches of psychodynamic foundations, cognitive-behavioral foundations, and existential/humanistic foundations. The fourth force involves multicultural counseling and therapy. Attending to multicultural issues is always important, but it is probably most important in the area of assessment. One of the most controversial issues in assessment is whether tests or assessment instruments are fair to individuals from different racial or ethnic groups (Padilla & Medina, 1996). Within the field of counseling, some debate exists about whether the term *multicultural* relates only to ethnic or cultural variations in groups, or if it is broader and incorporates variations from the dominant culture in terms of sexual preference, physical and mental disabilities, and other group differences (Pedersen, 1991; Reid, 2002).

In the first section of this chapter, consistent with the *Guidelines on Multicultural Education, Training, Research, Practice, and Organizational Change for Psychologists* (American Psychological Association, 2003), the term *multicultural* refers to "interactions between individuals from minority ethnic and racial groups in the United States and the dominant European-American culture. Ethnic and racial minority group membership includes individuals of Asian and Pacific Islander, sub-Saharan Black African, Latino/Hispanic, and Native American/American Indian descent" (p. 378). These guidelines also include assessment concerns with individuals from other nations, including international students, immigrants, and temporary workers in the United States. The second section of the chapter addresses some of the concerns related to assessment with individuals who have different physical disabilities.

Before beginning a discussion of racial differences in assessment, I need to acknowledge some of the thorny issues about discussing race. According to Helms, Jernigan, and Mascher (2005), racial groups or categories are not psychological constructs because they do not automatically result in explicit behaviors, traits, biological factors, or environmental conditions. As an example, someone who is depressed acts depressed but someone who is African American does not necessarily act African American. Helms et al. contended that racial categories are sociopolitical constructions that society uses to aggregate people on the basis of ostensible biological characteristics. There is substantial research that African Americans score almost a standard deviation below European Americans in intelligence or cognitive ability testing (Roth, Bevier, Bobko, Switzer, & Tyler, 2001). The average scores for Hispanics or Latinos on intelligence tests tend to fall between the average scores for African Americans and European Americans (Suzuki, Short, Pieterse, & Kugler, 2001). The pertinent issue concerns what conclusions are being drawn from these findings regarding racial group performance on assessments. As was indicated in Chapter 7, cognitive ability or intelligence assessment is not tapping some biological construct. Furthermore, as Helms et al. asserted, in counseling and psychological assessment, ascribed racial categories are typically associated with group-level socialization experiences that may or may not apply to the individual. For example, not all African American students attend inner-city schools with low achievement scores. Helms et al. (2005) contended that in counseling we should stop using race to categorize assessment results and use measures of constructs such as racial identity that have been found to explain significant differences in assessment of cognitive abilities and other areas of psychological assessment. Some measures of racial identity are sensitive to issues of oppression and privilege and can provide a better understand of why individuals may perform differently on various assessments.

Although there are problems associated with using race to categorize people, counselors cannot ignore that currently in our society there are racial differences in average performance on many psychological assessments. The impact of these differences is particularly noteworthy when we examine how assessments of cognitive ability, knowledge, and skills are currently being used. For example, there is substantial research that has found the overrepresentation of minority students in special education (Losen & Orfield, 2002; National Research Council, 2002). Moreover, Skiba, Poloni-Staudinger, Gallini, Simmons & Feggins-Azziz (2006) found that African-American students diagnosed with emotional disturbances, mild mental retardation, moderate mental retardation, learning disabilities, and speech and language difficulties were more likely to be placed in more restrictive educational environment than other students with comparable problems.

The *Standards for Educational and Psychological Testing* (AERA, APA, & NCME, 1999) indicates that the test user has a responsibility to examine the differential impact of test scores as part of the process of evaluating the validation evidence. Assessing clients from different ethnic and cultural backgrounds is complex and needs to be performed with professional care and consideration. Counselors need to be able to evaluate instruments that may be biased against certain groups and identify other methods for assessing these clients. In addition, counselors need to be competent in using assessment results appropriately with clients from diverse cultures. Using an instrument that is not culturally appropriate for clients can be problematic; there have been instances in which a lack of cultural sensitivity during the assessment process resulted in clients being harmed. Because counselors can expect to work with clients from cultures other than their own, they need to be skilled in cross-cultural assessment.

Types of Instrument Bias

As stated earlier, in appraisal, it is assumed that all individuals are given an equal opportunity to demonstrate their capabilities or level of functioning during the assessment process. However, even an instrument designed to be culturally sensitive and fair may be unfair, depending on the circumstances under which it is used or the groups of individuals with whom it is used. The term bias testing refers to the degree that construct-irrelevant factors systematically affect a group's performance. In other words, factors not related to the instrument's purpose either positively or negatively influence a group's performance. Given the potential consequences of using a biased instrument, it is important for counselors to know how to evaluate instruments for the various types of possible bias.

Content bias. Instruments may be biased in terms of the content being more familiar or appropriate for one group as compared with another group. As an example, let's imagine that an intelligence test has a question regarding what the state bird of Wyoming is. Many individuals would have difficulty remembering this piece of trivia; however, if you had attended school in Wyoming, you could probably answer that the Wyoming state bird is the meadowlark. Thus, individuals from Wyoming would have an advantage on this intelligence test over individuals from other states. The biased content of an instrument may be subtler than the Wyoming state bird question. For example, some groups could perceive certain items on an instrument as irrelevant or not engaging. Children living below the poverty level may see little relevance in a question concerning how long it will take an airplane to fly from Point A to Point B when these children cannot imagine ever having the financial resources to fly on an airplane. Children may be less likely to engage in questions when the names and circumstances on the test are always associated with the majority culture. Bracken and Barona (1991) found evidence to suggest that children from different cultural backgrounds interpret test items differently. As Sandoval (1998) argued, a basic issue in assessment concerns whether an ability or trait may be manifested differently in two different groups. If so, it is possible that even though a trait or ability is present in both groups, current testing methods may not assess the trait or ability in both groups.

In evaluating an instrument for content bias, the practitioner needs to examine the procedures used in developing the instrument. Haphazard selection of instrument content may result in an instrument with content bias. Specific attention needs to be paid to multicultural issues during the initial stages of instrument development. In the manual, instrument developers should document the steps they took to guard against content bias. Care in writing items that appear to be nonbiased may not be sufficient. A common procedure is to have a panel made up of diverse individuals review the instrument. Nevertheless, content bias can be difficult to uncover because subtle biases may not always appear by simply examining the instrument.

In addition, statistical methods are often employed to supplement review of the content. One statistical method for investigating item bias that has received increasing attention is differential item functioning (DIF). Differential item functioning is a method for analyzing the relative difficulty of individual items for different racial or ethnic groups. Although there are different methods for performing differential item functioning, all of them strive to examine differences in performance among individuals who are equal in ability but from different groups. If an item is found to have unequal probabilities for correct responses from certain groups with equal ability, then the item may be biased. Sometimes, however, statistical artifacts can result in group differences rather than the item being biased. In addition, more sophisticated models of DIF involve matching examinees across groups to control for group differences (Sireci & Geisinger, 1998). Although DIF techniques have been very useful in identifying and eliminating individual items on specific instruments, these techniques have not identified common themes or characteristics of items that are prone to bias. Advances are being made in this area, and, hopefully, research will soon shed light on methods for developing unbiased items.

Internal structure. Another method for detecting possible instrument bias is to examine the instrument's internal structure. For instance, an instrument's reliability coefficients for one ethnic group could be very high, whereas for another ethnic group, they could be significantly lower. Thus, an instrument can be a reliable measure for one client but not for another. Well-developed instruments will investigate this problem and, in the manual, present reliability information for different groups. Typically, researchers investigate differences between males and females and between different ethnic groups. The investigation of differences in reliability among different ethnic groups depends on the size and representation of the norming group. Hence, if there were problems with the makeup of the norming group in terms of minority participants, then it would be difficult to analyze differences in reliability.

Examination of internal structure as related to instrument bias can also involve the instrument's factor structure. As was discussed in Section II of this book, many instruments and tests used in counseling have subscales (e.g., Verbal and Performances IQs). It is important for researchers to determine if the dimensions or factors underlying the instrument vary for different groups. For example, in personality instruments, the factor structure for an ethnic group may not match the subscales of the instrument; thus, it would not be appropriate to interpret those subscales in the typical manner. Practitioners need to examine the research related to the factor structure of an instrument with subscales to determine if it is appropriate to interpret the scores of the subscales with clients from diverse backgrounds.

Instrument and criterion relationships. The analyses of possible bias should also include studies related to the relationship between the instrument and the criterion for different groups. For example, an instrument may be highly related to job performance for one ethnic group but may have a low relationship for another ethnic group. It is important to examine the differences among the validity coefficients, not simply whether the validity coefficients are statistically significant for one group and not significant for another group. Statistical significance is influenced by sample size; typically, the sample size is large for whites or European Americans and small for African Americans. With correlation, the smaller the sample, the larger the correlation coefficient needs to be in order to be significant. Therefore, the exact same validity coefficients for these two groups could be significant for European Americans and not significant for African Americans. For some of the more widely used employment selection instruments, Hunter, Schmidt, and Hunter (1979) found that the validity coefficients were not significantly different. Most of the research related to ethnic differences in validity coefficients has compared African Americans and European Americans. Very few studies, however, have examined the differences in validity coefficients for Hispanics and other ethnic groups.

Significant differences in validity coefficients can have a notable effect if the instrument is used for selection or predictive purposes. The statistical technique of regression is often used for selection, and when there are different validity coefficients, the instrument can vary in how well it predicts to the criterion for the different groups. If an instrument yields validity coefficients that are significantly different for two or more groups, then this difference is described as **slope bias.** Figure 15.1 reflects slope bias, because, as you can see, the same score on the instrument would predict *different* performance on the criterion depending on whether a client is in the green group or the blue group. In this example, a score of 20 by a green individual would predict a grade of a little over a C, whereas, for a blue individual, a score of 20 would predict a grade between D and F. In cases of slope bias, some experts in the field of assessment have suggested using separate regression equations for the different groups. As was discussed in Chapter 14, however, there are certain situations in which legislation has prohibited the use of separate regression equations for different ethnic groups.

Even instruments with the same validity coefficient can predict different criterion scores for members of different groups with the *same score.* If you examine Figure 15.2 on the following page, the regression lines for the green and the blue groups are parallel, which indicates that the validity coefficients are the same. The lines, however, differ in where they begin on the *y*-axis; hence, the **intercepts** are different. The first graph in Figure 15.2 indicates that a score of 20 on the instrument predicts a grade slightly above D for an individual from the blue group and that same score predicts a grade of almost a B for someone from the green group.

FIGURE 15.1
Slope bias

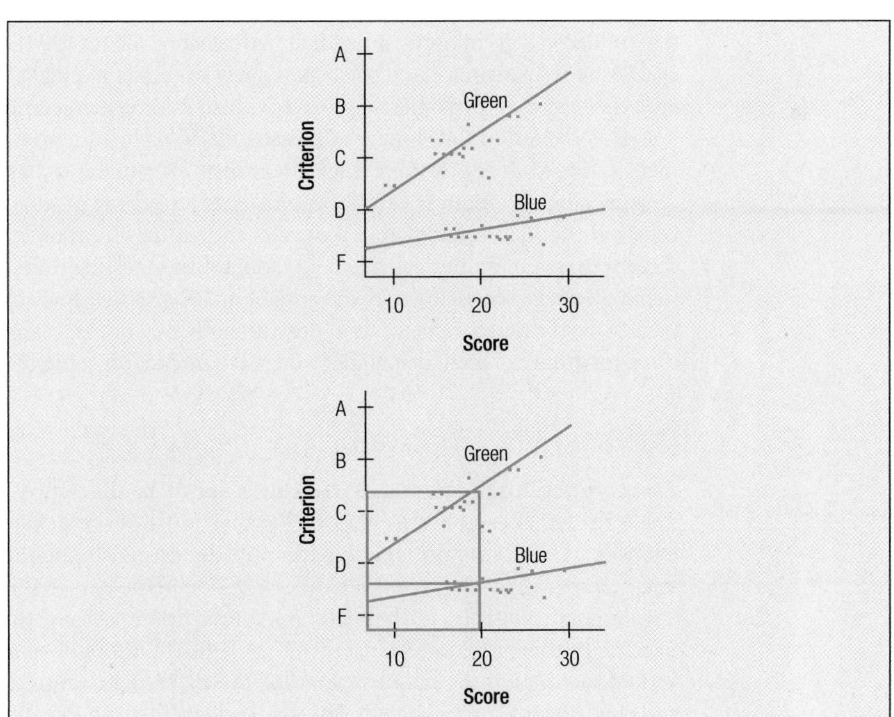

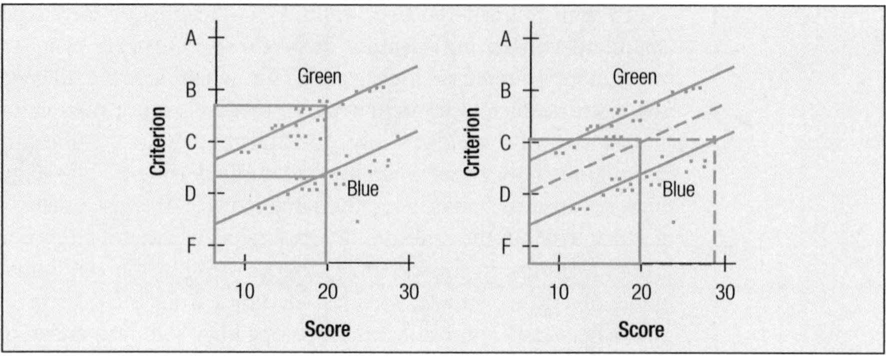

FIGURE 15.2
Intercept bias

Thus, using a cutoff score of 20 provides an advantage to the blue group. As the second graph in Figure 15.2 reflects, in using the intercept for the blue group, an individual from this group would need a score of almost 30 to be predicted to receive a grade of C. Numerous studies have found that there are no intercept differences among ethnic groups on many of the instruments in counseling (Anastasi & Urbina, 1997). Some researchers have found that when there are differences among majority and minority groups, majority group members tend to have higher intercepts than do minority members. Majority groups have also been found to have higher intercepts for some instruments that predict college grades (Duran, 1983) and job performance (Hunter et al., 1979). Thus, in Figure 15.2, the majority group members would be the green group and the minority members would be the blue group. Therefore, these instruments would overpredict, rather than underpredict, minority individual performance. Linn (1994), however, argued that evaluating instruments based solely on regression models is inadequate and that several artifacts of measurement affect this overprediction for certain ethnic groups.

This section of the chapter addressed methods for examining whether an instrument is biased. It is possible for an assessment instrument to have culturally sensitive content, almost identical validity coefficients for ethnic groups, and the same intercepts yet produce very different scores for individuals from different ethnic groups. In the discussion of ability, achievement, and aptitude testing, minority individuals tend to have average scores lower than those of majority individuals on many of the instruments. Even though some of these instruments may not be biased, the result of using these instruments has a disparate or negative impact on some minority individuals.

Differences in Test Performance and Culture

There are various opinions as to the causes for racial differences in test performance. The term *test* is used in this context because most of the debate has concerned differences in ability, achievement, and aptitude testing. It should be noted, however, that occasionally there are ethnic differences on some personality instruments. Some have argued that these differences are primarily innate and that little can be done to remedy this situation (Jensen, 1972, 1980). Others have argued that environmental factors are the major reason for the discrepant scores among racial groups and that unequal access to educational and stimulating experiences influences test performance. Those arguing for the latter perspective contend that tests highlight the unfairness of life, not the unfairness of tests.

For a time, some professionals in assessment focused on developing *culture-free* assessments. In general, experts in the field of assessment have concluded that, as of yet, there is *no* culture-free assessment device. Even with nonverbal tests, such as putting puzzles together or deciphering matrices, there are cultural components that influence performance. Because it has been impossible to develop an instrument devoid of cultural influences, attempts have been made to develop *culture-fair* instruments. Within the field of assessment, some individuals contend that culturally fair instruments already exist. Others, however, suggest that an instrument has yet to be developed that is culturally fair to all individuals. Stobart (2005) cogently argued that fairness in assessment cannot be separated from fairness in access opportunities and curriculum. He asserted that large-scale achievement tests highlight the sociocultural inequities in the U.S. educational system and testing should be used to examine the opportunities and curriculum of those students whose performance is weak.

Helms (2004) defined *fairness* as the removal from test scores systematic variance that is related to the test takers' psychological characteristics that were influenced by socialization practices or environmental conditions, that are "irrelevant to measurement of the construct of interest to the test user or assessor" (p. 87). Hence, Helms (2006) contended that test fairness or unfairness is often not due to the structure of the test but to the interaction among the examinees' internalized racial or cultural experiences, their environmental socialization, and the testing process. Consistent with how the profession now views reliability and validity, Helms argued that test fairness is not something that an instrument has or does not have from sample to sample. Her view of fairness in assessment is significant in that the counselor needs to consider the client's psychological characteristics and internalized racial or cultural experiences in interpreting test results. Consequently, individuals may have some similar experiences in life but how those experiences are internalized may be very different. Therefore, in testing, there may be construct-irrelevant variance for some individuals but not for others.

In discussing racial test score disparity, Helms (2002) presented the results from a study that examined her 1990 immersion-emersion racial identity scheme (e.g., idealization of one's blackness and black culture). Helms found that the difference between those not having any black culture and those having an average amount of black culture was around 129 points on the SAT-V. Interestingly, this difference of approximately 1 standard deviation is very similar to the difference typically found between white and minority student scores on the SAT. In a tongue-and-cheek manner, Helms suggested that these results mean that the remedy for improving black test scores is either to deliberately destroy positive racial identity development of black students or to socialize white students to idealize black identity, thus eliminating the automatic increase of 1 standard deviation of white cultural advantage per subtest.

Helms' (2002, 2006) writing reinforces the importance of not considering instruments as being either valid or not, because an instrument may be valid with one group but may have a very different meaning for individuals from another culture.

Recommendations for Practice

Counselors can expect to be involved in either formal or informal assessment of clients from cultures other than their own. The U.S. population is changing, and the percentage of minority individuals is increasing. Padilla and Medina (1996) suggested that practitioners may not be aware of how their linguistic, social class, and cultural experiences influence their construction of knowledge, selection of particular tests, and interpretation derived from assessment procedures. Thus, counselors need to find methods for effective cross-cultural assessment. One excellent resource for counselors is the *Standards for Multicultural Assessment* (Association for Assessment in Counseling, 2003b). This resource is a compilation of standards related to multicultural assessment from five source documents—the *Code of Fair Testing Practices in Education* (Joint Committee on Testing Practices, 2003), *Responsibilities of Users of Standardized Tests* (3rd ed., Association for Assessment in Counseling, 2003a), *Standards for Educational and Psychological Testing* (AERA, APA, & NCME, 1999), *Multicultural Competencies and Standards* (Sue, Arredondo, & McDavis, 1992), and the American Counseling Association's (2005a) *Code of Ethics.*

Even though an instrument may be of high quality, this does not automatically mean that it can be used with all ethnic or racial groups. There are unique issues in assessment with clients from diverse cultural backgrounds. Ridley, Li, and Hill (1998) proposed a multicultural assessment procedure with the following progressive phases: Phase 1: Identify Cultural Data; Phase 2: Interpret Cultural Data; Phase 3: Incorporate Cultural Data; and Phase 4: Arrive at a Sound Assessment Decision. This model is pragmatic and flexible. Clinicians do not just advance through this model sequentially; instead, they often recycle through the phases as needed. In Phase 1: Identify Cultural Data, the counselor gathers both overt and covert clinical data using multiple methods of data collection. In Phase 2: Interpret Cultural Data, the focus is on organizing and interpreting the cultural data, which results in the clinician forming working hypotheses. In Phase 3: Incorporate Cultural Data, the counselor tests these working hypotheses by integrating the cultural data with other clinical data. Ridley et al. (1998) encouraged clinicians to examine their assessment after each phase and to recycle through the phases, if necessary, before proceeding to Phase 4: Arrive at a Sound Assessment Decision. Ridley et al.'s model is similar to Sue's (1998) recommendation that cultural competence requires scientific-mindedness in therapists. In Sue's analysis of the research, he argued that culturally competent counselors form hypotheses, rather than conclusions, and then test those clinical hypotheses.

Practitioners should *not* attempt to evaluate clients with diverse backgrounds if the assessment process is outside the counselor's range of academic training or supervised experience. If the counselor is unable to refer or feels that referral would be detrimental to the client, then the counselor needs to gain both knowledge about assessment procedures and information about the client's background characteristics. Culturally sensitive assessment cannot be accomplished by following a few guidelines, because it requires careful deliberation on a number of factors. The following summary is an attempt to coalesce pertinent information related to culturally sensitive assessment in counseling; however, counselors should also closely adhere to the *Standards for Multicultural Assessment* (Association for Assessment in Counseling, 2003b), which are included in Appendix E of this book.

Selection of assessment instruments: Content and purpose. Counselors need to clearly understand a client's cultural identity and the purpose of the testing or assessment. Once counselors have acquired this information, they should thoroughly review available materials to determine the appropriate assessment procedures. In evaluating instruments, practitioners need to consider whether a common instrument or alternate instruments are required for accurate measurement. Counselors, however, should be aware that the use of alternate instruments for cultural, ethnic, and racial groups may not be effective in correcting for group differences. A thorough review, performed by counselors, should include evaluating the procedures used by the instrument developers to avoid potentially insensitive content or language. Furthermore, attention should be given to how the instrument handles variation in motivation, working speed, language facility, and individuals' experiential backgrounds, as well as to possible bias in responses to its content. The culturally competent counselor is able to evaluate the technical aspects of an instrument and use this information and cultural awareness to choose assessments that are in the best interest of clients from diverse cultural, racial, and ethnic groups. The *Standards for Multicultural Assessment* (AAC, 2003b) state that the culturally competent counselor is also knowledgeable about how race, culture, and ethnicity may influence personality formation, vocational choices, the manifestation of psychological disorders, help-seeking behaviors, and the appropriateness or inappropriateness of counseling approaches. Practitioners also need to consider language and the appropriate language for the assessment. If an instrument is recommended for linguistically diverse populations, then the counselor should expect to find in the manual appropriate information for the proper use and interpretation of that instrument (e.g., case studies and examples of interpretative material for diverse clients).

Selection of assessment instruments: Norming, reliability, and validity. The counselor is responsible for reviewing technical information to determine if the instrument's characteristics are appropriate for diverse individuals. The clinician also needs to evaluate, to the extent feasible, the degree to which performance may be affected by factors extraneous to the purpose of the assessment. Publishers are expected to publish, as soon as possible, reliability information, standard error of measurement, and other technical information for each major group that the instrument is intended to assess. Furthermore, when instruments are used for specific age groups (e.g., seventh graders, eighth graders) and separate norms are provided, then the publishers should also provide reliability information for the different age groups. In using a norm-referenced instrument with any client, a counselor needs to evaluate the suitability of the norming group; thus, norming groups should be clearly defined in the manual. The American Counseling Association's *Code of Ethics* (ACA, 2005a) states that a counselor should be cautious in interpreting results from clients who are not represented in the norming group on which an instrument was standardized.

As indicated earlier, instruments should be evaluated in terms of subgroup differences with regard to instrument content, internal structure, the relationship between scores and other pertinent variables, and the response processes. When credible research indicates that there are differences in scores for particular subgroups, then there should be separate, but parallel, analyses of the instrument's psychometric qualities for the different subgroups. When subgroup differences are found, the counselor should consider these differences when interpreting results. If construct-irrelevant variance is determined to be problematic for a subgroup, then the counselor should investigate whether construct-equivalent instruments can be used with different subgroups. However, it is not always possible to find alternative assessment resources that permit valid inferences across different subgroups.

Another issue related to subgroup differences concerns how the subgroups are identified. Counselors need to be careful with categories for race and ethnicity, because people from very similar backgrounds may categorize themselves quite differently. A self-report of group membership does not provide sufficient information, because the acculturation of individuals often varies greatly, even though they may report the same group membership (Dana, 2005). Often, with norm-referenced instruments, information about the norming group's ethnicity is gathered only through individuals reporting their racial background. Ridley et al. (1998) suggested that the assessment process should include an assessment of four constructs of psychocultural adjustment: acculturation, ethnic/racial identity, biculturalism, and worldview. *Acculturation* concerns the degree to which clients have integrated new cultural patterns into their original cultural patterns. *Ethnic/racial identity* is the degree of self-acceptance and acceptance of the social implications associated with clients' race or ethnicity. *Biculturalism* is slightly different and involves the capacity of clients to function within more than one culture and reconcile various cultural influences within themselves. As indicated earlier, *worldview* concerns the lens that people use to interpret their world.

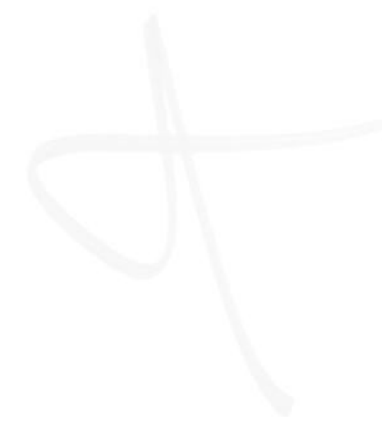

Administration and scoring of assessment instruments. Any assessment must be administered and scored appropriately for that specific instrument. Some assessments have very detailed instructions for administration, and any problems, irregularities, or accommodations must be noted. There are situations in which procedures for administering the assessment must be changed, and the counselor is responsible for knowing when accommodations should be made and what the professional literature indicates in terms of making those accommodations. The *Standards for Educational and Psychological Testing* (AERA, APA, & NCME, 1999) indicates that the assessment process should be performed so that test takers receive comparable and equitable treatment during all phases of the assessment process.

There has been substantial research examining the effects of an examiner's race on examinees' performance. There does not appear, however, to be general consensus about the degree to which the race of the examiner has an impact. Sattler (1993) found evidence that examiners who had stereotypes concerning Hispanic children assessed Hispanic children with heavily accented English to have slightly lower scores. In general, however, Sattler contended that the influence of the tester's race has a negligible effect on children's performance. On the other hand, Dana (1993) documented that the current Anglo American format for assessment services requires modification to take into account diverse cultural origins. Although Sattler found little evidence of bias, he further stated that examiners cannot be indifferent to the examinees' ethnicity and should be alert to any nuances in the testing situation.

Sometimes examinees' nonverbal behaviors influence the assessment process and therefore, differences in nonverbal behaviors across cultures need to be taken into account when performing assessments (Suzuki, Short, Pieterse, & Kugler, 2001). Certainly, it is important to have knowledge about an examinee's cultural group and about research related to using a specific instrument with that cultural group. To avoid having an unintended influence on the administration of the instrument, the examiner must be familiar with the administrative procedures and with research related to the administration of that particular instrument.

Before administering an assessment, a counselor has an ethical responsibility to explain to the client the nature and purposes of the assessment and how the results will be used. The counselor should do so in a language and manner that the client will understand. Counselors should consider the effects of examiner-examinee differences in ethnic and cultural background, attitudes, and values based on relevant research. They also need to be able to administer instruments using verbal clarity, calmness, empathy for the examinees, and impartiality toward all being assessed.

A number of researchers have explored the *expectancy effect*, which concerns whether examiners' expectations have an impact on examinees' performance. This is sometimes referred to as the Pygmalion effect, as coined by Rosenthal and Jacobson (1968) and has often been studied related to explaining differences among racial or ethnic groups. The degree to which the expectations have an influence on the examinees' performance is somewhat debatable, but, in general, the consensus is that examiner expectations have a small effect (Kaplan & Saccuzzo, 2005).

Whereas many of an examiner's attitudes and nonverbal behaviors during the administration of an instrument have been found to have a small and subtle influence on examinees' performance, the degree of rapport between the administrator and the examinee may be important and particularly important for individuals of color (Keitel, Kopala, & Adamson, 1996). In a meta-analysis, Fuchs and Fuchs (1986) found that, on average, test performance is about .28 of a standard deviation (about 4 IQ points) higher when the examiner was familiar to the test taker. The difference was slightly more for children from lower socioeconomic levels and for African American and Hispanic children, indicating the relationship may be more important for these examinees. Methods for establishing rapport vary depending on the client's cultural background. For example, Sue and Sue (1977) found that many Asian American women are uncomfortable with a clinician's efforts to make eye contact. Hence, multicultural assessment is more than simply selecting an unbiased instrument and extends to administering the assessment with sensitivity to the client's background and culture.

Interpretation and application of assessment results. With any assessment, the interpretation of the client's results must be based on validation evidence. Ridley, Hill, and Wiese (2001) defined *multicultural assessment competence* as the ability to consider and the committed intention of considering cultural data to formulate accurate, comprehensive, and impartial case conceptualizations. Thus, when interpreting assessment results, counselors must be knowledgeable about the instrument, but they must also have comprehensive knowledge about each client's culture (Hood & Johnson, 2007). Knowledge of a culture, however, does not mean viewing any client in a stereotypic manner. Enormous variation exists among individuals from different cultures.

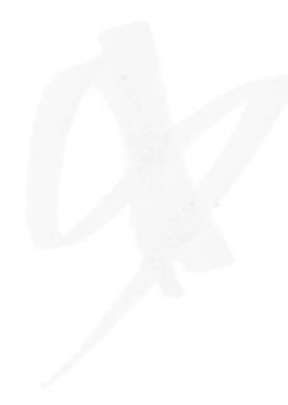

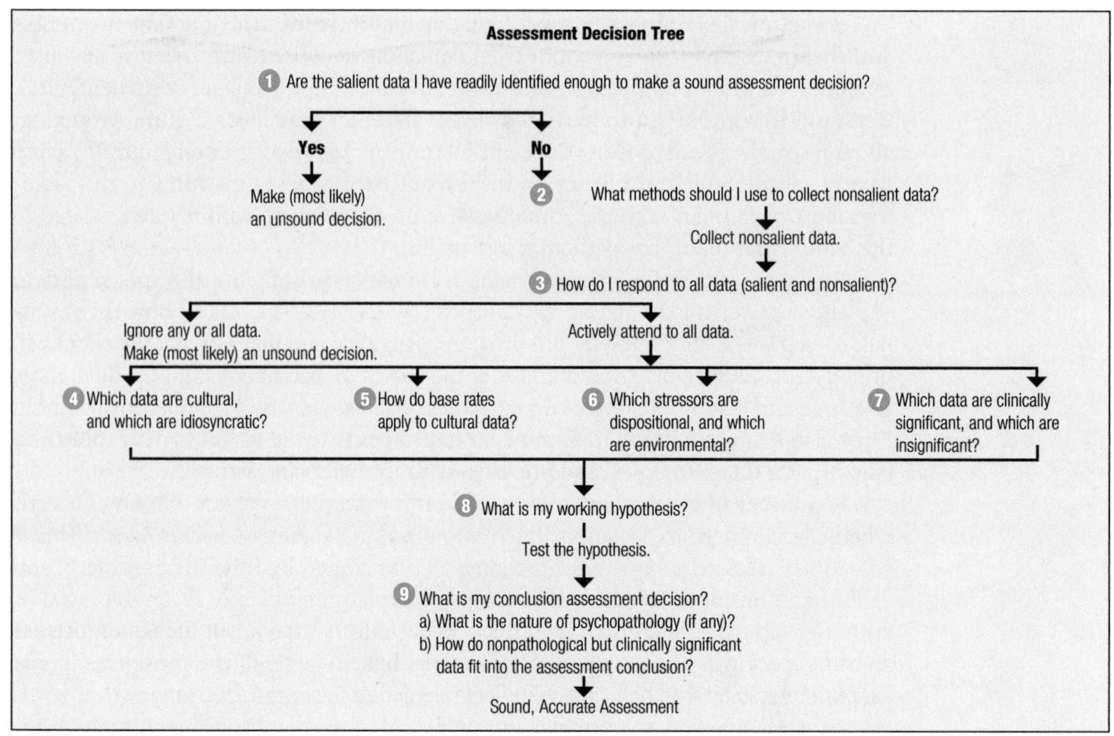

FIGURE 15.3
Ridley, Li, and Hill's Assessment Decision Tree
From Ridley, et al., 1998, "Multicultural assessment: Reexamination, reconceptualization, and practical application," The Counseling Psychologist, 26: 827–910. Reprinted by permission of Sage Publications, Inc.

Although culture is an important facet, appropriate assessment also involves analyzing comprehensive information to provide a more holistic view. Ridley et al. (1998) provided a decision tree (see Figure 15.3) to assist counselors in determining if they have sufficient information to make sound and accurate assessment.

Ultimately, the counselor is responsible for evaluating the impact of client gender, age, ethnicity, socioeconomic status, marital status, and other pertinent factors on assessment results. In a discussion of multicultural assessment, it is also valuable to note the significance of socioeconomic status and the importance of considering socioeconomic background in interpreting assessment results. Socioeconomic status is particularly critical because some researchers have found that it has more influence on test performance than either ethnicity or instrument bias (Bond, 1990; Groth-Marnat, 2003). Researchers have found that differences on intelligence tests (Loehelin, 1989) and on the MMPI (Timbrook & Graham, 1994) dissipate when African Americans and European Americans of equal socioeconomic status are compared.

When instruments are used for clinical purposes (e.g., diagnosis, placement in educational programs, treatment selection), there should be validation evidence for populations similar to the client (Dana, 2005). This is particularly important if the recommendations or decisions are considered to have an actuarial and clinical basis. If there seems to be predictive bias, as indicated by differences among groups, in the instrument's ability to predict performance, then there should also be investigations into the magnitude of the predictive bias. When instruments suggest or imply career options for clients, counselors need to examine information related to how the sample distributes in the actual occupational areas in terms of gender and racial or ethnic groups. Due to the limitations of many formal instruments, Goldman (1990, 1992) championed the use of qualitative techniques with diverse clients.

In interpreting assessment results to clients, counselors need to provide an orientation that includes an explanation of how the results function with other relevant factors (Allen, 2007). The intent is for clients to have a proper perspective on the results in connection with other factors, including recognizing the effects of socioeconomic, ethnic, and cultural factors on test scores. In some situations, clinicians should describe to clients, or their parents/guardians, the procedures for registering any complaints if they believe there has been a problem in the assessment process. Culturally skilled counselors interpret results with knowledge of potential bias, while keeping in mind the cultural and linguistic characteristics of the clients. As the previously mentioned guidelines suggest, counselors cannot be culturally competent in assessment unless they understand the client, the client's culture, and the strengths and limitations of using a particular assessment device with that client.

Linguistic Background and Appraisal

Issues related to cross-cultural assessment are already complex, but the issues increase in complexity when language and nonnative English speakers are considered in the assessment process. In 2005, 20% of school-aged children spoke a language at home other than English (Forum on Child and Family Statistics, 2007). Language skills almost always have some degree of influence on a person's performance on an assessment device. For example, reading or listening skills are typically needed to hear or read test instructions. Even with arithmetic or mathematical assessment, most tests require an examinee to read some items. There are also cultural differences in terms of language proficiency, and these differences may introduce irrelevant factors into the assessment process. For some examinees, their results on a test may be more a reflection of their proficiency with English than of their ability in mathematics. These linguistic factors become even more crucial when important decisions are made based on assessment results. The fact that the *Standards for Educational and Psychological Testing* (AERA, APA, & NCME, 1999) devotes an entire chapter to linguistic factors points to the topic's complexity and denotes its importance. Therefore, counselors need to be aware of concerns related to assessing those with limited proficiency in the dominant language. It should be noted that many of these issues pertain not only to nonnative speakers but also to those with unique linguistic backgrounds, such as clients who are deaf or those who have other disabilities that affect the development of language.

Counselors are responsible for ensuring that all examinees are given the same opportunities to demonstrate their level of competence on the attributes being assessed. In our culture, when English is a client's second language, the counselor needs to consider numerous factors to ensure fair assessment. One of the factors to consider is the purpose of the testing or assessment. If the purpose is to evaluate English proficiency, then there may be little need for adaptation of the testing situation. For example, if successful job performance in a position requires the ability to communicate in English (e.g., a technical writer), then it may be legitimate to use a test that assesses the ability to write in English. There are, however, a number of occupations for which the ability to communicate in English is not required. It is very rare that a clear distinction can be made concerning the influences of language and how to assess clients appropriately. Take, for example, the identification of a learning disability with a child whose dominant language is Spanish. It is sometimes difficult to decipher when the assessment results are related to language issues and when there is evidence of a learning disability. Assessment of individuals in a situation where there is a question of language proficiency requires special attention to administration, scoring, and interpretation.

Instrument translation, adaptation, and modification. Sometimes professionals will consider translating an existing instrument into the language of the nonnative speaker in order to assess the person fairly. A simple translation, however, usually does not suffice, because many issues need to be attended to in the translation. First, simple translations typically do not take into account different cultural considerations. As Bracken and Barona (1991) documented, there are several problems with translating instruments. First, test directions are often not easy to translate because they are often psychotechnical, stilted, and abstract. Second, practitioners rarely translate back to the original after translating the instrument to the second language, which can be a helpful step in determining if the meaning is retained in the translating process. Third, some of the psychological variables assessed in instruments are not universal across cultures. For example, an instrument could assess a person's ability to make decisions independently, which is not a value held by all cultures. Fourth, even for well-developed instruments, there are no universally accepted procedures or standards for evaluating translations. To translate an instrument properly, experts need to evaluate whether the translation is equivalent to the original version of the instrument in terms of content, difficulty level, and reliability. They also need to study the validity of the translation to see if it can be used in the same circumstances as the original instrument. In the instrument's manual, test publishers should describe the process of translating an instrument and provide information on the reliability and validity of the translated instrument. Even if care is taken in translating an instrument, counselors should not assume that clients' cultural experiences are comparable. For example, an item on an interest inventory concerning whether one "likes to go to the opera" may have little relevancy for an adolescent from rural Pakistan.

These same difficulties apply to attempts to adapt or modify an assessment for a nonnative speaker. Counselors should not attempt to adapt or modify an assessment on their own. Fernandez, Boccaccini, and Noland (2007) recommended the following four-step approach for identifying and selecting translated tests for Spanish-speaking clients. First, identify translated tests by examining assessment publishers' catalogs and websites. Second, identify research studies of translated tests. Fernandez et al., however, noted that the demand for translated instruments has outpaced the ability of test developers to evaluate the psychometric properties of these assessments. Their third step involved confirming that the research applies to the client who will be completing the assessment. The last step concerns determining the level of research supporting the use of the translated test with the client. Central to fair assessment is the concept of equivalence, and even minor modifications can sometimes alter what is being assessed. If a publisher recommends linguistic modifications, the research supporting these modifications and the modification methods should be described in detail in the manual (Association for Assessment in Counseling, 2003b). If research supports the modifications, practitioners should follow the procedures unless other research indicates that there are new procedures that are more appropriate. Potential problems can be avoided if practitioners thoroughly evaluate the existing research on assessment with nonnative speakers.

Issues related to instrument use and interpretation. Instruments are available in multiple languages, and with some multilingual individuals, it is difficult to determine which language is most appropriate to use in testing. According to the Individuals with Disabilities Education Act, which was last reauthorized in 2004, individuals should be assessed in the language with which they are most proficient. An exception is allowed when the assessment's purpose is to determine a level of proficiency in a certain language (e.g., English). It is important for counselors to remember that assessing individuals in their most proficient language does not guarantee a comprehensive and fair assessment.

The *Standards for Educational and Psychological Testing* (AERA, APA, & NCME, 1999) recommends that assessment should include consideration of both language dominance and language proficiency. In this process, the first step is to identify the examinee's dominant language and measure the individual's proficiency in that language. The second step is to administer the tests in the dominant language. Although this practice seems fair, the *Standards* goes on to say that testing individuals in their dominant language is no panacea, because bilingual individuals are likely to be specialized by domain (e.g., they use one language in home and social environments and another language in academic and work environments). Therefore, an assessment in either of the languages is likely to measure some domains but miss out on others that are primarily related to the other language. The *Standards* indicates that there may be times when individuals should be assessed in both languages; however, this is often a difficult practice to implement. Thus, interpretation of results from nonnative speakers should be done cautiously. Even with instruments that are designed for cross-cultural assessment, the counselor must be aware of appropriate uses and limitations.

Assessment of Individuals with Disabilities

In assessment, individuals with disabilities may be adversely affected by certain assessment procedures. For example, if a person has become quadriplegic, it would be difficult to perform the Block Design portion of the Wechsler Adult Intelligence Scale-Third Edition (WAIS-III) because of limitations with motor dexterity. The likelihood of a counselor having a client with a physical disability is high—about 20% of individuals in the United States have some type of physical disability and nearly 10% could be classified as having a severe disability (McNeil, 2001). According to the Individuals with Disabilities Education Act (IDEA), Public Law 101-476, there

TABLE 15.1
Thirteen separate categories of disabilities under which children may be eligible for special education and related services

- Autism
- Deafness
- Deaf-blindness
- Hearing impairment
- Mental retardation
- Multiple disabilities
- Orthopedic impairment
- Other health impairment
- Serious emotional disturbance
- Specific learning disability
- Speech or language impairment
- Traumatic brain injury
- Visual impairment

13 separate categories of disabilities under which children may be eligible for special education and related services. These are listed in Table 15.1. As was mentioned in Chapter 14, the Americans with Disabilities Act has legal implications related to the assessment of individuals with disabilities, and many counselors (particularly school counselors) need detailed knowledge about this legislation. As Helms and Ekstrom (2002) reported, counselors often have multiple roles when working with individuals with disabilities—empathic listener, advisor, educator, advocate, and intermediary; hence, knowledge of assessment and the difficult issues associated with "reasonable accommodations" are needed. Counselors may also be involved in documenting a disability or in documenting the accommodations that were implemented during a testing situation (see Vacc & Tippen, 2002).

Assessment of Individuals with Visual Impairments

The terms *visually impaired* and *visually handicapped* usually refer to individuals who require more than corrective lenses to function adequately (Bradley-Johnson & Ekstrom, 1998). Many of the assessment tools used in counseling involve reading; yet, for individuals with visual impairments, this type of assessment is problematic. In addition, Bertone, Bettinelli, and Faubert (2007) found even minimal loss of visual acuity (20/40) had some effect on the performance for certain nonverbal tests. With many types of instruments (e.g., personality assessments), the approach to assessing someone with a visual impairment is to have someone read the instrument to the client. Individuals who read assessment material for visually impaired individuals, however, can vary dramatically in terms of their tone, speed, and clarity of speech. These variations in reading can affect the reliability of the instrument and may have an impact on individuals' performance. Thus, as with other assessment practices, counselors need to research the procedures for using a specific assessment instrument with an individual who has a visual disability.

If counselors suspect that a visual impairment might be affecting the assessment process, they should refer their client to an optometrist or ophthalmologist for an initial screening. Some of the signs of a visual impairment are a client who rubs her eyes excessively; shuts or covers one eye, tilts her head, or leans forward; has difficulty in reading or loses her place while reading; blinks more than expected; is irritable when doing close visual work; has difficulty judging distances; or has recurring sties (Sattler, 2001). Sometimes counselors may need to determine if the assessment conducted with a client who has a visual impairment was comprehensive. In a comprehensive assessment, counselors would expect that the examiner observed the individual functioning in a naturalistic setting and conducted a functional vision evaluation. Kelley, Sanspree, and Davidson (2001) indicated that about 90% of children with visual impairments retain some vision. In assessment, it is important to consider the severity of the visual impairment and the age of onset of the disability. Individuals who lose their vision after the age of five usually retain some visual memories (Bradley-Johnson & Ekstrom, 1998). However, many conceptual factors (e.g., color, facial expressions) are difficult to teach to those who have never had vision. Furthermore, 30–50% of visually impaired children have other impairments (Kirchner, 1983) that need to be considered in the interpretation of the assessment results.

With many well-known instruments, researchers have studied the most effective methods for adapting the instrument for visually impaired individuals to eliminate potential sources of error. For example, for individuals with visual impairment, there are procedures for adapting the Wechsler Intelligence Scale for Children-Fourth Edition (WISC-IV) that use more of the subscales for Verbal Comprehension Index. Other instruments include prerecorded tapes that read the instruments in a systematic manner. In addition, many of the personality inventories have Braille or large-print versions. An adaptation of the Stanford-Binet is the Perkins-Binet Tests of Intelligence for the Blind, which is standardized on separate forms for partially sighted and blind children. One of the few instruments developed specifically for visually impaired individuals is the Blind Learning Aptitude Test.

When clients with a visual impairment are being assessed in the areas of personality and career interests, it is important that they answer the questions related to what they enjoy and like to do rather than what they are capable of doing. For achievement and aptitude assessments, Bradley-Johnson and Ekstrom (1998) found that common accommodations for individuals with visual impairments are the following: (a) the provision of special lighting; (b) changes in test scheduling, such as allowing extra time or allowing testing over several days; (c) revision of test directions, such as reading print directions aloud; (d) revision of test format, such as using Braille, large print, or audiotape; and (e) revision of response methods, such as dictating answers or using such low-vision aids as magnification devices, tactile accessories, or computers.

Assessment of Individuals with Hearing Impairments

Assessing individuals with hearing impairments involves a different set of problems than does assessing individuals with visual impairments. Hearing has a direct link to language acquisition, and verbal content is embedded in many of the methods by which individuals are assessed. In the past, counselors sometimes assessed hearing impaired children by using instruments that involved reading, but these counselors did not have an understanding of the connection between hearing and reading. It is often difficult to decipher aptitude and ability separately from the verbal handicap. In recent years, gains have been made in identifying children with hearing problems earlier and initiating beneficial educational interventions sooner.

In terms of understanding clients with hearing disabilities, counselors need to consider the magnitude of the hearing loss, the age of onset of the problem, the effects of the loss on language acquisition, and whether the loss is affecting adjustment. Hearing disabilities are often measured in terms of the decibel level (sound intensity) needed to recognize the presence of a sound at a given frequency (as measured in hertz; Brauer, Braden, Pollard, & Hardy-Braz, 1998). It is also important to realize that, with some individuals, hearing may fluctuate. Furthermore, some within the deaf community object to the terms *hearing-impaired* or *hearing loss* because of the pejorative nature or focus on loss. Instead, they prefer the term *deaf*.

Assessment of individuals with hearing disabilities should be conducted in the individual's preferred communication modality or language (e.g., American Sign Language). If a sign language translator is used, the individual's proficiency needs to be considered, and, typically, family members should not serve as translators. American Sign Language is a distinct language and not merely a translation of English into signs; hence, in assessment, the translator will need to make professional judgments that may influence the content of the assessment.

There are also more instruments with norms for individuals with hearing impairments than for those with visual impairments. The Wechlser scales have been used extensively with hearing-impaired children. For example, the WISC-R has established norms for individuals with hearing impairments. In general, performance subtests are usually considered the best estimate of cognitive ability for children with hearing disabilities (Sattler, 2002); however, Sullivan and Montoya (1997) maintained that verbal subtests should be used in estimating intelligence. It should also be noted that impairments of the vestibular system can affect balance, equilibrium, and other motor skills. In terms of assessment in the affective domain, counselors need to ensure that clients with hearing impairments comprehend the questions. Sometimes, particularly with children, clients may give the impression that they understand what is being discussed when, in fact, they are confused. There are also some indications that individuals with hearing impairments have a tendency to respond in concrete terms to projective techniques or to more abstract counseling questions.

Assessment of Individuals with Motor Disabilities

Imagine for a minute that even though you understand what is being asked of you on a test, you are unable to make your body physically respond and complete the required task. Individuals with motor disabilities are often faced with this exact situation, because they may immediately realize how to put the puzzle pieces together but are unable to do so quickly. The methods used to assess clients with motor impairment, as with those used for all clients, vary depending on the information needed. Sometimes the intent of the testing is to assess where a client's strengths and limitations are to determine possible careers and to identify areas where accommodations can be made. In cases such as this, clients may be compared with a normal sample rather than with a special norm, because they will be competing with people without disabilities for jobs.

Sometimes examiners will perform certain assessments with clients with motor disabilities twice; once, using the specified time limits and a second time, without time limits to determine if clients can perform the tasks. A well-written psychological report will identify any departures from the standardized procedures and will discuss how the violations might have influenced the results.

With assessment of individuals in rehabilitation settings, vocational evaluation can involve three approaches to assessment: psychological testing, use of work sample or related work activities, and actual on-the-job activities (Hood & Johnson, 2007). Because individuals with physical disabilities often tire more easily, accommodation often involves testing in time-limited intervals and over several days. Sampson (1990) discussed how computer technology can be used to adapt assessment devices so that individuals with disabilities can complete instruments with little outside assistance. Examples of computer technologies used are voice inputs, simplified keyboards, pneumatic controls, joysticks, head pointers, and Braille keyboards.

These devices can eliminate an intermediary who reads or responds to the test items for the examinee. As is discussed in Chapter 16, technological applications are having a significant influence on many aspects of assessment. For more information on assessment of individuals with physical disabilities, readers are directed to Frank and Elliott (2000).

There are a number of methods for assessing intelligence or general ability with individuals with motor disabilities. One commonly used method involves picture vocabulary tests, in which the individual simply points to the correct answer. The pictures eliminate the problems associated with reading, and the pointing is not timed and eliminates many of the problems associated with motor coordination difficulties. The *Peabody Picture Vocabulary Test-Fourth Edition* (PPVT-IV; Dunn & Dunn, 2007) is the most commonly used of these instruments. The PPVT-IV takes about 10 to 15 minutes to administer. The examinee is presented with a plate with four pictures. The examiner says a stimulus word, and the examinee responds by pointing to the appropriate picture. PPVT-IV scores are similar to other measures of intelligence, with a mean of 100 and a standard deviation of 15. Another instrument, the Expressive Vocabulary Test, measures expressive vocabulary and word retrieval and is co-normed with the PPVT-IV to allow for comparisons of receptive and expressive vocabulary.

An issue in assessment related to testing people with motor disabilities is the topic of *flagging*, which involves reporting any and all aspects of the test administration or interpretation that deviate from the standard procedure (Pratt & Moreland, 1998). On one side of the debate are those individuals with disabilities who argue that accommodation to the standard procedure is simply "leveling the playing field" and eliminating bias in the testing procedures. In comparison, some test developers and users argue that varying from the standard procedures violates the integrity of the results, and violations should be noted to inform professionals of these possible violations. Advocates for those with disabilities counter that this "flagging" perpetuates stereotypes and negative attitudes toward individuals with disabilities. In terms of admissions and employment testing, Mehrens and Ekstrom (2002) contended that accommodations and modifications used when assessing individuals with disabilities should be documented and that not doing so violates federal legislation. They also recommended that care should be taken to preserve the confidentiality of the individual and the accommodations that were made.

Assessment of Individuals with Cognitive Impairments

The assessment of individuals with mental retardation falls within the area of assessment of cognitive impairments. The term *mental retardation*, however, is being used less frequently because the American Association of Mental Retardation (AAMR) has recently changed its name to the American Association on Intellectual and Developmental Disabilities (AAIDD). Counselors usually do not perform testing related to the determination of intellectual disabilities or mental retardation, but it is important for them to have an understanding of this area. The American Association on Intellectual and Developmental Disabilities (2007) defined mental retardation as not being a medical or mental disorder, but rather a state of functioning that begins in childhood and is characterized by limitation in both intelligence and adaptive skills. In their view, mental retardation reflects the "fit" between the capabilities of individuals and expectation within their environment. The AAIDD definition of mental retardation is somewhat different from the *Diagnostic and Statistical Manual of Mental Disorders-Fourth Edition-Text Revision* (*DSM-IV-TR*; American Psychiatric Association, 2000) criteria for mental retardation (see Chapter 12). Using the *DSM-IV-TR* criterion, mental retardation is characterized by significantly subaverage intellectual functioning (typically an IQ of approximately 70 or below), with onset before the age of 18 years. The subaverage intelligence must be accompanied by concurrent deficits or impairments in adaptive functioning.

In both definitions of mental retardation, there is consensus that limitations must be evident in both intelligence and adaptive functioning. The assessment of mental retardation typically involves an individual test of intelligence (e.g., the WISC-IV or the Stanford-Binet) and a measure of *adaptive* behavior. Psychologists often used an earlier version of the *Vineland Adaptive Behavior Scales-Second Edition* (Vineland-II) to measure adaptive behavior. There are three versions of the recently published Vineland-II that can be used in combination or alone: the Survey Interview Form, Parent/Caregiver Rating Form, and the Teacher Rating Form. The Extended Interview Form should be released in 2008. The major domains assessed in the Vineland-II are Communication, Daily Living Skills, Socialization, and Motor Skills. There is also an option to score an Adaptive Behavior Composite Index. Other measures of adaptive behavior are the *AAMR Adaptive Behavior Scale-School, Second Edition* and the *AAMR Adaptive Behavior Scale-Residential and Community, Second Edition*. Recently, the AAIDD has published the *Supports Intensity Scale*, which is designed to assess the practical support requirements of an individual with intellectual disability. This assessment is somewhat unique in that it focuses on what the individual may need to best function rather than on identifying deficits.

In terms of both assessment and supportive services for individuals with mental retardation, the American Association on Intellectual and Developmental Disabilities (AAIDD) recommends the following:

1. Evaluate limitations in present functioning within the context of the individual's age peers and culture.
2. Take into account the individual's cultural and linguistic differences as well as communication, sensory, motor, and behavioral factors.
3. Recognize that within an individual, limitations often coexist with strengths.
4. Describe limitations so that an individualized plan of needed supports can be developed.
5. Provide appropriate personalized supports to improve the functioning of a person with mental retardation.

Another major area of assessment related to cognitive impairments is **neuropsychological assessment,** which concerns assessing the behavioral effects of possible brain injury or damage. Brain damage can result from injury or disease, or it can be organic. Insults to the nervous system are often associated with cognitive dysfunctions, such as memory difficulties, but they can also have an effect on personality and temperament. Once again, although counselors will not be performing neuropsychological testing, they do need an overview of the typical process to know when to refer clients for neuropsychological assessment. Clients who display abrupt mental or behavioral changes should be referred for a neuropsychological assessment. An evaluation is also probably warranted if the changes are more subtle, such as individuals exhibiting mild memory changes, borderline EEG (electroencephalograph) results, attention lapses, speech disturbances, and motor dysfunction (Swiercinsky, 1978). It is also wise for a client to be evaluated if there is any suspected trauma to the brain resulting from illness or injury. For instance, clients should be referred for a neurological screening if an injury resulted in loss of consciousness.

Neuropsychologists often administer a battery of tests to clients because no single test can detect the diversity of brain dysfunctions. These batteries were designed to systematically assess a broad spectrum of neurological functioning. Two of the most commonly used assessment batteries for neuropsychological testing are the *Halstead-Reitan Neuropsychological Test Battery* and the *Luria-Nebraska Neuropsychological Battery.* The Halstead-Reitan takes about 6 to 8 hours to administer and typically involves administering either the WISC-IV or the WAIS-III. The Luria-Nebraska takes about 2.5 hours to administer and is designed to assess a broad range of neurological impairments. These specifically designed neuropsychological batteries are not the only methods used in this area. Neuropsychologists will also often use individual measures of intelligence or specific subscales (e.g., the Digit Span of the WAIS-III) as part of the assessment process. Another commonly used instrument is the *Bender Visual Motor Gestalt Test,* usually referred to as the Bender-Gestalt Test. The Bender-Gestalt Test consists of nine cards, each of which contains an abstract design that the examinee is asked to copy. The Bender-Gestalt may reveal visual-motor difficulties indicative of neurological impairments. There are different methods of administering the Bender-Gestalt, many of which require that the examiner show the examinee each card for a specific period of time so that information on memory deficits can be obtained. In addition to neurological assessment, the Bender-Gestalt is also frequently used to assess possible learning disabilities.

Recent medical advances have also contributed to the assessment of brain injury and damage. Techniques such as magnetic resonance imaging (MRI) and positron emission tomography (PET) provide better insight into the brain's functioning than ever before. These medical techniques, however, cannot provide the entire picture, and often neurologists and neuropsychologists work together, both in diagnosing the impairments and determining appropriate treatment. Sometimes the treatment involves counseling, either for the victim of the neurological impairment or for the family coping with the disability.

Summary

Counselors can expect to work with clients from various backgrounds; therefore, they need to be skilled in cross-cultural assessment. When selecting an instrument, counselors need to consider the client's ethnic or racial background and select an instrument appropriate for that client. Counselors also work in locations (e.g., schools) where they do not choose the assessment instruments (e.g., achievement tests) but are still the ones responsible for administering and interpreting the results. In all assessment situations, counselors need to evaluate the assessment instruments for possible bias. One area counselors should consider is whether the instrument has been evaluated for possible content bias. Content bias concerns whether the content of the instrument is more familiar or appropriate to one group as compared with another group or groups. Another area counselors should examine is the instrument's internal structure for different ethnic groups. Instruments can differ in the degree to which they are reliable for different groups, and the factor structure may vary depending on the ethnic group. The analysis of possible bias should also include studies related to the relationship between the instrument and the criterion for different groups. It is important to examine differences among the validity coefficients and possible slope bias. Another area to examine is whether there are differences in the intercepts for different ethnic groups.

Some of the instruments counselors use may not be biased but may still produce results that have a disparate or negative impact on some minority individuals. There is debate about whether differences in ability, achievement, and aptitude testing are primarily genetic, social, or cultural. Helms (1992) argued that researchers should also examine cultural equivalence; that is, whether the constructs have similar meanings within and across cultures. Presently, it is impossible to develop a culture-free instrument, but many professionals are committed to developing instruments that attempt to be more culturally fair. There are also multicultural assessment standards to which counselors should adhere to provide competent services to clients from diverse backgrounds.

Counselors also need to consider clients with physical disabilities. In assessing clients with disabilities, counselors need to review the research on the most appropriate methods for adapting the assessment for these individuals. In many settings, a counselor may be on a multi-disciplinary treatment team that will be involved with developing treatments for individuals with disabilities. The client may have been assessed by a vocational rehabilitation specialist or a psychologist and the counselor will need to understand the psychological assessment report. A well-written psychological report will identify any departures from the standardized procedures and will discuss how the violations may influence the results. The results from any significant departure from standard procedures should be viewed with concern. Assessment with a special population can provide useful information if it is carefully performed and conservatively interpreted.

In conclusion, assessment with individuals from diverse backgrounds and cultures is a complex topic and it is anticipated that this topic will continue to be debated in the next 10 or more years. The goal of any assessment is to provide pertinent information that is meaningful, fair, and accurate. This is often a challenging goal because the constructs counselors are attempting to assess are typically multifaceted and our culture is becoming less homogeneous. There are, however, many dedicated professionals who are attempting to address topics related to assessment with diverse individuals and it is anticipated that strides will be made in leveling the playing field related to many types of assessments.

CHAPTER 16

Technological Applications and Future Trends

As we approach the end of this book, it may be wise to direct our attention to future trends in appraisal in counseling. Previous chapters addressed both the history of and current practices in assessment. This chapter identifies some future trends in assessment that practitioners need to consider when providing counseling services to clients. Many changes have occurred in the area of appraisal in counseling over the past 50 years; however, we can expect even greater changes in the next 50 years. Almost every aspect of our lives is being affected by changes in technology. Certainly, the field of assessment has been affected by computers and technology and will continue to be affected by technological changes in the future. The intent of this chapter is to examine current trends in terms of the use of computers and technology and to consider future trends in the general field of appraisal.

Technological Applications

Currently in the field of assessment, technology and computers have had a major influence on how assessment services are delivered. Technology and computer applications are not a new phenomenon in this area; the Strong Vocational Interest Blank used electromechanical scoring as early as the 1930s. Computers continued to be used primarily for scoring, and sometimes interpretation, until the late 1970s and early 1980s. The expansion of computer usage in assessment coincided with the widespread use of microcomputers or personal computers. Computers are now intimately involved in the administration, scoring, and interpretation of many assessment instruments in counseling.

Almost 10 years ago, Sampson (1998) projected that in the field of counseling, the Internet would have a profound impact on ways in which counselors conduct assessments. Sampson's prophecy was accurate—in the past five years, the Internet and other types of technology have influenced the manner in which many counselors conduct assessments in. Using a common search engine, I recently entered the words *assessment in counseling*, which produced more than a million matches. In perusing the matches, I found a multitude of topics, such as overviews of professional organizations (e.g., Association for Assessment in Counseling and Education), counseling agencies and centers, syllabi for courses in assessment in counseling, books on assessment, and articles on such diverse topics as assessments related to cancer risks. The Internet enables individuals to easily access information from various locations, including many individuals' homes and workplaces. It is logical to assume that both counselors and clients will want to access assessment information through this medium that is becoming part of daily life for millions of people throughout the world.

It is not difficult to understand the growth of Internet assessment. A new instrument with appropriate translations can be made available to counselors around the world instantly (Naglieri et al., 2004). Revising an Internet instrument often can be done less expensively than paper-and-pencil versions because there is not a need to make printed copies nor are there mailing costs. Also, as Naglieri et al. explained, the Internet is more scalable, which in the vernacular of the Internet means adding volume with very little expense. For example, if an assessment is a paper-and-pencil assessment there are significant costs related to printing and mailing additional instruments, whereas, there is very little cost in publishing additional versions of Internet-based assessment. Of course, for some assessments, additional hardware, such as servers, are probably needed as the volume increases; however, these costs are typically less than costs associated with increased production of a paper-and-pencil assessment. In addition to the Internet, other technological resources have made the gathering, collating, and analyzing of assessment data enormously easier than it was in the 1940s and 1950s when some assessments were first developed.

The Internet also makes assessment easier for counselors to find and use formal assessments. Clinicians might identify areas where they would like to use formal instruments to supplement their clinical decision making (e.g., screening tools for groups, suicide potential measures, measures related to certain problems) but may not be familiar with assessments in this area. Search engines make it easy for clinicians to search for assessments that may correspond to their clinical needs. A very helpful resource is the Buros Institute website (http://buros.unl.edu/). Through the Test Review Online feature, counselors enter topics (e.g., eating disorders, career interests, achievement) into the keyword search and the program identifies instruments in that area. The Buros Institute's database is comprised of the more than 2,500 tests that have been reviewed. In using the website, counselors both identify potential assessment instruments and purchase reviews of those assessments from the *Mental Measurements Yearbooks*. The information contained in the *Mental Measurements Yearbooks* also includes the publisher of the instrument so counselors can then go to the publisher's website.

Most established assessment publishers have websites, many of which include extensive information about assessments. Not only can counselors get descriptions of counseling assessment instruments and sometimes samples of interpretation reports, they can also access information on the costs of potential instruments and order assessment materials over the Internet. For many of the publishers of psychological assessments, clinicians will first have to submit a user's qualification form indicating that they have the sufficient background and training to administer the particular instrument they are ordering. A word of caution concerning ordering any materials over the Internet: It is advisable to order materials only through reputable publishers and *secure* online sites.

According to Naglieri et al. (2004), psychological Internet tests and assessments can be classified into three broad categories according to their goals. First, many Internet tests, instruments, and surveys are designed for personal development and growth, and may or may not be scientifically based. These assessments are designed for the layperson and involve personality, career issues, relationship styles, or other characteristics. The second category of assessments is psychodiagnostic measures such as the Minnesota Multiphasic Personality Inventory-2 (MMPI-2) and Beck inventories that are now available on the Internet. Finally, cognitive ability tests, certification tests, and licensing exams are beginning to be administered via the Internet. Barak (2003) proposed two categories of online assessments: (1) assessments conducted by professionals in which various online means are used to develop a psychological evaluation and (2) online tests published throughout the Internet that provide surfers with a means of evaluating various personal characteristics. The distinction between professional assessments and nonprofessionally-based assessments is an important distinction and one that I will return to for a more in-depth analysis.

Technology and Terminology

Advances in technology are having significant influences on assessment in counseling and the future course of these rapid advancements is difficult to predict. Fifteen years ago, the cutting-edge in assessment was downloading software to desktop computers, which enabled the computer to administer the assessment, score it, and provide an interpretative report. It is difficult to describe current methods that are influenced by technology in regards to the administration, scoring, and interpretation because advances are being made on a daily basis. There is a movement from computer-based assessment to Internet-based assessment, but many of the issues that applied to computer-based assessment also apply to Internet or other technology-based applications. In this discussion of terms, I am going to use the term *technology* often to address both computer- and Internet-based applications because many topics and issues apply to both applications. In addition, many publishers offer both computer-based scoring and interpretation packages and Internet packages; thus, the term *technology-based* can describe both applications. There will be times, however, that I will separate computer-based from Internet-based assessments because some situations present issues unique to using software that is downloaded to a computer and is stored on a hard drive that are different from assessment applications that involve the Internet. In those situations, I will use the terms *computer* or *Internet* to highlight the topics or issues that are unique to the specified format.

In terms of technological applications in assessment or appraisal, two terms need to be defined. **Technology-assisted assessment** concerns the use of computers or other technologies that assist in the administration, scoring, or interpretation of any assessment tool. The manner in which the technology assists in the assessment process can vary from using a computer that simply scores the instrument to an Internet-based system that scores a client's answers, interprets the results, and writes a detailed report. With technology-assisted assessment, the instrument may be accessed on the Internet, or software may be downloaded to a computer. In contrast, the term **technology-adapted assessment** indicates that there is an *interactive* process between the individual and the computer. One example of technology-adapted assessment is sometimes called *item branching*, which involves different sets of items or test questions that are administered to different individuals and vary according to each individual's responses. As an example, if an answer or answers to test questions indicate that a fifth grader does not comprehend material at the fifth-grade level, the software would adapt the questions and select questions at a fourth-grade level. If another student, however, comprehends the fifth-grade questions, then the software would be programmed to select items at the sixth-grade level. This adaptive process is mostly used in achievement tests, but it can also be used in other types of assessments. For example, if a client reports that he or she has never experienced any auditory hallucinations or hearing of voices when no one actually appears to be talking, the technology-adapted system could then eliminate the items that ask about when the voices are heard and what types of messages the voices are giving. Technology-adapted assessments can be efficient because, for most clients, the time needed to complete the instrument is reduced when the administration of the assessment is programmed to eliminate inappropriate items. For instance, the computerized version of the Graduate Record Examination (GRE) is a technology-adapted assessment, and studies indicate that most people spend less time taking it as compared with the time spent on the paper-and-pencil version of the GRE (Educational Testing Service, 1997).

Advantages of Using Technology in Assessment

There are many advantages to computer and Internet applications in client assessment. Computers can be patient in gathering information and substantial amounts of data can be retrieved, analyzed, and stored. In addition, because of advancements in technology, there is often a negligible time lag between the administration, scoring, and interpretation of the instrument. Technology has made it possible to receive results and offer interpretation of those results instantaneously. Rather than having to mail answer sheets to publishers and wait for the results to be mailed back, clinicians can often get results by a simple click on a computer. These technological applications in assessment have helped professionals save time, because when computers are used to monitor, score, and interpret results, practitioners can spend more time on other duties. Using technology enables instruments to be designed to see whether an individual understands the instructions. For example, on an analogies test, the computer can determine if the individual understands the premise of the test by giving sample items involving simple analogies. If the person answers the sample items incorrectly, then additional instructions can be provided. Moreover, computer- or Internet-based assessments respond solely to the information that is entered and do not have any preconceived notions about individuals based on physical appearance or the color of their skin. Computers and online assessments are unbiased and do not react to the individual's gender, race, age, or demeanor. Using existing technologies, computers that are programmed correctly do not make the types of scoring errors that can occur with hand scoring. The programming can also involve complex scoring and interpretations that the computer can perform in minutes but that would take counselors hours to perform. Examples of instruments involving complicated scoring procedures are the Millon Clinical Multiaxial Inventory and the Strong Interest Inventory®.

Another advantage of Internet assessment is the Internet makes it easier to recruit participants and expand the number of individuals in norming groups. In the past, many norming groups were composed of samples that were not particularly diverse because of the time and expense of gathering a representative sample. Through the Internet, instrument developers and publishers can more easily gather data from a larger number of individuals and access a more diverse and representative sample. Publishers can download a new assessment to their website quickly and easily and then can send out emails to customers who might use this new instrument.

In addition, Internet assessment enables some individuals who might not normally have access to assessments to be able to take an assessment. For example, someone living in rural North Dakota might take a depression screening assessment online and decide that they should drive 120 miles to the nearest mental health center. A school district can purchase the use of an online career assessment series and a school counselor can have students take it either at home or at the public library over the weekend as a part of a guidance curriculum program. Buchanan (2002) contended that online personality assessments also enable more people to complete assessments than previously would have been possible. One of the arguments for cyber-counseling is that individuals who had been unable to access mental health services either because of geographical or financial limitations, may now have easier access to these services.

Internet assessment also facilitates technological advances in assessment theory and practice, such as item response theory (Naglieri et al., 2004). As addressed in Chapter 4, item response theory requires individuals with different traits or levels of achievement to answer multiple items and the responses are analyzed using a complex modeling program. The interactive nature of computers and Internet are just beginning to be recognized and this in leading to new types of assessments. For example, Drasgow, Olson-Buchanan, and Moberg (1999) developed an assessment of individuals' conflict-resolution skills that uses an interactive program involving video clips.

Considerations and Caveats in Using Technology in Assessment

Although current technologies are leading to exciting developments in educational and psychological assessment, some aspects of this technology must be closely scrutinized to assess clients in an ethical, sound, and meaningful manner. The following sections highlight some crucial topics related to using technology to take assessments (i.e., inputting information), using results and interpretation (i.e., output information), and using technology in an ethical manner.

Issues related to inputting information. Using technology-based assessments involves using a technological device, such as a computer, to take the assessment, which is followed by receiving assessment results and/or interpretation. Many of these instruments that use technology to administer the assessment have been adapted from paper-and-pencil formats. For example, the Beck Depression Inventory-II has a paper-and-pencil version, a computer-administered version, and a version that can be taken on-line. In addition to paper-and-pencil assessments that have been adapted for the computer or on-line, there are instruments that been developed to be available only on-line or via a computer (e.g., some career assessments).

Another limitation of computer-administered assessment is that clients' behaviors during the process are typically not observed by professionals. In psychological reports, examiners' behavioral observations of clients are traditionally used in the interpretation of the testing results. Behavioral observations during the administration of an instrument can provide insight into the client's degree of motivation and level of anxiety. Another issue pertinent to computer-administered assessment concerns the effects on the results of individual differences in comfort level, amount of experience, and attitudes toward computers. Surveys have indicated that most people have favorable attitudes toward computerized test administration. There are, however, differences in experience level—for example, some clients may think the term *mouse* applies only to an animal, whereas other clients have carpal tunnel syndrome from the extensive use of their computer's keyboard and mouse. Counselors should consider client experiences with and attitudes toward computerized assessment when deciding whether to use a computer-administered instrument and when interpreting the results from such an instrument. Barak (2003) noted some research studies indicate that, in general, females tend to score lower on online assessments.

Another issue pertains to the psychometric qualities of computer-administered or online instruments. Some people erroneously view a computer-administered instrument as being scientifically sound simply because it is computerized. In the beginning of computer-administered assessment, there were few investigations into the psychometric qualities of these instruments. With increased usage, professional organizations, such as the American Counseling Association and the American Psychological Association, revised their ethical codes and standards to address many of the issues related to computer-assisted assessment (see Appendix C for the ACA *Code of Ethics* related to assessment). If the instrument is an adaptation of a paper-and-pencil instrument, then the evaluation of the psychometric qualities must include an analysis of the *equivalency* of the two forms of the instrument. Research indicates that the item type or format influences whether the computer-administered version is equivalent to the instrument's conventional form. Instruments containing multiple-choice or true/false items are more likely to be equivalent (Hoffman & Lundberg, 1976) as compared with matching items or checklist items (Allred & Harris, 1984). Allred and Harris found individuals tend to check more items on a computer-administered version as compared with those who take a paper-and-pencil version. In a meta-analysis of studies related to the MMPI, Finger and Ones (1999) found little difference in scores between the computer-administered and paper-and-pencil version.

An additional issue in this area concerns the different levels of self-disclosure and honesty in responses on computer-administered assessment and those on methods that are more conventional. Researchers have hypothesized that, with instruments that contain personally sensitive information, computer administration may increase the honesty of the disclosures because test takers may perceive the computer as offering greater anonymity and less judgmental responses. The opposite, however, can also be hypothesized—individuals may be more likely to disclose personally sensitive information to a skilled and empathic clinician than to a computer. Although the research is not overwhelming, some studies have found that individuals are more likely to disclose more information about themselves to a computer than to another person. Turner et al. (1998) found adolescents were more likely to report violence, sexual behavior, and drug use if they were using a computer survey with an audio computer-assisted interviewing program than with traditional methods. Joinson and Buchanan (2001) found that, in general, people were more self-disclosing with web-based assessments. Garb (2007) argued that, in general, computer-based interviews and rating scales tend to be more reliable, less biased, and more comprehensive than interviews conducted in clinical practice. Garb, however, concluded his article by indicating computer-based interviews are not always appropriate and using only computer-based assessments can lead to more false positives (i.e., people appearing to have more pathology than they actually have).

Issues related to outputting information. A major issue related to output received from online assessment is that instruments could be developed and marketed by entrepreneurs with little or no background in counseling or psychological assessment. Individuals taking these pseudo assessments may place more confidence in these results, as compared with magazine personality tests, because, by being on the Internet, the instruments have the illusion of technological sophistication. The possibility of making a profit from marketing psychological instruments through the Internet appears to exist, because many sites charge for various types of assessments (e.g., career, personality, relationship profiles). The possibility exists that individuals could purchase online assessments that are neither reliable nor valid. A possibly more hazardous outcome is that individuals could make crucial decisions based on these faulty assessments. For example, a depressed client could take a psychometrically unsound instrument indicating that she was not depressed. This client may continue to suffer from depression unnecessarily when personal treatment could have possibly helped her. Currently, no formal or informal oversight exists for these online instruments, some of which may appear to be very professional to the layperson.

The ease of using technology in assessment and instantaneously receiving results may be appealing to many clinicians, but practitioners should evaluate the results or output of any computer-generated assessment before using that information with a client. Concerning computer or online assessments, the old adage "garbage in/garbage out" often applies. Although a computer may accurately score any instrument, if the instrument is lacking in terms of reliability and validity evidence, then it does not really matter if the scoring was performed accurately. In terms of assessment, computer- or technology-generated outputs can vary from simple scoring to extensive and complex interpretations. Increasingly, interpretations of assessment results are done by computers rather than clinicians. Rubenzer (1992) found that clinicians could not tell the difference between a computer-generated report and one written by a clinician.

Interpretative reports can be anything from elementary descriptions to complex clinical interpretations involving diagnostic decisions. A counselor using computer-generated reports must always evaluate the quality of these reports. Eyde and Kowal (1987) found differences among interpretative reports for the same personality assessment that were generated by different software programs. It is possible for some interpretative reports to be programmed by individuals who have no counseling or assessment experience. Furthermore, the computer programs used to produce the reports can vary. For example, some programs use simple cookbook approaches with little examination of the interrelationship of answers or, even worse, online assessments can provide outputs that may appear to be descriptive of individuals' personality but may have little or any validation evidence.

With the proliferation of online assessments, counselors should consider the **Barnum effect** when evaluating the reports from these assessment websites. The term *Barnum effect* is related to the showman P. T. Barnum's statement "There's a sucker born every minute." The Barnum effect applies to *all* types of personality reports but is particularly relevant to online results. As an example of the Barnum effect, let us pretend that you have just taken a personality inventory online and the following is the interpretation of your results:

> You are a person that some people are drawn to; yet, there are a few people who do not see your strengths. You tend to be warm and friendly at times but need to be by yourself at other times. People tend to see you as someone they can trust. You can be critical of yourself, particularly when you do not function to your full capacity. Presently, you are unsure of all of your skills and abilities. You are energetic when it comes to important matters. It is difficult for you to attain a balance in your life because you have a tendency to be pulled in different directions. You seek a certain amount of change and variation in your activities. While you are generally honest with others, you are most honest with those who know you very well. You can also be honest with yourself, which sometimes causes you to doubt some of your decisions.

For many people, the preceding description would probably fit because it is somewhat vague and general. The Barnum effect occurs when a report is written so vaguely that it applies to most individuals. A number of research studies have used similar Barnum effect statements and found that many participants thought the description was a good or excellent description of their personality (Snyder, Shenkel, & Lowery, 1977; Ulrich, Stachnik, & Stainton, 1963). Merrens and Richards (1970) found that individuals could not discriminate between bogus interpretations and bona fide interpretations. Because the Internet is not regulated, individuals can easily set up websites in which assessments appear legitimate and reports can be written so that they apply to most individuals. Most generalized personality descriptions tend to include *double-headed* sentences (e.g., "You tend to be warm and friendly at times but need to be by yourself at other times."); *modal* statements, descriptive of virtually anyone (e.g., "You seek a certain amount of change and variation in your activities."); *vague* statements (e.g., "Presently, you are unsure of all of your skills and abilities."); and *favorable* statements (e.g., "People tend to see you as someone they can trust."). When counselors begin to see a number of these types of statements in a report, they should examine it more carefully to see if a Barnum effect may be present.

Another issue to consider with online assessments is the makeup of the norming group. For some online assessments, there is little information available regarding the norming group. In some cases, the norming group is continually evolving as new examinees become part of the norming group after they have completed the online assessment. Although online-based assessments may make it easier to recruit participants, it does not mean the norming groups are appropriate for all clients. Some researchers devote substantial time and resources to obtaining a norming sample that is more representative than simply using people who can afford to take an assessment on-line. In addition, computers are still not in every household and recruiting online volunteers for a norming sample may exclude low-income individuals.

Nonprofessionals can develop websites that feature instruments that have not been researched and interpretative results that may appear legitimate to most readers. In addition, nonprofessionals can establish faulty websites that appear to be generating sound interpretative reports of established instruments but, in fact, are programmed to generate results that are not based on the validation evidence of the instrument. In evaluating whether to use an online or computer-generated report, a counselor should find answers to the following questions:

1. What is the basis for the programming of the report?
2. Who was involved in the writing of the computer programs, and what are his or her professional credentials?
3. Were the individuals knowledgeable about the instrument, and did they have extensive experience in interpreting the results?
4. Is the interpretation based on sound research and validation information?
5. Is there evidence that the technology-generated reports are comparable to clinician-generated reports?
6. Is the interpretative information in the report helpful and appropriate for the client with whom the counselor is working?
7. Is the cost of the technology-generated report (e.g., software, hardware) worth the information produced by the report?
8. Are supplemental resources, such as a hotline number, available for questions?

With the ease of computer-generated reports, clinicians may be lulled into a false sense of security and may use the computer-generated results without becoming educated about the instrument. Instruments used in counseling are validated for specific purposes; therefore, a counselor cannot use a general computer-generated report in isolation. The American Counseling Association's (2005a) *Code of Ethics* states that counselors confirm the validity of assessment scoring and interpretation if they use such assessment services. Furthermore, the offering of automated test interpretation services is considered a professional-to-professional consultation, and the overriding and ultimate responsibility is to the client; hence, counselors bear the ultimate responsibility for ensuring that the scoring and interpretation of an assessment is accurate and legitimate. Simply using a computer-generated report without knowledge of the instrument's strengths and limitations would be considered by the courts to be negligent and unprofessional. Computer-generated reports are designed to supplement or complement the clinician's interpretation of the results, not replace them. Sampson, Purgar, and Shy (2003) advocated that the following competencies are necessary for the ethical use of a computer-based test interpretation (CBTI):

- An understanding of the construct or behavior.
- An understanding of the test including the theoretical basis (if any), item selection and scale construction, standardization, reliability, validity, and utility.
- An understanding of the test interpretation including scale interpretations and recommended interventions based on scale scores.
- An understanding of the CBTI including the equivalence of test forms (if interpretations from an original form are used) and the evidence of CBTI validity.
- Initial supervised experience in using the test and CBTI (with supervision provided by an appropriately qualified practitioner) (p. 27).

Sampson et al.'s suggestions are consistent with the American Counseling Association's (2005a) *Code of Ethics*, which conveys that counselors who use technology-assisted test interpretations are trained in the construct being measured and are qualified to use the instrument.

Although reviews of computer-based test interpretation programs may be helpful, they are not as easy to access as reviews of more traditional instruments. The publishers of the *Mental Measurements Yearbooks* considered including such reviews but abandoned that effort (Kramer & Conoley, 1992). Reviews of computer-based test interpretation programs are, however, sometimes published in professional journals such as *Computers in Human Behavior, Computers and Education,* and, occasionally, other counseling journals.

Computers, the Internet, and other technologies are influencing both ways individuals are taking assessments and the manner in which the assessment results are scored, interpreted, and used. Counselors should be aware of the ways in which technology can assist them in gathering information about assessments and in assessing clients. On the other hand, these technologies also introduce into the assessment process unique complications and ethical issues.

Ethical considerations. In the American Counseling Association's (2005a) *Code of Ethics*, Section A.12 is entitled "Technology Applications" and it addresses the uses of technology in various counseling-related actives. This section on technological applications begins by clearly stating that "Counselors inform clients of the benefits and limitations of using information technology applications in the counseling process and in business/billing procedures" (p. 6). As in paper-and-pencil assessments, informed consent applies to computer and online assessment. The ACA *Code of Ethics* provides detailed guidance on technology and informed consent (see A.12.g). Counselors should not rely on the informed consent procedure being a part of the computer or online assessment and should plan accordingly.

Confidentiality is another issue that is relevant in technological applications in assessment. Practitioners should have clients take only assessments in which the clinicians are sure of how the assessment information will be used. Reputable sites will provide information related to the degree to which clients' results are secure and they will make it clear that the results will not be disclosed to a third party. Buchanan (2002) argued that the risk of confidentiality being breached using online assessments is probably less than it was with "old-fashioned" file cabinets and other storage methods used in counselors' offices. This may be true if the clinician thoroughly explores potential online assessments and evaluates the safeguards the site uses to ensure assessment results are kept confidential.

Counselors not only need to ensure that the websites clients use are secure, but they must also consider confidentiality issues regarding how clients take assessments and how that information may be stored on a hard drive or a server within the counselor's office. For example, for some secondary or postsecondary schools, a computerized career guidance program is available to students in an unsupervised location (e.g., library, resources center, or computer lab). In many cases, the career guidance programs contain multiple assessments (see Chapter 9) and students often progress through the program during multiple sessions. They often have passwords that enable them to access previous results and integrate results from different assessments (e.g., interest inventory, skills assessment, and values instrument). Though these programs may be password-protected, other students with time and "hacking skills" could access this confidential information. Some of these programs enable students to enter quite sensitive information such as grades and ACT scores. Hence, counselors have an ethical obligation to ensure that these types of assessments are supervised and only the counselor and the client have access to the assessment results and sensitive information.

In addressing Internet assessment, we should also consider issues related to protecting the public. For some individuals, it may be difficult to determine if a website is secure and whether the information they disclose is being kept confidential. For example, some pharmaceutical companies might be interested in the email addresses of individuals whose scores on a web-based depression inventory indicated depressive symptoms. In addition, there is also a hidden commercial agenda with some websites. I recently took an online intelligence test, which provided an IQ score and an advertisement for a book that was guaranteed to increase my intellectual capabilities.

The ease of taking tests through the Internet and the lack of preliminary screening may contribute to individuals taking instruments they should not have taken (Barak, 2003). Problems may occur if individuals who take Internet assessments receive distressing feedback or misinterpret results in isolation and without the support and assistance provided by a counselor. Oliver and Chartrand (2000) noted that the quality of the interpretative materials used on Internet assessment sites is critical, because there is no practitioner to ensure that the client understands the results.

Barak (2003) argued that public education related to the strengths and limitations of Internet assessment is crucial. In particular, individuals need to be made aware of the risks related to solicitation, exploitation, lack of confidentiality and privacy, and misuse of personal information. It might also be helpful for professional organizations to evaluate assessment sites and provide information to the public regarding Internet assessments that have met some professional standards and those that have not. This procedure could be analogous to the "Good Housekeeping Seal of Approval," in which the public would know that the assessment they are considering taking had been positively evaluated. As advances in technology affect the field of assessments, counselors need to consider clients' well-being and ensure that these advances are helpful to clients. They also must consider possible ramifications that may negatively impact individuals.

Future Trends and Directions

When we speculate about upcoming trends in assessment in counseling, it would be helpful to find a crystal ball, because there are conflicting opinions concerning those future directions. In the educational community, some individuals contend that educational reform can best be accomplished by more assessment of students, whereas others contend that less intrusion and assessment is the wave of the future. Even within counseling, some argue that testing is no longer relevant to counseling practice (Goldman, 1994), whereas others argue that assessment will continue to play an important role in the services provided to clients (Hood & Johnson, 2007). Certainly, social, economic, and political developments have influenced assessment practices in the past and will continue to influence assessment in the future. Current practices and trends in appraisal can also provide some insight into future directions and developments.

Increased Use of Technology

In examining future trends in appraisal in counseling, I would be negligent not to mention, again, the rapidly evolving influence that technology is having on this field. It may be that our grandchildren will laugh when we tell them how we once took tests using paper and pencils. The Internet is increasingly being used in assessment and more publishers are offering testing through the Internet. Individuals can take personality tests, aptitude assessments, and even intelligence tests on-line. Due to the unregulated status of the Internet, however, there are no controls on who publishes these instruments and whether assessment instruments comply with any established standards. The possibility exists that individuals could take instruments that are unreliable or invalid. Whether professional organizations should monitor the use of psychological assessments on the Internet is the subject of some debate. In either case, this is certainly a topic that will be discussed in future professional forums. Although there are ethical guidelines for Internet- or web-based counseling, it would be helpful if detailed professional guidelines existed to guide practitioners in the appropriate use of Internet assessment with clients.

The Internet is not the only area related to technology that probably will influence assessment in counseling, for technological advances may incorporate a wide spectrum of developments. Computer scanners are beginning to be used so that more original works can be entered into the computer. In addition, sophistication in computer programming will allow for more intricate and complex scoring. These developments will permit the scoring of less-structured assessments, such as analysis of drawings, essays, or stories. Other technologies, such as the expansion of video analysis, may influence appraisal methods in counseling. In this case, the initial interview could be videotaped and analyzed by computers. Maruish (2004) suggested IVR technology could be used in assessment, particularly in terms of an initial screening of clients. IVR is short for interactive voice response, in which someone either uses a touch-tone telephone or speaks into the telephone in response to cues. This technology could enable clients to call a counseling center and if they answered questions indicating that they were in crisis, then the call could be directed to an appropriate referral (e.g., crisis unit at a local hospital) or to a counselor who is on-call and who could assess the level of client distress. There is little doubt that technological applications will be incorporated into assessment procedures; the questions surround what new technologies will be developed in the coming decades.

Garb (2000) argued that more sophisticated computer assessment programs will increase psychological assessment accuracy in predicting client behavior. Garb further contended that computer programs are already better at predicting client behavior than are clinicians. There is the possibility that these computer programs could increase the accuracy of psychodiagnosis and behavioral prediction (e.g., suicidal behavior), which could result in clinicians making better treatment decisions because they would be working with better client information.

More Concise Measures

According to Beutler et al. (2004), to capitalize on the empirical advantage that psychological tests have over unstandardized clinical methods, psychological assessments must change in accordance with the changes in clinical practice. Rather than lengthy, broad range assessments, assessment procedures need to be short, practical, and treatment-centered. They asserted that researchers can develop psychological instruments with sound psychometric qualities and sophisticated scoring methods that can truly assist clinicians in selecting appropriate treatments. Maruish (2004) agreed with this analysis and maintained that the field of psychological assessment is moving away from lengthy and time consuming batteries to "brief, inexpensive, yet well-validated instruments" (p. 45). These brief problem-oriented assessments have the potential to be used in not only identifying client problems, but also for monitoring treatment progress and outcome assessment.

Increasing Demands for Accountability

Indications are that, in the future, practitioners will continue to need to provide sound accountability information that documents the effectiveness of counseling. In all likelihood, administrators of managed health care organizations, school boards, and even clients will increasingly want proof that the services counselors provide are worth the cost. Researchers are refining methods of outcome assessment, and clinicians may be wise to incorporate these methods into their practice. Whiston (2002b) urged school counselors to start using standardized outcome measures, because the field of school counseling has only recently begun to see the need to collect systematic accountability information. As compared to other areas of counseling (e.g., individual counseling or career counseling), school counseling has very few outcome instruments that have much evidence of reliability and validity. For counselors in community and mental health settings, there are also new directions in accountability assessment. In the future, there is probably going to be less focus on statistical significance and more emphasis on clinical significance (i.e., evidence that people are feeling and behaving differently). There will also probably be increasing scrutiny of costs and pressures to show that counseling not only helps people but is also cost effective.

Advances in technology may also change how accountability information is gathered. Some publishers are developing computer-assisted assessment programs that provide treatment planning information and accountability data. The assessment of counseling outcomes does not only produce accountability data, it also provides information that clinicians can use to increase their own effectiveness. It is anticipated that there will be increasing demands for accountability information and, hopefully, counselors will use technology, clinical experience, and creativity to identify efficient and sound methods for gathering this essential information.

Alternative Methods for Multicultural Assessment

In many sections of this book, issues related to multicultural assessment have been discussed. As we move toward a more global society, the issues in multicultural assessment become even more complex. Developing instruments that may be appropriate for children in China, Sri Lanka, Poland, and Uganda is especially difficult. Yet, as the field of counseling becomes more international, issues related to multicultural assessment must continue to be studied. One issue related to multicultural assessment concerns the development of appropriate norming groups. The determination of whether to use separate norms or combined norms is complex and has no simple solutions. Counselors must look at the situation and the type of information needed to determine the appropriate norming group. In addition, there may be times when an appropriate norming group is not available. In this case, the practitioner must sort out what information can be appropriately inferred from the client's results. Refinement of testing techniques, such as instruments based on item response theory, may provide better methods for assessing clients from diverse backgrounds. On the other hand, counselors must recognize and respect differences in culture and worldview and not assume there is homogeneity in all psychological constructs.

Future research may help guide practitioners in the complicated clinical decisions associated with multicultural assessment. Additional research may aid clinicians in understanding different cultures and in deciding which instruments provide the most pertinent information. Research may also assist practitioners by identifying other information germane to the interpretation of assessment results of clients from certain cultures. There are many individuals in the field of assessment that are dedicated to providing practitioners with better methods of assessing *all* clients.

Assessment of Older Clients

The term *multicultural* is often applied to many differences among people (e.g., sexual orientation) and many counselors would say that acknowledging ageism would fall under the umbrella of multicultural assessment. There are popular magazine articles in which 60 is labeled the new 40, and stereotypes about the physical and mental health of older adults are debated. With people living longer and with the baby boomer generation now in their 50s and 60s, a growing number of counselors need assessment skills related to older clients. It is important to note that assessments of neurological impairments are complex and should be conducted by individuals with substantial training in neuropsychology; counselors will need more training in assessment of older individuals and to understand when referral to a neuropsychologist is warranted.

In attempting to assess older adults, some counselors may have difficulty in distinguishing between grief, loss and loneliness, and depression. According to Bartels, Blow, Brockmann, and Van Citters (2005) one in four older adults has a mental disorder and the most prevalent disorders are depression, anxiety, and dementia. The Drug and Alcohol Services Information System (2007) found that around 10% of those admitted to substance abuse treatment facilities were aged 50 or older. In addition, Bartels et al. found high rates of co-occuring mental health and substance use disorders and projected that these numbers will increase as the baby boomers age. Bartels et al. called for the development of innovative and effective screening methods for mental health and substance misuse among older individuals.

Expansion of Authentic/Performance Assessment

The 1990s movement toward authentic or performance-based assessment is directly related to the concept that better assessment is performed through the gathering of multiple measures of an individual's performance. The intent of these strategies is to assess the individual in a real or authentic manner; hence, the assessment strategy should match the skill or process being measured. In addition, performance-based or authentic assessment employs context-sensitive strategies focusing on higher-order or more complex skills. Researchers are beginning to explore methods for evaluating the psychometric qualities of these assessment strategies. It is anticipated that researchers will develop standardized authentic/performance assessments. These standardized assessments will be psychometrically sound and will have established criteria for evaluating the aspects of the assessment. Attempting to measure in a real or authentic manner does not guarantee that the assessment is valid. In all likelihood, however, there will be well-established and well-researched authentic/performance assessments in the future.

Performance or authentic assessment has had a significant influence on assessment in the area of achievement (Baker, O'Neil, & Linn, 1993). This philosophy of assessment may influence other areas of assessment, such as personality and intelligence. In counseling, it may be helpful to systematically gather context-sensitive or real-life information. In many ways, counselors have attempted to implement various concepts of authentic or performance assessment for many years. In the future, however, researchers may provide more insights into how to systematically use authentic assessment in counseling.

Positive Psychology

Assessment in counseling is often associated with identifying clients' issues, limitations, or psychopathology. Lopez et al. (2003) argued that this focus on weakness is an unbalanced approach to assessment that ignores vital client characteristics that are particularly important in the therapeutic process. Substantial research indicates that a sense of optimism has many positive effects on individuals' abilities to cope with and address difficult situations (Seligman, 1998). Other strengths that could be assessed include hope or a sense of hopefulness, courage, love, empathy, and a sense of gratitude. In many ways, this focus on strengths is the antithesis of traditional diagnosis and of the *DSM*, which focuses on the identification of disorders. A positive psychology approach to assessment does not ignore problems in functioning; rather, it strives to achieve a "vital balance" that incorporates client resources and assets. Snyder et al. (2003) contended that positive assessment can foster a constructive counseling process in which there is a sense of healing and buoyancy that begins in the initial sessions.

Rise of New Ethical and Legal Issues

Although it would be desirable to predict that all assessment instruments will be used in an ethical manner in the future, the history of assessment does not support this prediction. Even as far back as 2,000 years ago, there is evidence that there were concerns about the ethical use of the Chinese civil service examination (Bowman, 1989). As technology becomes more intertwined in many types of testing, new ethical issues will probably arise. For example, as mentioned earlier, online assessment poses new dilemmas related to privacy and confidentiality.

Assessment training and competencies may be a focus of ethical concerns in the coming years. It is anticipated that there will be continued efforts to legally restrict counselors' use of assessment measures. Therefore, counselors need to document that they have received adequate training and are competent. However, little research has established what constitutes adequate training. There is research (e.g., Moreland et al., 1995) that provides some insight into assessment competencies, yet additional inquiry is needed in this area. In the future, we may know more about the skills necessary for assessing clients effectively. Additional research is also needed on communicating assessment results to clients. As a general guideline for interpreting results to clients, counselors should encourage a therapeutic dialogue between themselves and the client, with both participants exploring and investigating possible meanings and the applicability of the results (Martin, Prupas, & Sugarman, 1999). We, however, need additional research comparing methods of providing assessment results and determining if there are interactions among methods of providing information and types of clients (e.g., males as compared to females).

Summary

This chapter explored current practices in using computers and other technologies in assessment and examined future trends in the field. In this chapter, the term *technology* is used to include both computer- and Internet-based applications. In the past five years, more publishers of formal psychological assessments have made many assessments available on-line. With many of these assessments, the client can take the assessment on-line and then the clinician receives the results in a matter of seconds.

In considering whether to use a technology-based assessment, clinicians need to consider the advantages and disadvantages of the technology in the assessment process. Computer-administered assessments can sometimes save time for clients and clinicians may be able to access a wider spectrum of assessments more easily by using the Internet. In addition, computers can perform complex scoring and interpretation functions quickly, without the errors to which humans are prone. When using technology, such as computer-administered assessments, these approaches often reduce bias because computer scoring does not typically vary based on an individual's race, gender, or sexual orientation. Furthermore, Internet-based assessments often can assist researchers in gathering larger and more diverse samples and may facilitate the gathering of complex reliability and validity evidence. New technology may lead to instruments with better psychometric characteristics and more inventive and informative methods of assessment.

There are, however, some limitations in using technological applications in appraisal and often clinicians need to be more vigilant in using such an assessment. Often some information is lost when a clinician does not observe clients while they are taking computer-administered assessments. The psychometric qualities of any instrument must be evaluated before it is used (this also applies to a computerized instruments). If the instrument is an adaptation of a paper-and-pencil version, then the equivalence of the two forms must be evaluated. Computers are increasingly being used not only to provide results but also to provide interpretive reports. A counselor viewing a computer-generated report must evaluate the quality and content of that report. Many community and school counselors have demanding schedules, and they may be tempted to rely on computer-generated results and interpretations without knowing the strengths and limitations of the instrument. This is the type of situation that may lead to clients not understanding the results or more onerous outcomes where clients make ill-informed decisions or flawed decisions are made about a client (e.g., hospitalization or misdiagnosis of a learning disability). Moreover, in using technology-based assessments, clinicians also need to consider confidentiality and electronic security. Once again, a clinician must take the time to ensure that the assessment system complies with professional standards and that there is adequate oversight of the computer to deter any attempted nonprofessional hacking into the assessment system.

An issue in Internet assessment concerns counselors' roles in protecting the public and the marketing of assessments that may appear professional but are not psychometrically sound assessments. The possibility exists that people are using unsound instruments, and the field needs to consider developing methods to protect the public from fraudulent instruments.

The second segment of this chapter concerned future trends and directions in the field of appraisal. Technological changes will probably affect the delivery of assessment services in the future. Some of those changes may involve more sophisticated computer software and advances in video technology. It is clear that in the coming years, technological advances will continue to have a significant influence on assessment in counseling. Professionals need to ensure that these advances are used in the best interests of clients. It is anticipated that multicultural assessment will be the focus of future research. Given our increasingly global society and the changing demographics in the United States, there will probably be more demands for effective methods of assessing clients from diverse cultures. Counselors also need to be aware of the changing demographics in terms of age and the likelihood that they will be working with older clients. There is some speculation that authentic or performance-based assessment will continue to be influential and will affect other assessment areas. Some of the ideas from authentic or performance-based assessment may have an impact on the methods used in assessment in counseling. The ethical delivery of assessment services will continue to be a professional issue in the coming decades. It is hoped that research will provide insight into ethical practices and needed competencies.

Concluding Remarks

In this book, I have argued that assessment is an integral part of the counseling process and that counselors need to be skilled assessors. To provide effective counseling services, counselors must first assess the client. For counselors, competency in both formal and informal assessment techniques is a necessity in today's mental health care environment. Often formal and informal assessment strategies can complement each other, resulting in assessments that are more effective. Informal assessments are subject to counselor bias and typically lack reliability and validation evidence. Formal assessment instruments, though typically objective, are often narrow in focus and cannot measure all client factors. The purpose of this book is to assist counseling students, counselors, and others in the helping professions to become skillful consumers of assessment measures. By using assessment measures effectively, practitioners can assist clients in making decisions, solving problems, functioning more effectively, and achieving their potential.

As I close this book, I want to encourage readers to consider their future clients. In terms of assessment skills, each counselor has strengths and limitations, and it is important for you to consider what your strengths and limitations are in this area. In considering your professional future, you need to look at methods for expanding those strengths in assessment and identify avenues for remediating your limitations. All of your clients deserve professional and ethical counseling services, which can be facilitated by the development of competent assessment skills. Therefore, I want to encourage you to continue to expand your assessment skills.

APPENDIX A

Table of Areas under the Normal Curve

z	.00	.01	.02	.03	.04	.05	.06	.07	.08	.09
−3.0	.0013	.0013	.0013	.0012	.0012	.0011	.0011	.0011	.0010	.0010
−2.9	.0019	.0018	.0018	.0017	.0016	.0016	.0015	.0015	.0014	.0014
−2.8	.0026	.0025	.0024	.0023	.0023	.0022	.0021	.0021	.0020	.0019
−2.7	.0035	.0034	.0033	.0032	.0031	.0030	.0029	.0028	.0027	.0026
−2.6	.0047	.0045	.0044	.0043	.0041	.0040	.0039	.0038	.0037	.0036
−2.5	.0062	.0060	.0059	.0057	.0055	.0054	.0052	.0051	.0049	.0048
−2.4	.0082	.0080	.0078	.0075	.0077	.0071	.0069	.0068	.0066	.0064
−2.3	.0107	.0104	.0102	.0099	.0096	.0094	.0091	.0089	.0087	.0084
−2.2	.0139	.0136	.0132	.0129	.0125	.0122	.0119	.0116	.0113	.0110
−2.1	.0179	.0174	.0170	.0166	.0162	.0158	.0154	.0150	.0146	.0143
−2.0	.0228	.0222	.0217	.0212	.0207	.0202	.0197	.0192	.0188	.0183
−1.9	.0287	.0281	.0274	.0268	.0262	.0256	.0250	.0244	.0239	.0233
−1.8	.0359	.0351	.0344	.0336	.0329	.0322	.0314	.0307	.0301	.0294
−1.7	.0446	.0436	.0427	.0418	.0409	.0401	.0392	.0384	.0375	.0367
−1.6	.0548	.0537	.0526	.0516	.0505	.0495	.0485	.0475	.0465	.0455
−1.5	.0668	.0655	.0643	.0630	.0618	.0606	.0594	.0582	.0571	.0559
−1.4	.0808	.0793	.0778	.0764	.0749	.0735	.0721	.0708	.0694	.0681
−1.3	.0968	.0951	.0934	.0918	.0901	.0885	.0869	.0853	.0838	.0823
−1.2	.1151	.1131	.1112	.1093	.1075	.1056	.1038	.1020	.1003	.0985
−1.1	.1357	.1335	.1314	.1292	.1271	.1251	.1230	.1210	.1190	.1170
−1.0	.1587	.1562	.1539	.1515	.1492	.1469	.1446	.1423	.1401	.1379
−0.9	.1841	.1814	.1788	.1762	.1736	.1711	.1685	.1660	.1635	.1611
−0.8	.2119	.2090	.2061	.2033	.2005	.1977	.1949	.1922	.1894	.1867
−0.7	.2420	.2389	.2358	.2327	.2296	.2266	.2236	.2206	.2177	.2148
−0.6	.2743	.2709	.2676	.2643	.2611	.2578	.2546	.2514	.2483	.2451
−0.5	.3085	.3050	.3015	.2981	.2946	.2912	.2877	.2843	.2810	.2776
−0.4	.3446	.3409	.3372	.3336	.3300	.3264	.3228	.3194	.3156	.3121
−0.3	.3821	.3783	.3745	.3707	.3669	.3632	.3594	.3557	.3520	.3483
−0.2	.4207	.4168	.4129	.4090	.4052	.4013	.3974	.3936	.3897	.3859
−0.1	.4602	.4562	.4522	.4483	.4443	.4404	.4364	.4325	.4286	.4247
−0.0	.5000	.4960	.4920	.4880	.4840	.4801	.4761	.4721	.4681	.4641
0.0	.5000	.5040	.5080	.5120	.5160	.5199	.5239	.5279	.5319	.5359
0.1	.5398	.5438	.5478	.5517	.5557	.5596	.5636	.5675	.5714	.5753
0.2	.5793	.5832	.5871	.5910	.5948	.5987	.6026	.6064	.6103	.6141
0.3	.6179	.6217	.6255	.6293	.6331	.6368	.6406	.6443	.6480	.6517
0.4	.6554	.6591	.6628	.6664	.6700	.6736	.6772	.6808	.6844	.6879
0.5	.6915	.6950	.6985	.7019	.7054	.7088	.7123	.7157	.7190	.7224

z	.00	.01	.02	.03	.04	.05	.06	.07	.08	.09
0.6	.7257	.7291	.7324	.7357	.7389	.7422	.7454	.7486	.7517	.7549
0.7	.7580	.7611	.7642	.7673	.7704	.7734	.7764	.7794	.7823	.7852
0.8	.7881	.7910	.7939	.7967	.7995	.8023	.8051	.8078	.8106	.8133
0.9	.8159	.8186	.8212	.8238	.8264	.8289	.8315	.8340	.8365	.8389
1.0	.8413	.8438	.8461	.8485	.8508	.8531	.8554	.8577	.8599	.8621
1.1	.8643	.8665	.8686	.8708	.8729	.8749	.8770	.8790	.8810	.8830
1.2	.8849	.8869	.8888	.8907	.8925	.8944	.8962	.8980	.8997	.9015
1.3	.9032	.9049	.9066	.9082	.9099	.9115	.9131	.9147	.9162	.9177
1.4	.9192	.9207	.9222	.9236	.9251	.9265	.9279	.9292	.9306	.9319
1.5	.9332	.9345	.9357	.9370	.9382	.9394	.9406	.9418	.9429	.9441
1.6	.9452	.9463	.9474	.9484	.9495	.9505	.9515	.9525	.9535	.9545
1.7	.9554	.9564	.9573	.9582	.9591	.9599	.9608	.9616	.9625	.9633
1.8	.9641	.9649	.9656	.9664	.9671	.9678	.9686	.9693	.9699	.9706
1.9	.9713	.9719	.9726	.9732	.9738	.9744	.9750	.9756	.9761	.9767
2.0	.9772	.9778	.9783	.9788	.9793	.9798	.9803	.9808	.9812	.9817
2.1	.9821	.9826	.9830	.9834	.9838	.9842	.9846	.9850	.9854	.9857
2.2	.9861	.9864	.9868	.9871	.9875	.9878	.9881	.9884	.9887	.9890
2.3	.9893	.9896	.9898	.9901	.9904	.9906	.9909	.9911	.9913	.9916
2.4	.9918	.9920	.9922	.9925	.9927	.9929	.9931	.9932	.9934	.9936
2.5	.9938	.9940	.9941	.9943	.9945	.9946	.9948	.9949	.9951	.9952
2.6	.9953	.9955	.9956	.9957	.9959	.9960	.9961	.9962	.9963	.9964
2.7	.9965	.9966	.9967	.9968	.9969	.9970	.9971	.9972	.9973	.9974
2.8	.9974	.9975	.9976	.9977	.9977	.9978	.9979	.9979	.9980	.9981
2.9	.9981	.9982	.9982	.9983	.9984	.9984	.9985	.9985	.9986	.9986
3.0	.9987	.9987	.9987	.9988	.9988	.9989	.9989	.9989	.9990	.9990

APPENDIX B

Code of Fair Testing Practices in Education

The Code of Fair Testing Practices in Education (Code) is a guide for professionals in fulfilling their obligation to provide and use tests that are fair to all test takers regardless of age, gender, disability, race, ethnicity, national origin, religion, sexual orientation, linguistic background, or other personal characteristics. Fairness is a primary consideration in all aspects of testing. Careful standardization of tests and administration conditions helps to ensure that all test takers are given a comparable opportunity to demonstrate what they know and how they can perform in the area being tested. Fairness implies that every test taker has the opportunity to prepare for the test and is informed about the general nature and content of the test, as appropriate to the purpose of the test. Fairness also extends to the accurate reporting of individual and group test results. Fairness is not an isolated concept, but must be considered in all aspects of the testing process.

The Code has been prepared by the Joint Committee on Testing Practices, a cooperative effort among several professional organizations. The aim of the Joint Committee is to act, in the public interest, to advance the quality of testing practices. Members of the Joint Committee include the American Counseling Association (ACA), the American Educational Research Association (AERA), the American Psychological Association (APA), the American Speech-Language-Hearing Association (ASHA), the National Association of School Psychologists (NASP), the National Association of Test Directors (NATD), and the National Council on Measurement in Education (NCME).

The *Code* applies broadly to testing in education (admissions, educational assessment, educational diagnosis, and student placement) regardless of the mode of presentation, so it is relevant to conventional paper-and-pencil tests, computer-based tests, and performance tests. It is not designed to cover employment testing, licensure or certification testing, or other types of testing outside the field of education. The *Code* is directed primarily at professionally developed tests used in formally administered testing programs. Although the *Code* is not intended to cover tests prepared by teachers for use in their own classrooms, teachers are encouraged to use the guidelines to help improve their testing practices.

The *Code* addresses the roles of test developers and test users separately. Test developers are people and organizations that construct tests, as well as those that set policies for testing programs. Test users are people and agencies that select tests, administer tests, commission test development services, or make decisions on the basis of test scores. Test developer and test user roles may overlap, for example, when a state or local education agency commissions test development services, sets policies that control the test development process, and makes decisions on the basis of the test scores.

Many of the statements in the *Code* refer to the selection and use of existing tests. When a new test is developed, when an existing test is modified, or when the administration of a test is modified, the *Code* is intended to provide guidance for this process.*

The *Code* provides guidance separately for test developers and test users in four critical areas:

A. Developing and Selecting Appropriate Tests

B. Administering and Scoring Tests

C. Reporting and Interpreting Test Results

D. Informing Test Takers

The *Code* is intended to be consistent with the relevant parts of the Standards for Educational and Psychological Testing (American Educational Research Association [AERA], American Psychological Association [APA], and National Council on Measurement in Education [NCME], 1999). The *Code* is not meant to add new principles over and above those in the Standards or to change their meaning. Rather, the *Code* is intended to represent the spirit of selected portions of the Standards in a way that is relevant and meaningful to developers and users of tests, as well as to test takers and/or their parents or guardians. States, districts, schools, organizations and individual professionals are encouraged to commit themselves to fairness in testing and safeguarding the rights of test takers. The *Code* is intended to assist in carrying out such commitments.

---

* The Code is not intended to be mandatory, exhaustive, or definitive, and may not be applicable to every situation. Instead, the Code is intended to be aspirational, and is not intended to take precedence over the judgment of those who have competence in the subjects addressed.

A. Developing and Selecting Appropriate Tests

Test Developers

Test developers should provide the information and supporting evidence that test users need to select appropriate tests.

1. Provide evidence of what the test measures, the recommended uses, the intended test takers, and the strengths and limitations of the test, including the level of precision of the test scores.
2. Describe how the content and skills to be tested were selected and how the tests were developed.
3. Communicate information about a test's characteristics at a level of detail appropriate to the intended test users.
4. Provide guidance on the levels of skills, knowledge, and training necessary for appropriate review, selection, and administration of tests.
5. Provide evidence that the technical quality, including reliability and validity, of the test meets its intended purposes.
6. Provide to qualified test users representative samples of test questions or practice tests, directions, answer sheets, manuals, and score reports.
7. Avoid potentially offensive content or language when developing test questions and related materials.
8. Make appropriately modified forms of tests or administration procedures available for test takers with disabilities who need special accommodations.
9. Obtain and provide evidence on the performance of test takers of diverse subgroups, making significant efforts to obtain sample sizes that are adequate for subgroup analyses. Evaluate the evidence to ensure that differences in performance are related to the skills being assessed.

Test Users

Test users should select tests that meet the intended purpose and that are appropriate for the intended test takers.

1. Define the purpose for testing, the content and skills to be tested, and the intended test takers. Select and use the most appropriate test based on a thorough review of available information.
2. Review and select tests based on the appropriateness of test content, skills tested, and content coverage for the intended purpose of testing.
3. Review materials provided by test developers and select tests for which clear, accurate, and complete information is provided.
4. Select tests through a process that includes persons with appropriate knowledge, skills, and training.
5. Evaluate evidence of the technical quality of the test provided by the test developer and any independent reviewers.
6. Evaluate representative samples of test questions or practice tests, directions, answer sheets, manuals, and score reports before selecting a test.

7. Evaluate procedures and materials used by test developers, as well as the resulting test, to ensure that potentially offensive content or language is avoided.
8. Select tests with appropriately modified forms or administration procedures for test takers with disabilities who need special accommodations.
9. Evaluate the available evidence on the performance of test takers of diverse subgroups. Determine to the extent feasible which performance differences may have been caused by factors unrelated to the skills being assessed.

B. Administering and Scoring Tests

Test Developers

Test developers should explain how to administer and score tests correctly and fairly.

1. Provide clear descriptions of detailed procedures for administering tests in a standardized manner.
2. Provide guidelines on reasonable procedures for assessing persons with disabilities who need special accommodations or those with diverse linguistic backgrounds.
3. Provide information to test takers or test users on test question formats and procedures for answering test questions, including information on the use of any needed materials and equipment.
4. Establish and implement procedures to ensure the security of testing materials during all phases of test development, administration, scoring, and reporting.
5. Provide procedures, materials, and guidelines for scoring the tests and for monitoring the accuracy of the scoring process. If scoring the test is the responsibility of the test developer, provide adequate training for scorers.
6. Correct errors that affect the interpretation of the scores and communicate the corrected results promptly.
7. Develop and implement procedures for ensuring the confidentiality of scores.

Test Users

Test users should administer and score tests correctly and fairly.

1. Follow established procedures for administering tests in a standardized manner.
2. Provide and document appropriate procedures for test takers with disabilities who need special accommodations or those with diverse linguistic backgrounds. Some accommodations may be required by law or regulation.
3. Provide test takers with an opportunity to become familiar with test question formats and any materials or equipment that may be used during testing.
4. Protect the security of test materials, including respecting copyrights and eliminating opportunities for test takers to obtain scores by fraudulent means.
5. If test scoring is the responsibility of the test user, provide adequate training to scorers and ensure and monitor the accuracy of the scoring process.

6. Correct errors that affect the interpretation of the scores and communicate the corrected results promptly.
7. Develop and implement procedures for ensuring the confidentiality of scores.

C. Reporting and Interpreting Test Results

Test Developers

Test developers should report test results accurately and provide information to help test users interpret test results correctly.

1. Provide information to support recommended interpretations of the results, including the nature of the content, norms or comparison groups, and other technical evidence. Advise test users of the benefits and limitations of test results and their interpretation. Warn against assigning greater precision than is warranted.
2. Provide guidance regarding the interpretations of results for tests administered with modifications. Inform test users of potential problems in interpreting test results when tests or test administration procedures are modified.
3. Specify appropriate uses of test results and warn test users of potential misuses.
4. When test developers set standards, provide the rationale, procedures, and evidence for setting performance standards or passing scores. Avoid using stigmatizing labels.
5. Encourage test users to base decisions about test takers on multiple sources of appropriate information, not on a single test score.
6. Provide information to enable test users to accurately interpret and report test results for groups of test takers, including information about who were and who were not included in the different groups being compared and information about factors that might influence the interpretation of results.
7. Provide test results in a timely fashion and in a manner that is understood by the test taker.
8. Provide guidance to test users about how to monitor the extent to which the test is fulfilling its intended purposes.

Test Users

Test users should report and interpret test results accurately and clearly.

1. Interpret the meaning of the test results, taking into account the nature of the content, norms or comparison groups, other technical evidence, and benefits and limitations of test results.
2. Interpret test results from modified test or test administration procedures in view of the impact those modifications may have had on test results.

3. Avoid using tests for purposes other than those recommended by the test developer unless there is evidence to support the intended use or interpretation.
4. Review the procedures for setting performance standards or passing scores. Avoid using stigmatizing labels.
5. Avoid using a single test score as the sole determinant of decisions about test takers. Interpret test scores in conjunction with other information about individuals.
6. State the intended interpretation and use of test results for groups of test takers. Avoid grouping test results for purposes not specifically recommended by the test developer unless evidence is obtained to support the intended use. Report procedures that were followed in determining who were and who were not included in the groups being compared and describe factors that might influence the interpretation of results.
7. Communicate test results in a timely fashion and in a manner that is understood by the test taker.
8. Develop and implement procedures for monitoring test use, including consistency with the intended purposes of the test.

D. Informing Test Takers

Under some circumstances, test developers have direct communication with the test takers and/or control of the tests, testing process, and test results. In other circumstances the test users have these responsibilities.

Test developers or test users should inform test takers about the nature of the test, test taker rights and responsibilities, the appropriate use of scores, and procedures for resolving challenges to scores.

1. Inform test takers in advance of the test administration about the coverage of the test, the types of question formats, the directions, and appropriate test-taking strategies. Make such information available to all test takers.
2. When a test is optional, provide test takers or their parents/guardians with information to help them judge whether a test should be taken—including indications of any consequences that may result from not taking the test (e.g., not being eligible to compete for a particular scholarship)—and whether there is an available alternative to the test.
3. Provide test takers or their parents/guardians with information about rights test takers may have to obtain copies of tests and completed answer sheets, to retake tests, to have tests rescored, or to have scores declared invalid.
4. Provide test takers or their parents/guardians with information about responsibilities test takers have, such as being aware of the intended purpose and uses of the test, performing at capacity, following directions, and not disclosing test items or interfering with other test takers.
5. Inform test takers or their parents/guardians how long scores will be kept on file and indicate to whom, under what circumstances, and in what

manner test scores and related information will or will not be released. Protect test scores from unauthorized release and access.

6. Describe procedures for investigating and resolving circumstances that might result in canceling or withholding scores, such as failure to adhere to specified testing procedures.
7. Describe procedures that test takers, parents/guardians, and other interested parties may use to obtain more information about the test, register complaints, and have problems resolved.

Working Group

Note: The membership of the working group that developed the Code of Fair Testing Practices in Education and of the Joint Committee on Testing Practices that guided the working group is as follows:

Peter Behuniak, PhD
Lloyd Bond, PhD
Gwyneth M. Boodoo, PhD
Wayne Camara, PhD
Ray Fenton, PhD
John J. Fremer, PhD (Cochair)
Sharon M. Goldsmith, PhD
Bert F. Green, PhD
William G. Harris, PhD
Janet E. Helms, PhD
Stephanie H. McConaughy, PhD
Julie P. Noble, PhD
Wayne M. Patience, PhD
Carole L. Perlman, PhD
Douglas K. Smith, PhD
Janet E. Wall, EdD (Cochair)
Pat Nellor Wickwire, PhD
Mary Yakimowski, PhD
Lara Frumkin, PhD, of the APA, served as staff liaison.

The Joint Committee intends that the *Code* be consistent with and supportive of existing codes of conduct and standards of other professional groups who use tests in educational contexts. Of particular note are the Responsibilities of Users of Standardized Tests (Association for Assessment in Counseling and Education, 2003), APA Test User Qualifications (2000), ASHA Code of Ethics (2001), Ethical Principles of Psychologists and Code of Conduct (1992), NASP Professional Conduct Manual (2000), NCME Code of Professional Responsibility (1995), and Rights and Responsibilities of Test Takers: Guidelines and Expectations (Joint Committee on Testing Practices, 2000).

APPENDIX C

American Counseling Association Code of Ethics

Section E: Evaluation, Assessment, and Interpretation

Introduction

Counselors use assessment instruments as one component of the counseling process, taking into account the client personal and cultural context. Counselors promote the well-being of individual clients or groups of clients by developing and using appropriate educational, psychological, and career assessment instruments.

E.1. General

E.1.a. Assessment

The primary purpose of educational, psychological, and career assessment is to provide measurements that are valid and reliable in either comparative or absolute terms. These include, but are not limited to, measurements of ability, personality, interest, intelligence, achievement, and performance. Counselors recognize the need to interpret the statements in this section as applying to both quantitative and qualitative assessments.

E.1.b. Client welfare

Counselors do not misuse assessment results and interpretations, and they take reasonable steps to prevent others from misusing the information these techniques provide. They respect the client's right to know the results, the interpretations made, and the bases for counselors' conclusions and recommendations.

E.2. Competence to Use and Interpret Assessment Instruments

E.2.a. Limits of competence

Counselors utilize only those testing and assessment services for which they have been trained and are competent. Counselors using technology assisted test interpretations are trained in the construct being measured and the specific instrument being used prior to using its technology based application. Counselors take reasonable measures to ensure the proper use of psychological and career assessment techniques by persons under their supervision. *(See A.12.)*

E.2.b. Appropriate use

Counselors are responsible for the appropriate application, scoring, interpretation, and use of assessment instruments relevant to the needs of the client, whether they score and interpret such assessments themselves or use technology or other services.

E.2.c. Decisions based on results

Counselors responsible for decisions involving individuals or policies that are based on assessment results have a thorough understanding of educational, psychological, and career measurement, including validation criteria, assessment research, and guidelines for assessment development and use.

E.3. Informed Consent in Assessment

E.3.a. Explanation to clients

Prior to assessment, counselors explain the nature and purposes of assessment and the specific use of results by potential recipients. The explanation will be given in the language of the client (or other legally authorized person on behalf of the client), unless an explicit exception has been agreed upon in advance. Counselors consider the client's personal or cultural context, the level of the client's understanding of the results, and the impact of the results on the client. *(See A.2., A.12.g., F.1.c.)*

E.3.b. Recipients of results

Counselors consider the examinee's welfare, explicit understandings, and prior agreements in determining who receives the assessment results. Counselors include accurate and appropriate interpretations with any release of individual or group assessment results. *(See B.2.c., B.5.)*

E.4. Release of Data to Qualified Professionals

Counselors release assessment data in which the client is identified only with the consent of the client or the client's legal representative. Such data are released only to persons recognized by counselors as qualified to interpret the data. *(See B.1., B.3., B.6.b.)*

E.5. Diagnosis of Mental Disorders

E.5.a. Proper diagnosis

Counselors take special care to provide proper diagnosis of mental disorders. Assessment techniques (including personal interview) used to determine client care (e.g., locus of treatment, type of treatment, or recommended follow-up) are carefully selected and appropriately used.

E.5.b. Cultural sensitivity

Counselors recognize that culture affects the manner in which clients' problems are defined. Clients' socioeconomic and cultural experiences are considered when diagnosing mental disorders. *(See A.2.c.)*

E.5.c. Historical and social prejudices in the diagnosis of pathology

Counselors recognize historical and social prejudices in the misdiagnosis and pathologizing of certain individuals and groups and the role of mental health professionals in perpetuating these prejudices through diagnosis and treatment.

E.5.d. Refraining from diagnosis

Counselors may refrain from making and/or reporting a diagnosis if they believe it would cause harm to the client or others.

E.6. Instrument Selection

E.6.a. Appropriateness of instruments

Counselors carefully consider the validity, reliability, psychometric limitations, and appropriateness of instruments when selecting assessments.

E.6.b. Referral information

If a client is referred to a third party for assessment, the counselor provides specific referral questions and sufficient objective data about the client to ensure that appropriate assessment instruments are utilized. *(See A.9.b., B.3.)*

E.6.c. Culturally diverse populations

Counselors are cautious when selecting assessments for culturally diverse populations to avoid the use of instruments that lack appropriate psychometric properties for the client population. *(See A.2.c., E.5.b.)*

E.7. Conditions of Assessment Administration

(See A.12.b., A.12.d.)

E.7.a. Administration conditions

Counselors administer assessments under the same conditions that were established in their standardization. When assessments are not administered under standard conditions, as may be necessary to accommodate clients with disabilities, or when unusual behavior or irregularities occur during the administration, those conditions are noted in interpretation, and the results may be designated as invalid or of questionable validity.

E.7.b. Technological administration

Counselors ensure that administration programs function properly and provide clients with accurate results when technological or other electronic methods are used for assessment administration.

E.7.c. Unsupervised assessments

Unless the assessment instrument is designed, intended, and validated for self-administration and/or scoring, counselors do not permit inadequately supervised use.

E.7.d. Disclosure of favorable conditions

Prior to administration of assessments, conditions that produce most favorable assessment results are made known to the examinee.

E.8. Multicultural Issues/Diversity in Assessment

Counselors use with caution assessment techniques that were normed on populations other than that of the client. Counselors recognize the effects of age, color, culture, disability, ethnic group, gender, race, language preference, religion, spirituality, sexual orientation, and socioeconomic status on test administration and interpretation, and place test results in proper perspective with other relevant factors. *(See A.2.c., E.5.b.)*

E.9. Scoring and Interpretation of Assessments

E.9.a. Reporting

In reporting assessment results, counselors indicate reservations that exist regarding validity or reliability due to circumstances of the assessment or the inappropriateness of the norms for the person tested.

E.9.b. Research instruments

Counselors exercise caution when interpreting the results of research instruments not having sufficient technical data to support respondent results. The specific purposes for the use of such instruments are stated explicitly to the examinee.

E.9.c. Assessment services

Counselors who provide assessment scoring and interpretation services to support the assessment process confirm the validity of such interpretations. They accurately describe the purpose, norms, validity, reliability, and applications of the procedures and any special qualifications applicable to their use. The public offering of an automated test interpretations service is considered a professional-to-professional consultation. The formal responsibility of the consultant is to the consultee, but the ultimate and overriding responsibility is to the client. *(See D.2.)*

E.10. Assessment Security

Counselors maintain the integrity and security of tests and other assessment techniques consistent with legal and contractual obligations. Counselors do not appropriate, reproduce, or modify published assessments or parts thereof without acknowledgment and permission from the publisher.

E.11. Obsolete Assessments and Outdated Results

Counselors do not use data or results from assessments that are obsolete or outdated for the current purpose. Counselors make every effort to prevent the misuse of obsolete measures and assessment data by others.

E.12. Assessment Construction

Counselors use established scientific procedures, relevant standards, and current professional knowledge for assessment design in the development, publication, and utilization of educational and psychological assessment techniques.

E.13. Forensic Evaluation: Evaluation for Legal Proceedings

E.13.a. Primary obligations

When providing forensic evaluations, the primary obligation of counselors is to produce objective findings that can be substantiated based on information and techniques appropriate to the evaluation, which may include examination of the individual and/or review of records. Counselors are entitled to form professional opinions based on their professional knowledge and expertise that can be supported by the data gathered in evaluations. Counselors will define the limits of their reports or testimony, especially when an examination of the individual has not been conducted.

E.13.b. Consent for evaluation

Individuals being evaluated are informed in writing that the relationship is for the purposes of an evaluation and is not counseling in nature, and entities or individuals who will receive the evaluation report are identified. Written consent to be evaluated is obtained from those being evaluated unless a court orders evaluations to be conducted without the written consent of individuals being evaluated. When children or vulnerable adults are being evaluated, informed written consent is obtained from a parent or guardian.

E.13.c. Client evaluation prohibited

Counselors do not evaluate individuals for forensic purposes they currently counsel or individuals they have counseled in the past. Counselors do not accept as counseling clients individuals they are evaluating or individuals they have evaluated in the past for forensic purposes.

E.13.d. Avoid potentially harmful relationships

Counselors who provide forensic evaluations avoid potentially harmful professional or personal relationships with family members, romantic partners, and close friends of individuals they are evaluating or have evaluated in the past.

APPENDIX D

Responsibilities of Users of Standardized Tests (RUST) (3rd Edition)

Prepared by the Association for Assessment in Counseling (AAC)

Many recent events have influenced the use of tests and assessment in the counseling community. Such events include the use of tests in the educational accountability and reform movement, the publication of the *Standards for Educational and Psychological Testing* (American Educational Research Association [AERA], American Psychological Association [APA], National Council on Measurement in Education [NCME], 1999), the revision of the *Code of Fair Testing Practices in Education* (Joint Committee on Testing Practices [JCTP], 2002), the proliferation of technology-delivered assessment, and the historic passage of the *No Child Left Behind Act* (HR1, 2002) calling for expanded testing in reading/language arts, mathematics, and science that are aligned to state standards.

The purpose of this document is to promote the accurate, fair, and responsible use of standardized tests by the counseling and education communities. RUST is intended to address the needs of the members of the American Counseling Association (ACA) and its Divisions, Branches, and Regions, including counselors, teachers, administrators, and other human service workers. The general public, test developers, and policy makers will find this statement useful as they work with tests and testing issues. The principles in RUST apply to the use of testing instruments regardless of delivery methods (e.g., paper/pencil or computer administered) or setting (e.g., group or individual).

The intent of RUST is to help counselors and other educators implement responsible testing practices. The RUST does not intend to reach beyond or reinterpret the principles outlined in the *Standards for Educational and Psychological Testing* (AERA et al., 1999), nor was it developed to formulate a basis for legal action. The intent is to provide a concise statement useful in the ethical practice of testing. In addition, RUST is intended to enhance the guidelines found in ACA's *Code of Ethics and Standards of Practice* (ACA, 1997) and the *Code of Fair Testing Practices in Education* (JCTP, 2002).

Organization of Document: This document includes test user responsibilities in the following areas:

- Qualifications of Test Users
- Technical Knowledge
- Test Selection
- Test Administration
- Test Scoring
- Interpreting Test Results
- Communicating Test Results

Qualifications of Test Users

Qualified test users demonstrate appropriate education, training, and experience in using tests for the purposes under consideration. They adhere to the highest degree of ethical codes, laws, and standards governing professional practice. Lack of essential qualifications or ethical and legal compliance can lead to errors and subsequent harm to clients. Each professional is responsible for making judgments in each testing situation and cannot leave that responsibility either to clients or others in authority. The individual test user must obtain appropriate education and training, or arrange for professional supervision and assistance when engaged in testing in order to provide valuable, ethical, and effective assessment services to the public. Qualifications of test users depend on at least four factors:

- **Purposes of Testing:** A clear purpose for testing should be established. Because the purposes of testing direct how the results are used, qualifications beyond general testing competencies may be needed to interpret and apply data.
- **Characteristics of Tests:** Understanding of the strengths and limitations of each instrument used is a requirement.
- **Settings and Conditions of Test Use:** Assessment of the quality and relevance of test user knowledge and skill to the situation is needed before deciding to test or participate in a testing program.
- **Roles of Test Selectors, Administrators, Scorers, and Interpreters:** The education, training, and experience of test users determine which tests they are qualified to administer and interpret.

Each test user must evaluate his or her qualifications and competence for selecting, administering, scoring, interpreting, reporting, or communicating test results. Test users must develop the skills and knowledge for each test he or she intends to use.

Technical Knowledge

Responsible use of tests requires technical knowledge obtained through training, education, and continuing professional development. Test users should be conversant and competent in aspects of testing including:

- **Validity of Test Results:** Validity is the accumulation of evidence to support a specific interpretation of the test results. Since validity is a characteristic of test results, a test may have validities of varying degree, for different purposes. The concept of instructional validity relates to how well the test is aligned to state standards and classroom instructional objectives.

- **Reliability:** Reliability refers to the consistency of test scores. Various methods are used to calculate and estimate reliability depending on the purpose for which the test is used.
- **Errors of Measurement:** Various ways may be used to calculate the error associated with a test score. Knowing this and knowing the estimate of the size of the error allows the test user to provide a more accurate interpretation of the scores and to support better-informed decisions.
- **Scores and Norms:** Basic differences between the purposes of norm-referenced and criterion-referenced scores impact score interpretations.

Test Selection

Responsible use of tests requires that the specific purpose for testing be identified. In addition, the test that is selected should align with that purpose, while considering the characteristics of the test and the test taker. Tests should not be administered without a specific purpose or need for information. Typical purposes for testing include:

- **Description:** Obtaining objective information on the status of certain characteristics such as achievement, ability, personality types, etc. is often an important use of testing.
- **Accountability:** When judging the progress of an individual or the effectiveness of an educational institution, strong alignment between what is taught and what is tested needs to be present.
- **Prediction:** Technical information should be reviewed to determine how accurately the test will predict areas such as appropriate course placement; selection for special programs, interventions, and institutions; and other outcomes of interest.
- **Program Evaluation:** The role that testing plays in program evaluation and how the test information may be used to supplement other information gathered about the program is an important consideration in test use.

Proper test use involves determining if the characteristics of the test are appropriate for the intended audience and are of sufficient technical quality for the purpose at hand. Some areas to consider include:

- **The Test Taker:** Technical information should be reviewed to determine if the test characteristics are appropriate for the test taker (e.g., age, grade level, language, cultural background).
- **Accuracy of Scoring Procedures:** Only tests that use accurate scoring procedures should be used.
- **Norming and Standardization Procedures:** Norming and standardization procedures should be reviewed to determine if the norm group is appropriate for the intended test takers. Specified test administration procedures must be followed.

- **Modifications:** For individuals with disabilities, alternative measures may need to be found and used and/or accommodations in test taking procedures may need to be employed. Interpretations need to be made in light of the modifications in the test or testing procedures.
- **Fairness:** Care should be taken to select tests that are fair to all test takers. When test results are influenced by characteristics or situations unrelated to what is being measured. (e.g., gender, age, ethnic background, existence of cheating, unequal availability of test preparation programs), the use of the resulting information is invalid and potentially harmful. In achievement testing, fairness also relates to whether or not the student has had an opportunity to learn what is tested.

Test Administration

Test administration includes carefully following standard procedures so that the test is used in the manner specified by the test developers. The test administrator should ensure that test takers work within conditions that maximize opportunity for optimum performance. As appropriate, test takers, parents, and organizations should be involved in the various aspects of the testing process including.

Before administration it is important that relevant persons

- are informed about the standard testing procedures, including information about the purposes of the test, the kinds of tasks involved, the method of administration, and the scoring and reporting;
- have sufficient practice experiences prior to the test to include practice, as needed, on how to operate equipment for computer-administered tests and practice in responding to tasks;
- have been sufficiently trained in their responsibilities and the administration procedures for the test;
- have a chance to review test materials and administration sites and procedures prior to the time for testing to ensure standardized conditions and appropriate responses to any irregularities that occur;
- arrange for appropriate modifications of testing materials and procedures in order to accommodate test takers with special needs; and
- have a clear understanding of their rights and responsibilities.

During administration it is important that

- the testing environment (e.g., seating, work surfaces, lighting, room temperature, freedom from distractions) and psychological climate are conducive to the best possible performance of the examinees;
- sufficiently trained personnel establish and maintain uniform conditions and observe the conduct of test takers when large groups of individuals are tested;
- test administrators follow the instructions in the test manual; demonstrate verbal clarity; use verbatim directions; adhere to verbatim directions; follow exact sequence and timing; and use materials that are identical to those specified by the test publisher;

- a systematic and objective procedure is in place for observing and recording environmental, health, emotional factors, or other elements that may invalidate test performance and results; deviations from prescribed test administration procedures, including information on test accommodations for individuals with special needs, are recorded; and
- the security of test materials and computer-administered testing software is protected, ensuring that only individuals with a legitimate need for access to the materials/software are able to obtain such access and that steps to eliminate the possibility of breaches in test security and copyright protection are respected.

After administration it is important to

- collect and inventory all secure test materials and immediately report any breaches in test security; and
- include notes on any problems, irregularities, and accommodations in the test records.

These precepts represent the basic process for all standardized tests and assessments. Some situations may add steps or modify some of these to provide the best testing milieu possible.

Test Scoring

Accurate measurement necessitates adequate procedures for scoring the responses of test takers. Scoring procedures should be audited as necessary to ensure consistency and accuracy of application.

- Carefully implement and/or monitor standard scoring procedures.
- When test scoring involves human judgment, use rubrics that clearly specify the criteria for scoring. Scoring consistency should be constantly monitored.
- Provide a method for checking the accuracy of scores when accuracy is challenged by test takers.

Interpreting Test Results

Responsible test interpretation requires knowledge about and experience with the test, the scores, and the decisions to be made. Interpretation of scores on any test should not take place without a thorough knowledge of the technical aspects of the test, the test results, and its limitations. Many factors can impact the valid and useful interpretations of test scores. These can be grouped into several categories including psychometric, test taker, and contextual, as well as others.

- **Psychometric Factors:** Factors such as the reliability, norms, standard error of measurement, and validity of the instrument are important when interpreting test results. Responsible test use considers these basic concepts and how each impacts the scores and hence the interpretation of the test results.

- **Test Taker Factors:** Factors such as the test taker's group membership and how that membership may impact the results of the test is a critical factor in the interpretation of test results. Specifically, the test user should evaluate how the test taker's gender, age, ethnicity, race, socioeconomic status, marital status, and so forth, impact on the individual's results.
- **Contextual Factors:** The relationship of the test to the instructional program, opportunity to learn, quality of the educational program, work and home environment, and other factors that would assist in understanding the test results are useful in interpreting test results. For example, if the test does not align to curriculum standards and how those standards are taught in the classroom, the test results may not provide useful information.

Communicating Test Results

Before communication of test results takes place, a solid foundation and preparation is necessary. That foundation includes knowledge of test interpretation and an understanding of the particular test being used, as provided by the test manual.

Conveying test results with language that the test taker, parents, teachers, clients, or general public can understand is one of the key elements in helping others understand the meaning of the test results. When reporting group results, the information needs to be supplemented with background information that can help explain the results with cautions about misinterpretations. The test user should indicate how the test results can be and should not be interpreted.

Closing

Proper test use resides with the test user—the counselor and educator. Qualified test users understand the measurement characteristics necessary to select good standardized tests, administer the tests according to specified procedures, assure accurate scoring, accurately interpret test scores for individuals and groups, and ensure productive applications of the results. This document provides guidelines for using tests responsibly with students and clients.

References and Resource Documents

American Counseling Association. (1997). *Code of ethics and standards of practice.* Alexandria, VA: Author.

American Counseling Association. (2003). *Standards for qualifications of test users.* Alexandria, VA: Author.

American Educational Research Association, American Psychological Association, & National Council on Measurement in Education. (1999). *Standards for educational and psychological testing.* Washington, DC: American Educational Research Association.

American School Counselor Association & Association for Assessment in Counseling. (1998). *Competencies in assessment and evaluation for school counselors.* Alexandria, VA: Author.

Joint Committee on Testing Practices. (2000). *Rights and responsibilities of test takers: Guidelines and expectations.* Washington, DC: Author.

Joint Committee on Testing Practices. (2002). *Code of fair testing practices in education.* Washington, DC: Author.

RUST Committee

Janet Wall, Chair
James Augustin
Charles Eberly
Brad Erford
David Lundberg
Timothy Vansickle

APPENDIX E

Standards for Multicultural Assessment (2nd Ed.)

Preface

The Association for Assessment in Counseling (AAC) is an organization of counselors, counselor educators, and other professionals that advances the counseling profession by providing leadership, training, and research in the creation, development, production, and use of assessment and diagnostic techniques.

The increasing diversity in our society offers a special challenge to the assessment community, striving always to assure fair and equitable treatment of individuals regardless of race, ethnicity, culture, language, age, gender, sexual orientation, religion or physical ability. This is especially important given the increased emphasis place on assessment spawned by national and state legislation and educational reform initiatives.

This document, *Standards for Multicultural Assessment*, is an attempt to create and maintain an awareness of the various assessment standards that have been produced by various professional organizations. It is a compilation of standards produced by several professional associations.

This publication is based on a study completed by the Committee on Diversity in Assessment under the direction of the AAC Executive Council. The first version of this document was published in 1992, and was also published as an article in *Measurement and Evaluation in Counseling and Development* (Prediger, 1994). The original publication was prompted by a request from Jo-Ida Hansen, Chair of the 1991–1992 Committee on Testing of the American Association for Counseling and Development (now ACA). The original publication was prepared by Dale Prediger under the direction of the AAC Executive Council.

Because of advances in professional standards in the past decade, it was necessary to update and expand upon the first version. This revised document was created by a committee of members from the AAC, chaired by Dr. Wendy Charkow-Bordeau along with committee members, Drs. Debbie Newsome and Marie Shoffner. This publication was commissioned by the Executive Council of the Association for Assessment in Counseling.

AAC also wishes to thank Drs. Pat Nellor Wickwire and Janet Wall for their care and assistance in finalizing this document and coordinating its production.

AAC hopes that all counselors, teachers, and other assessment professionals find this document to be useful in improving their assessment practices.

Purpose

The Association for Assessment in Counseling (AAC), a division of the American Counseling Association (ACA), presents this revised compilation of professional standards. Although AAC believes that tests, inventories, and other assessment instruments can be beneficial for members of all populations, AAC recognizes that the increasing diversity in client backgrounds presents special challenges for test users. The standards assembled here address many of these challenges that are specifically related to the assessment of multicultural populations.

Although a number of standards in this compilation have relevance for the use of assessment instruments in psychological screening, personnel selection, and placement, they were selected because they have special relevance for counseling and for multicultural and diverse populations. Standards that apply in the same way for all populations (e.g., general standards for norming, scaling, reliability, and validity) are not included. Readers may consult the source documents and other publications for universal testing standards.

AAC urges all counselors to subscribe to these standards and urges counselor educators to include this compilation in programs preparing the "culturally competent counselor" (Sue, Arredondo, & McDavis, 1992, p. 447). Finally, AAC supports other professional organizations in advocating the need for a multicultural approach to assessment, practice, training, and research.

Definition of Multicultural and Diverse Populations

A precise definition of multicultural and diverse populations is evolving. The multicultural competencies outlined by Sue et al. (1992), and then revised by Arredondo and Toporek (1996), define the following five major cultural groups in the United States and its territories: African/Black, Asian, Caucasian/European, Hispanic/Latino, and Native

American. Arredondo and Toporek differentiated between these cultural groups, which are based on race and ethnicity, and diversity, which applies to individual differences based on age, gender, sexual orientation, religion, and ability or disability.

In revising the *Standards for Multicultural Assessment*, an inclusive definition of multiculturalism and diversity was used. For the purposes of this document, multicultural and diverse populations include persons who differ by race, ethnicity, culture, language, age, gender, sexual orientation, religion, and ability.

Source Documents

Five documents which include professional standards for assessment in counseling were used as sources for this compilation.

1. ***Code of Fair Testing Practices in Education*** (2nd ed.) (CODE). (Joint Committee on Testing Practices [JCTP], 2002). Available for download at http://aac.ncat.edu.
2. ***Responsibilities of Users of Standardized Tests*** (3rd ed.) (RUST). (ACA & AAC, 2003). Available for download at http://aac.ncat.edu.
3. ***Standards for Educational and Psychological Testing*** (2nd ed.) (SEPT). (American Educational Research Association, APA, & National Council on Measurement in Education, 1999). Ordering information is available from APA, 750 First Street, NE, Washington, DC 20002-4242 or online at http://www.apa.org/science/standards.html.
4. ***Multicultural Counseling Competencies and Standards*** (COMPS). (Association for Multicultural Counseling and Development, 1992). These standards can be viewed in the 1996 article by Arredondo and Toporek. Full reference information is listed below in the reference section.
5. ***Code of Ethics and Standards of Practice of the American Counseling Association*** (ETHICS). (ACA, 1996). Ordering information can be obtained from ACA, 5999 Stevenson Avenue, Alexandria, VA, 22304-3300. The ethical code and standards of practice may also be viewed online at [http://www.counseling.org/Files/FD.ashx?guid=ab7c1272-71c4-46cf-848c-f98489937dda]

Classification of Standards

Sixty-eight standards specifically relevant to the assessment of multicultural and diverse populations were identified in a reading of the five source documents. The content and intent of these standards were analyzed and classified. Assessment roles, functions, and tasks cited in these standards were clustered into three major groups.

Selection of Assessment Instruments

- Content and Purpose (n = 13)
- Norming, Reliability, and Validity (n = 18)

Administration and Scoring of Assessment Instruments (n = 16)

- Interpretation and Application of Assessment Results (n = 21)

The Standards

The 68 standards are listed below by cluster and source.

Selection of Assessment Instruments: Content and Purpose

1. Evaluate procedures and materials used by test developers, as well as the resulting test, to ensure that potentially offensive content or language is avoided. (CODE, Section A-7)
2. Select tests with appropriately modified forms or administration procedures for test takers with disabilities who need special accommodations. (CODE, Section A-8)
3. For individuals with disabilities, alternative measures may need to be found and used.
4. Care should be taken to select tests that are fair to all test takers. (RUST)
5. Test developers should strive to identify and eliminate language, symbols, words, phrases, and content that are generally regarded as offensive by members of racial, ethnic, gender, or other groups, except when judged to be necessary for adequate representation of the domain. (SEPT 7.4)
6. In testing applications where the level of linguistic or reading ability is not part of the construct of interest, the linguistic or reading demands of the test should be kept to the minimum necessary for the valid assessment of the intended construct. (SEPT, Standard 7.7)
7. Linguistic modifications recommended by test publishers, as well as the rationale for modifications, should be described in detail in the test manual. (SEPT, Standard 9.4)
8. In employment and credentialing testing, the proficiency language required in the language of the test should not exceed that appropriate to the relevant occupation or profession. (SEPT, Standard 9.8)
9. Inferences about test takers' general language proficiency should be based on tests that measure a range of language features, and not on a single linguistic skill. (SEPT, Standard 9.10)
10. Tests selected for use in individual testing should be suitable for the characteristics and background of the test taker. (SEPT, Standard 12.3)
11. Culturally competent counselors understand how race, culture, and ethnicity may affect personality formation, vocational choices, manifestation of psychological disorders, help-seeking behavior, and the appropriateness or inappropriateness of counseling approaches. (COMPS, 13)
12. Culturally competent counselors have training and expertise in the use of traditional assessment and testing instruments. They not only understand the technical aspects of the instruments but also are aware of the cultural limitations. This allows them to use test instruments for the welfare of clients from diverse cultural, racial, and ethnic groups. (COMPS, 29)
13. Counselors are cautious when selecting tests for culturally diverse populations to avoid inappropriateness of testing that may be outside of socialized behavioral or cognitive patterns. (ETHICS, Section III.C.5)

Selection of Assessment Instruments: Norming, Reliability, and Validity

1. Evaluate the available evidence on the performance of test takers of diverse subgroups. Determine to the extent feasible which performance differences may have been caused by factors unrelated to skills being assessed. (CODE, Section A-9).
2. Technical information should be reviewed to determine if the test characteristics are appropriate for the test taker (e.g., age, grade level, language, cultural background). (RUST)
3. Where there are generally accepted theoretical or empirical reasons for expecting that reliability coefficients, standard errors of measurement, or test information functions will differ substantially for various subpopulations, publishers should provide reliability data as soon as feasible for each major population for which the test is recommended. (SEPT, Standard 2.11)
4. If a test is proposed for use in several grades or over a range of chronological age groups and if separate norms are provided for each grade or age group, reliability data should be provided for each age or grade population, not solely for all grades or ages combined. (SEPT, Standard 2.12)
5. When significant variations are permitted in test administration procedures, separate reliability analyses should be provided for scores produced under each major variation if adequate sample sizes are available. (SEPT, Standard 2.18)
6. Norms, if used, should refer to clearly described populations. These populations should include individuals or groups to whom test users will ordinarily wish to compare their own examinees. (SEPT, Standard 4.5)
7. When credible research reports that test scores differ in meaning across examinee subgroups for the type of test in question, then to the extent feasible, the same forms of validity evidence collected for the examinee population as a whole should also be collected for each relevant subgroup. Subgroups may be found to differ with respect to appropriateness of test content, internal structure of test responses, the relation of test scores to other variables, or the response processes employed by the individual examinees. Any such findings should receive due consideration in the interpretation and use of scores as well as in subsequent test revisions. (SEPT, Standard 7.1)
8. When credible research reports differences in the effects of construct-irrelevant variance across subgroups of test takers on performance on some part of the test, the test should be used if at all only for the subgroups for which evidence indicates that valid inferences can be drawn from test scores. (SEPT, Standard 7.2)
9. When empirical studies of differential prediction of a criterion for members of different subgroups are conducted, they should include regression equations (or an appropriate equivalent) computed separately for each group or treatment under

consideration or an analysis in which group or treatment variables are entered as moderator variable. (SEPT, Standard 7.6)

10. When a construct can be measured in different ways that are approximately equal in their degree of construct representation and freedom from construct-irrelevant variance, evidence of mean score differences across relevant subgroups of examinees should be considered in deciding which test to use. (SEPT, Standard 7.11)
11. When credible research evidence reports that test scores differ in meaning across subgroups of linguistically diverse test takers, then to the extent feasible, test developers should collect for each linguistic group studied the same form of validity evidence collected for the examinee population as a whole. (SEPT, Standard 9.2)
12. When a test is translated from one language to another, the methods used in establishing the adequacy of translation should be described, and empirical and logical evidence should be provided for score reliability and the validity of the translated test's score inferences for the uses intended in the linguistic groups to be tested. (SEPT, Standard 9.7)
13. When multiple language versions of a test are intended to be comparable, test developers should report evidence of test comparability. (SEPT, Standard 9.9)
14. When feasible, tests that have been modified for use with individuals with disabilities should be pilot tested on individuals who have similar disabilities to investigate the appropriateness and feasibility of the modifications. (SEPT, Standard 10.3)
15. When sample sizes permit, the validity of inferences made from test scores and the reliability of scores on tests administered to individuals with various disabilities should be investigated and reported by the agency or publisher that makes the modification. Such investigations should examine the effects of modifications made for people with various disabilities on resulting scores, as well as the effects of administering standard unmodified tests to them. (SEPT, Standard 10.7)
16. When relying on norms as a basis for score interpretation in assisting individuals with disabilities, the norm group used depends upon the purpose of testing. Regular norms are appropriate when the purpose involves the test taker's functioning relative to the general population. If available, normative data from the population of individuals with the same level or degree of disability should be used when the test taker's functioning relative to individuals with similar disabilities is at issue. (SEPT, Standard 10.9)
17. When circumstances require that a test be administered in the same language to all examinees in a linguistically diverse population, the test user should investigate the validity of the score interpretations for test takers believed to have limited proficiency in the language of the test. (SEPT, Standard 11.22)
18. Counselors carefully consider the validity, reliability, psychometric limitations, and appropriateness of instruments when selecting tests for use in a given situation or with a particular client. (ETHICS, Section E.6.a)

Administration and Scoring of Assessment Instruments

1. Provide and document appropriate procedures for test takers with disabilities who need special accommodations or those with diverse linguistic backgrounds. Some accommodation may be required by law or regulation. (CODE, Section B-2)
2. For individuals with disabilities, accommodations in test taking procedures may need to be employed. Appropriate modifications of testing materials and procedures in order to accommodate test takers with special needs are to be arranged. (RUST)
3. Include notes on any problems, irregularities, and accommodations in the test records. (RUST)
4. A systematic and objective procedure is in place for observing and recording environmental, health, emotional factors, or other elements that may invalidate test performance and results; deviations from prescribed test administration procedures, including information on test accommodations for individuals with special needs, are recorded. Carefully observe, record, and attach to the test record any deviation from the prescribed test administration procedures. Include information on test accommodations for individuals with special needs. (RUST)
5. The testing or assessment process should be carried out so that test takers receive comparable and equitable treatment during all phases of the testing or assessment process. (SEPT, Standard 7.12)
6. Testing practice should be designed to reduce threats to the reliability and validity of test score inferences that may arise from language differences. (SEPT, Standard 9.1)
7. When testing an examinee proficient in two or more languages for which the test is available, the examinee's relative language proficiencies should be determined. The test generally should be administered in the test taker's most proficient language, unless proficiency in the less proficient language is part of the assessment. (SEPT, Standard 9.3)
8. When an interpreter is used in testing, the interpreter should be fluent in both the language of the test and the examinee's native language, should have expertise in translating, and should have a basic understanding of the assessment process. (SEPT, Standard 9.11)
9. People who make decisions about accommodations and test modifications for individuals with disabilities should be knowledgeable of existing research on the effects of the disabilities in question on test performance. Those who modify tests should also have access to psychometric expertise for so doing. (SEPT, Standard 10.2)
10. If a test developer recommends specific time limits for people with disabilities, empirical procedures should be used, whenever possible, to establish time limits for modified forms of timed tests rather than simply allowing test takers with disabilities a multiple of the standard time. When possible, fatigue should be investigated as a potentially important factor when time limits are extended. (SEPT, Standard 10.6)

11. Those responsible for decisions about test use with potential test takers who may need or may request specific accommodations should (a) possess the information necessary to make an appropriate selection of measures, (b) have current information regarding the availability of modified forms of the test in question, (c) inform individuals, when appropriate, about the existence of modified forms, and (d) make these forms available to test takers when appropriate and feasible. (SEPT, Standard 10.8)
12. Any test modifications adopted should be considered appropriate for the individual test taker, while maintaining all feasible standardized features. A test professional needs to consider reasonably available information about each test taker's experiences, characteristics, and capabilities that might impact test performance, and document the grounds for the modification. (SEPT, Standard 10.10)
13. If a test is mandated for persons of a given age or all students in a particular grade, users should identify individuals whose disabilities or linguistic background indicates the need for special accommodations in test administration and ensure that those accommodations are employed. (SEPT, Standard 11.23)
14. Counselors provide for equal access to computer applications in counseling services. (ETHICS, Section A.12.c)
15. When computer applications are used in counseling services, counselors ensure that: (1) the client is intellectually, emotionally, and physically capable of using the computer application; (2) the computer application is appropriate for the needs of the client; (3) the client understands the purpose and operation of the computer applications; and (4) a follow-up of client use of a computer application is provided to correct possible misconceptions, discover inappropriate use, and assess subsequent needs. (ETHICS, Section A.12.a)
16. Prior to assessment, counselors explain the nature and purposes of assessment and the specific use of results in language the client (or other legally authorized person on behalf of the client) can understand, unless an explicit exception to this right has been agreed upon in advance. (ETHICS, Section E.3.a)

Interpretation and Application of Assessment Results

1. Interpret the meaning of the test results, taking into account the nature of the content, norms or comparison groups, other technical evidence, and benefits and limitations of test results. (CODE, Section C-1)
2. Review the procedures for setting performance standards or passing scores. Avoid using stigmatizing labels. (CODE, Section C-4)
3. For individuals with disabilities, interpretations need to be made in light of the modifications in the test or testing procedures. (RUST)
4. When test results are influenced by irrelevant test taker characteristics (e.g., gender, age, ethnic background, cheating, availability of test preparation programs) the use of the resulting information is invalid and potentially harmful. (RUST)

5. Factors such as the test taker's group membership and how that membership may impact the results of the test is a critical factor in the interpretation of test results. Specifically, the test user should evaluate how the test taker's gender, age, ethnicity, race, socioeconomic status, marital status, and so forth, impact on the individual's results. (RUST)
6. If local examinees differ materially from the population to which the norms refer, a user who reports derived scores based on the published norms has the responsibility to describe such differences if they bear upon the interpretation of the reported scores. (SEPT, Standard 4.7)
7. In testing applications involving individualized interpretations of test scores other than selection, a test taker's score should not be accepted as a reflection of standing on a characteristic being assessed without consideration of alternate explanations for the test taker's performance on that test at that time. (SEPT, Standard 7.5)
8. When scores are disaggregated and publicly reported for groups identified by characteristics such as gender, ethnicity, age, language proficiency, or disability, cautionary statements should be included whenever credible research reports that test scores may not have comparable meaning across different groups. (SEPT, Standard 7.8)
9. When tests or assessments are proposed for use as instruments of social, educational, or public policy, the test developers or users proposing the test should fully and accurately inform policymakers of the characteristics of the tests as well as any relevant and credible information that may be available concerning the likely consequences of test use. (SEPT, Standard 7.9)
10. When the use of a test results in outcomes that affect the life chances or educational opportunities of examinees, evidence of mean test score differences between relevant subgroups of examinees should, where feasible, be examined for subgroups for which credible research reports mean differences for similar tests. Where mean differences are found, an investigation should be undertaken to determine that such differences are not attributable to a source of construct underrepresentation or construct-irrelevant variance. While initially the responsibility of the test developer, the test user bears responsibility for users with groups other than those specified by the developer. (SEPT, Standard 7.10).
11. When score reporting includes assigning individuals to categories, the categories should be chosen carefully and described precisely. The least stigmatizing labels, consistent with accurate representation, should always be assigned. (SEPT, Standard 8.8)
12. When there is credible evidence of score comparability across regular and modified administrations, no flag should be attached to a score. When such evidence is lacking, specific information about the nature of the modification should be provided, if permitted by law, to assist test users properly to interpret and act on test scores. (SEPT, Standard 9.5 and 10.11)
13. In testing persons with disabilities, test developers, test administrators, and test users should take steps to ensure that the test score inferences accurately reflect the intended construct rather than any disabilities and their associated characteristics extraneous to the intent of the measurement. (SEPT, Standard 10.1)

14. In testing individuals with disabilities for diagnostic and intervention purposes, the test should not be used as the sole indicator of the test taker's functioning. Instead, multiple sources of information should be used. (SEPT, Standard 10.12)
15. Agencies using tests to conduct program evaluations or policy studies, or to monitor outcomes, should clearly describe the population the program or policy is intended to serve and should document the extent to which the sample of test takers is representative of that population. (SEPT, Standard 15.5)
16. Reports of group differences in average test scores should be accompanied by relevant contextual information, where possible, to enable meaningful interpretation of these differences. Where appropriate contextual information is not available, users should be cautioned against misinterpretation. (SEPT, Standard 15.12)
17. Culturally competent counselors possess knowledge about their social impact on others. They are knowledgeable about communication style differences, how their style may clash or facilitate the counseling process with minority clients, and how to anticipate the impact it may have on others. (COMPS, 7)
18. Culturally competent counselors have knowledge of the potential bias in assessment instruments and use procedures and interpret findings keeping in mind the cultural and linguistic characteristics of the clients. (COMPS, 22)
19. Counselors recognize that culture affects the manner in which clients' problems are defined. Clients' socioeconomic and cultural experience is considered when diagnosing mental disorders. (ETHICS, Section E.5.b)
20. Counselors are cautious in using assessment techniques, making evaluations, and interpreting the performance of populations not represented in the norm group on which an instrument was standardized. They recognize the effects of age, color, culture, disability, ethnic group, gender, race, religion, sexual orientation, and socioeconomic status on test administration and interpretation and place test results in proper perspective with other relevant factors. (ETHICS, Section E.8)
21. In reporting assessment results, counselors indicate any reservations that exist regarding validity or reliability because of the circumstances of the assessment or the inappropriateness of the norms for the person tested. (ETHICS, Section E.9.a)

References

American Counseling Association. (1996). *Code of ethics and standards of practice*. Alexandria, VA: Author.

American Counseling Association and Association for Assessment in Counseling. (2003). *Responsibilities of users of standardized tests*. Alexandria, VA: Author.

American Educational Research Association, American Psychological Association, and National Council on Measurement in Education. (1999). *Standards for educational and psychological testing* (2nd ed.). Washington, DC: American Educational Research Association.

Arredondo, P., & Toporek, R. (1996). Operationalization of the multicultural counseling Competencies. [Electronic version]. *Journal of Multicultural Counseling and Development, 24*, 42–79.

Association for Multicultural Counseling and Development. (1992). *Multicultural counseling competencies and standards*. Alexandria, VA: American Counseling Association.

Joint Committee on Testing Practices. (2002). *Code of fair testing practices in education*. Washington, DC: Author.
Prediger, D. J. (1992). *Standards for multicultural assessment*. Alexandria, VA: Association for Assessment in Counseling.
Prediger, D. J. (1994). Multicultural assessment standards: A compilation for counselors. *Measurement and Evaluation in Counseling and Development, 27*, 68–73.
Sue, D. W., Arredondo, P., & McDavis, R. (1992). Multicultural counseling competencies and standards: A call to the profession. *Journal of Counseling and Development, 70*, 477–486.

AAC Executive Council

President—Dr. Janet Wall, Sage Solutions
Past President—Mrs. Patricia Jo McDivitt, Data Recognition Corporation
President-Elect—Dr. Brad Erford, Loyola College of Maryland
Secretary—Dr. Debbie Newsome, Wake Forest University
Treasurer—Dr. Brian Glaser, University of Georgia
Member-at-Large Publications—Dr. David Jepsen, University of Iowa
Member-at-Large Awards—Dr. Claire Miner, Assessment and Counseling Services
Member-at-Large Membership—Dr. Donna Gibson, The Citadel
Governing Council Representative—Dr. F. Robert Wilson, University of Cincinnati

Association for Assessment in Counseling

Vision: The Association for Assessment in Counseling (AAC) is an organization of counselors, counselor educators, and other professionals that advances the counseling profession by providing leadership, training, and research in the creation, development, production, and use of assessment and diagnostic techniques.
Mission: The mission of AAC is to promote and recognize scholarship, professionalism, leadership, and excellence in the development and use of assessment and diagnostic techniques in counseling.
Purposes: AAC is positioned to fulfill seven fundamental purposes:

- **Administration and Management:** to provide long range planning, policies, organizational structure, operating procedures, and resources to fulfill AAC's missions;
- **Professional Development:** to promote professional development which enhances competence in assessment, evaluation, measurement, and research for counselors, counselor educators, and other professionals who develop or use assessment and diagnostic tools and techniques;
- **Professionalization:** to promote the professionalization of counseling through the appropriate use of assessment;
- **Research and Knowledge:** to promote the development and dissemination of knowledge regarding assessment procedures used in counseling;

- **Human Development:** to promote concern for human rights as integral to all assessment activities and to serve as a resource to counselors, counselor educators, and other professionals concerning the assessment aspects of human development;
- **Public Awareness and Support:** to promote and support public policies and legislation that advance the appropriate use of assessment in optimizing human potential;
- **International and Interprofessional Collaboration:** to promote communication and collaboration between AAC and other professional organizations (national and international) in order to address common, assessment-related concerns.

Contact: 3gibsond@citadel.edu for membership information

GLOSSARY

Achievement test An assessment in which the person has "achieved" either knowledge, information, or skills through instruction, training, or experience. Achievement tests measure acquired knowledge and do not make any predictions about the future.

Age or grade equivalent scores Scores used to compare individuals with other individuals at the same age that are calculated by item response theory or by using a norm-referenced approach.

Alternate or parallel forms Two forms of an instrument that can be correlated, resulting in an estimate of reliability.

Appraisal Another term for *assessment*.

Aptitude test A test that provides a prediction about the individual's future performance or ability to learn based on his or her performance on the test. Aptitude tests often predict either future academic or vocational/career performance.

Assessment A procedure for gathering client information that is used to facilitate clinical decisions, provide clients with information, or for evaluative purposes.

Authentic assessments Performance assessments that involve the performance of "real" or authentic applications rather than proxies or estimators of actual learning.

Barnum effect A personality description that appears to be authentic but is written so vaguely that it applies to everyone.

Bias testing A term that refers to the degree to which construct-irrelevant factors systematically affect a specific group's performance.

Coefficient of determination This statistic estimates the percent of shared variance between two sets of variables that have been correlated. The coefficient of determination (r^2) is calculated by squaring the correlation coefficient.

Concurrent validity A type of criterion-related validity in which there is no delay between the time the instrument is administered and the time the criterion information is gathered.

Construct validity One of the three traditional forms of validity that is broader than either content or criterion-related validity. Many experts in assessment now argue that evidence of construct validity, which includes the other traditional forms of validity, applies in all types of psychological and educational assessment. This type of validation involves the gradual accumulation of evidence. Evidence of construct validity is concerned with the extent to which the instrument measures some psychological trait or construct and how the results can be interpreted.

Content-related validity One of the three traditional forms of validity, in which the focus was on whether the instrument's content adequately represented the domain being assessed. Evidence of content-related validity is often reflected in the steps the authors used in developing the instrument.

Convergent evidence Validation evidence that indicates the measure is positively related with other measures of the construct.

Correlation A statistic that provides an indication of the degree to which two sets of scores are related. A *correlation coefficient* (r) can range from -1.00 to $+1.00$ and, thus, provides an indicator of both the strength and direction of the relationship. A correlation of $+1.00$ represents a perfect positive relationship; a correlation of -1.00 represents a perfect negative or inverse relationship. A correlation coefficient of .00 indicates the absence of a relationship.

Correlational method A statistical tool often used in providing validation evidence related to an instrument's relationship with other variables.

Criterion-referenced instrument Instruments designed to compare an individual's performance to a stated criterion or standard. Often criterion-referenced instruments provide information on specific knowledge or skills and on whether the individual has "mastered" that knowledge or skill. The focus is on what the person knows rather than how he or she compares to other people.

Criterion-related validity One of the three types of validity in which the focus is the extent to which the instrument confirms (concurrent validity) or predicts (predictive validity) a criterion measure.

Cronbach's Alpha Also known as *coefficient alpha*, it is one of the methods of estimating reliability through the examination of the interna consistency of the instrument. This method is appropriate when the instrument is *not* dichotomously scored, such as an instrument that uses a Likert-scale.

Decision theory A method that examines the relationship between an instrument and a criterion or predictor variable, which usually involves an expectancy table. Expectancy tables frequently are used to determine cut-off scores or to provide clients with information regarding the probability of a certain performance on the criterion based on scores on the assessment.

Differential item functioning (DIF) A statistical method for investigating item bias that examines differences in performance among individuals who are equal in ability but are from different groups (e.g., different ethnic groups).

Discriminant evidence Validation evidence that indicates the measure is not related to measures of different psychological constructs.

Domain sampling theory Another term for *generalizability theory*.

Expectancy table A method of providing criterion-related validity evidence that involves charting performance on the criterion based on the instrument's score. It is often used to predict who would be expected to fall in a certain criterion category (e.g., who is likely to succeed in graduate school) and to determine cutoff scores.

Factor analysis A term that covers various statistical techniques that are used to study the patterns of relationship among variables with the goal of explaining the common underlying dimensions (factors). In assessment, factor analysis is often used to examine if the intended internal structure of an instrument is reflected mathematically. For example, a researcher would analyze whether all items on each subscale "load" with the other items on the appropriate subscale (factor) and not with another factor.

False negative In decision theory, a term used to describe when the assessment procedure is incorrect in predicting a negative outcome on the criterion.

False positive In decision theory, a term used to describe when the assessment procedure is incorrect in predicting a positive outcome on the criterion.

Formative evaluation A continuous or intermediate evaluation typically performed to examine the counseling services process.

Frequency distribution A chart that summarizes the scores on an instrument and the frequency or number of people receiving that score. Scores are often grouped into intervals to provide an easy-to-understand chart that summarizes overall performance.
Frequency polygon A graphic representation of the frequency of scores. The number or frequency of individuals receiving a score or falling within an interval of scores is plotted with points that are connected by straight lines.

General ability test Another term for intelligence test.
Generalizability theory An alternative model to the true score model of reliability. The focus of this theory is on estimating the extent to which specific sources of variation under defined conditions influence scores on an instrument.
Grade equivalent norms Norms that are typically used in achievement tests and provide scores in terms of grade equivalents. In some instruments, grade equivalent scores are not validated on each specific grade but are extrapolated scores based on group performance at each grade level.
Group separation table Another term for an *expectancy table*.

Histogram A graphic representation of the frequency of scores in which columns are utilized.

Individualized Education Plan (IEP) An educational plan that is developed for each student who is receiving special education and related services. The plan is developed by a team of educators and the child's parents or guardians.
Instrument An assessment tool that typically is not related to grading. In this book, instruments includes tests, scales, checklists, and inventories.
Intelligence tests Instruments that are designed to measure the mental capabilities of an individual. These assessments are also referred to as general ability tests.
Interval scale A type of measurement scale in which the units are in equal intervals. Many of the statistics used to evaluate an instrument's psychometric qualities require an interval scale.
Item difficulty An item analysis method in which the difficulty of individual items is determined. The most common item difficulty index (p) is the percentage of people who get the item correct.
Item discrimination A form of item analysis that examines the degree to which an individual item discriminates on some criterion. For example, in achievement testing, item discrimination would indicate whether the item discriminates between people who know the information and people who do not.
Item response theory (IRT) A measurement approach in which the focus is on each item and on establishing items that measure the individual's ability or level of a latent trait. This approach involves examining the item characteristic function and the calibration of each individual item.

Kuder-Richardson formulas Two formulas (KR 20 and KR 21) that were developed to estimate reliability. Both of these methods are measures of internal consistency. KR 20 has been shown to approximate the average of all possible split-half coefficients. KR 21 is easier to compute, but the items on the instrument must be homogeneous.

Latent trait theory Another term for *item response theory*.

Mean The arithmetic average of the scores. It is calculated by adding the scores together and dividing by the number in the group.
Median The middle score, with 50% of the scores falling below it and 50% of the scores falling above it.
Mental status examination An examination used to describe a client's level of functioning and self-presentation. It is generally conducted during the initial session or intake interview and is a statement of how a person appears, function, and behaves during the initial session.

Mode The most frequent score in a distribution.
Multitrait-multimethod matrix A matrix that includes information on correlations between the measure and traits that it should be related to and traits that it should not theoretically be related to. The matrix also includes correlations between the measure of interest and other same-methods measures and measures that use different assessment methods.

Neuropsychological assessment An assessment of cognitive impairments, specifically the behavioral effects of possible brain injury or damage.
Nominal scale A scale of measurement characterized by assigning numbers to name or representing mutually exclusive groups (e.g., 1 = male, 2 = female).
Normal curve A bell-shaped, symmetrical, and unimodal curve. The majority of cases are concentrated close to the mean, with 68% of the individual scores falling between one standard deviation below the mean and one standard deviation above the mean.
Normal distribution A distribution of scores with certain specific characteristics.
Norm-referenced instruments Instruments in which the interpretation of performance is based on the comparison of an individual's performance with that of a specified group of people.

Ordinal scale Type of measurement scale in which the degree of magnitude is indicated by the rank ordering of the data.

Percentile rank A ranking that provides an indication of the percent of scores that fall at or below a given score. For example: "Mary's percentile of 68 means that if there were 100 people who had taken this instrument, 68 of them would have a score at or below Mary's."
Performance assessments An alternate method of assessing individuals, other than through multiple-choice types of items, in which the focus is on evaluating the performance of tasks or activities.
Performance tests Tests which require the manipulation of objects with minimal verbal influences.
Predictive validity A type of criterion-related validity in which there is a delay between the time the instrument is administered and the time the criterion information is gathered.
Projective techniques A type of personality assessment that provides the client with a relatively ambiguous stimulus, thus encouraging a nonstructured response. The assumption underlying these techniques is that the individual will project his or her personality into the response. The interpretation of projective techniques is subjective and requires extensive training in the technique.
Psychological report A summary of a client's assessment results that is geared toward other professionals. Often written by a psychologist, a typical report includes background information, behavioral observations, test results and interpretations, recommendations, and a summary.
Psychosocial interview A detailed interview that gathers background information and information about the client's current psychological and social situation.

Ratio scale A scale of measurement that has both interval data and a meaningful zero (e.g., weight, height). Because ratio scales have a meaningful zero, ratio interpretations can be made.
Raw scores Raw scores are the unadjusted scores on an instrument before they are transformed into standard scores. An example of a raw score is the number of answers an individual gets correct on an achievement test.
Regression A commonly used statistical technique in which the researcher examines whether independent variables predict to a criterion or independent variable. Regression is used to determine if there is a linear relationship among the variables or a line of best fit.
Regression equation An equation that describes the linear relationship between the predictor variable(s) and the criterion variable. These equations are often used to determine if it

is possible to predict the criterion based on the instrument's scores.

Reliability Concerns the degree to which a measure or a score is free of unsystematic error. In classical test theory, it is the ratio of true variance to observed variance.

Reliability generalization A meta-analytic method which combines estimates of reliability across studies in order to calculate an estimate based on multiple indicators of reliability.

Restructured clinical (RC) scales Clinical scales of the MMPI-2 or MMPI-A that are based on combining factor-analytic methods with construct-oriented scale development in order to measure more focused and clinically relevant elements. Currently included in the MMPI-2 Extended Score Report.

Score A number or letter that is the product of a client taking an assessment. A score cannot be interpreted without additional information about the assessment.

Semi-structured interview An interview that is a combination of a structured and unstructured format in which there are a set of established questions and the clinician can also ask additional questions for elaboration or to gather additional information.

Sequential processing The use of mental abilities to arrange stimuli in sequential, or serial, order in order to process the information.

Simultaneous processing The use of mental abilities to integrate information in a unified manner, with the individual integrating fragments of information in order to comprehend the whole.

Skewed distributions Distributions in which the majority of scores are either high or low. Skewed distributions are not asymmetrical and the mean, mode, and median are different. In *positively skewed distributions*, the majority of scores are on the lower end of the distribution; in *negatively skewed distributions*, the majority of scores are on the upper end of the distribution.

Slope bias A term referring to a situation in which a test yields significantly different validity coefficients for different groups, resulting in different regression lines.

Spearman-Brown formula A formula for correcting a split-half reliability coefficient that estimates what the coefficient would be if the original number of items were used.

Spearman's model A two-factor theory of intelligence that postulates everyone has a *general ability factor* influencing their performance on intellectual tasks, and also specific factors correlated to g that influence performance in specific areas.

Specifiers Certain diagnoses in the DSM-IV-TR require that clinicians provide more information that specify certain characteristics of the disorder.

Split-half reliability One of the internal consistency measures of reliability in which the instrument is administered once and then split into two halves. The scores on the two halves are then correlated to provide an estimate of reliability. Often the split-half reliability coefficients are corrected using the Spearman-Brown formula. This formula adjusts the coefficient for using only half of the total number of items to provide an estimate of what the correlation coefficient would be if the original number of items were used.

Standard deviation The most common statistic used to describe the variability of a set of measurements. It is the square root of the variance.

Standard error of difference A measure used by a counselor to examine the difference between two scores and determine if there is a significant difference.

Standard error of estimate A numerical result that indicates the margin of expected error in the individual's predicted criterion score as a result of imperfect validity.

Standard error of measurement This deviation provides an indication of what an individual's true score would be if he or she took the instrument repeated times. Counselors can use standard error of measurement to determine the range of scores 68%, 95%, or 99.5% of the time.

Structured interview An interview that is conducted using a predetermined set of questions that is asked in the same manner and sequence for every client.

Structured personality instruments Formalized assessments in which clients respond to a fixed set of questions or items.

Substance Abuse A maladaptive pattern of substance use leading to clinically significant impairments or distress occurring repeatedly over a 12-month period.

Substance Dependence Occurs when regular substance use leads to the development of impaired control over the substance use and the continued use of the substance despite adverse consequences. Typically includes a pattern resulting in tolerance, withdrawal, and compulsive drug-taking behaviors over a 12-month period.

Summative evaluation A cumulative evaluation of services that are typically completed at the endpoint of the service. These types of evaluation are designed to provide an overall indication of the effectiveness of the services.

Technology-adapted assessment A term that applies to an interactive process between the individual and typically the computer, in which the computer adapts the items on the test based on the individual's answers to other items.

Technology-assisted assessment An assessment in which some sort of technology, usually a computer, is used to assist in the administration, scoring, or interpretation of the assessment.

Test An individual instrument in which the focus is on evaluation.

Test-retest reliability One in which the reliability coefficient is obtained by correlating a group's performance on the first administration of an instrument with the same group's performance on the second administration of that same instrument.

Unstructured interview An interview in which the clinician gears the questions toward each individual client and there is no established set of questions.

Validity coefficient The correlation between the scores on an instrument and the criterion measure.

Validity generalization A term applied to findings indicating that the validity of cognitive ability tests can be generalized and that cognitive ability is highly related to job performance.

Variance The average of the squared deviation from the mean. It is a measure of variability and its square root is the standard deviation of the set of measurements.

REFERENCES

Ackerman, S. J., Hilsenroth, M. J., Baity, M. R., & Blagys, M. D. (2000). Interaction of therapeutic process and alliance during psychological assessment. *Journal of Personality Assessment, 75,* 82–109.

ACT. (2001). *DISCOVER a world of possibilities: Research support for DISCOVER assessment components.* Iowa City: Author.

ACT. (2003). *Content validity evidence in support of ACT's educational achievement tests: ACT national curriculum study.* Iowa City, IA: Author.

ACT. (2005). *Your guide to the ACT.* Iowa City, IA: Author.

ACT. (2007). *Using your ACT results.* Iowa City, IA: Author.

Adesso, V. J., Cisler, R. A., Larus, B. J., & Haynes, B. B. (2004). Substance abuse. In M. Herson (Ed.), *Psychological assessment in clinical practice* (pp. 147–174). New York: Brunner-Routledge.

Æquisdótti. S., White, M. J., Spengler, P. M., Maugherman, A. S., Anderson, L. A., Cook, R. S., Nichols, C. N., Lampropoulos, G. K., Walker, B. S., Cohen, G., & Rush, J. D. (2006). The meta-analysis of clinical judgment project: Fifty-six years of accumulated research on clinical versus statistical prediction. *The Counseling Psychologist, 34,* 341–382.

Agresti, A., & Finlay, B. (1997). *Statistical methods for the social sciences.* Englewood Cliffs, NJ: Prentice Hall.

Aiken, L. R. (1999). *Personality assessment: Methods and practice* (3rd ed.). Kirkland, WA: Hogrefe & Huber.

Aiken, L. R., & Groth-Marnat, G. (2005). *Psychological testing and assessment* (12th ed.). Boston: Allyn & Bacon.

Airasian, P. W. (2000). *Classroom assessment* (4th ed.). New York: McGraw-Hill.

Allen, J. (2007). Multicultural assessment supervision model to guide research and practice. *Professional Psychology: Research and Practice, 38,* 248–258.

Allred, L. J., & Harris, W. G. (1984). *The non-equivalence of computerized and conventional administration of the Adjective Checklist.* Unpublished manuscript, Johns Hopkins University, Baltimore, MD.

American Association of Suicidoloy. (2006). *U.S.A. suicide: 2004 official data.* Retrieved August 23, 2006, from http://www.suicidology.org/associations/1045/files/2004datapgv1.pdf

American Association on Intellectual and Developmental Disabilities. (2007). *Definition of mental retardation.* Retrieved December 2, 2007, from http://www.aamr.org/Policies/faq_mental_retardation.shtml

American Counseling Association. (1999). *Ethical standards for Internet on-line counseling.* Alexandria, VA: Author.

American Counseling Association. (2003). *Standards for qualifications of test users.* Alexandria, VA: Author.

American Counseling Association. (2005a). *ACA code of ethics.* Alexandria, VA: Author.

American Counseling Association. (2005b). *ACA Policies and procedures for processing complaints of ethical violations.* Alexandria, VA: Author.

American Educational Research Association. (2000). *AERA position statement concerning high-stakes testing in pre-K–12 education.* Washington, DC: Author.

American Educational Research Association, American Psychological Association, & National Council on Measurement in Education. (1999). *Standards for educational and psychological testing.* Washington, DC: American Educational Research Association.

American Psychiatric Association. (2000). *Diagnostic and statistical manual of mental disorders*—fourth edition-text revision. Washington, DC: Author.

American Psychological Association. (2001). *Appropriate use of high stakes testing in our nation's schools.* Retrieved

October 27, 2007, from http://www.apa.org/pubinfo/testing.html

American Psychological Association. (2002). Ethical principles of psychologists and code of conduct. *American Psychologist, 57,* 1060–1073.

American Psychological Association. (2003). Guidelines on multicultural education, training, research, practice, and organizational change for psychologists. *American Psychologist, 58,* 377–402.

American School Counselor Association. (2003). *The ASCA national model: A framework for school counseling programs.* Alexandria, VA: Author.

American School Counselor Association. (2004). *Ethical standards for school counselors.* Alexandria, VA: Author.

Anastasi, A. (1981). Coaching, test sophistication, and developed abilities. *American Psychologist, 36,* 1086–1093.

Anastasi, A. (1988). *Psychological testing* (6th ed.). New York: Macmillan.

Anastasi, A. (1992). What counselors should know about the use and interpretation of psychological tests. *Journal of Counseling & Development, 70,* 610–616.

Anastasi, A. (1993). A century of psychological testing: Origins, problems and progress. In T. K. Fagen & G. R. VandenBos (Eds.), *Exploring applied psychology: Origins and critical analyses* (pp. 3–36). Washington, DC: American Psychological Association.

Anastasi, A., & Urbina, S. (1997). *Psychological testing* (7th ed.). Upper Saddle River, NJ: Prentice Hall.

Anderson, B. S. (1996). *The counselor and the law* (4th ed.). Alexandria, VA: American Counseling Association.

Anderson, W. (1995). Ethnic and cross-cultural differences on the MMPI-2. In J. C. Duckworth & W. P. Anderson (Eds.), *MMPI and MMPI-2 interpretation manual for counselors and clinicians* (pp. 382–395). Bristol, PA: Accelerated Press.

Archer, R. P. (1992). Review of the Minnesota Multiphasic Personality Inventory 2. In J. C. Conoley & J. J. Kramer (Eds.), *Eleventh mental measurements yearbook* (pp. 558–562). Lincoln, NE: The University of Nebraska Press.

Archer, R. P., & Krishnamurthy, R. (1996). The Minnesota Multiphasic Personality Inventory—Adolescent. In C. S. Newmark (Ed.), *Major psychological assessment instruments* (pp. 59–107). Boston: Allyn & Bacon.

Archer, R. P., Maruish, M., Imhof, E. A., & Piotrowski, C. (1991). Psychological test usage with adolescent clients: 1990 survey findings. *Professional Psychology: Research and Practice, 22,* 247–252.

Archer, R. P., & Newsom, C. R. (2000). Psychological test usage with adolescent clients: Survey update. *Assessment, 7,* 227–235.

Association for Assessment in Counseling. (2002). *Applying the standards for educational and psychological testing: what counselors need to know.* Alexandria, VA: Author.

Association for Assessment in Counseling. (2003a). *Responsibilities of users of standardized tests (RUST)* (3rd ed.). Alexandria, VA: Author.

Association for Assessment in Counseling. (2003b). *Standards for multicultural assessment.* Alexandria, VA: American Counseling Association.

Athanasou, J. A., & Cooksey, R. W. (1993). Self-estimates of vocational interests. *Australian Psychologist, 28,* 118–127.

Austin, J. T. (1994). Test review: Minnesota Multiphasic Personality Inventory 2. *Measurement and Evaluation in Counseling and Development, 27,* 178–185.

Baghurst, P. A., McMichael, A. J., Wigg, N. R., Vimpani, G. V., Robertson, E. F., Roberts, R. J., & Ton, S. L. (1992). Environmental exposure to lead and children's intelligence at the age of seven years: The Port Pirie cohort study. *New England Journal of Medicine, 327,* 1279–1284.

Baker, E. L., O'Neil, H. F., & Linn, R. L. (1993). Policy and validity prospects for performance-based assessment. *American Psychologist, 48,* 1210–1218.

Baker, S. B. (2000). *School counseling for the 21st century* (3rd ed.). New York: Prentice Hall.

Baldwin, A. L., Kalhorn, J., & Breese, F. H. (1945). Patterns of parent behavior. *Psychological Monographs, 58* (Whole No. 268).

Bandura, A. (1977). Self-efficacy: Toward a unifying theory of behavioral change. *Psychological Review, 84,* 191–215.

Barak, A. (2003). Ethical and professional issues in career assessment on the Internet. *Journal of Career Assessment, 11,* 3–21.

Barak, A. & English, N. (2002). Prospects and limitations of psychological testing on the Internet. *Journal of Technology in Human Services, 19,* 65–89.

Bartels, S. J., Blow, F. C., Brockmann, L. M., & Van Citters, A. D. (2005). *Substance abuse and mental health among older Americans: The state of the knowledge and future directions.* Retrieved January 6, 2008, from http://www.samhsa.gov/OlderAdultsTAC/SA_MH_%20AmongOlderAdultsfinal102105.pdf

Barthlow, D. L., Graham, J. R., Ben-Porath, Y. S., & McNulty, J. L. (1999). Incremental validity of the MMPI-2 Content Scales in an outpatient mental health setting. *Professional Assessment, 11,* 39–47.

Bayley, N., & Oden, M. H. (1955). The maintenance of intellectual ability in gifted adults. *Journal of Gerontology, 10,* 91–107.

Beck, A. T., & Steer, R. A. (1991). *Beck Scale for Suicide Ideation.* San Antonio, TX: Psychological Corporation.

Beck, A. T., & Steer, R. A. (1993). *Beck Hopelessness Scale.* San Antonio, TX: Psychological Corporation.

Beck, A. T., Steer, R. A., & Brown, G. K. (1996). *Beck Depression Inventory II.* San Antonio, TX: Psychological Corporation.

Becker, K. A. (2003). History of the Stanford-Binet Intelligence scales: Content and psychometrics. *Stanford-Binet Intelligence Scales, Fifth Edition Assessment Service Bulletin*. Itasca, IL: Riverside.

Beevers, C. G., Strong, D. R., Meyer, B., Pilkonis, P. A., & Miller, I. W. (2007). Efficiently assessing negative cognition in depression: An item response theory analysis of the Dysfunctional Attitude Scale. *Psychological Assessment, 19,* 199–200.

Bennett, G. K., Seashore, H. G., & Wesman, A. G. (1990). *Differential Aptitude Tests* (5th ed.). San Antonio, TX: Psychological Corporation.

Ben-Porath, Y. F. (1997). Use of personality assessment instruments in empirically guided treatment planning. *Psychological Assessment, 9,* 361–367.

Benziman, H., & Toder, A. (1993). The psychodiagnostic experience: Reports of subjects. In B. Nevo & R. S. Jager (Eds.), *Educational and psychological testing: The test taker's outlook* (pp. 287–299). Toronto: Hogrefe & Huber.

Berk, R. A. (1984). Selecting the index of reliability. In R. A. Berk (Ed.), *A guide to criterion-referenced test construction* (pp. 231–266). Baltimore, MD: Johns Hopkins University Press.

Bernstein, R. (2007). *More than 300 counties now "majority-minority."* Retrieved November 25, 2007, from http://www.census.gov/Press-Release/www/releases/archives/population/010482.html

Bernt, F. (2001). Review of the Marital Satisfaction Inventory—Revised. In B. Plake & J. Impara (Eds.), *The fourteenth mental measurements yearbook* (pp. 711–712). Lincoln, NE: Buros Institute of Mental Measures.

Bertone, A., Bettinelli, L., & Faubert, J. (2007). The impact of blurred vision on cognitive assessment. *Journal of Clinical and Experimental Neuropsychology, 29,* 467–476.

Betsworth, D. G., & Fouad, N. A. (1997). Vocational interests: A look at the past 70 years and a glance at the future. *The Career Development Quarterly, 46,* 23–41.

Betz, N. E. (1988). The assessment of career development and maturity. In W. B. Walsh & S. H. Osipow (Eds.), *Career decision making* (pp. 77–136). Hillsdale, NJ: Erlbaum.

Betz, N. E. (1992). Career assessment: A review of critical issues. In S. D. Brown & R. W. Lent (Eds.), *Handbook of counseling psychology* (2nd ed., pp. 453–484). New York: Wiley.

Betz, N. E. (1994). Basic issues and concepts in career counseling for women. In W. B. Walsh & S. H. Osipow (Eds.), *Career counseling for women* (pp. 1–42). Hillsdale, NJ: Erlbaum.

Betz, N. E. (2000). Self-efficacy theory as a basis for career assessment. *Journal of Career Assessment, 8,* 205–222.

Betz, N. E., Borgen, F. H., & Harmon, L. W. (2005). *Skills Confidence Inventory: Research, development, and strategies for interpretation.* Mountain View CA: CPP, Inc.

Betz, N. E., Borgen, F. H., Kaplan, A., & Harmon, L. W. (1998). Gender and Holland type as moderators of validity and interpretative utility of the Skills Confidence Inventory. *Journal of Vocational Behavior, 53,* 281–299.

Betz, N. E., Borgen, F. H., Rottinghaus, P., Paulsen, A., Halper, C. R., & Harmon, L. W. (in press). The Expanded Skills Confidence inventory: Measuring basic dimensions of vocational activity. *Journal of Vocational Behavior.*

Betz, N. E., & Taylor, K. M. (1994). *Manual for the Career Decision-Making Self-Efficacy Scale.* Columbus, OH: Ohio State University Department of Psychology.

Beutler, L. E., Albanese, A. L., Fisher, D., Karno, M., Sandowicz, M., & Williams, O. B. (1999, June). *Selecting and matching to patient variables.* Paper presented at the annual meeting of the Society for Psychotherapy Research, Braga, Portugal.

Beutler, L. E., & Clarkin, J. F. (1990). *Systematic treatment selection.* New York: Brunner/Mazel.

Beutler, L. E., & Harwood, T. M. (2000). *Prescriptive psychotherapy: A guide to systematic treatment selection.* New York: Oxford University Press.

Beutler, L. F., Malik, M., Alimohamed, S., Harwood, T. M., Talebi, H., Noble, S., & Wong, E. (2004). Therapist variables. In M. J. Lambert (Ed.), *Bergin and Garfield's handbook of psychotherapy and behavior change* (5th ed., pp. 227–306). New York; Wiley.

Beutler, L. F., Malik, M., Talebi, H., Fleming, J., & Moleiro, C. (2004). Use of psychological tests/instruments for treatment planning. In M. E. Maruish (Ed.), *The use of psychological testing for treatment planning and outcome assessment: Third edition volume 1* (pp. 111–145). Mahwah, NJ: Erlbaum.

Bickman, L., Rosof-Williams, J., Salzer, M. S., Summerfelt, W. T., Noser, K., Wilson, S. J., & Karver, M. S. (2000). What information do clinicians value for monitoring adolescent client progress and outcomes? *Professional Psychology: Research and Practice, 31,* 70–74.

Bjorklund, D. F. (2005). *Children's thinking: Developmental function and individual differences* (4th ed.). Belmont, CA: Brooks/Cole.

Bond, L. (1989). The effects of special preparation on measures of scholastic ability. In R. L. Linn (Ed.), *Educational measurement* (3rd ed., pp. 429–444). New York: Macmillan.

Bond, L. (1990). Understanding the Black-White student gap on measures of qualitative reasoning. In F. C. Serafica, A. I. Schwebel, R. K. Russes, P. D. Issac, & L. B. Myers (Eds.), *Mental health of ethnic minorities* (pp. 89–107). New York: Praeger.

Bonner, M. (2005). Review of the Kaufman Test of Educational Achievement-Second Edition Comprehensive Form. In R. A. Spies & B. S. Plake (Eds.), *The sixteenth mental measurements yearbook* (pp. 523–526). Lincoln, NE: Buros Institute of Mental Measurements.

Bornstein, R. F., Rossner, S. C., Hill, E. L., & Stephanian, M. L. (1994). Face validity and fakability of objective and projective measures of dependency. *Journal of Personality Assessment, 63,* 363–386.

Bowen, M. (1978). *Family therapy in clinical practice.* New York: Jason Aronson.

Bowman, M. L. (1989). Testing individual differences in ancient China. *American Psychologist, 41,* 1059–1068.

Boyle, G. J. (1995). Review of the Rotter Incomplete Sentences Blank. In J. C. Conoley & J. J. Kramer (Eds.), *Twelfth mental measurements yearbook* (pp. 880–882). Lincoln, NE: The University of Nebraska Press.

Bracken, B. A., & Barona, A. (1991). State of the art procedures for translating, validating, and using psychoeducational tests in cross-cultural assessment. *School Psychology International, 12,* 119–132.

Braden, J. P., & Ouzts, S. M. (2005). Review of the Kaufman Assessment Battery for Children, Second Edition. In R. A. Spies & B. S. Plake (Eds.). *The sixteenth mental measurements yearbook* (pp. 117–123). Lincoln, NE: Buros Institute of Mental Measurements.

Bradley, R., Danielson, L., & Hallahan D. P. (2002). *Identification of learning disabilities.* Mahwah, NJ: Erlbaum.

Bradley-Johnson, S., & Ekstrom, R. (1998). Visual impairments. In J. Sandoval, C. L. Frisby, K. F. Geisinger, J. D. Scheuneman, & J. R. Grenier (Eds.), *Test interpretation and diversity: Achieving equity in assessment* (pp. 271– 295). Washington, DC: American Psychological Association.

Brauer, B. A., Braden, J. P., Pollard, R. Q., & Hardy-Braz, S. T. (1998). Deaf and hard of hearing people. In J. Sandoval, C. L. Frisby, K. F. Geisinger, J. D. Scheuneman, & J. R. Grenier (Eds.), *Test interpretation and diversity: Achieving equity in assessment* (pp. 297–315). Washington, DC: American Psychological Association.

Bray, D. W. (1982). The assessment center and the study of lives. *American Psychologist, 37,* 180–189.

Brewer, C. A., & Suchan, T. A. (2001). *Mapping Census 2000: The geography of U.S. diversity*. Washington, DC: U.S. Census Bureau.

Brooke, S. L., & Ciechalski, J. C. (1994). Minnesota Importance Questionnaire. In J. T. Kapes, M. M. Mastie, & E. A. Whitfield (Eds.), *A counselor's guide to career assessment instruments* (pp. 222–225). Alexandria, VA: National Career Development Association.

Brown, J., Dreis, S., & Nace, D. K. (1999). What really makes a difference in psychotherapy outcome? Why does managed care want to know? In M. A. Hubble, B. L. Duncan, & S. D. Miller (Eds.), *The heart & soul of change: What works in therapy* (pp. 389–406). Washington, DC: American Psychological Association.

Brown, L., Sherbenou, R. J., & Johnsen, S. K. (1997). *Test of Nonverbal Intelligence,* Third Edition. Los Angeles: Western Psychological Services.

Brown, M. B. (2001). Review of the Self-Directed Search: 4th edition. In B. Plake & J. Impara (Eds), *The fourteenth mental measurements yearbook* (pp. 1105–1107). Lincoln, NE: Buros Institute of Mental Measures.

Bubenzer, D. L., Zimpfer, D. G., & Mahrle, C. L. (1990). Standardized individual appraisal in agency and private practice: A survey. *Journal of Mental Health Counseling, 12,* 51–66.

Buchanan, T. (2002). Online assessment: Desirable or dangerous? *Professional Psychology: Research and Practice, 33,* 148–154.

Buck, J. (1948). The H-T-P. *Journal of Clinical Psychology, 4,* 151–159.

Buck, J. (1992). *The House-Tree-Person projective drawing technique: Manual and interpretive guide.* (Revised by W. L. Warren). Los Angeles: Western Psychological Services.

Bujold, C. (2004). Constructing career through narrative. *Journal of Vocational Behavior, 64,* 470–484.

Burlingame, G. M., Wells, M. G., Hoag, M. J., Hope, C. A., Nebeker, R. S., Konkel, K., M., McCollam, P., Peterson, G., Lambert, M. J., Latkowski, M., Ferre, R., & Resinger, C. W. (1996). *Youth Outcome Questionnaire (Y-OQ-2.01).* Salt Lake City, UT: OQ Measures LLC.

Burns, R. (1982). *Self-growth in families: Kinetic Family Drawings (K-F-D) research and application.* New York: Brunner/Mazel.

Burns, R. (1987). *Kinetic-House-Tree-Person Drawings (K-H-T-P).* New York: Brunner/Mazel.

Burns, R., & Kaufman, S. (1970). *Kinetic Family Drawings (K-F-D): An introduction to understanding children through kinetic drawings.* New York: Brunner/Mazel.

Burns, R., & Kaufman, S. (1972). *Action, styles, symbols in Kinetic Family Drawings (K-F-D).* New York: Brunner/Mazel.

Busby, D. M., Holman, T. B., & Taniguchi N. (2001). RELATE: Relationship evaluation of the individual, family, cultural, and couple contexts. *Family Relations, 50,* 308–316.

Busch, J. C. (1995). Review of the Strong Interest Inventory. In J. C. Conoley & J. J. Kramer (Eds.), *Twelfth mental measurements yearbook* (pp. 997–999). Lincoln, NE: The University of Nebraska Press.

Burton, N. W. & Wang, M. (2005). *Predicting long-term success in graduate school: A collaborative validity study*. GRE Board Report No. 99-14R. Retrieved October 18, 2007, from http://www.ets.org/Media/Research/pdf/RR-05-03.pdf

Butcher, J. N. (1995). Clinical personality assessment: An overview. In J. N. Butcher (Ed.), *Clinical personality assessment: Practical approaches* (pp. 3–9). New York: Oxford University Press.

Butcher, J. N. (1998). *Butcher Treatment Planning Inventory*. San Antonio, TX: The Psychological Corporation.

Butcher, J. N., Cabiya, J., Lucio, E., & Garrido, M. (2007). *Assessing Hispanic clients using the MMPI-2 and MMPI-A.* Washington, DC: American Psychological Association.

Butcher, J. N., Dahlstrom, W. G., Graham, J. R., Tellegen, A., & Kraemmer, B. (1989). *Minnesota Multiphasic Personality Inventory-2 (MMPI-2): Manual for administration and scoring.* Minneapolis: University of Minnesota Press.

Butcher, J. N., & Williams, C. L. (2000). *Essentials of the MMPI-2 and MMPI-A interpretation* (2nd ed.). Minneapolis: University of Minnesota Press.

Butcher, J. N., Williams, C. L., Graham, J. R., Archer, R., Tellegen, A., Ben-Porath, Y. S., & Kraemmer, B. (1992). *MMPI: A manual for administration, scoring, and interpretation.* Minneapolis: University of Minnesota Press.

Callaghan, G. M. (2001). Demonstrating clinical effectiveness for individual practitioners and clinics. *Professional Psychology: Research & Practice, 32,* 289–297.

Camara, W. J., Nathan, J. S., & Puente, A. E. (2000). Psychological test usage: Implications in professional psychology. *Professional Psychology: Research and Practice, 31,* 141–154.

Campbell, C. A., & Dahir, C. A. (1997). *Sharing the vision: The national standards for school counseling programs.* Alexandria, VA: American School Counselor Association.

Campbell, D. P. (1992). *Campbell Interest and Skills Survey manual.* Minneapolis: National Computer Systems.

Campbell, D. T., & Fiske, D. W. (1959). Convergent and discriminant validation by the multi-trait multimethod matrix. *Psychological Bulletin, 56,* 81–105.

Campbell, J. P. (1994). Alternative models of job performance and their implications for selection and classification. In M. G. Rumsey, C. B. Walker, & J. H. Harris (Eds.), *Personnel selection and classification* (pp. 33–51). Hillsdale, NJ: Erlbaum.

Campbell, V. L. (2000). A framework for using tests in counseling. In C. E. Watkins & V. L. Campbell (Eds.), *Testing and assessment in counseling practice* (2nd ed., pp. 3–11). Mahwah, NJ: Erlbaum.

Caprara, G. V., Barbaranelli, C., & Comfrey, A. L. (1995). Factor analysis of the NEO-PI Inventory and the Comfrey Personality Scales in an Italian sample. *Personality and Individual Differences, 18,* 193–200.

Capraro, R. M., & Capraro, M. M. (2002). Myers-Briggs Type Indicator score reliability across: Studies: A meta-analytic reliability generalization study. *Educational and Psychological Measurement, 62,* 590–602.

Carroll, J. B. (1997). The three-stratum theory of cognitive abilities. In D. P. Flanagan, J. L. Genshaft, & P. L. Harrison (Eds.), *Contemporary intellectual assessment: Theories, tests, and issues* (pp. 122–130). New York: Guilford.

Carter, E. A., & McGoldrick, M. (1998). *The expanded family life cycle: Individual, family, and social perspectives* (3rd ed.). Boston: Allyn & Bacon.

Cattell, R. B. (1971). *Abilities: Their structure, growth, and action.* Boston: Houghton Mifflin.

Cattell, R. B. (1979). Are culture fair intelligence tests possible and necessary? *Journal of Research and Development in Education, 12*(2), 3–13.

Cattell, R. B., Cattell, A. K., & Cattell, H. E. (1993). *Sixteen Personality Factor Questionnaire,* Fifth Edition. Champaign, IL: Institute for Personality and Ability Testing.

CBT/McGraw-Hill (2004). *Guidelines for inclusive test administration.* Monterey, CA: Author.

Ceci, S. J. (1990). *On intelligence—more or less: A bioecological treatise on intellectual development.* Englewood Cliffs, NJ: Prentice Hall.

Ceci, S. J. (1991). How much does school influence general intelligence and its cognitive components: A reassessment of the evidence. *Developmental Psychology, 27,* 703–723.

Ceci, S. J. (1993). Contextual trends in intellectual development. *Developmental Review, 13,* 403–435.

Chartrand, J. M., & Walsh, W. B. (2001). Career assessment: Changes and trends. In F. T. L. Leong & A. Barak (Eds.), *Contemporary models in vocational psychology* (pp. 231–256). Mahwah, NJ: Lawrence Erlbaum.

Chipuser, H. M., Rovine, M., & Plomin, R. (1990). LISREL modeling: Genetic and environmental influences on IQ revisited. *Intelligence, 14,* 11–29.

Ciechalski, J. C. (2002). Self-Directed Search. In J. T. Kapes, M. M. Mastie, & E. A. Whitfield (Eds.), *A counselor's guide to career assessment instruments* (4th ed., pp. 276–287). Tulsa, OK: National Career Development Association.

Cierpka, M. (2005a). Introduction to family assessment. In M. Cierpka, V. Thomas, & D. H. Sprenkle (Eds.), *Family assessment: Integrating multiple perspectives* (pp. 3–14). Cambridge, MA: Hogrefe.

Cierpka, M. (2005b). The three-level model of family assessment. In M. Cierpka, V. Thomas, & D. H. Sprenkle (Eds.), *Family assessment: Integrating multiple perspectives* (pp. 15–32). Cambridge, MA: Hogrefe.

Cizek, G. J. (2003). Review of the Woodcock-Johnson III. In B. S. Plake & J. C. Impara (Eds.). *The fifteenth mental measurements yearbook* (pp. 1020–1024). Lincoln, NE: Buros Institute of Mental Measures.

Cizek, G. J. (2005). Review of the TerraNova, second edition. In R. A. Spies & B. Plake (Eds.), *The sixteenth mental measurements yearbook* (pp. 1025–1030). Lincoln, NE: Buros Institute of Mental Measures.

Clair, D., & Prendergast, D. (1994). Brief psychotherapy and psychological assessment: Entering a relationship, establishing a focus, and providing feedback. *Professional Psychology: Research and Practice, 25,* 46–49.

Clark, D. A. (1999). Case conceptualization and treatment failure: A commentary. *Journal of Cognitive Psychotherapy: An International Quarterly, 13,* 331–337.

Clark, D. C., & Fawcett, J. (1992). Review of empirical risk factors for evaluation of the suicidal patient. In B. Bongar (Ed.), *Suicide: Guidelines for assessment, management, and treatment* (pp. 16–48). New York: Oxford University Press.

Clarkin, J. F., & Levy, K. N. (2004). The influence of client variables on psychotherapy. In M. J. Lambert (Ed.), *Bergin and Garfield's handbook of psychotherapy and behavior change* (5th ed., pp. 227–306). New York: Wiley.

Clawson, T. W. (1997). Control of psychological testing: The threat and a response. *Journal of Counseling & Development, 76,* 90–93.

Cohen, L., Duberly, J., Mallon, M. (2004). Social constructionism in the study of career: Accessing the parts that other approaches cannot reach. *Journal of Vocational Behavior, 64,* 979–1006.

Cohen, R. J., & Swerdlik, M. E. (2005). *Psychological testing and assessment: An introduction to tests and measurement* (6th ed.). Columbus, OH: McGraw-Hill.

College Board (2002). *Guidelines on the uses of College Board scores and related data.* Retrieved October 17, 2007, from http://www.collegeboard.com/prod_downloads/research/RDGuideUseCBTest020729.pdf

College Board SAT (2007). *SAT program handbook.* Miami, FL: Author.

Commission of Rehabilitation Counselor Certification. (2001). *Code of professional ethics for rehabilitation counselors.* Rolling Meadows, IL: Author.

Conners, C. K. (1996). *Conners' Rating Scales—Revised.* Minneapolis: Pearson Assessments.

Cormier, S., & Nurius, P. S. (2003). *Interviewing and change strategies for helpers: Fundamental skills and cognitive behavioral interventions.* Belmont, CA: Brooks/Cole.

Costa, P. T., & McCrae, R. R. (1992). *Revised NEO Personality Inventory (NEO-PI-R) and NEO Five-Factor Inventory (NEO-FFI) professional manual.* Odessa, FL: Psychological Assessment Resources.

Council for Accreditation of Counseling and Related Educational Programs. (2001). *CACREP accreditation manual of the Council for Accreditation of Counseling and Related Educational Programs.* Alexandria, VA: Author.

Coupland, S. K., Serovic, J., & Glenn, J. E. (1995). Reliability in constructing genograms: A study among marriage and family therapy doctoral students. *Journal of Marital and Family Therapy, 21,* 251–263.

Craig, R. J. (1993). *The Millon Clinical Multiaxial Inventory: A clinical research information synthesis.* Hillsdale, NJ: Erlbaum.

Crew, J. A., & Hill, N. R. (2005). Diagnosis in marriage and family counseling: An ethical double bind. *The Family Journal, 13,* 63–66.

Crites, J. O. (1999). Operational definitions of vocational interests. In M. L. Savicakas & A. R. Spokane (Eds.), *Vocational interests: Meaning, measurement, and counseling use.* Palo Alto, CA: Davies-Black.

Crites, J. O., & Savickas, M. L. (1995). *Career Maturity Inventory: Sourcebook.* Oroville, WA: Bridges.com.

Crocker, L., & Algina, J. (1986). *Introduction to classical and modern test theory.* Fort Worth, TX: Harcourt Brace Jovanovich.

Cromwell, R., Fournier, D., & Kvebaek, D. (1980). *The Kvebaek Family Sculpture Technique: A diagnostic and research tool in family therapy.* Jonesboro, TN: Pilgrimage.

Cronbach, L. J. (1951). Coefficient alpha and internal structure of tests. *Psychometrika, 16,* 297–334.

Cronbach, L. J. (1990). *Essentials of psychological testing* (5th ed.). New York: HarperCollins.

Cronbach, L. J., & Gleser, G. C. (1965). *Psychological tests and personnel decisions* (2nd ed.). Champaign, IL: University of Illinois Press.

Cronbach, L. J., Gleser, G. C., Rajaratnam, N., & Nanda, H. (1972). *The dependability of behavioral measurements.* New York: Wiley.

CTB/McGraw-Hill. (2000). *TerraNova: The measure of success.* [Brochure]. Monterey, CA: Author.

CTB/McGraw-Hill. (2001). *TerraNova, the second edition: Teacher's guide.* Monterey, CA: Author.

CTB/McGraw-Hill. (2002). *TerraNova, the second edition: CAT technical bulletin 1.* Monterey, CA: Author.

CTB/McGraw-Hill. (2004). *CTB assessment accommodations guide.* Monterey, CA: Author.

Cull, J. G., & Gill, W. S. (1992). *Suicide Probability Scale.* Los Angeles: Western Psychological Services.

Dahir, C. A., & Stone, C. B. (2003). Accountability: A M.E.A.S.U.R.E. of impact school counselors have on student achievement. *Professional School Counseling, 6,* 214–221.

Dahlstrom, W. G. (1995). Pigeons, people, and pigeon holes. *Journal of Personality Assessment, 64,* 2–20.

Dana, R. H. (1993). *Multicultural assessment perspectives for professional psychology.* Boston: Allyn & Bacon.

Dana, R. H. (2005). *Multicultural assessment: Principles, applications, and examples.* Mahwah, NJ: Erlbaum.

Dana, R. H. (1998). *Understanding cultural identity in intervention and assessment.* Thousand Oaks, CA: Sage.

Daniels, M. H. (1994). Self-Directed Search. In J. T. Kapes, M. M. Mastie, & E. A. Whitfield (Eds.), *A counselor's guide to career assessment instruments* (pp. 206–212). Alexandria, VA: National Career Development Association.

Danzinger, P. R., & Welfel, E. R. (2001). The impact of managed care on mental health counselors: A survey of perceptions, practices, and compliance with ethical standards. *Journal of Mental Health Counseling, 23,* 137–151.

Dawes, R. M. (1994). *House of cards: Psychology and psychotherapy built on myths.* New York: Free Press.

Dawes, R. M., Faust, D., & Meehl, P. E. (1989). Clinical and actuarial judgment. *Science, 243,* 1668–1674.

Day, S. X., & Rounds, J. (1998). Universality of vocational interest structure among racial and ethnic minorities. *American Psychologist, 53,* 728–736.

Derogatis, L. R. (1993). *The Brief Symptom Inventory (BSI) administration, scoring, and procedures.* Minneapolis: Pearson Assessments.

Derogatis, L. R. (1994). *Administration, scoring, and procedures manual for the SCL-90-R* (3rd ed.). Minneapolis: Pearson Assessments.

Derogatis, L. R. (2000). *Brief Symptoms Inventory-18.* Minnetonka, MN: NCS Assessments.

Digman, J. M. (1990). Personality structure: Emergence of the five-factor model. *Annual Review of Psychology, 41,* 417–440.

Digman, J. M., & Takemoto-Chock, N. K. (1981). Factors in the natural language of personality: Re-analysis, comparison, and interpretation of six major studies. *Multivariate Behavioral Research, 16,* 149–170.

Doll, B. J. (2003). Review of the Wechsler Individual Achievement Test-Second Edition. In B. S. Plake, J. C. Impara, & R. A. Spies (Eds.), *The fifteenth mental measurements yearbook* (pp. 996–999). Lincoln, NE: Buros Institute of Mental Measurements.

Dollarhide, C. T., & Lemberger, M. E. (2006). No Child Left Behind: Implications for school counselors. *Professional School Counseling, 9,* 295–304.

Donlon, T. F. (Ed.). (1984). *The College Board technical handbook for the Scholastic Aptitude Test and achievement testing.* New York: College Board Publications.

Donnay, D. A. C., & Borgen, F. H. (1999). The incremental validity of vocational self-efficacy: An examination of interest, self-efficacy, and occupation. *Journal of Counseling Psychology, 49,* 432–447.

Donnay, D. A. C., Morris, M. L., Schaubhut, N. A., & Thompson, R. C. (2005). *Strong Interest Inventory manual.* Mountain View, CA: Consulting Psychologists Press.

Dorr, D. (1981). Conjoint psychological testing in marriage therapy: New wine in old skins. *Professional Psychology, 12,* 549–555.

Dowd, E. T., Milne, C. R., & Wise, S. L. (1991). The Therapeutic Reactance Scale: A measure of psychological reactance. *Journal of Counseling & Development, 69,* 541–545.

Dozois, D. J. A., Dobson, K. S., & Ahnberg, J. L. (1998). A psychometric evaluation of the Beck Depression Inventory—II. *Psychological Assessment, 10,* 83–89.

Drasgow, F., Olson-Buchanan, J. B., & Moberg, P. J. (1999). Development of an interactive video assessment: Trials and tribulations. In F. Drasgow & J. B. Olson-Buchanan (Eds.), *Innovations in computer assessment* (pp. 177–196). Mahwah, NJ: Erlbaum.

Druckman, J. M., Fournier, D. F., Robinson, R., & Olson, D. H. (1980). *Effectiveness of five types of premarital preparation programs.* Minneapolis: PREPARE-ENRICH, Inc.

Drug and Alcohol Services Information System. (2007). *The DASIS report: Older Adults in substance abuse treatment: 2005.* Retrieved January 8, 2008, from http://www.oas.samhsa.gov/2k7/older/older.pdf

Drummond, R. J. (2000). *Appraisal procedures for counselors and helping professionals* (4th ed.). Upper Saddle River, NJ: Merrill.

Duckworth, J. C. (1990). The counseling approach to the use of testing. *The Counseling Psychologist, 18,* 198–204.

Duckworth, J. C., & Anderson, W. P. (1997). *MMPI and MMPI-2: Interpretation manual for counselors and clinicians.* Muncie, IN: Accelerated Press.

Duffy, M., & Chenail, R. J. (2004). Qualitative strategies in couple and family assessment. In L. Sperry (Ed.), *Assessment of couples and families: Cutting-edge strategies* (pp. 33–64). New York: Brunner-Routledge.

Duley, S. M., Cancelli, A. A., Kratochwill, T. R., Bergan, J. R., & Meredith, K. E. (1983). Training and generalization of motivational analysis interview assessment skills. *Behavioral Assessment, 5,* 281–293.

Dunn, L. M., & Dunn, D. M. (2007). *Peabody Picture Vocabulary Test* (4th ed.). Minneapolis: Pearson.

Duran, R. P. (1983). *Hispanics' education and background: Predictors of college achievement.* New York: College Entrance Examination Board.

Educational Testing Service. (1997). *GRE 1997–98 Guide to the use of scores.* Princeton, NJ: Author.

Eells, T. D. (1997). *Handbook of psychotherapy case formulation.* New York: Guilford.

Egan, G. (2001). *The skilled helper: A problem-management and opportunity-development approach to helping* (7th ed.). Belmont, CA: Brooks/Cole.

Ekstrom. R. B., Elmore, P. B., Schafer, W. D., Trotter, T. V., & Webster, B. (2004). A survey assessment and evaluation activities of school counselors. *Professional School Counseling, 8,* 24–30.

Elliot, C. D. (2006). *Differential Ability Scale-Second Edition: Technical manual.* San Antonio, TX: The Psychological Corporation.

Elmore, P. B., Ekstrom, R., Diamond, E. E., & Whittaker, S. (1993). School counselors' test use patterns and practices. *The School Counselor, 41,* 73–80.

Elmore, P. B., Ekstrom, R., Shafer, W., & Webster, B. (1998, January). *School counselors' activities and training in assessment and evaluations.* Presented at the Assessment 1998, Assessment for Change—Changes in Assessment, St. Petersburg, FL.

Embretson, S. E. (1996). The new rules of measurement. *Psychological Assessment, 8,* 341–349.

Embretson, S. E., & Hershberger, S. L. (1999). *The new rules of measurement: What every psychologist and educator should know.* Mahwah, NJ: Erlbaum.

Engelhard, G. (2005). Review of the Wide Range Achievement Test-Expanded Edition. In R. A. Spies, & B. S. Plake (Eds.). *The sixteenth mental measurements yearbook* (pp. 1136–1138). Lincoln, NE: Buros Institute of Mental Measurements.

Epperson, D. L., Bushway, D. J., & Warman, R. E. (1983). Client self-termination after one session: Effects of problem recognition, counselor gender, and counselor experience. *Journal of Counseling Psychology, 30,* 307–315.

Erford, G. T., Klein, L., & McNinch, K. (2007). Assessment of intelligence. In B. T. Erford (Ed.), *Assessment for counselors* (pp. 45–98). Boston: Lahaska.

Erford, B. T., Moore-Thomas, C., & Linde, L. (2007). Foundations of assessment: Historical, legal, ethical, and diversity perspectives. In B. T. Erford (Ed.), *Assessment for counselors* (pp. 45–98). Boston: Lahaska.

Essau, C. A., Conradt, J., & Petermann, F. (2000). Frequency, comorbidity, and psychosocial impairment of depressive disorders in adolescents. *Journal of Adolescent Research, 15,* 470–481.

Evans, J. J., Floyd, R. G., McGrew, K. S., & Leforgee, M. H. (2002). The relations between measures of Cattell-Horn-Carroll (CHC) cognitive abilities and reading achievement during childhood and adolescence. *School Psychology Review, 31,* 246–262.

Eyde, L. D., & Kowal, D. M. (1987). Computerized test interpretation services: Ethical and professional concerns regarding U.S. producers and users. *Applied Psychology: An International Review, 36,* 401–417.

Eyde, L. D., Robertson, G. J., Moreland, K. L., Robertson, A. G., Shewan, C. M., Harrison, P. L., Porch, B. E., Hammer, A. L., & Primoff, E. S. (1993). *Responsible test use: Case studies for assessing human behavior.* Washington, DC: American Psychological Association.

Fassinger, R. E., & O'Brien, K. M. (2000). Career counseling with college women: A scientist-practitioner advocate model of intervention. In D. A. Luzzo (Ed.), *Career counselor of college students* (pp. 253–265). Washington, DC: American Psychological Association.

Fernandez, K., Boccaccini, M. T., & Noland, R. M. (2007). Professionally responsible test selection for Spanish-speaking clients: A four-step approach for identifying and selecting translated tests. *Professional Psychology: Research and Practice, 38,* 363–374.

Finger, M. S., & Ones, D. S. (1999). Psychometric equivalence of the computer and booklet form of the MMPI: A meta-analysis. *Psychological Assessment, 11,* 58–66.

Finn, S. E., & Tonsager, M. E. (1992). Therapeutic effects of providing MMPI-2 test feedback to college students awaiting therapy. *Psychological Assessment, 4,* 278–287.

Finn, S. E., & Tonsager, M. E. (1997). Information gathering and therapeutic models of assessment: Complementary paradigms. *Psychological Assessment, 9,* 374–385.

First, M. B., Gibbon, M., Spitzer, R. L., Williams, J. B. W., & Benjamin, L. (1997). *User's guide for the Structured Clinical Interview for* DSM-IV *Axis II Personality Disorders.* Washington, DC: American Psychiatric Press.

First, M. B., Spitzer, R. L., Gibbon, M., & Williams, J. B. W. (1997). *User's guide for the Structured Clinical Interview for* DSM-IV *Axis I Disorders.* Washington, DC: American Psychiatric Press.

Fisher, C. F., & King, R. M. (1995). *Authentic assessment: A guide to implementation.* Thousand Oaks, CA: Corwin.

Fisher, L., & Sorenson, G. P. (1996). *School law for counselors, psychologists, and social workers.* White Plains, NY: Longman.

Fiske, A. P., Kitayama, S., Markus, H. R., & Nisbett, R. E. (1998). The cultural matrix of social psychology. In D. T. Gilbert & S. T. Fiske (Eds.), *Handbook of social psychology: Vol. 2* (4th ed., pp. 915–981). New York: McGraw-Hill.

Fitts, W. H., & Warren, W. L. (1997). *Tennessee Self-Concept Scale: Second Edition (TSCS:2).* Los Angeles: Western Psychological Services.

Fitzpatrick, C. (2001). Review of the PREPARE-ENRICH. In B. Plake & J. Impara (Eds.), *The fourteenth mental measurements yearbook* (pp. 951–953). Lincoln, NE: Buros Institute of Mental Measures.

Flanagan, D. P. (1995). Review of the Kaufman Adolescent and Adult Intelligence Test. In J. C. Conoley & J. J. Kramer (Eds.), *Twelfth mental measurements yearbook* (pp. 527–530). Lincoln, NE: The University of Nebraska Press.

Flanagan, R. (2005). Review of the Achenbach System of Empirically Based Assessment. In Spies, R. A., & Plake, B. S. (Eds.). *The sixteenth mental measurements yearbook* (pp. 10–13). Lincoln, NE: Buros Institute of Mental Measurements.

Fleenor, J. W. (2001). Review of the Myers-Briggs Type Indicator. In B. Plake & J. Impara (Eds), *The fourteenth mental measurements yearbook* (pp. 816–818). Lincoln, NE: Buros Institute of Mental Measures.

Fletcher, J. M., Francis, D. J., Morris, R. D., & Lyon, G. R. (2005). Evidence-based assessment of learning disabilities in children and adolescents. *Journal of Clinical and Adolescent Psychology, 34,* 506–522.

Fletcher, J. M., Lyon, G. R., Fuchs, L. S., & Barnes, M. A. (2007). *Learning disabilities: From identification to intervention.* New York: Guilford.

Flores, L. Y., Spanerman, L. B., & Obasi, E. M. (2003). Ethical and professional issues in career assessment with diverse racial and ethnic groups. *Journal of Career Assessment, 11,* 76–95.

Flynn, J. R. (1984). The mean IQ of Americans: Massive gains 1932 to 1978. *Psychological Bulletin, 95,* 29–51.

Flynn, J. R. (1987). Massive IQ gains in 14 nations: What IQ tests really measure. *Psychological Bulletin, 101,* 171–191.

Flynn, J. R. (1991). *Asian-Americans: Achievement beyond IQ.* Hillsdale, NJ: Erlbaum.

Folstein, M. F., Folstein, S. E., & McHugh, P. R. (1975). Mini-mental state: A practical method for grading the cognitive state of patients for the clinician. *Journal of Psychiatric Research, 12,* 189–198.

Fong, M. L. (1993). Teaching assessment and diagnosis within a *DSM-III-R* framework. *Counselor Education and Supervision, 32,* 276–286.

Fong, M. L. (1995). Assessment and *DSM-IV* diagnosis of personality disorders: A primer for counselors. *Journal of Counseling and Development, 73,* 635–639.

Fortier, L. M., & Wanlass, R. L. (1984). Family crisis following the diagnosis of a handicapped child. *Family Relations, 33,* 13–24.

Forum on Child and Family Statistics (2007). *America's children: Key national indicators of well-being, 2007.* Retrieved December 1, 2007, from http://www.childstats.gov/americaschildren/famsoc5.asp

Fouad, N., Harmon, L. W., & Borgen, F. H. (1997). The structure of interests in employed adult members of U.S. racial/ethnic minority groups and nonminority groups. *Journal of Counseling Psychology, 44,* 339–345.

Fowers, B. J. (1983). *PREPARE as a predictor of marital satisfaction.* Unpublished master's thesis, University of Minnesota, St. Paul, MN 55108.

Frank, R. G., & Elliott, T. R. (2000). *Handbook of rehabilitation psychology.* Washington, DC: American Psychological Association.

Frauenhoffer, D., Ross, M. J., Gfeller, J., Searight, H. R., & Piotrowski, C. (1998). Psychological test usage among licensed mental health practitioners: A multidisciplinary survey. *Journal of Psychological Practice, 4,* 28–33.

Fredman, N., & Sherman, R. (1987). *Handbook of measurements for marriage and family therapy.* New York: Brunner/Mazel.

Frisch, M. B. (1994). *Quality of Life Inventory.* Minneapolis: Pearson Assessments.

Fuchs, D., & Fuchs, L. S. (1986). Test procedure bias: A meta-analysis of examiner familiarity effects. *Review of Educational Research, 56,* 243–262.

Garb, H. N. (2000). Computers will become increasingly important for psychological assessment: Not that there's anything wrong with that! *Psychological Assessment, 12,* 31–39.

Garb, H. N. (2007). Computer-administered interview and rating scales. *Psychological Assessment, 19,* 4–13.

Gardner, H. (1993). *Frames of mind: The theory of multiple intelligences* (10th anniversary ed.). New York: Basic Books.

Garis, J. W., & Niles, S. G. (1990). The separate and combined effects of SIGI and DISCOVER and a career planning course on undecided university students. *Career Development Quarterly, 39,* 261–274.

Gati, I. (1994). Computer-assisted career counseling: Dilemmas, problems, and possible solutions. *Journal of Counseling and Development, 73,* 51–56.

Gati, I., Krausz, M., & Osipow, S. H. (1996). A taxonomy of difficulties in career decision-making. *Journal of Counseling Psychology, 43,* 510–526.

Gati, I., Osipow, S. H., Krausz, M., & Saka, N. (2000). Validity of the Career Decision-Making Questionnaire: Counselee versus career counselor perceptions. *Journal of Vocational Behavior, 56,* 99–113.

Gati, I., Saka, N., & Krausz, M. (2001). Should I use a computer-assisted career guidance system? It depends on where your career decision-making difficulties lie. *British Journal of Guidance & Counseling, 29,* 301–321.

Geisinger, K. F. (1994). Psychometric issues in testing students with disabilities. *Applied Measurement in Education, 72,* 121–140.

Gergen, K. J. (1985). The social constructionist movement in modern psychology. *American Psychologist, 34,* 127–140.

Giordano, F. G., & Schwiebert, V. L. (1997). School counselors' perceptions of the usefulness of standardized tests, frequency of their use, and assessment training needs. *School Counselor, 44,* 198–206.

Glass, G. V., McGaw, B., & Smith, M. L. (1981). *Meta-analysis in social science research.* Thousand Oaks, CA: Sage.

Goldberg, L. R. (1992). The development of markers of the Big-Five factor structure. *Psychological Assessment, 4,* 26–42.

Goldberg, L. R. (1994). The structure of phenotypic personality traits. *American Psychologist, 48,* 26–34.

Goldman, B. A. & Mitchell, D. F. (2002). *Directory of unpublished experimental mental measures: Volume 8.* Washington, DC: American Psychological Association.

Goldman, L. (1990). Qualitative assessment. *The Counseling Psychologist, 18,* 205–213.

Goldman, L. (1992). Qualitative assessment: An approach for counselors. *Journal of Counseling & Development, 70,* 616–621.

Goldman, L. (1994). The marriage is over for most of us. *Measurement and Evaluation in Counseling and Development, 26,* 217–218.

Goodyear, R. K. (1990). Research on the effects of test interpretation: A review. *The Counseling Psychologist, 18,* 240–257.

Goodyear, R. K., & Lichtenberg, J. W. (1999). A scientist-practitioner perspective on test interpretation. In J. W. Lichtenberg & R. K. Goodyear (Eds.), *Scientist-practitioner perspectives on test interpretation* (pp. 1–14). Boston: Allyn & Bacon.

Gordon, H. W., & Lee, P. (1986). A relationship between gonadotroins and visuospatial function. *Neuropsycholia, 24,* 563–576.

Gottfredson, L. S. (1994). The science and politics of race norming. *American Psychologist, 49,* 955–963.

Gough, H. G., & Bradley, P. (1996). *CPI manual* (3rd ed.). Palo Alto, CA: CPP, Inc.

Graduate Record Examination Board. (2007). Graduate Record Examinations: Guide to the use of scores 2007–2008: Princeton, NJ: Educational Testing Service.

Graham, J. M., Liu, Y. J., & Jeziorski, J. L. (2006). The Dyadic Adjustment Scale: A reliability generalization meta-analysis. *Journal of Marriage and Family, 68,* 701–717.

Graham, J. R. (1999). *MMPI-2: Assessing personality and psychopathology* (3rd ed.). New York: Oxford University Press.

Graham, J. R. (2006). *MMPI-2: Assessing personality and psychopathology* (4th ed.). New York: Oxford University Press.

Grant, B. F., Dawson, D. A., Stinson, F. S., Chou, S. P., Dufour, M. C., & Pickering, R. P. (2004). The 12-month prevalence and trends in *DSM-IV* alcohol abuse and dependence: United States, 1991–1992 and 2001–2002. *Drug and Alcohol Dependence, 74,* 223–234.

Greene, R. L., & Banken, J. A. (1995). Assessing alcohol/drug abuse problems. In J. N. Butcher (Ed.), *Clinical personality assessment: Practical approaches* (pp. 460–474). New York: Oxford University Press.

Greenspan, S. I., & Greenspan, N. T. (1981). *The clinical interview of the child.* New York: McGraw-Hill.

Gronlund, N. E. (1998). *Assessment of student achievement* (6th ed.). Boston: Allyn & Bacon.

Groth-Marnat, G. (2003). *Handbook of psychological assessment* (4th ed.). New York: Wiley.

Grove, W. M., Zald, D. H., Lebow, B. S., Snitz, B. E., & Nelson, C. (2000). Clinical versus mechanical prediction: A meta-analysis. *Psychological Assessment, 12,* 19–30.

Guilford, J. B. (1988). Some changes in the structure of the intellect model. *Educational and Psychological Measurement, 48,* 1–4.

Hackett, G., & Lonborg, S. D. (1993). Career assessment for women: Trends and issues. *Journal of Career Assessment, 3,* 197–216.

Hackett, G., & Lonborg, S. D. (1994). Career assessment and counseling for women. In W. B. Walsh & S. H. Osipow (Eds.), *Career counseling for women* (pp. 43–86). Hillsdale, NJ: Erlbaum.

Hackett, G., & Watkins, C. E. (1995). Research in career assessment: Abilities, interests, decision making, and career development. In W. B. Walsh & S. H. Osipow (Eds.), *Handbook of vocational psychology: Theory, research, and practice* (2nd ed., pp. 181–215). Hillsdale, NJ: Erlbaum.

Hagen, J. W., & Hagen, W. W. (1995). What employment counselors need to know about employment discrimination and the Civil Rights Act of 1991. *Journal of Employment Counseling, 32,* 2–10.

Hallahan, D. P., & Kauffman, J. M. (2002). *Exceptional learners: Introduction to special education* (9th ed.). Boston: Allyn & Bacon.

Hambleton, R. K., Swaminathan, H., & Rogers, J. H. (1991). *Fundamentals of item response theory.* Thousand Oaks, CA: Sage.

Handler, L. (1996). The clinical use of figure drawings. In C. S. Newmark (Ed.), *Major psychological assessment instruments* (2nd ed., pp. 206–293). Boston: Allyn & Bacon.

Hansen, J. C. (2005). Assessment of interest. In S.D. Brown & R. W. Lent (Eds.), *Career development and counseling: Putting theory and research to work* (pp. 281–304). Hoboken, NJ: Wiley.

Hansen, J. C, & Leuty, M. E. (2007). Evidence of validity for the Skills Scale scores of the Campbell Interest and Skills Survey. *Journal of Vocational Behavior, 71,* 23–44.

Hanson, W. E. (2001). Review of the Butcher Training Planning Inventory. In B. Plake & J. Impara (Eds.), *The fourteenth mental measurements yearbook* (pp. 711–712). Lincoln, NE: Buros Institute of Mental Measures.

Hanson, W. E., & Claiborn, C. D. (1998). Providing test feedback to clients: What really matters. In C. Claiborn (Chair), *Test interpretation in counseling—Recent research and practice.* Symposium conducted at the conference of the American Psychological Association, San Francisco.

Hanson, W. E., & Claiborn, C. D. (2006). Effects of test interpretation style and favorability in the counseling process. *Journal of Counseling & Development, 84,* 349–357.

Hanson, W. E., Claiborn, C. D., & Kerr, B. (1997). Differential effects of two test-interpretation styles in counseling: A field study. *Journal of Counseling Psychology, 44,* 400–405.

Harmon, L. W. (1994). Career Decision Scale (CDS). In J. T. Kapes, M. M. Mastie, & E. A. Whitfield (Eds.), *A counselor's guide to career assessment instruments* (pp. 258–262). Alexandria, VA: National Career Development Association.

Harmon, L. W. (1997). Do gender differences necessitate separate career development theories and measures? *Journal of Career Assessment, 5,* 463–470.

Hartigan, J. A., & Wigdor, A. K. (1989). *Fairness in employment testing: Validity generalization minority issues and the General Aptitude Test Battery.* Washington, DC: National Academy Press.

Hartung, P. J. (1999). Interest assessment using card sorts. In M. L. Savickas & A. R. Spokane (Eds.), *Vocational interests: Meaning, measurement, and counseling use* (pp. 235– 252). Palo Alto, CA: Davies-Black.

Hattie, J. (1998). Review of the Tennessee Self-Concept Scale, Second Edition. In C. W. Conoley & J. Impara (Eds.), *The thirteenth mental measurements yearbook* (pp. 1011–1012). Lincoln, NE: Buros Institute of Mental Measures.

Haynes, S., Follingstad, T., & Sullivan, J. (1979). Assessment of marital satisfaction and interaction. *Journal of Consulting and Clinical Psychology, 47,* 789–791.

Hedges, L. V., & Olkin, I. (1985). *Statistical methods for meta-analysis.* Orlando, FL: Academic Press.

Helms, J. E. (2002). A remedy for the Black-white test score disparity. *American Psychologist, 57,* 30–35.

Helms, J. E. (2004). Fair and valid use of educational testing in grades K-12. In J. E.Wall & G. R.Walz (Eds.), *Measuring up: Assessment issues for teachers, counselors, and administrators* (pp. 81–88). Greensboro, NC: CAPS Press.

Helms, J. E. (2006). Fairness is not validity or cultural bias in racial-group assessment: A quantitative perspective. *American Psychologist, 61,* 845–859.

Helms, J. E., & Ekstrom, R. B. (2002). Counseling assessment. In R. B. Ekstrom & D. K. Smith (Eds.), *Assessing individuals with disabilities in education, employment, and counseling settings* (pp.121–132). Washington, DC: American Psychological Association.

Helms, J. E., Jernigan, M., & Mascher, J. (2005). The meaning of race in psychology and how to change it. *American Psychologist, 60,* 27–36.

Henard, D. H. (2000). Item response theory. In L. G. Grimm & P. R. Yarnold (Eds.), *Reading and understanding more multivariate statistics* (pp. 67–97). Washington, DC: American Psychological Association.

Henson, R. W., & Hwang, D. (2002). Variability and predication of measurement error in Kolb's Learning Styles Inventory scores: A reliability generalization study. *Educational and Psychological Measurement, 62,* 712–727.

Heppner, P. P., & Claiborn, C. D. (1989). Social influence research in counseling: A review and critique. *Journal of Counseling Psychology, 36,* 365–387.

Hernstein, R. J., & Murray, C. A. (1994). *The bell curve: Intelligence and class structure in American life.* New York: Free Press.

Herr, E. L., & Cramer, S. H. (1996). *Career guidance and counseling through the life span: Systematic approaches.* New York: HarperCollins.

Herr, E. L., Cramer, S. H., & Niles, S. G. (2004). *Career guidance and counseling through the lifespan: Systematic approaches* (6th ed.). Boston: Allyn & Bacon.

Hess, A. K. (2001). Review of the Wechsler Adult Intelligence Scale, Third Edition. In B. Plake & J. Impara (Eds), *The fourteenth mental measurements yearbook* (pp. 1332–1336). Lincoln, NE: Buros Institute of Mental Measures.

Hill, C. E., & Lambert, M. J. (2004). Methodological issues in studying psychotherapy processes and outcome. In M. J. Lambert (Ed.), *Bergin and Garfield's handbook of psychotherapy and behavior change* (5th ed., pp. 84–135). New York: Wiley.

Hill, C. E., & O'Brien, K. M. (2004). *Helping skills: Facilitating exploration, insight, and action* (2nd ed.). Washington, DC: American Psychological Association.

Hiller, J. B., Rosenthal, R., Bornstein, R. F., Berry, D. T. R., & Brunell-Neuleib, S. (1999). A comparative meta-analysis of Rorschach and MMPI validity. *Psychological Assessment, 11,* 278–296.

Hines, M. (1990). Gonadal hormones and human cognitive development. In J. Balthazart (Ed.), *Hormones brains, and behaviors in vertebrates: Sexual differentiation, neuroanatomical aspects, neurotransmitters, and neuropeptides* (pp. 51–63). Basel, Switzerland: Karger.

Hoffman, K. I., & Lundberg, G. D. (1976). A comparison of computer monitored group tests and paper-and-pencil tests. *Educational and Psychological Measurement, 36,* 791–809.

Hoffman, M. A., Spokane, A. R., & Magoon, T. M. (1981). Effects of feedback mode on counseling outcomes using the Strong-Campbell Interest Inventory: Does the counselor really matter? *Journal of Counseling Psychology, 28,* 119–125.

Hogan, R., Hogan, J., & Roberts, B. W. (1996). Personality measurement and employment: Questions and answers. *American Psychologist, 51,* 469–477.

Hoge, R. D. (1985). The validity of direct observation measures of pupil classroom behavior. *Review of Educational Research, 55,* 469–483.

Hohenshil, T. H. (1993). Teaching the *DSM-III-R* in counselor education. *Counselor Education and Supervision, 32,* 267–275.

Hohenshil, T. H. (1996). Editorial: Role of assessment and diagnosis in counseling. *Journal of Counseling and Development, 75,* 64–67.

Holland, J. L. (1997). *Making vocational choices: A theory of vocational personalities and work environments* (3rd ed.). Odessa, FL: Psychological Assessment Resources.

Holland, J. L., Daiger, D., & Power, P. G. (1980). *My Vocational Situation.* Odessa, FL: Psychological Assessment Resources.

Holland, J. L., Fritzsche, B. A., & Powell, A. B. (1994). *The Self-Directed Search (SDS) technical manual—1994 edition.* Odessa, FL: Psychological Assessment Resources.

Holland, J. L., Powell, A. B., & Fritzsche, B. A. (1997). *Self-Directed Search professional user's guide.* Odessa, FL: Psychological Assessment Resources.

Hombo, C. M. (2003). NAEP and No Child Left Behind: Technical challenges and practical solutions. *Theory into Practice, 42,* 60–65.

Honzik, M. P. (1967). Environmental correlates of mental growth: Predictions from the family setting at 21 months. *Child Development, 38,* 323–337.

Hood, A. B., & Johnson, R. W. (2007). *Assessment in counseling: A guide to the use of psychological assessment procedures* (4th ed.). Alexandria, VA: American Counseling Association.

Horn, C. (2003). High-stakes testing and students: Stopping or perpetuating a cycle of failure? *Theory into Practice, 4,* 30–41.

Horn, J. L., & Cattell, R. B. (1966). Refinement and test of the theory of fluid and crystallized general intelligences. *Journal of Educational Psychology, 57,* 253–270.

Horn, J. L. (1985). Remodeling old models of intelligence: G-Gc theory. In B. B. Wolman (Ed.), *Handbook of intelligence* (pp. 267–300). New York: Wiley.

Hughes, D. K., & James, S. H. (2001). Using accountability data to protect a school counseling program: One counselor's experience. *Professional School Counseling, 4,* 306–310.

Hummel, T. J. (1999). The usefulness of tests in clinical decisions. In J. W. Lichtenberg & R. K. Goodyear (Eds.), *Scientist-practitioner perspectives on test interpretation* (pp. 59–112). Boston: Allyn & Bacon.

Hunsley, J., & Bailey, J. M. (1999). The clinical utility of the Rorschach: Unfulfilled promises and an uncertain future. *Psychological Assessment, 11,* 266–277.

Hunter, J. E. (1980). *Validity generalization for 12,000 jobs: An application of synthetic validity and validity generalization to the General Aptitude Test Battery (GATB).* Washington, DC: U.S. Department of Labor.

Hunter, J. E. (1982). *The dimensionality of the General Aptitude Test Battery and the dominance of general factors over specific factors in the prediction of job performance.* Washington, DC: U.S. Department of Labor.

Hunter, J. E. (1986). Cognitive ability, cognitive aptitudes, job knowledge, and job performance. *Journal of Vocational Behavior, 29,* 340–362.

Hunter, J. E., & Schmidt, F. L. (1983). Quantifying the effects of psychological interventions on employee performance and work-force productivity. *American Psychologist, 38,* 473–478.

Hunter, J. E., Schmidt, F. L., & Hunter, R. (1979). Differential validity of employment tests by race: A comprehensive review and analysis. *Psychological Bulletin, 86,* 721–735.

Impara, J. C., & Plake, B. S. (1995). Comparing counselors', school administrators', and teachers' knowledge about student assessment. *Measurement and Evaluation in Counseling and Development, 28,* 78–87.

Ivey, A. E., Ivey, M. B., & Simek-Morgan, L. (1993). *Counseling and psychotherapy: A multicultural perspective* (3rd ed.). Boston: Allyn & Bacon.

Jackson, D. N. (1996). *Jackson Vocational Interest Survey.* Port Huron, MI: Sigma Assessment Systems.

Jackson, D. N. (1997). *Jackson Personality Inventory—Revised.* London, Ontario: Research Psychologists Press.

Jackson, D. N. (1998). *Multidimensional Aptitude Battery-II.* Port Huron, MI: Sigma Assessment System.

Jastak, J. F., & Jastak, S. (1979). *Wide Range Interest-Opinion Test.* Wilmington, DE: Jastak Associates.

Jensen, A. R. (1969). How much can we boost IQ and scholastic achievement? *Harvard Educational Review, 39,* 1–23.

Jensen, A. R. (1972). *Genetics and education.* New York: Harper & Row.

Jensen, A. R. (1980). *Bias in mental testing.* New York: Free Press.

Jensen, A. R. (1985). The nature of black-white differences on various psychometric tests: Spearman's hypothesis. *The Behavioral and Brain Sciences, 8,* 192–263.

Johansson, C. B. (1984). *Manual for the Career Assessment Inventory* (2nd ed.). Minneapolis: National Computer Systems.

Johansson, C. B. (1986). *Manual for the Career Assessment Inventory: The enhanced version.* Minneapolis: National Computer Systems.

Johnson, R. L., & Mazzie, D. (2005). Review of the TerraNova, second edition. In R. A. Spies & B. Plake (Eds.), *The Sixteenth Mental Measurements Yearbook* (pp.1030–1035). Lincoln, NE: Buros Institute of Mental Measures.

Joinson, A. N., & Buchanan, T. (2001). Doing educational psychology research on the Web. In C. Wolfe (Ed.), *Teaching and learning on the World Wide Web* (pp. 221– 242). San Diego, CA: Academic Press.

Joint Committee on Testing Practices. (1998). *Rights and responsibilities of test takers: Guidelines and expectations.* Washington, DC: Author.

Joint Committee on Testing Practices. (2004). *Code of fair testing practices in education.* Washington, DC: Author. (Mailing address: Joint Committee on Testing Practices, American Psychological Association, 750 First Avenue, NE, Washington, DC, 20002-4242.)

Jones, A. S., & Gelso, C. J. (1988). Differential effects of style of interpretation: Another look. *Journal of Counseling Psychology, 35,* 363–369.

Juni, S. (1995). Review of the revised NEO Personality Inventory. In J. C. Conoley & J. J. Kramer (Eds.), *Twelfth mental measurements yearbook* (pp. 863–868). Lincoln, NE: The University of Nebraska Press.

Kahne, J. (1996). The politics of self-esteem. *American Educational Research Journal, 33,* 3–22.

Kamphaus, R. W. (2000). *Clinical assessment of child and adolescent intelligence* (2nd ed.). Boston: Allyn & Bacon.

Kapes, J. T., Borman, C. A., & Frazier, F. D. (1989). An evaluation of SIGI and DISCOVER microcomputer-based career guidance systems. *Measurement and Evaluation in Counseling and Development, 22,* 126–136.

Kaplan, R. M., & Saccuzzo, D. P. (2005). *Psychological testing: Principles, applications, and issues* (6th ed.). Belmont, CA: Wadsworth.

Kaufman, A. S. (1990). *Assessing adolescents and adults in intelligence.* Boston: Allyn & Bacon.

Kaufman, A. S. (1994). *Intelligent testing with the WISC-III.* New York: Wiley.

Kaufman, A. S., & Kaufman, N. L. (2004). *Kaufman Test of Educational Achievement, Second Edition.* Circle Pines, MN: AGS Publishing.

Kaufman, A. S., & Kaufman, N. L. (1993). *Kaufman Adolescent and Adult Intelligence test manual.* Circle Pines, MN: American Guidance Service.

Kavale, K. A. (1995). Setting the record straight on learning disability and low achievement: The tortuous path of ideology. *Learning Disabilities Research and Practice, 10,* 145–152.

Keitel, M. A., Kopala, M., & Adamson, W. S. (1996). Ethical issues in multicultural assessment. In L. A. Suzuki, P. J. Meller, & J. G. Ponterotto (Eds.), *Handbook of multicultural assessment: Clinical, psychological, and educational applications* (pp. 29–50). San Francisco: Jossey-Bass.

Kelley, P. A., Sanspree, M. J., & Davidson, R.C. (2001). Visual impairment in children and youth. In B. Siverstone, M. A. Lang, B. Rosenthal, & E. E. Faye (Eds.),

The Lighthouse handbook on visual impairment and visual rehabilitation (pp. 1137–1151). New York: Oxford University Press.

Kelley, T. L. (1939). The selection of upper and lower group. *Journal of Educational Psychology, 30,* 17–24.

Kelley, M. L. (2005). Review of the Piers-Harris Children's Self-Concept Scale, Second Edition, In R. A. Spies, & B. S. Plake (Eds.). *The sixteenth mental measurements yearbook* (pp. 789–790). Lincoln, NE: Buros Institute of Mental Measurements.

Kelly, K. E. (2002). *Kuder Occupational Interest Survey Form DD and Kuder Career Search with Person Match.* In J. T. Kapes, M. M. Mastie, & E. A. Whitfield (Eds.), *A counselor's guide to career assessment instruments* (4th ed., pp. 269–275). Tulsa, OK: National Career Development Association.

Kent, N., & Davis, D. R. (1957). Discipline in the home and intellectual development. *British Journal of Medical Psychology, 30,* 27–33.

Kerig, P., & Lindhal, K. M. (2001). *Family observational coding systems: Resources for systematic research.* Mahwah, NJ: Erlbaum.

Kessler, R. C., & Ustün, T. B. (2004). The World Mental Health (WMH) Survey initiative version of the World Health Organization (WHO) Composite International Diagnostic Interview (CIDI). *International Journal of Methods in Psychiatric Research, 13,* 93–121.

Keyser, D. J., & Sweetland, R. C. (Eds.) (1994). *Test critiques: Volume X.* Austin, TX: PRO-ED.

King, K. (2001). A critique of behavioral observational coding systems of couples' interaction: CISS and RCISS. *Journal of Social and Clinical Psychology, 20,* 1–23.

Kinston, W., Loader, P., & Sullivan, J. (1985). *Clinical assessment of family health.* London: Hospital for Sick Children, Family Studies Group.

Kirchner, C. (1983). Special education for visually handicapped children: A critique of data on numbers served and costs. *Journal of Visual Impairment & Blindness, 77,* 219–223.

Kiresuk, T. J., Smith, A., & Cardillo, J. E. (1994). *Goal Attainment Scaling: Application, theory, and measurement.* Hillsdale, NJ: Erlbaum.

Kivlighan, D. M., & Shapiro, R. M. (1987). Holland type as a predictor of benefit from self-help career counseling. *Journal of Counseling Psychology, 34,* 326–329.

Knoff, H. M., & Prout, H. T. (1993). *Kinetic drawing system for family and school: A handbook* (5th ed.). Los Angeles: Western Psychological Services.

Knutson, L., & Olson, D. H. (2003). *Effectiveness of PREPARE Program (Version 2000) with premarital couples in a community setting.* Retrieved August 8, 2004, from http://www.lifeinnovations.com

Kovacs, M. (2003). *Children's Depression Inventory (2003 update).* North Tonawanda, NY: Multi-Health Systems.

Kramer, J. J., & Conoley, J. C. (Eds.). (1992). *Eleventh mental measurements yearbook.* Lincoln, NE: Buros Institute of Mental Measures.

Krivasty, S. E., & Magoon, T. M. (1976). Differential effects of three vocational counseling treatments. *Journal of Counseling Psychology, 23,* 112–117.

Kuder, F. (1988). *Kuder General Interest Survey Form E: General manual* (preliminary edition). Adel, IA: National Career Assessment Services.

Kuder, F., & Zytowski, D. G. (1991). *Kuder Occupational Interest Survey Form DD: General manual* (3rd ed.). Adel, IA: National Career Assessment Services.

Kuncel, N. R., Hezlett, S. A., & Ones, D. S. (2001). A comprehensive meta-analysis of the predictive validity of the Graduate Record Examinations: Implication for graduate selection and performance. *Psychological Bulletin, 127,* 162–181.

Kupper, L. (2007). *The top 10 basics of special education (Module 1). Building the legacy: IDEA training curriculum.* Retrieved November 23, 2007, from www.nichcy.org/training/contents.asp

L' Abate, L. (1994). *Family evaluation: A psychological approach.* Thousand Oaks, CA; Sage.

Lachar, D., & Gruber, C. P. (1995). *Personality Inventory for Youth (PIY).* Los Angeles: Western Psychological Services.

Lachar, D., & Gruber, C. P. (2001). *Personality Inventory for Children—Second Edition.* Los Angeles: Western Psychological Services.

LaCrosse, M. B. (1980). Perceived counselor social influence and counseling outcome: Validity of the Counselor Rating Form. *Journal of Counseling Psychology, 27,* 320–327.

Lambert, M. J. (2007). Presidential address: What we have learned from a decade of research aimed at improving psychotherapy outcome in routine care. *Psychotherapy Research, 17,* 1–14.

Lambert, M. J., Hansen, N. B., & Finch, A. E. (2001). Patient-focused research: Using patient outcome data to enhance treatment effects. *Journal of Consulting and Clinical Psychology, 69,* 159–172.

Lambert, M. J., Morton, J. S., Hatfield, D., Harmon, C., Hamilton, S. Reid, R. C., Shimokawa, K., Christopherson, C., & Burlingame, G. M. (1996). *OQ45.2 Outcome questionnaire.* Salt Lake City, UT: OQ Measures LLC.

Lambert, M. J., Okiishi, J. C., Finch, A. E., & Johnson, L. D. (1998). Outcome assessment: From conceptualization to implementation. *Professional Psychology: Research and Practice, 29,* 63–70.

Lambert, M. J., Whipple, J. L., Hawkins, E. J., Vermeersch, D. A., Nielsen, S. L., & Smart, D. W. (2003). Is it time for clinicians to routinely track patient outcome? A meta-analysis. *Clinical Psychology: Science and Practice, 10,* 288–301.

Lambert, M. J., Whipple, J. L., Smart, D. W., Vermeersch, D. A., Nielsen, S. L., & Hawkins, E. J. (2001). The effects of providing therapists with feedback on client progress during psychotherapy: Are outcomes enhanced? *Psychotherapy Research, 11,* 49–68.

Lapan, R. T. (2001). Results-based comprehensive guidance and counseling programs: A framework for planning and evaluation. *Professional School Counseling, 4,* 289–299.

Lapan, R. T., & Kosciulek, J. F. (2001). Toward a community career system program evaluation framework. *Journal of Counseling & Development, 79,* 3–16.

Larson, J. H. (2002). *Consumer update: Marriage preparation.* [Brochure]. Alexandria, VA: American Association of Marriage and Family Therapists.

Lees-Haley, P. R., English, L. T., & Glenn, W. J. (1991). A Fake Bad Scale on the MMPI-2 for personal injury claimants. *Psychological Reports, 68,* 203–210.

Lent, R. W., Brown, S. D., & Hackett, G. (1994). Toward a unifying social cognitive theory of career and academic interest, choice, and performance. *Journal of Vocational Behavior, 45,* 79–122.

Lenz, J. G., Reardon, R. C., & Sampson, J. P. (1993). Holland's theory and effective use of computer-assisted career guidance systems. *Journal of Career Development, 19,* 245–253.

Leong, F. T. L., & Hartung, P. J. (2000). Cross-cultural career assessment: Review and prospects for the new millennium. *Journal of Career Assessment, 8,* 391–401.

Lerner, B. (1981). The minimum competence testing movement: Social, scientific, and legal implications. *American Psychologist, 36,* 1056–1066.

Lichtenberg, J. W., & Hummel, T. J. (1998). The communication of probabilistic information through test interpretation. In C. Claiborn (Chair), *Test interpretation in counseling—Recent research and practice.* Symposium conducted at the conference of the American Psychological Association, San Francisco.

Lichtenberger, E. O., & Smith, D. R. (2005). *Essentials of the WIAT-II and KTEA-II assessments.* Hoboken, NJ: Wiley.

Lindzey, G. (1959). On the classification of projective techniques. *Psychological Bulletin, 56,* 158–168.

Linn, R. L. (1994). Fair test use: Research and policy. In M. G. Rumsey, C. B. Walker, & J. H. Harris (Eds.), *Personnel selection and classification* (pp. 363–375). Hillsdale, NJ: Erlbaum.

Linn, R. L., Baker, E. L., & Betebenner, D. W. (2002). Accountability systems: Implications of requirements of the No Child Left Behind Act of 2001. *Educational Researcher, 31,* 3–16.

LinnLocke, H., & Wallace, K. (1959). Short marital adjustment and predictions tests: Their reliability and validity. *Marriage and Family Living, 2,* 251–255.

Loehlin, J. C. (1989). Partitioning environmental and genetic contributions to behavioral development. *American Psychologist, 10,* 1285–1292.

Loehlin, J. C., Lindzey, G., & Spuhler, J. N. (1975). *Race differences in intelligence.* San Francisco: Freeman.

Long, K. A., Graham, J. R., & Timbrook, R. E. (1994). Socioeconomic status and MMPI-2 interpretation. *Measurement and Evaluation in Counseling and Development, 27,* 159–177.

Lopez, S. J., & Snyder, C. R. (2003). *Positive psychological assessment: A handbook of models and measures.* Washington, DC: American Psychological Association.

Lopez, S. J., Snyder, C. R., & Rasmussen, H. N. (2003). Striking a vital balance: Developing a complementary focus on human weakness and strength through positive psychological assessment. In S. J. Lopez & C. R. Snyder (Eds.), *Positive psychological assessment: A handbook of models and measures* (pp. 3–20). Washington, DC: American Psychological Association.

Lord, F. M. (1980). *Applications of item response theory to practical testing problems.* Hillsdale, NJ: Erlbaum.

Losen, D. J., & Orfield, G. (2002). *Racial inequality in special education.* Cambridge, MA: Harvard Education Press.

Luria, A. R. (1966). *Human brain and psychological processes.* New York: Harper & Row.

MacCluskie, K. C., Welfel, E. R., & Toman, S. M. (2002). *Using test data in clinical practice: A handbook of mental health professionals.* Thousand Oaks, CA: Sage.

Machover, K. (1949). *Personality projection in the drawings of the human figure: A method of personality investigation.* Springfield, IL: Charles C. Thomas.

Maddox, T. (2003). *Tests: A comprehensive reference for assessment in psychology, education, and business.* Austin, TX: PRO-ED.

Mahoney, M. J. (2000). A changing history of efforts to understand and control change: The case of psychotherapy. In C. R. Snyder & R. E. Ingram (Eds.), *Handbook of psychological change: Psychotherapy processes and practice for the 21st century* (pp. 2–12). New York: Wiley.

Maller, S. J. (2005). Review of the Wechsler Intelligence Scale for Children-Fourth Edition. In R. A. Spies & B. S. Plake (Eds.), *The sixteenth mental measurements yearbook* (pp. 1093–1096). Lincoln, NE: Buros Institute of Mental Measurements.

Manges, K. J. (2001). Review of the Family Assessment Measure, Version III. In B. Plake & J. Impara (Eds.), *The fourteenth mental measurements yearbook* (pp. 480–482). Lincoln, NE: Buros Institute of Mental Measures.

Manuele-Adkins, C. (1989). Review of the Self-Directed Search. In J. C. Conoley & J. J. Kramer (Eds.), *Tenth mental measurements yearbook* (pp. 738–740). Lincoln, NE: The University of Nebraska Press.

Maraist, C. C., & Russell, M. T. (2002). *16PF Fifth Edition norm supplement, release 2002.* Champaign, IL: Institute for Personality and Ability Testing.

Martin, J., Prupas, L., & Sugarman, J. (1999). Test interpretation as the social-cognitive construction of therapeutic change. In J. W. Lichtenberg &

R. K. Goodyear (Eds.), *Scientist-practitioner perspectives on test interpretation* (pp. 132–150). Needham Heights, MA: Allyn & Bacon.

Masters, M. S., & Sanders, B. (1993). Is the gender difference in mental rotation disappearing? *Behavior Genetics, 23,* 337–341.

Mastrangelo, P. M. (2001). Review of the Myers-Briggs Type Indicator. In B. Plake & J. Impara (Eds.), *The fourteenth mental measurements yearbook* (pp. 714–715). Lincoln, NE: Buros Institute of Mental Measures.

Maruish, M. E. (2004). Introduction. In M. E. Maruish (Ed.), *The use of psychological testing for treatment planning and outcomes assessment: Volume 1 general considerations* (3rd ed., pp. 1–64). Mahwah, NJ: Erlbaum.

Mayfield, D. G., McLeod, G., & Hall, P. (1974). The CAGE questionnaire: Validation of a new alcoholism screening instrument. *American Journal of Psychiatry, 131,* 1121–1123.

McClure, E. B., Kubiszyn, T., & Kaslow, N. J. (2002). Advances in the diagnosis and treatment of childhood mood disorders. *Professional Psychology: Research and Practice, 33,* 125–134.

McConnaughy, E. A., DiClemente, C. C., Prochaska, J. O., & Velicer, W. F. (1989). Stages of change in psychotherapy: A follow-up report. *Psychotherapy, 26,* 494–503.

McConnaughy, E. A., Prochaska, J. O., & Velicer, W. F. (1983). Stages of change in psychotherapy: Measurement and sample profiles. *Psychotherapy: Theory, Research, and Practice, 20,* 368–375.

McCrae, R. R., & Costa P. T. (1997). Personality trait structure as a human universal. *American Psychologist, 52,* 509–516.

McCrae, R. R., & John, O. P. (1992). An introduction to the five-factor model and its applications. *Journal of Personality, 60,* 175–215.

McGhee, R.L., Ehrler, D. J., & Buckhalt, J. A. (2007). *FFPI-C: Five Factors Personality Inventory-Children examiner's manual.* Austin, TX: PRO-ED.

McGoldrick, M., Gerson, R., & Shellenberger, S. (1999). *Genograms: Assessment and intervention* (2nd ed.). New York: W. W. Norton.

McGrew, K. S. (1997). Analysis of major intelligence batteries according to a proposed comprehensive Gc-Gf framework. In D. P. Flanagan, J. L. Genshaft, & P. L. Harrison (Eds.), *Contemporary intellectual assessment: Theories, tests, and issues* (pp. 151–180). New York: Guilford.

McGrew, K. S., & Flanagan, D. P. (1998). *The intelligence test desk reference: Gf-Gc cross battery assessment.* Boston: Allyn & Bacon.

McGrew, K. S., & Woodcock, R. W. (2001). *Woodcock-Johnson III: Technical manual.* Itasca, IL: Riverside.

McGue, M., Bouchard, T. J., Jr., Iacono, W. G., & Lykken, D. T. (1993). Behavioral genetics of cognitive ability: A life-span perspective. In R. Plomin & G. E. McClearn (Eds.), *Nature, nurture, & psychology* (pp. 59–76). Washington, DC: American Psychological Association.

McIntosh, J. L. (1992). Methods of suicide. In R. W. Maris, A. L. Berman, & J. T. Maltsberger (Eds.), *Assessment and prediction of suicide* (pp. 381–397). New York: Guilford.

McMahon, M., Patton, W., & Watson, M. (2003). Developing qualitative career assessment processes. *Career Development Quarterly, 51,* 194–202.

McMichael, A. J., Baghurst, P. A., Wigg, N. R., Vimpani, G. V., Robertson, E. F., & Roberts, R. J. (1988). Port Pirie cohort study: Environmental exposure to lead and children's abilities at the age of four years. *New England Journal of Medicine, 319,* 468–475.

McNamara, K. (1992). Depression assessment and intervention: Current status and future direction. In S. D. Brown & R. W. Lent (Eds.), *Handbook of counseling psychology* (2nd ed., pp. 691–718). New York: Wiley.

McNeil, J. M. (2001, February). *Americans with disabilities: 1997* (Publication No. 70–73). Washington, DC: U.S. Department of Education.

McShane, D. A., & Plas, J. M. (1984). The cognitive functioning of American Indian children: Moving from the WISC to the WISC-R. *School Psychology Review, 13,* 61–73.

Mead, M. A., Hohenshil, T. H., & Singh, S. (1997). How the *DSM* system is used by clinical counselors: A national study. *Journal of Mental Health Counseling, 19,* 383–395.

Meehl, P. E. (1956). Wanted: A good cookbook. *American Psychologist, 11,* 263–272.

Mehrens, W. A., & Ekstrom, R. B. (2002). Score reporting issues in the assessment of people with disabilities: Policies and practices. In R. B. Ekstrom & D. K. Smith (Eds.), *Assessing individuals with disabilities in education, employment, and counseling settings* (pp. 87–100). Washington, DC: American Psychological Association.

Meir, S. T. (2003). *Bridging case conceptualization, assessment, and intervention.* Thousand Oaks, CA: Sage.

Merenda, P. F. (1995). Substantive issues in the *Soroka v. Dayton-Hudson* case. *Psychological Reports, 77,* 595–606.

Merrell, K. W. (2007). *Behavioral, social, and emotional assessment of children and adolescents* (3rd ed.). Mahwah, NJ: Erlbaum.

Merrens, M. R., & Richards, W. S. (1970). Acceptance of generalized versus "bona fide" personality interpretations. *Psychological Reports, 27,* 691–694.

Messick, S. (1995). Validity of psychological assessment: Validation of inferences from persons' responses and performances as scientific inquiry into score meaning. *American Psychologist, 50,* 741–749.

Meyer, G. J., Finn, S. E., Eyde, L. D., Kay, G. G., Moreland, K. L., Dies, R. R., Eisman, E., Kubiszyn, T. W., & Reed G. M. (2001). Psychological testing and psychological assessment: A review of evidence and issues. *American Psychologist, 56,* 128–165.

Michel, D. M. (2002). Psychological assessment as a therapeutic intervention in patients hospitalized with eating disorders. *Professional Psychology: Research and Practice, 33,* 470–477.

Miller, G. A. (1997). *The Substance Abuse Subtle Screening Inventory 3 (SASSI-3).* Springville, IN: The SASSI Institute.

Miller, G. A. (2001). *The Adolescent Substance Abuse Subtle Screening Inventory-A2 (SASSI-A2).* Springville, IN: The SASSI Institute.

Millon, T. (1969). *Modern psychological pathology: A biosocial approach to maladaptive learning and functioning.* Philadelphia: Saunders.

Millon, T. (1994). *Millon Index of Personality Styles (MIPS) manual.* San Antonio, TX: Psychological Corporation.

Millon, T. (2006). *Millon Clinical Multiaxial Inventory III manual* (3rd ed.). Minneapolis: Pearson Assessments.

Millon, T., Davis, R., & Millon, C. (1997). *Millon Clinical Multiaxial Inventory III manual* (2nd ed.). Minneapolis: National Computer Systems.

Millon, T., Millon, C., & Davis, R. (1994). *Millon Adolescent Clinical Inventory.* Minneapolis: National Computer Systems.

Miner, C. U., & Sellers, S. T. (2002). Career Assessment Inventory. In J. T. Kapes, M. M. Mastie, & E. A. Whitfield (Eds.), *A counselor's guide to career assessment instruments* (4th ed., pp. 204–209).Tulsa, OK: National Career Development Association.

Minuchin, S. (1974). *Families and family therapy.* Cambridge, MA: Harvard University Press.

Mitchell, R. R., & Friedman, H. (1994). *Sandplay: Past, present, and future.* New York: Routledge.

Mohr, D. C. (1995). Negative outcome in psychotherapy: A critical review. *Clinical Psychology: Science and Practice, 2,* 1–27.

Moos, R. H. (1973). Conceptualizing human environments. *American Psychologist, 28,* 652–665.

Moos, R. H., & Moos, B. S. (1994). *Family Environment Scale manual: Development, application, research.* Palo Alto, CA: CPP, Inc.

Moreland, K. L., Eyde, L. D., Robertson, G. J., Primoff, E. S., & Most, R. B. (1995). Assessment of test user qualifications: A research-based measurement procedure. *American Psychologist, 50,* 14–23.

Morera, O. F., Johnson, T. P., Freels, S., Parsons, J., Crittenden, K. S., Play, B. R., & Warnecke, R. B. (1998). The measure of stage of readiness to change: Some psychometric considerations. *Psychological Assessment, 10,* 182–186.

Morris, T. M. (1990). Culturally sensitive family assessment: An evaluation of the Family Assessment Device with Hawaiian-American and Japanese-American families. *Family Process, 29,* 105–116.

Morrison, J. (2007). *Diagnosis made easier: Principles and techniques for mental health clinicians.* New York: Guilford.

Munoz-Sandoval, A. F., Cummins, J., Alvarado, C. G., & Ruef, M. L. (1998). *Bilingual Verbal Ability Tests.* Itasca, IL: Riverside.

Murphy, E., & Meisgeier, C. (1987). *Murphy-Meisgeier Type Indicatory for Children.* Palo Alto, CA: CPP, Inc.

Murphy, L. L., Plake, B. S., & Spies, R. A. (2006). *Tests in Print VII.* Lincoln, NE: Buros Institute of Mental Measures.

Murray, H. A. (1943). *Thematic Apperception Test.* Cambridge, MA: Harvard University Press.

Myers, I. B., McCaulley, M. H., Quenk, N. L., & Hammer, A. L. (1998). *MBTI manual: A guide to the development and use of the Myers-Briggs Type Indicator.* Palo Alto, CA: CPP, Inc.

Myers, I. B., with Myers, P. B. (1980). *Gifts differing.* Palo Alto, CA: CPP, Inc.

Myrick, R. D. (2003). Accountability: Counselors count. *Professional School Counseling, 6,* 174–179.

Naglieri, J. A. (1997). *Naglieri Nonverbal Ability Test.* San Antonio, TX: Harcourt Educational Measurement.

Naglieri, J. A., Drasgow, F., Schmit, M., Handler, L., Prifitera, A., Margolis, A., & Velasquez, R. (2004). Psychological testing on the Internet: New problems, old issues. *American Psychologist, 59,* 150–162.

Nairn, A. (1980). *The reign of ETS: The corporation that makes up minds.* New York: Ralph Nader.

National Board for Certified Counselors. (1998). *Standards for the ethical practice of Web counseling.* Greensboro, NC: Author.

National Board for Certified Counselors. (2001). *The practice of Internet counseling.* Greensboro, NC: Author.

National Career Development Association. (1997). *NCDA guidelines for the use of the Internet for the provision of career information and planning services.* Columbus, OH: Author.

National Career Development Association (2007). *National Career Development Association code of ethics.* Broken Arrow, OK: Author.

National Center for Education Statistics. (2003). *Overview: The nation's report card.* Retrieved July 29, 2003, from http://nces.ed.gov/nationsreportcard/about/

National Institutes of Health (2007). *Rates of bipolar diagnosis in youth rapidly climbing, treatment patterns similar to adults.* Retrieved September 30, 2007, from http://www.nih.gov/news/pr/sep2007/nimh-03.htm

National Institute of Mental Health (2006). *Suicide in the U.S.: Statistics and prevention.* Retrieved August 23, 2007, from http://www.nimh.nih.gov/publicat/harmsway.cfm

National Institute of Mental Health (2007). *The number count: Mental disorders in American.* Retrieved October 28, 2007, from http://www.nimh.nih.gov/health/publications/the-numbers-count-mental-disorders-in-america.shtml

National Research Council (2001). *Knowing what students know: The science and design of educational assessment.* Washington, DC: National Academy Press.

National Research Council (2002). *Minority students in special and gifted education.* Washington, DC: National Academy Press.

Needleman, P. E. (1999). *Cognitive case conceptualization.* Mahwah, NJ: Erlbaum.

Neisser, U., Boodoo, G., Bouchard, T. J., Boykin, A. W., Brody, N., Ceci, S. J., et al. (1996). Intelligence: Knowns and unknowns. *American Psychologist, 51,* 77–98.

Nelson, R. O. (1983). Behavioral assessment: Past, present, and future. *Behavioral Assessment, 5,* 196–206.

Nevill, D. D., & Super, D. E. (1986). *The Salience Inventory: Theory, application, and research.* Palo Alto, CA: CPP, Inc.

Nevill, D. D., & Super, D. E. (1989). *The Values Scale: Theory, application, and research.* Palo Alto, CA: CPP, Inc.

New Freedom Commission on Mental Health (2003). *Achieving the promise: Transforming mental health care in America.* Retrieved September 6, 2003, from http://www. mentalhealthcommission.gov/reports/FinalReport/down loads/downloads.html

Newman, M. L., & Greenway, P. (1997) Therapeutic effects of providing MMPI-2 test feedback to clients at a university counseling service: A collaborative approach. *Psychological Assessment, 9,* 122–131.

Newmark, C. S., & McCord, D. M. (1996). The Minnesota Multiphasic Personality Inventory 2. In C. S. Newmark (Ed.), *Major psychological assessment instruments* (2nd ed., pp. 1–58). Boston: Allyn & Bacon.

Newsome, D. (2000). Test review: The Skills Confidence Inventory (SCI). *AAC Newsnotes, 36,* 3–4.

Nguyen, T. D., Attkisson, C. C., & Stegner, B. L. (1983). Assessment of patient satisfaction: Development and refinement of a Service Evaluation Questionnaire. *Evaluation and Program Planning, 6,* 299–313.

Nichols, D. S. (1992). Review of the Minnesota Multiphasic Personality Inventory 2. In J. C. Conoley & J. J. Kramer (Eds.), *Eleventh mental measurements yearbook* (pp. 562–565). Lincoln, NE: The University of Nebraska Press.

Nicholson, C. L., & Hibpshman, T. H. (1990). *Slosson Intelligence Test for Children and Adults, Revised.* East Aurora, NY: Slosson Educational Publications.

Nurse, A. R. (1999). *Family assessment: Effective uses of personality tests with couples and families.* New York: Wiley.

Nurse, A. R., & Sperry, L. (2004). Effective use of psychological tests with couples and families. In L. Sperry (Ed.), *Assessment of couples and families: Cutting-edge strategies* (p. 65–89). New York: Brunner-Routledge.

Oetting, E. R., & Beauvais, F. (1990). Adolescent drug use: Findings of national and local surveys. *Journal of Consulting and Clinical Psychology, 58,* 385–394.

Ogles, B. M., Lambert, M. J., & Fields, S. A. (2002). *Essentials of outcome assessment.* New York: Wiley.

Okun, B. F., & Kantrowitz, R. E. (2007). *Effective helping: Interviewing and counseling techniques* (7th ed.). Belmont, CA: Brooks/Cole.

Oliver, L. W., & Chartrand, J. M. (2000). Strategies for career assessment research on the Internet. *Journal of Career Assessment, 8,* 95–103.

Oliver, L. W., & Spokane, A. R. (1988). Career intervention outcome: What contributes to client gain? *Journal of Counseling Psychology, 35,* 447–462.

Oliver, L. W., & Zack, J. S. (1999). Career assessment on the Internet: An exploratory study. *Journal of Career Assessment, 7,* 323–356.

Olson, D. H. (1983). *Inventories of premarital, marital, parent-child, and parent-adolescent conflict.* St. Paul, MN: University of Minnesota, Department of Family Social Science.

Olson, D. H., & DeFrain, J. (2002). *Marriages and families: Intimacy, diversity, and strengths* (4th ed.). McGraw-Hill.

Olson, D. H., Gorall, D. M., & Tiesel, J. (2004). *Family Adaptability and Cohesion Evaluation Scale IV.* Roseville, MN: Life Innovations.

Olson, D. H., & Gorall, D. M. (2006). *FACES IV and the Circumplex Model.* Retrieved November 3, 2007, from http://www.facesiv.com/pdf/3.innovations.pdf

Olson, D. H., & Ryder, R. (1978). *Marital and Family Interaction Coding System (MFICS): Abbreviated coding manual.* St. Paul, MN: University of Minnesota, Department of Family Social Science.

Oosterhof, A. (1994). *Classroom application of educational measurement* (2nd ed.). Merrill: New York.

Oosterhof, A. (2000). *Classroom application of educational measurement* (3rd ed.). Upper Saddle River, NJ: Merrill Prentice-Hall.

Orlinsky, D. E., Ronnestad, M. H., & Willutzki, U. (2004). Fifty years of psychotherapy process-outcome research: Continuity and change. In M. J. Lambert (Ed.), *Bergin and Garfield's handbook of psychotherapy and behavior change* (5th ed., pp. 307–389). New York: Wiley.

Osborne, W. L., Brown, S., Niles, S., & Miner, C. U. (1997). *Career development, assessment, and counseling: Applications of the Donald E. Super C-DAC approach.* Alexandria, VA: American Counseling Association.

Osipow, S. H. (1987). *Career Decision Scale manual.* Odessa, FL: Psychological Assessment Resources.

Osipow, S. H., & Gati, I. (1998). Construct and concurrent validity of the Career Decision-Making Difficulties Questionnaire. *Journal of Career Assessment, 6,* 347–364.

Oster, G. D., & Crone, P. G. (2004). *Using drawings in assessment and therapy: A guide for mental health professionals* (2nd ed.). New York: Brunner-Routledge.

Oswald, D. P. (2005). Review of the Piers-Harris Children's Self-Concept Scale, Second Edition, In R. A. Spies, & B. S. Plake (Eds.). *The sixteenth mental measurements yearbook* (pp. 790–792). Lincoln, NE: Buros Institute of Mental Measurements.

Ownby, R. L. (1997). *Psychological reports: A guide to report writing in professional psychology* (3rd ed.). New York: Wiley.

Padilla, A. M. (2001). Issues of culturally appropriate assessment. In L. A. Suzuki, J. G. Ponterotto, & P. J. Meller (Eds.), *Handbook of multicultural assessment: Clinical, psychological, and educational applications* (2nd ed., pp. 5–27). San Francisco: Jossey-Bass.

Padilla, A. M., & Medina, A. (1996). Cross-cultural sensitivity in assessment: Using tests in culturally appropriate ways. In L. A. Suzuki, P. J. Meller, & J. G. Ponterotto (Eds.), *Handbook of multicultural assessment: Clinical, psychological, and educational applications* (pp. 3–28). San Francisco: Jossey-Bass.

Page, E. B. (1985). Review of Kaufman Assessment Battery for Children. In J. V. Mitchell (Ed.), *Ninth mental measurements yearbook* (pp. 773–777). Highland Park, NJ: Gryphon.

Parsons, F. (1909). *Choosing a vocation*. Boston: Houghton Mifflin.

Pearlman, K., Schmidt, F. L., & Hunter, J. E. (1980) Validity generalization results for tests used to predict training success and job proficiency. *Journal of Applied Psychology, 65,* 373–406.

Pedersen, P. B. (1991). Multiculturalism as a generic approach to counseling. *Journal of Counseling & Development, 70,* 6–12.

Pfeiffer, S. I. (2005). Review of the OQ-45 (Outcome Questionnaire). In Spies, R. A., & Plake, B. S. (Eds.), *The sixteenth mental measurements yearbook* (pp. 740–742). Lincoln, NE: Buros Institute of Mental Measurements.

Phillips, S. E. (2000). *GI Forum v. Texas Education Agency*: Psychometric evidence. *Applied Measurement in Education, 13,* 343–385.

Piaget, J. (1972). *The psychology of intelligence*. Totowa, NJ: Littlefield Adams.

Piers, E. V., Harris, D. B., & Herzberg, D. S. (2002). *Piers-Harris Children's Self-Concept Scale*–Second Edition. Los Angeles: Western Psychological Services.

Piotrowski, C. (1999). Assessment practices in the era of managed care: Current status and future directions. *Journal of Clinical Psychology, 55,* 787–796.

Pittenger, D. J. (1993). The utility of the Myers-Briggs Type Indicator. *Review of Educational Research, 63,* 467–488.

Plake, B. S., Impara, J. C., & Spies, R. A. (2003). *The fifteenth mental measurements yearbooks*. Lincoln, NE: Buros Institute of Mental Measures.

Pledge, D. S., Lapan, R. T., Heppner, P. P., Kivlighan, D., & Roehlke, H. J. (1998). Stability and severity of presenting problems at a university counseling center: A 6-year analysis. *Professional Psychology: Research and Practice, 29,* 396–399.

Polanski, P. J., & Hinkle, J. S. (2000). The mental status examination: Its use by professional counselors. *Journal of Counseling & Development, 78,* 357–364.

Ponterotto, J. G., Pace, J. A., & Kavan, K. (1989). A counselor's guide to the assessment of depression. *Journal of Counseling and Development, 67,* 301–309.

Pope, M. (2002). *Kuder General Interest Survey Form G*. In J. T. Kapes, M. M. Mastie, & E. A. Whitfield (Eds.), *A counselor's guide to career assessment instruments* (4th ed., pp. 256–263). Tulsa, OK: National Career Development Association.

Powers, D. E. (1993). Coaching for the SAT: A summary of the summaries and an update. *Educational Measurement Issues and Practice, 12*(2), 24–30.

Poznanski, E. O., & Mokros, H. B. (1996). *Children's Depression Rating Scale, Revised*. Los Angeles: Western Psychological Services.

Pratt, S. L., & Moreland, K. L. (1998). Individuals with other characteristics. In J. Sandoval, C. L. Frisby, K. F. Geisinger, J. D. Scheuneman, & J. R. Grenier (Eds.), *Test interpretation and diversity: Achieving equity in assessment* (pp. 349–371). Washington, DC: American Psychological Association.

Prediger, D. J. (1999). Integrating interests and abilities for career exploration: General considerations. In M. L. Savickas & A. R. Spokane (Eds.), *Vocational interests: Meaning, measurement, and counseling use* (pp. 295–325). Palo-Alto, CA: Davies-Black.

Prince, J. P., & Heiser, L. J. (2000). *Essentials of career interest assessment*. New York: John Wiley.

Prochaska, J. (2000). Change at differing stages. In C. R. Snyder, & R. Ingram (Eds.), *Handbook of psychological change* (pp. 109–127). New York: Wiley.

Prochaska, J. M., Prochaska, J. O., & Johnson, S. S. (2006). Assessing readiness for adherence to treatment. In W. T. O'Donohue & E. R. Lenensky (Eds.), *Promoting treatment adherence: A practical handbook for health care providers* (pp. 35–46). Thousand Oaks, CA: Sage.

Prochaska, J. O., & DiClemente, C. C. (1992). Stages of change in modification of problem behaviors. In M. Hersen, R. M. Eisler, & P. M. Miller (Eds.), *Progress in behavior modification* (pp. 184–214). Sycamore, IL: Sycamore Press.

Prochaska, J. O., DiClemente, C. C., & Norcross, J. C. (1992). In search of how people change: Applications to addictive behaviors. *American Psychologist, 47,* 1102–1114.

Prochaska, J. O., & Norcross, J. C. (2001). Stages of change. *Psychotherapy: theory, research, practice, and training, 38,* 443–448.

Prochaska, J. O., & Norcross, J. C. (2002). *Systems of psychotherapy: A transtheoretical analysis* (5th ed.). Belmont, CA: Brooks/Cole.

Prochaska, J. O., Velicer, W. F., Fava, J. L., Rossi, J. S., & Tsoh, J. Y. (2001). Evaluating a population-based recruitment approach and a stage-based expert system intervention for smoking cessation. *Addictive Behaviors, 26,* 583–602.

Pryor, R. G. L., & Taylor, N. B. (1986). On combining scores from interest and values measures in counseling. *Vocational Guidance Quarterly, 34,* 178–187.

Psychological Corporation (1991). *Differential Aptitude Tests (5th ed.) Career Interest Inventory counselors' manual.* San Antonio, TX: Author.

Pugh, R. C. (1998). Review of the Campbell Interest and Skill Inventory. In C. W. Conoley & J. Impara (Eds.), *The thirteenth mental measurements yearbook* (pp. 167–170). Lincoln, NE: Buros Institute of Mental Measures.

Rada, R. (2003). *HIPAA@IT reference, 2003 edition: Health information transactions, privacy, and security.* [Electronic resource]. Norwood, MA: Hypermedia Solutions Limited.

Rahdert, E. R. (1997). *Adolescent assessment referral manual* (NIH No. 27189–8252). Rockville, MD: National Institute of Drug Abuse.

Raven, J. C., Court, J. H., & Raven, J. (1983). *Manual for Raven's Progressive Matrices and Vocabulary Scales: Standard progressive matrices.* London: Lewis.

Reid, P. T. (2002). Multicultural psychology: Bringing together gender and ethnicity. *Cultural Diversity and Ethnic Minority Psychology, 8,* 103–114.

Reivich, K., & Gillham, J. (2003). Learned optimism: The measurement of explanatory style. In S. J. Lopez & C. R. Snyder (Eds.), *Positive psychological assessment: A handbook of models and measures* (pp. 57–74). Washington, DC: American Psychological Association.

Reynolds, C. R., Chastain, R. L., Kaufman, A. S., & McLean, E. (1987). Demographic characteristics and IQ among adults: Analysis of the WAIS-R standardization sample as a function of the stratification variables. *Journal of School Psychology, 25,* 323–342.

Reynolds, W. M. (1988). *Suicidal Ideation Questionnaire.* Odessa, FL: Psychological Assessment Resources.

Reynolds, W. M. (1989). *Reynolds Child Depression Scale.* Lutz, FL: Psychological Assessment Resources.

Reynolds, W. M. (1991). *Adult Suicidal Ideation Questionnaire.* Lutz, FL: Psychological Assessment Resources.

Reynolds, W. M. (2002). *Reynolds Depression Scale* (2nd ed.). Lutz, FL: Psychological Assessment Resources.

Reynolds, W. M., & Kobak, K. A. (1995). *Hamilton Depression Inventory.* Odessa, FL: Psychological Assessment Resources.

Ridley, C. R., Hill, C. L., & Wiese, D. L. (2001). Ethics in multicultural assessment: A model of reasoned application. In L. A. Suzuki, J. G. Ponterotto, & P. J. Meller (Eds.), *Handbook of multicultural assessment: Clinical, psychological and educational applications* (2nd ed., pp. 29–45). San Francisco: Jossey-Bass.

Ridley, C. R., Li, L. C., & Hill, C. L. (1998). Multicultural assessment: Reexamination, reconceptualization, and practical application. *The Counseling Psychologist, 26,* 827–910.

Robertson, G. J. (2002). *Wide Range Achievement Test-Expanded.* Lutz, FL: Psychological Assessment Resources.

Rogers, J. E. (2002). Armed Services Vocational Aptitude Battery (ASVAB). In J. T. Kapes, M. M. Mastie, & E. A. Whitfield (Eds.), *A counselor's guide to career assessment instruments* (4th ed., pp. 93–101). Tulsa, OK: National Career Development Association.

Rogers, J. R., Guelulette, C. M., Abbey-Hines, J., Carney, J. V., & Werth, J. L., Jr. (2001). Rational suicide: An empirical investigation of counselor attitudes. *Journal of Counseling & Development, 79,* 365–372.

Rogers, R., Sewell, K. W., Harrison, K. S., & Jordan, M. J. (2006). The MMPI-2 restructured clinical scales: A paradigmatic shift in scale development. *Journal of Personality Assessment, 87,* 139–147.

Rohrbraugh, M., Rogers, J. C., & McGoldrick, M. (1992). How do experts read family genograms? *Family Systems Medicine, 10,* 79–89.

Roid, G. H. (2003). *Stanford-Binet Intelligence Scale, Fifth Edition.* Itasca, IL: Riverside Publishing.

Rosenthal, R. (1991). *Meta-analytic procedures for social research.* Thousand Oaks, CA: Sage.

Rosenthal, R., & Jacobson, L. (1968). *Pygmalion in the classroom.* New York: Holt, Rinehart & Winston.

Rosenzweig, S. (1977). *Manual for the children's form of the Rosenzweig Picture-Frustration Study.* St. Louis, MO: Rana House.

Rosenzweig, S. (1978). *The Rosenzweig Picture-Frustration Study: Basic manual.* St. Louis, MO: Rana House.

Rosenzweig, S. (1988). Revised norms for the Children's Form of the Rosenzweig Picture-Frustration Study, with updated reference list. *Journal of Clinical Child Psychology, 17,* 326–328.

Roszkowski, M. J. (2001). Review of the Jackson Vocational Interest Survey [1995 Revision]. In B. Plake & J. Impara (Eds), *The fourteenth mental measurements yearbook* (pp. 615–618). Lincoln, NE: Buros Institute of Mental Measures.

Roth, P. L., Bevier, C. A., Bobko, P., Switzer, F. S., & Tyler, P. (2001). Ethnic group differences in cognitive ability in employment and educational settings: A meta-analysis. *Personnel Psychology, 54,* 297–330.

Rotter, J. B., Lah, M. I., & Rafferty, J. E. (1992). *Rotter Incomplete Sentence Blank,* Second Edition. San Antonio, TX: The Psychology Corporation.

Rounds, J. B. (1990). The comparative and combined utility of work value and interest data in career counseling with adults. *Journal of Vocational Behavior, 37,* 32–45.

Rounds, J. B., & Armstrong, P. I. (2005). Assessment of needs and values. In S. D. Brown & R. W. Lent, (Eds.), *Career development and counseling* (pp. 305–329). Hoboken, NJ: Wiley.

Rounds, J., & Tracey, T. J. (1996). Cross-cultural structural equivalence of RIASEC models and measures. *Journal of Counseling Psychology, 43,* 310–330.

Rubenzer, S. (1992). A comparison of traditional and computer-generated psychological reports in an adolescent inpatient setting. *Journal of Clinical Psychology, 48,* 817–827.

Ryan Krane, N. E., & Tirre, W. C. (2005). Ability assessment in career counseling. In S. D. Brown & R. W. Lent (Eds.), *Career development and counseling: Putting theory and research to work* (pp. 330–352). Hoboken, NJ: Wiley.

Sackett, P. R., & Wilk, S. L. (1994). Within-group norming and other forms of scoring adjustment in preemployment testing. *American Psychologist, 49,* 929–954.

Sampson, J. P., Jr. (1990). Computer-assisted testing and the goals of counseling psychology. *The Counseling Psychologist, 18,* 227–239.

Sampson, J. P., Jr. (1998, January). *Assessment and the Internet.* Paper presented at the Assessment 1998 Conference, St. Petersburg, FL.

Sampson, J. P., Jr. (2000). Using the Internet to enhance testing in counseling. *Journal of Counseling & Development, 78,* 348–356.

Sampson, J. P. Jr., Lumsden, J. A., & Carr, D. L. (2002). Computer-assisted career assessment. In J. T. Kapes, M. M. Mastie, & E. A. Whitfield (Eds.), *A counselor's guide to career assessment instruments* (4th ed., pp. 47–63). Tulsa, OK: National Career Development Association.

Sampson, J. P. Jr., Purgar, M. P., & Shy, J. D. (2003). Computer-based test interpretation in career assessment: Ethical and professional issues. *Journal of Career Assessment, 11,* 22–39.

Sampson, J. P. Jr., Vacc, N. A., & Loesch, L. C. (1998). The practice of career counseling by specialist and counselors in general practice. *The Career Development Quarterly, 46,* 404–415.

Sanchez, H. B. (2001). Risk factor model for suicide assessment and intervention. *Professional Psychology: Research and Practice, 32,* 351–358.

Sanderson, W. C. (2003). Why empirically supported psychological treatments are important. *Behavioral Modification, 27,* 290–299.

Sandoval, J. (1998). Testing in a changing world: An introduction. In J. Sandoval, C. L. Frisby, K. F. Geisinger, J. D. Scheuneman, & J. R. Grenier (Eds.), *Test interpretation and diversity: Achieving equity in assessment* (pp. 3–16). Washington, DC: American Psychological Association.

Sandoval, J. (2003). Review of the Woodcock-Johnson III. In B. S. Plake & J. C. Impara (Eds.). *The fifteenth mental measurements yearbook* (pp. 1024–1028). Lincoln, NE: Buros Institute of Mental Measures.

Sattler, J. M. (1993). *Assessment of children* (3rd ed. revised reprint). San Diego, CA: Jerome M. Sattler Publisher.

Sattler, J. M. (2001). *Assessment of children* (4th ed.). San Diego, CA: Jerome M. Sattler Publisher.

Sattler, J. M. (2002). *Assessment of children: Behavioral and clinical applications* (4th ed.). San Diego, CA: Jerome M. Sattler.

Savickas, M. L. (1993). Career counseling in the postmodern era. *Journal of Cognitive Psychotherapy: An International Quarterly, 7,* 205–215.

Savickas, M. L. (2001). Toward a comprehensive theory of career development: Dispositions, concerns, and narratives. In F. L. T. Leong & A. Barak (Eds.), *Contemporary models of vocational psychology: A volume in honor of Samuel H. Osipow* (pp. 295–320). Mahwah, NJ: Erlbaum.

Savickas, M. L., Taber, B. J., & Spokane, A. R. (2002). Convergent and discriminant validity of five interest inventories. *Journal of Vocational Behavior, 61,* 139–184.

Savin, H. A., & Kiesling, S. S. (2000). *Accountable systems of behavioral health care: A provider's guide.* San Francisco: Jossey-Bass.

Scarr, S. (1992). Developmental theories for the 1990s: Developmental and individual differences. *Child Development, 63,* 1–19.

Scarr, S. (1993). Biological and cultural diversity: The legacy of Darwin for development. *Child Development, 64,* 1333–1354.

Schaefer, C. E., Gitlin, K., & Sandgrund, A. (Eds.). (1991). *Play diagnosis and assessment.* New York: Wiley.

Schaie, K. W., & Strother, C. R. (1968). A cross-sequential study of age changes in cognitive behavior. *Psychological Bulletin, 70,* 671–680.

Schmidt, F. L., & Hunter, J. E. (1977). Development of a general solution to the problem of validity generalization. *Journal of Applied Psychology, 62,* 529–540.

Schmidt, F. L., Hunter, J. E., & Caplan, J. R. (1981). Validity generalization results for two jobs in the petroleum business. *Journal of Applied Psychology, 66,* 261–273.

Schoenrade, P. (2002). *Values Scale*. In J. T. Kapes, M. M. Mastie, & E. A. Whitfield (Eds.), *A counselor's guide to career assessment instruments* (4th ed., pp. 299–302). Tulsa, OK: National Career Development Association.

Schuerger, J. M. (2001). *16PF Adolescent Personality Questionnaire.* Champaign, IL: Institute for Personality and Ability Testing.

Schultheiss, D. E. P. (2005). Qualitative relational career assessment: A constructivist paradigm. *Journal of Career Assessment, 13,* 381–394.

Schwab, D. P., & Packard, G. L. (1973). Response set distortion on the Gordon Personal Inventory and the Gordon Personal Profile in the selection context: Some implications for predicting employee behavior. *Journal of Applied Psychology, 58,* 372–374.

Seligman, L. (2004). *Diagnosis and treatment planning in counseling.* New York: Springer.

Seligman, M. E. P. (1998). Optimism: The difference it makes. *Science and Spirit, 9,* 6–19.

Sireci, S. G., & Geisinger, K. F. (1998). Equity issues in employment testing. In J. Sandoval, C. L. Frisby, K. F. Geisinger, J. D. Scheuneman, & J. R. Grenier (Eds.), *Test interpretation and diversity: Achieving equity in assessment* (pp.105–140). Washington, DC: American Psychological Association.

Sexton, T. L. (1996). The relevance of counseling outcome research: Current trends and practical implications. *Journal of Counseling & Development, 74,* 590–600.

Skiba, R. J., Poloni-Staudinger, L., Gallini, S., Simmons, A. D., & Feggins-Azziz, R. (2006). The disproportionality of African American students with disabilities across educational environments. *Exceptional Children, 72,* 411–424.

Skinner, H. A., Steinhauer, P. D., & Santa-Barbara, J. (1995). *The Family Assessment Measure.* North Tonawanda, NY: Multi-Health Systems.

Slaney, R. B., & MacKinnon-Slaney, F. (1990). The use of vocational card sorts in career counseling. In M. L. Savickas & W. B. Walsh (Eds.), *Handbook of career counseling theory and practice* (pp. 317–371). Palo Alto, CA: Davies-Black.

Slaney, R. B., & Suddarth, B. H. (1994). The Values Scale (VS). In J. T. Kapes, M. M. Mastie, & E. A. Whitfield (Eds.), *A counselor's guide to career assessment instruments* (pp. 236–240). Alexandria, VA: National Career Development Association.

Snyder, C. R. (1997). *Marital Satisfaction Inventory, Revised manual.* Los Angeles: Western Psychological Services.

Snyder, C. R., Lopez, S. J., Edwards, L. M., Pedrotti, J. T., Prosser, E. C., Walton, S. L., Spalitto, S. V., & Ulven, J. C. (2003). Measuring and labeling the positive and the negative. In S. J., Lopez & C. R., Snyder (Eds.), *Positive psychological assessment: A handbook of models and measures* (pp. 21–39). Washington, DC: American Psychological Association.

Snyder, C. R., Shenkel, R. J., & Lowery, C. R. (1977). Acceptance of personality interpretations: The "Barnum effect" and beyond. *Journal of Consulting and Clinical Psychology, 45,* 104–114.

Spanier, G. B. (1976). Measuring dyadic adjustment: New scales for assessing the quality of marriage or similar dyads. *Journal of Marriage and the Family, 38,* 15–28.

Spearman, C. (1927). *The abilities of man.* New York: Macmillan.

Spengler, P. M., Strohmer, D. C., Dixon, D. N., & Shivy, V. A. (1995). A scientist-practitioner model of psychological assessment: Implications for training, practice, research. *The Counseling Psychologist, 23,* 506–534.

Spillane, S. A. (2001). Review of the Family Assessment measure Version III. In B. Plake & J. Impara (Eds.), *The fourteenth mental measurements yearbook* (pp. 482). Lincoln, NE: Buros Institute of Mental Measures.

Spitzer, R. L., Gibbon, M., Skodol, A. E., Williams, J. B. W., & First, M. B. (2002). *DSM-IV-TR casebook: A learning companion to the Diagnostic and Statistical Manual of Mental Disorders, fourth edition, text revision.* Washington, DC: American Psychiatric Association.

Spokane, A. R. (1991). *Career interventions.* Englewood Cliffs, NJ: Prentice Hall.

Spokane, A. R., & Jacob, E. J. (1996). Career and vocational assessment 1993–1994: A biennial review. *Journal of Career Assessment, 4,* 1–32.

Steer, R. A., & Clark, D. A. (1997). Psychometric characteristics of the Beck Depression Inventory II. *Measurement and Evaluation in Counseling and Development, 30,* 128–136.

Stelmachers, Z. T. (1995). Assessing suicidal clients. In J. N. Butcher (Ed.), *Clinical personality assessment: Practical approaches* (pp. 367–379). New York: Oxford University Press.

Sternberg, R. J. (1985). *Beyond IQ: A triarchic theory of human intelligence.* New York: Cambridge University Press.

Sternberg, R. J. (1988). *The triarchic mind: A new theory of human intelligence.* New York: Viking.

Sternberg, R. J., Conway, B. E., Ketron, J. L., & Bernstein. M. (1981). People's conceptions of intelligence. *Journal of Personality and Social Psychology, 41,* 37–55.

Stiles, W. B., Gordon, L. E., & Lani, J. A. (2002). Session evaluation and the Session Evaluation Questionnaire. In G. S. Tyron (Ed.), *Counseling based on process research: Applying what we know* (pp. 325–343). Boston: Allyn & Bacon.

Stinnett, T. A. (2001). Review of the Naglieri Nonverbal Ability Test. In B. Plake & J. Impara (Eds.), *The fourteenth mental measurements yearbook* (pp. 819–822). Lincoln, NE: Buros Institute of Mental Measures.

Straabs, G. V. (1991). *The Scenotest.* Toronto: Hegrefe & Huber.

Stratton, K., Howey, C., & Battaglia, F. (1996). *Fetal alcohol syndrome: Diagnosis, epidemiology, prevention, and treatment.* Washington, DC: National Academy Press.

Stobart, G. (2005). Fairness in multicultural assessment systems. *Assessment in Education, 13,* 275–287.

Strickler, L. J. (1969). "Test-wiseness" on personality scales. *Journal of Applied Psychology Monograph, 53*(3).

Strong, S. R. (1968). Counseling: An interpersonal influence process. *Journal of Counseling Psychology, 15,* 215–224.

Strupp, H. H., Horowitz, L. M., & Lambert, M. J. (1997). *Measuring patient changes: Mood, anxiety, and personality disorders.* Washington, DC: American Psychological Association.

Stuart, R. B., & Jacobsen, B. (1987). *Couple's Pre-Counseling Inventory, Revised Edition.* Champaign, IL: Research Press.

Subkoviak, M. J. (1984). Estimating the reliability of mastery-nonmastery classifications. In A. S. Bellack & M. Hersen (Eds.), *A guide to criterion-referenced test construction* (pp. 267–291). Baltimore: Johns Hopkins University Press.

Substance Abuse and Mental Health Services Administration (2005). *Assessing suicide risk: Initial tips for counselors.* Retrieved August 21, 2007, from http://download.ncadi.samhsa.gov/ken/pdf/SVP06-0153/SVP06-0153.pdf

Substance Abuse and Mental Health Services Administration, Office of Applied Studies (2007). *The NSDUH report: Worker substance use by industry.* Retrieved August 27, 2007, from http://www.drugabusestatistics.samhsa.gov/2k7/industry/worker.pdf

Sue, D. W., Arredondo, P., & McDavis, R. (1992). Multicultural competencies and standards: A call to the profession. *Journal of Counseling & Development, 70,* 477–486.

Sue, D. W., & Sue, D. (1977). Barriers to effective cross-cultural counseling. *Journal of Counseling Psychology, 24,* 420–429.

Sue, S. (1998). In search of cultural competence in psychotherapy and counseling. *American Psychologist, 53,* 440–448.

Sullivan, P. M., & Montoya, L. A. (1997). Factor analysis of the WISC-III with deaf and hard-of-hearing children. *Psychological Assessment, 9,* 317–321.

Super, D. E. (1980). A life-span approach to career development. *Journal of Vocational Behavior, 16,* 282–298.

Super, D. E., Thompson, A. S., Lindeman, R. H., Jordaan, J. P., & Myers, R. A. (1988a). *Adults Career Concerns Inventory.* Palo Alto, CA: Consulting Psychologists Press.

Super, D. E., Thompson, A. S., Lindeman, R. H., Jordaan, J. P., & Myers, R. A. (1988b). *Career Development Inventory.* Palo Alto, CA: CPP, Inc.

Suzuki, L. A., Short, E. L., Pieterse, A., & Kugler, J. (2001). Multicultural issues and the assessment of aptitude. In L. A. Suzuki, J. G. Ponterotto, & P. J. Mellers (Eds.), *Handbook of multicultural assessment: Clinical, psychological, and educational applications* (2nd ed., pp. 359–382). San Francisco: Jossey-Bass.

Swanson, J. L. (1995). The process and outcome of career counseling. In W. B. Walsh & S. H. Osipow (Eds.), *Handbook of vocational psychology: Theory, research, and practice* (pp. 217–259). Hillsdale, NJ: Erlbaum.

Swenson, C. H. (1968). Empirical evaluations of human figure drawings: 1957–1966. *Psychological Bulletin, 70,* 20–44.

Swiercinsky, D. (1978). *Manual for the adult neurological evaluation.* Springfield, IL: Thomas.

Taylor, R. M., & Morrison, L. D. (1996). *Taylor-Johnson Temperament Analysis test manual.* Thousand Oaks, CA: Sigma Assessment Systems.

Tellegen, A., Ben-Porath, Y. S., McNulty, J. L., Arbisi, P. A., Graham, J. R., & Kaemmer, B. (2003). *The MMPI-2 restructured clinical (RC) scales: Development, validation, and interpretation.* Minneapolis: University of Minnesota Press.

Texas Education Agency (2006). *Texas student assessment program:Interpreting assessment reports.* Austin, TX: Author.

Thompson, B., & Snyder, P. A. (1998). Statistical significance and reliability analyses in recent *Journal of Counseling and Development* research articles. *Journal of Counseling and Development, 76,* 436–441.

Thorndike, R. M. (2005a). *Measurement and evaluation in psychology and education* (7th ed.).

Thorndike, R. M. (2005b). Review of the Kaufman Assessment Battery for Children, Second Edition. In Spies, R. A., & Plake, B. S. (Eds.). *The sixteenth mental measurements yearbook* (pp.). Lincoln, NE: Buros Institute of Mental Measurements.

Thurstone, L. L. (1938). Primary mental abilities. *Psychometric Monographs,* No. 1.

Timbrook, R. E., & Graham, J. R. (1994). Ethnic differences on the MMPI-2? *Psychological Assessment, 6,* 212–217.

Timm, T., & Blow, A. (2005). The family life cycle and the genogram. In M. Cierpka, V. Thomas, & D. H. Sprenkle (Eds.), *Family assessment: Integrating multiple perspectives* (pp.159–181). Cambridge, MA: Hogrefe

Tindal, G. (2002). Large-scale assessments for all students: Issues and options. In G. Tindal & T. M. Haladyna (Eds.), *Large-scale assessment programs for all students.* Mahwah, NJ: Erlbaum.

Touliatos, J., Perlmutter, B. F., & Straus, M. A. (2001). *Handbook of family measurement techniques: Abstracts* (Vol. I, II, III). Thousand Oaks, CA: Sage.

Tracey, T. J. G., & Hopkins, N. (2001). Correspondence of interests and abilities with occupational choice. *Journal of Counseling Psychology, 48,* 178–189.

Tracey, T. J. G., & Rounds, J. (1999). Inference and attribution errors in test interpretation. In J. W. Lichtenberg & R. K. Goodyear (Eds.), *Scientist-practitioner perspectives on test interpretation* (pp. 113–131). Boston: Allyn & Bacon.

Transberg, M., Slane, S., & Ekeberg, S. E. (1993). The relation between interest congruence and satisfaction: A meta-analysis. *Journal of Vocational Behavior, 42,* 253–264.

Trull, T., & Widiger, T. A. (1997). *Structured Interview for the Five-Factor Model of Personality.* Odessa, FL: Psychological Assessment Resources.

Trzepacz, P. T., & Baker, R. W. (1993). *The psychiatric mental status examination.* New York: Oxford.

Tuddenham, R. D., Blumenkrantz, J., & Wilken, W. R. (1968). Age changes on AGCT: A longitudinal study of average adults. *Journal of Consulting and Clinical Psychology, 32,* 659–663.

Turner, C. F., Ku, L., Rogers, S. M., Lindberg, L. D., Pleck, J. H., & Sonenstein, F. L. (1998). Adolescent sexual behavior, drug use, and violence: Increased reporting with computer survey technology. *Science, 280,* 867–873.

Turner, S. M., DeMers, S. T., Fox, H. R., & Reed, G. (2001). APA's guidelines for test user qualifications: An executive summary. *American Psychologist, 56,* 1099–1113.

Ulrich, R. E., Stachnik, T. J., & Stainton, N. R. (1963). Student acceptance of generalized personality interpretations. *Psychological Report, 13,* 831–834.

U.S. Bureau of Census. (2001). *2000 census data sampler.* Washington, DC: Author.

U.S. Census Bureau. (2004). *More diversity, slower growth.* Retrieved February 27, 2008, from http://www.census.gov/Press-Release/www/releases/archives/population/001720.html

U.S. Department of Defense. (2007). *ASVAB career exploration program: Counselor manual.* Washington, DC: Author.

U.S. Department of Education. (1999). 34 CFR Parts 300 and 303: Assistance to the states for the education of children with disabilities. Final regulations. *Federal Register, 64,* 12406–12672.

U.S. Department of Health and Human Services. (1999). *Mental health: A report of the surgeon general.* Rockville, MD: U.S. Department of Health and Human Services, Substance Abuse and Mental Health Services Administration, Center for Mental Health Services, National Institutes of Health, National Institute of Mental Health.

U.S. Department of Health and Human Services. (2005). *Basic facts about mental health.* Rockville, MD: U.S. Department of Health and Human Services, Substance Abuse and Mental Health Services Administration, Center for Mental Health Services, National Institutes of Health, National Institute of Mental Health.

U.S. Department of Labor, Employment and Training Administration. (2002). *O*NET Ability Profiler: Users' guide.* Washington, DC: U.S. Government Printing Office.

Vacc, N. A., & Juhnke, G. A. (1997). The use of structured clinical interviews for assessment in counseling. *Journal of Counseling and Development, 75,* 470–480.

Vacc, N. A., & Tippen, N. (2002). Documentation. In R. B. Ekstrom & D. K. Smith (Eds.), *Assessing individuals with disabilities in education, employment, and counseling settings* (pp. 59–70). Washington, DC: American Psychological Association.

Vacha-Haase, T. (1998). Reliability Generalization: Exploring variance in measurement error affecting score reliability across studies. *Educational and Psychological Measurement, 58,* 6–20.

Vaacha-Haase, T., Kogan, L. R., Tani, C. R., & Woodall, R. A. (2001). Reliability generalization: Exploring variation of reliability coefficients of MMPI clinical scales scores. *Educational and Psychological Measurement, 61,* 45–59.

van der Linden, W. J., & Hambleton, R. K. (1997). Item response theory: Brief history, common models, and extensions. In W. J. van der Linden & R. K. Hambleton (Eds.), *Handbook of modern item response theory* (pp. 1–28). New York: Springer.

Verhaeghen, P. (2003). Aging and vocabulary scores. A meta-analysis. *Psychology and Aging, 18,* 332–339.

Vernon, P. E. (1950). *The structure of human abilities.* New York: Wiley.

Waiswol, N. (1995). Projective techniques as psychotherapy. *American Journal of Psychotherapy, 49,* 244–259.

Wampold, B. E., Lichtenberg, J. W., & Waehler, C. A. (2002). Principles of empirically supported interventions in counseling psychology. *The Counseling Psychologist, 30,* 197–217.

Wang, L. (2002) Differential Aptitude Tests & Career Interest Inventory. In J. T. Kapes, M. M. Mastie, & E. A. Whitfield (Eds.), *A counselor's guide to career assessment instruments* (4th ed., pp. 93–101). Tulsa, OK: National Career Development Association.

Ware, J. E. (2007). *User manual for the SF-36v2 Health Survey-Second Edition.* Lincoln, RI: Quality Metric.

Warren, W. L. (1994). *Revised Hamilton Rating Scale for Depression.* Los Angeles: Western Psychological Services.

Watkins, C. E., Campbell, V. L., & Nieberding, R. (1994). The practice of vocational assessment by counseling psychologists. *The Counseling Psychologist, 22,* 115–128.

Watts-Jones, D. (1997). Toward an African American genogram. *Family Process, 36,* 375–383.

Wechsler, D. (1992). *Wechsler Individual Achievement Test.* San Antonio, TX: The Psychological Corporation.

Wechsler, D. (1997a). *Wechsler Adult Intelligence Scale-Third Edition.* San Antonio, TX: The Psychological Corporation.

Wechsler, D. (1997b). *Wechsler Memory Scale-Third Edition.* San Antonio, TX: The Psychological Corporation.

Wechsler, D. (2001). *Wechsler Individual Achievement Test-Second Edition.* San Antonio, TX: The Psychological Corporation.

Wechsler, D. (2002). *Wechsler Preschool and Primary Scale of Intelligence-Third Edition.* San Antonio, TX: The Psychological Corporation.

Wechsler, D. (2003). *Wechsler Intelligence Scale for Children-Fourth Edition.* San Antonio, TX: The Psychological Corporation.

Wechsler, D., Kaplan, E., Fein, D., Kramer, J., & Morris, R., Delis, D., & Maelender, A. (2004). *Wechsler Intelligence Scale for Children-Fourth Edition Integrated.* San Antonio, TX: The Psychological Corporation.

Weiss, D. J., Dawis, R. V., & Lofquist, L. H. (1981). *Minnesota Importance Questionnaire.* Minneapolis: Vocational Psychology Research.

Westbrook, B. W., Sanford, E., Gilleland, K., Fleenor, J., & Merwin, J. (1988). Career maturity in grade 9: The relationship between accuracy of self-appraisal and ability to appraise the career-relevant capabilities of others. *Journal of Vocational Behavior, 32,* 269–283.

Whipple, J. L., Lambert, M. J., Vermeersch, D. A., Smart, D. W., Nielsen, S. L., & Hawkins, E. J. (2003). Improving the effects of psychotherapy: The use of early identified treatment failure and problem-solving strategies in routine practice. *Journal of Counseling Psychology, 50,* 59–68.

Whiston, S. C. (1996). Accountability through action research: Research methods for practitioners. *Journal of Counseling & Development, 74,* 616–623.

Whiston, S. C. (2001). Selecting career outcome assessments: An organizational scheme. *Journal of Career Assessment, 9* (3), 215–228.

Whiston, S. C. (2002a). Application of the principles: Career counseling and interventions. *The Counseling Psychologist, 30,* 218–237.

Whiston, S. C. (2002b). Response to the past, present, and future of school counseling: Raising some issues. *Professional School Counseling, 5,* 148–155.

Whiston, S. C., & Aricak, T. (in press). Development and initial investigation of the School Counseling Program Evaluation Scale. *Professional School Counseling.*

Whiston, S. C., Brecheisen, B. K., & Stephens, J. (2003). Does treatment modality affect career counseling effectiveness? *Journal of Vocational Behavior, 62,* 390–410.

Whiston, S. C., & Oliver, L. (2005). Career counseling process and outcome. In W. B. Walsh & M. Savickas (Eds.), *Handbook of vocational psychology* (3rd ed., pp. 155–194). Hillsdale NJ: Erlbaum.

Whiston, S. C., & Rahardja, D. (2005). Qualitative career assessment: An overview and analysis. *Journal of Career Assessment, 13,* 371–380.

Whiston, S. C., & Sexton, T. L. (1998). A review of school counseling outcome research: Implications for practice. *Journal of Counseling & Development, 76,* 412–426.

Whiston, S. C., Sexton, T. L., & Lasoff, D. L. (1998). Career-intervention outcome: A replication and extension of Oliver and Spokane. *Journal of Counseling Psychology, 45,* 150–165.

Wickwire, P. N. (2002). COPSystem. In J. T. Kapes, M. M. Mastie, & E. A. Whitfield (Eds.), *A counselor's guide to career assessment instruments* (4th ed., pp. 212–217). Tulsa, OK: National Career Development Association.

Widiger, T. A. (1992). Review of the NEO Personality Inventory. In J. C. Conoley & J. J. Kramer (Eds.), *Eleventh mental measurements yearbook* (pp. 605–606). Lincoln, NE: The University of Nebraska Press.

Wiggins, J. S. (1966). Social desirability estimation and "faking good" well. *Educational and Psychological Measurement, 26,* 329–341.

Wiggins, J. S. (1989). Review of the Myers-Briggs Type Indicator. In J. C. Conoley & J. J. Kramer (Eds.), *Tenth mental measurements yearbook* (pp. 536–538). Lincoln, NE: University of Nebraska Press.

Wilkinson, G. S, & Robertson, G. J. (2007). *Wide Range Achievement Test 4.* Lutz, FL: Psychological Assessment Resources.

Williams, S. K. (1978). The vocational card sort: A tool for vocational exploration. *The Vocational Guidance Quarterly, 48,* 237–243.

Willson, V. L., & Stone, E. (1994). Differential Aptitude Tests. In J. T. Kapes, M. M. Mastie, & E. A. Whitfield (Eds.), *A counselor's guide to career assessment instruments* (pp. 90–98). Alexandria, VA: National Career Development Association.

Wilson, M. (2005). *Constructing measures: An item response model approach.* Mahwah, NJ: Erlbaum.

Wonderlic Personnel Test, Inc. (1998). *Wonderlic Personnel Test user's manual.* Libertyville, IL: Author.

Worthington, E. L., McCullough, M. E., Shortz, J. L. Mindes, E. J., Sandage, S. J., & Chartrand, J. M. (1995). Can couples assessment and feedback improve relationships? Assessment as a brief relationship enrichment procedure. *Journal of Counseling Psychology, 42,* 466–475.

Wright, B. A., & Lopez, S. J. (2002). Widening the diagnostic focus: A case for including human strengths and environmental resources. In C. R. Snyder & S. J. Lopez (Eds.), *Handbook of positive psychology* (pp. 26–44). New York: Oxford University Press.

Zytowski, D. G. (2001). Kuder Career Search with Person Match: Career Assessment for the 21st century. *Journal of Career Assessment, 9,* 229–241.

Zytowski, D. G. (2006). *Super's Work Values Inventory-revised: Technical manual version 1.0.* Retrieved November 8, 2007, from https://www.kuder.com/PublicWeb/swv_manual.aspx

Zytowski (nd). *Kuder® Career Search with Person Match: Technical manual version 1.1.* Retrieved November 8, 2007, from https://www.kuder.com/PublicWeb/kcs_manual.aspx

Zytowski, D. G., & Luzzo, D. A. (2002). Developing the Kuder Skills Assessment. *Journal of Career Assessment, 10,* 190–199.

Zytowski, D. G., Rottinghaus, P. J., & D'Archiardi, C. (2007). *Kuder® Skills Assessment: User's manual version 2.0.* Retrieved November 8, 2007, from https://www.kuder.com/PublicWeb/ksa_manual.aspx

INDEX

A

E

J

Q

R

T

Y

Z